Molecular Diagnostics in Cancer Patients

Kamla Kant Shukla • Praveen Sharma
Sanjeev Misra
Editors

Molecular Diagnostics in Cancer Patients

Springer

Editors
Kamla Kant Shukla
Department of Biochemistry
All India Institute of Medical Sciences
Jodhpur
India

Praveen Sharma
Department of Biochemistry
All India Institute of Medical Sciences
Jodhpur
India

Sanjeev Misra
Department of Surgical Oncology
All India Institute of Medical Sciences
Jodhpur
India

ISBN 978-981-13-5876-0 ISBN 978-981-13-5877-7 (eBook)
https://doi.org/10.1007/978-981-13-5877-7

Library of Congress Control Number: 2019934726

This Springer imprint is published by the registered company Springer Nature Singapore Pte Ltd.
The registered company address is: 152 Beach Road, #21-01/04 Gateway East, Singapore 189721, Singapore

Contents

About the Editors

Kamla Kant Shukla is Assistant Professor of Biochemistry in All India Institute of Medical Sciences, Jodhpur. He passed his Masters in Biochemistry with first division and was awarded Ph.D. in Medical Biochemistry from King George's Medical University, Lucknow, in May, 2010. He has worked as Post-doctoral Fellow at Chung Ang University, South Korea, and visited Canada, Japan, South Korea and Australia for international scientific interactions and conferences. He has published more than 25 research papers in reputed international journals in the area of reproductive and cancer biology and has written a book. His work has been cited more than 1000 times with an H-index of 18. He has received several international and national awards like Post-doctoral scholar of Kyushu University, Japan, and Chung Ang University, South Korea. He is an associate editor of *Frontiers in Genetics* and *Frontiers in Endocrinology*. He has delivered various guest lectures in international and national conferences. He is a member of national and international regulatory bodies and several scientific societies.

Praveen Sharma is Professor and Head of Biochemistry Department, Dean (Research) and Controller of Examination at All India Institute of Medical Sciences, Jodhpur. He has done M.Sc and Ph.D. in (Med) Biochemistry from S.M.S. Medical College, Jaipur, India. He has more than 37 years of experience teaching Clinical Biochemistry and Laboratory Management. He has more than 100 research publications and 8 book chapters in various prestigious journals and has interest in diabetes, metabolic syndrome, atherosclerosis, antioxidants and lead toxicity. He has delivered invited lectures at various national and international meetings. He is a recipient of G S Seth Medical College Oration Award (2004), Pattabiraman Oration Award (2010), Awadhesh Saran Memorial Oration Awards (2013) and A.J. Thakur-ACBI Award (2015) for distinguished service and significant contribution to the field of clinical biochemistry. He has been awarded with merit award by Rajasthan Government in 2002. He has been twice President of ACBI and Fellow of the Association of Clinical Biochemists of India (FACBI). He is Editor-in-Chief of the *Indian Journal of Clinical Biochemistry* (IJCB) and Chairman of the Corporate Wing of ACBI. He has also served as member of Accreditation Committee of National Accreditation Board for Testing and Calibration Laboratories (NABL) and also NABL Assessor. Dr. Sharma is a Director of National Referral Center of Lead Project India, Jodhpur. He was ACBI Representative to Asia Pacific Federation of Clinical Biochemistry and

Laboratory Medicine (APFCB) and International Federation of Clinical Chemistry and Lab Medicine (IFCC). Dr. Sharma is Chair of the Communication Committee of APFCB and also Chief Editor of APFCB News. Besides he is organizing chairman of the forthcoming APFCB Congress 2019 Jaipur.

Sanjeev Misra is the Director and CEO of All India Institute of Medical Sciences, Jodhpur. He passed his MBBS and MS in General Surgery from KGMC, Lucknow, India. He has been a sectional Editor of the Oncology Section of the *Indian Journal of Surgery* and Honorary Secretary (2007–2008), Vice President (2011), President-Elect (2012) and President (2013) of the Indian Association of Surgical Oncology. He is a postgraduate teacher recognized by the MCI and NBE and examiner for M.Ch. and DNB. He is a Fellow of the National Academy of Medical Sciences, India, Fellow of the National Academy of Sciences, India, Fellow of the American College of Surgeons, USA, and Fellow of the International College of Surgeons, USA. He has received several international and national awards like Commonwealth fellowship and International Guest Scholar of American College of Surgeons. He has been a visiting professor to King's College, London, Mayo Clinic, Rochester, USA, John Hopkins Medical Center, USA, and University of Pittsburgh Medical Center, USA. For his contribution to surgery, he was awarded FRCS, England and Glasgow (Ad eundem). He was awarded fellowships at MSKCC, New York, MD Anderson Cancer Center, Houston, and Cancer Institute Hospital, Tokyo. He has published extensively and has over 105 published papers and 20 chapters in several international and national journals. He is an associate editor of the *Indian Journal of Surgical Oncology* and is on the editorial board of the *International Journal of Surgical Oncology*. He is a member of the Executive committee of Asian Clinical Oncology Society. He has delivered various guest lectures and orations in international and national conferences. He is the founder member of Indian Breast Group and Indian Liver Group. He has been involved with medical education and is dedicated to the teaching, training and practice of surgery and its growth for close to two decades.

Recent Advances in Molecular Diagnostic Approaches for Cancer

1

Kamla Kant Shukla,
Shrimanjunath Sankanagoudar,
Barkha Singhal Sanganeria, Puneet Pareek,
Jeevan Ram, Sanjeev Misra, and Praveen Sharma

1.1 Introduction

Cancer is one of the most common human diseases, which occurs due to abnormal growth and proliferation of cells undergoing sporadic or familial mutations. These cancer cells have potential to break away from the tumor mass and spread through the lymphatic system or bloodstream in body leading to metastasis [1]. Cancer is caused by changes in genes controlling the functions of cells, especially the growth and cell division [2]. Genes carry the instructions for synthesis of proteins and certain changes may alter protein production leads to cancer development such as increase production of a protein responsible for cell growth, resulting in uncontrolled cell division, or production of nonfunctional proteins of cellular damage repair [3]. The abnormal cell division is also due to the breakdown in the regulation of cell cycle signaling pathway leading to tumor formation [4, 5].

K. K. Shukla (✉) · S. Sankanagoudar · P. Sharma
Department of Biochemistry, All India Institute of Medical Sciences, Jodhpur, Rajasthan, India
e-mail: shuklakk@aiimsjodhpur.edu.in

B. S. Sanganeria
Centre for Transplant and Renal Research, Westmead Institute for Medical Research, Westmead, NSW, Australia

P. Pareek
Department of Radiation Oncology, All India Institute of Medical Sciences, Jodhpur, Rajasthan, India

J. Ram · S. Misra
Department of Surgical Oncology, All India Institute of Medical Sciences, Jodhpur, Rajasthan, India

1.2 Causes of Cancer

To determine the causative factors of cancer is a complex process as many factors are known to increase the risk of cancer. Cancer is caused by changes in normal cellular DNA known as mutations [6]. These mutations may alter gene expression and mRNA production and also result in uncontrolled cell growth mainly by the following three mechanisms.

- ***Mutation of normal genes***: These mutations make cells to grow and divide more rapidly creating many new cells that all have the same mutations. For example, KRAS is a gene that acts as an on/off switch in cell signaling and functions normally by controlling cell proliferation. If it is mutated, it leads to continuous cell proliferation.
- ***Mutation of tumor suppressor genes***: Tumor suppressor genes normally regulate the cell growth but due to a mutation, cells lose inhibition and grow uncontrollably. For example, tumor suppressor p53 protein is encoded by the TP53 gene and loss of p53 have been found in more than half of human cancers. Li-Fraumeni syndrome (LFS), an inherited p53

K. K. Shukla et al. (eds.), *Molecular Diagnostics in Cancer Patients*,
https://doi.org/10.1007/978-981-13-5877-7_1

mutation increases the risk of developing various types of cancers.

- ***Mutation of genes involved in repair mechanism***: Mutations occurring during normal cell growth are recognized and repaired by DNA repair mechanism and if, this fails, leads to cancer development. For example, hereditary non-polyposis colon cancer is caused by mutation in one of the DNA repair genes like MLH1, MSH2 and PMS2.

The full sequential events of human cancer development is not yet completely understood, but role of oncogenes (genes promoting cell growth and reproduction) and tumor suppressor genes (genes inhibiting cell division and survival) are critical in tumor initiation and progression (Fig. 1.1).

1. **Hereditary (genetic factor):** Genetic changes that promote cancer can be inherited from parents if it is present in germ cells, like reproductive cells of the body (egg and sperm). These germ-line changes would present in every cell of the offspring [7] and carried to the next generations [8]. However, these types of mutations account for small percentages of cancers.
2. **Mutations that occur after birth (environmental factor)**: Genetic changes that occur after conception is called somatic mutations [9]. There are many reasons, which cause these mutations such as carcinogen (tobacco and alcohol), radiation, certain infections, sedentary lifestyle, obesity and environmental pollutants [10]. These type of cancer even being non-hereditary sometimes appear to run in families e.g., tobacco use in family leading to the development of similar cancers among family members [11].

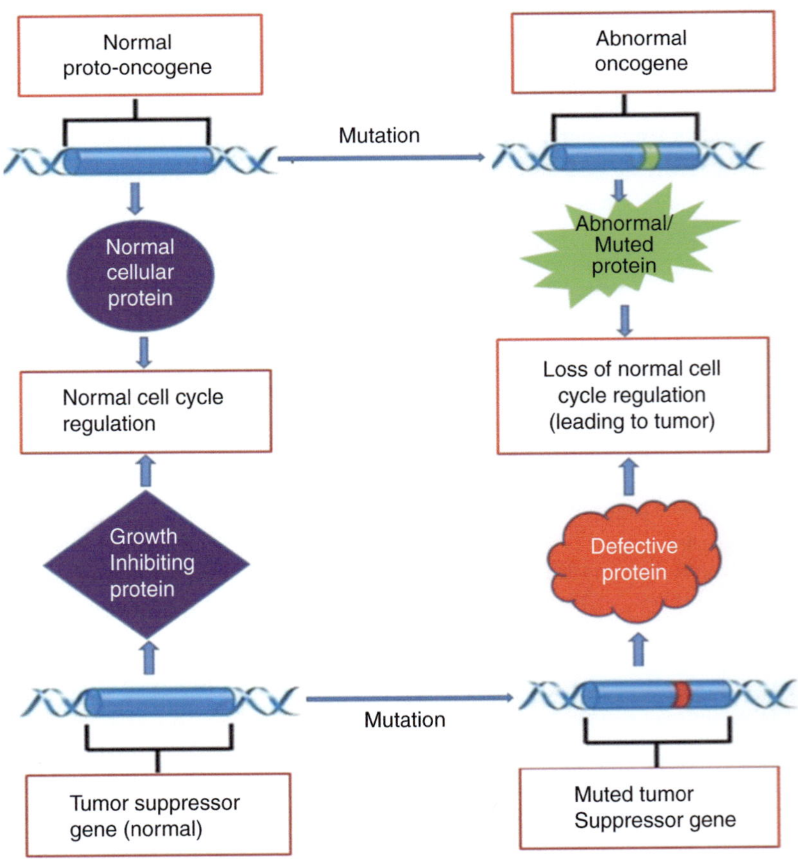

Fig. 1.1 Mechanism of cancer development

1.3 Classification of Cancers

There are around 200 different known cancers that affect humans and their types are often described by the body part or tissue of origination. However, some body parts contain multiple types of tissue, so for greater precision, cancers are additionally classified by type of cell of origination [12]. These types include:

- ***Carcinoma*:** These are of epithelial origin and most common cancer of older age. Cancer developing in the breast, prostate, lung, pancreas and colon are mostly carcinomas.
- ***Sarcoma*:** Cancers arising from connective tissue (i.e. bone, cartilage, fat, nerve), develop from cells originating in mesenchymal cells outside the bone marrow.
- ***Lymphoma and leukemia*:** Cancers of hematopoietic system and leukemia is most commonly seen in children.
- ***Germ cell tumor*:** Originating from pluripotent cells, these are most commonly seen in the testicle or the ovary i.e. seminoma and dysgerminoma, respectively.
- ***Blastoma*:** Cancers derived from immature "precursor" cells or embryonic tissue are called blastomas. They are more common in children.

There are some cancers which are named based on the size and shape of the cells as seen under a microscope, such as giant cell carcinoma, spindle cell carcinoma and small cell carcinoma.

1.4 Screening of Cancer

Cancers which are detected and treated early may have better long-term survival but unfortunately, there are no effective screening tests for early cancer detection in most cases.

There have been some important successes in screening and early detection [13]. Deaths from carcinoma cervix reduced significantly in the United States after the annual screening with the "pap" test became a common practice; screening for colorectal and breast cancer have also been shown to reduce mortality caused by these cancers (Fig. 1.2).

1.5 Diagnosis

Molecular diagnostic tests can help in the diagnosis and classification of cancers and these tests can help to know specific mutations causing cancer. Similarly, the molecular profile of the tumor

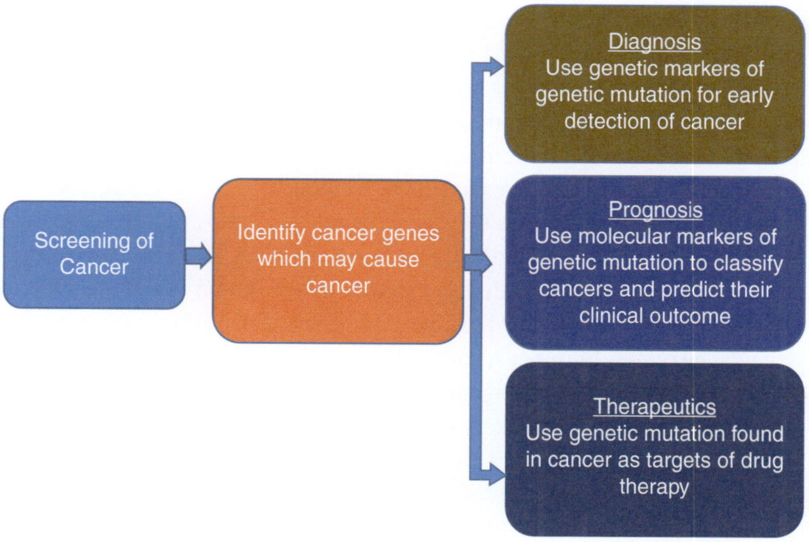

Fig. 1.2 Cancer patients screening via molecular diagnostics

cells is increasingly being used for the classification and choice of personalised treatment of cancer. Family history and genetic information may identify people at risk of cancer which may serve as the first step in identification of an inherited cancer [13]. For an increasing number of diseases, DNA-based testing can be used to identify a specific pathogenic variant. The proportion of individuals carrying a pathogenic variant who will manifest the disease is referred to as penetrance. In general, common genetic variants that are associated with cancer susceptibility have a lower penetrance than rare genetic variants [14].

Companion diagnostics is the relatively new term describing the tests, often molecular, which are used to determine whether a specific therapy would likely be effective for a specific patient. These tests improve patient outcomes and can reduce health care costs. The molecular diagnostics helps at every stage of care, make them one of the most dynamic and transformative areas of diagnostics in health care system.

1.6 Molecular Biomarkers

Biomarkers have many potential applications in oncology, including risk assessment, screening, differential diagnosis, prognosis, prediction of response to treatment, and monitoring of progression of disease [15, 16]. Because of the critical role that biomarkers play at all stages of disease, it is important that they must undergo rigorous evaluation, including analytical validation, clinical validation, and assessment of clinical utility, prior to incorporation into routine clinical care.

Molecular alterations also serve as convenient "markers" of disease. Since they are carried in the coded elements contained within tumor cells, their detection in biological fluids or tissues indicates the presence of tumour [17]. Several genes, proteins, enzymes, hormones, carbohydrate moieties and a few oncofetal antigens have been recognized as potential biomarkers. There are some specific genomic biomarkers proposed such as *TP53*, a protein that suppresses the growth of tumors, has been found to be a commonly mutated gene in almost all cancer types [18]. Germline mutations in this gene cause Li-Fraumeni syndrome, a rare, inherited disorder that leads to a higher risk of developing certain cancers. Inherited mutations in the *BRCA1* and *BRCA2* genes are associated with an increased lifetime risk of hereditary breast and ovarian cancer syndrome in women [19]. Several other cancers such as pancreatic and prostate cancers, as well as male breast cancer have also been associated with this syndrome [20]. PTEN is another gene that produces a protein suppressing the growth of tumors. Mutations in PTEN are associated with Cowden syndrome, an inherited disorder that increases the risk of breast, thyroid, endometrial, and other types of cancers [21].

1.7 Various Techniques Used in Molecular Diagnostics

Various promising technologies and diagnostic applications of structural genomics are currently producing a large database of cancer-genes by mutation scanning and DNA chip technology [22]. A variety of methods can be used to study genetic aberrations includes fluorescent *in situ* hybridization (FISH), allele-specific polymerase chain reaction (PCR), quantitative real-time (qPCR), gene sequencing, gene expression using microarrays and next generation sequencing (NGS) and proteomic analysis through mass spectrometry (SELDI TOF MS) and peptide receptors.

1.7.1 Polymerase Chain Reaction (PCR)

PCR is the most frequently used molecular technique in a molecular genetic laboratory. Using a pair of priming complementary sequences (oligonucleotide primers) flanking to a location of interest, together with unique heat-resistant polymerases, multiple copies of a targeted gene can be obtained. PCR is a very sensitive molecular technique that can detect mutations in even a small cell population [23]. For example, in leukemia patients who have received bone marrow transplants, PCR may be used to test for residual malignant cells present in very low levels in the circulation. Therefore, PCR can precisely detect the success of therapy in the course of illness.

1.7.2 Real-Time PCR

Quantitative PCR (qPCR) is of great utility in the assessment of minimal residual disease following novel targeted therapy against specific molecular defects as well as bone marrow transplantation for myelogenous leukemia [24]. Along with detecting the presence or absence of leukemia cells carrying the target translocation, qPCR can be used to evaluate a series of blood samples (or bone marrow aspirates) after transplantation and determine if the number of BCR-ABL–positive cells in these samples is stable or is increasing. Results can be obtained in 2 h and, depending on the instrument used, as many as 384 samples can be tested in a single run [25].

1.7.3 DNA Sequencing

DNA sequencing is the method of detecting the precise order of nucleotides within a DNA molecule or segment. This technology is used to determine the order of the four nitrogenous bases such as adenine, guanine, cytosine and thymine in a DNA strand. The advent of rapid DNA sequencing methods has greatly accelerated biological and medical research in cancer diagnosis [26].

The only drawback of DNA sequencing is the time and cost. Today, methods are available that sequence DNA much more quickly and inexpensively. The most popular method used currently is called next-generation sequencing (NGS). In this method, up to 500 million separate sequencing reactions are run at the same time on a slide the size of a Band-Aid®. This slide is put into a machine which analyzes each reaction separately and stores the DNA sequences in a computer. The reaction is a copying procedure similar to the one described for the Sanger method but does not require the use of altered nucleotide bases [27].

1.7.4 Microarrays

DNA microarrays can be used to compare the gene expression patterns in two different cell populations, such as a population of cancer cells with normal cells and in this case, two different fluorescent dyes are used [28]. The results obtained from microarray are dramatically changing cancer-treatment decisions [29]. Microarrays can also be used to detect differences in patterns of gene expression even within the same tumor type. However, one of the major challenges is to effectively select a few informative genes to construct accurate cancer prediction models from thousands to ten thousands of gene expression profiles.

1.7.5 Cytogenetic Testing

Cytogenetic test involves examining the number and structure of chromosomes. The conventional cytogenetic tests involve culturing of nucleated cells, allowing for division and their metaphase arrest. It is essential in cytogenetics testing that the cells must be in dividing stage so that the chromosome can be easily visualized by microscope [30]. The dividing cells are then placed on a microscope slide and evaluated in multiple cells (usually at least 20). Cytogenetics is mainly used for the typing of blood cancers such as leukemia [31]. One of the drawbacks of conventional cytogenetics is time-consuming cell culture step and using only fresh tissue samples.

1.7.6 Fluorescent In Situ Hybridization (FISH)

FISH, also known as molecular cytogenetic testing, is a way to visualize and document the location of genetic material, including specific genes or DNA sequences within genes. FISH exploits the binding of fluorescence-labeled oligonucleotide probes to its specific complementary DNA sequence target on the genome and highlights that region with fluorescence color (e.g., Texas red, FITC green, acridine orange). Firstly, DNA in the chromosomes is denatured then DNA probe is introduced where it can bind to complementary DNA sequences in the sample [32]. Once the probes have hybridized, they viewed under a fluorescent microscope. Unlike conventional cytogenetic techniques, FISH does not have to be performed on cells that are actively dividing which makes it more versatile and also offers great advantages over conventional cytogenetics in the study of chromosomal deletions, translocations and gene amplification. This great adaptability, in addition to the topographic identification by fluorescent microscopic examination, which allows distinction between signals from tumorous and non-tumorous cells, has fueled the field of "interphase cytogenetics" in both tumor and prenatal settings. FISH is particularly helpful in identifying copy number variations, especially translocation and amplification, for example frequency of HER2 in breast and gastric cancers [33].

1.7.7 Surface-Enhanced Laser Desorption/Ionization Time-of-Flight Mass Spectrometry (SELDI-TOF-MS)

Surface-enhanced laser desorption/ionization (SELDI) is an ionization method in mass spectrometry that is used for the analysis of protein mixtures [34]. Typically, SELDI is used with time-of-flight mass spectrometers (TOF-MS) to detect proteins in tissue samples, blood, urine, or other clinical samples. SELDI-TOF MS is the technology used to acquire the proteomic patterns to be used in the diagnostic setting [35, 36]. The high sensitivity and specificity achieved by this method show a great potential for the early detection of cancer and facilitation of discovering new and improved biomarkers (Fig. 1.3).

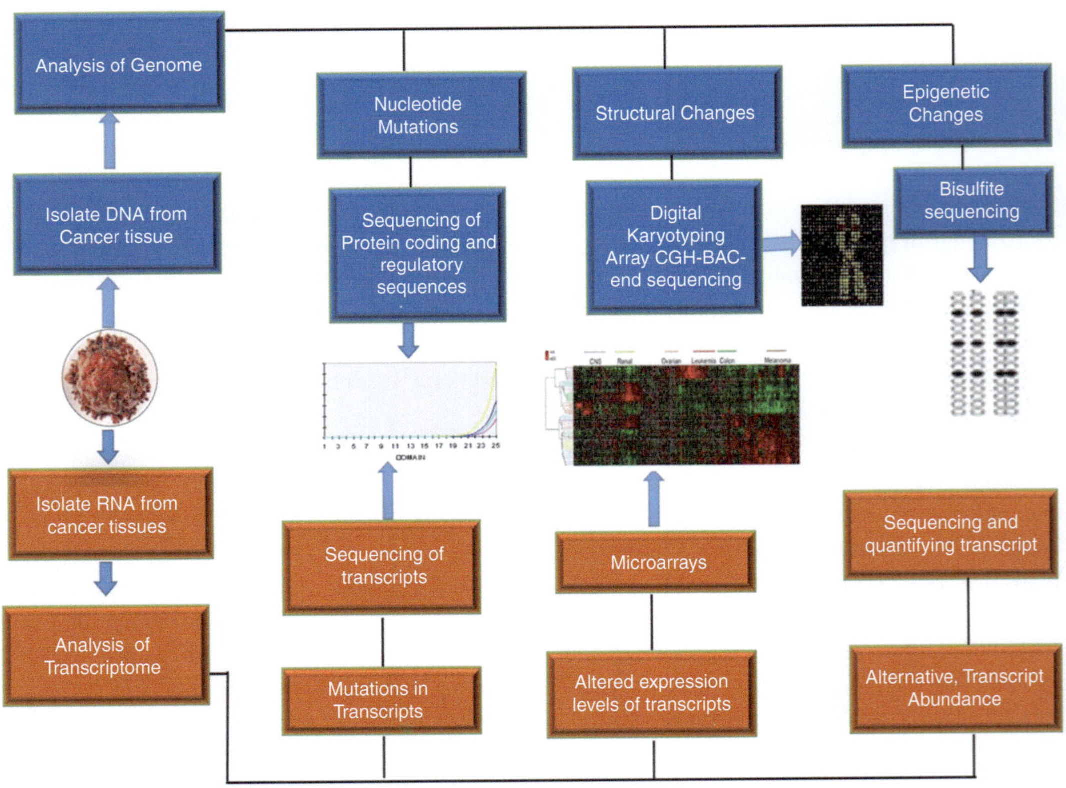

Fig. 1.3 Molecular diagnostics tools for cancer patients

1.8 Prognosis

Prognostication is integral component of decision making in cancer care. It usually combines the cancer diagnosis with considering the efficacy, toxicity, and risks of treatment. The advancement of molecular evaluation in the early twenty-first century, there is possibility of decoding the complete full-length sequence of the human genome [37]. This gave a remarkable impulse to the development of DNA sequencing technologies and computational approaches to analyze large volumes of data. There are two important areas that have been drastically transformed, such as the ability to prognosticate cancer outcome and the ability to predict tumor response to a specific drug.

Molecular diagnostics play an important role in prognosis by evaluating the likelihood of cancer recurrence after treatment. Several molecular diagnostics are available to predict the likelihood of breast cancer recurrence in women with early-stage, node-negative, estrogen receptor-positive, invasive breast cancer which can be treated with hormone therapy.

1.9 Pharmacokinetics and Pharmacodynamics

Pharmacokinetics (PK) and pharmacodynamics (PD) are reciprocal terms often described in cancer drug discovery and development, where PK is the measurement of change in drug concentration with time and PD is the measurement of the biological effects of the drug at different concentrations over different time periods. Cancer biomarkers can be used to determine the most effective treatment regime for personalized patient care. Some people metabolize drugs differently because of the differences in their genetic makeup. In certain cases, reduced metabolism of certain drugs can create threatening conditions in which high levels of the drug accumulate in the body [38]. The drug dosing decisions in particular cancer treatments can be benefited by the screening of the biomarkers. An example is a gene encoding the enzyme thiopurine methyl-transferase (TPMT) in which individuals with TPMT gene mutations are unable to metabolize large amounts of a chemotherapeutic drug against leukemia such as mercaptopurine, which potentially causes a fatal drop in white blood count for such patients. For safety considerations, patients with TPMT mutations are recommended a lower dose of mercaptopurine [39].

1.10 Conclusion

This chapter brings together excerpts from various techniques of molecular diagnostics in cancer patients. In the current chapter, we highlighted many aspects of molecular diagnostics, use of biomarkers for diagnosis, prognosis and their role in pharmacokinetics and pharmacodynamics of cancer treatment. Molecular diagnostics is a fast-evolving area of research and medicine, with newer emerging technologies. The applications of these techniques being continually used for rapid diagnosis of cancer before its advanced stage. The technologies that come under the broad category of molecular diagnosis include cancer genetics study using PCR, real time PCR, gene sequencing and FISH; profiling of gene expression using microarrays, miRNAs and proteomic analysis through mass spectrometry (SELDI TOF MS). In near future, nanotechnology will have a pivotal role in the area of molecular diagnosis of cancer by employing technologies involving nanodevices, micro fluidic systems, newer generation biochips etc. for an early diagnosis and effective management of cancer.

The knowledge of cancer genetics and molecular diagnostics applications are rapidly improving our understanding of cancer biology, offering great help to identify at-risk individuals (screening) and diagnosis, furthering the ability to characterize malignancies (classification of different types of cancer). All these techniques offer a great promise for development of tailored treatment to the molecular fingerprint of the disease and have led to the discovery of numerous therapeutic molecules for cancer treatment, and the optimization of drug therapy. Undoubtedly molecular diagnosis will take a major role in improvements in care for cancer patients in the not-too-distant future.

References

1. World Health Organization. Cancer Fact sheet N°297. February 2018. Accessed 21 Mar 2018.
2. National Cancer Institute. Defining cancer. Accessed 28 Mar 2018.
3. Nebbioso A, Tambaro FP, Dell'Aversana C, Altucci L. Cancer epigenetics: moving forward. PLoS Genet. 2018;14(6):e1007362.
4. Balmain A, Gray J, Ponder B. The genetics and genomics of cancer. Nat Genet. 2003;33:238–44.
5. McClelland SE. Role of chromosomal instability in cancer progression. Endocr Relat Cancer. 2017;24(9):T23–31.
6. Tomasetti C, Li L, Vogelstein B. Stem cell divisions, somatic mutations, cancer etiology, and cancer prevention. Science. 2017;355(6331):1330–4.
7. Emery J, Barlow-Stewart K, Metcalfe SA. There's cancer in the family. Aust Fam Physician. 2009;38(4):194–8.
8. Rhine CL, Cygan KJ, Soemedi R, Maguire S, Murray MF, Monaghan SF, Fairbrother WG. Hereditary cancer genes are highly susceptible to splicing mutations. PLoS Genet. 2018;14(3):e1007231.
9. Forbes SA, Beare D, Gunasekaran P, Leung K, Bindal N, Boutselakis H, Ding M, Bamford S, Cole C, Ward S, Kok CY, Jia M, De T, Teague JW, Stratton MR, McDermott U, Campbell PJ. COSMIC: exploring the world's knowledge of somatic mutations in human cancer. Nucleic Acids Res. 2015;43:D805–D81.
10. Simonati C1, Limina RM, Gelatti U, Indelicato A, Scarcella C, Donato F, Nardi G. Cancer incidence and mortality in some health districts in Brescia area 1993–1995. Ann Ig. 2004;16(6):767–75.
11. Boroughs LK, DeBerardinis RJ. Metabolic pathways promoting cancer cell survival and growth. Nat Cell Biol. 2015;17:351–9.
12. Idikio HA. Human cancer classification: a systems biology-based model integrating morphology, cancer stem cells, proteomics, and genomics. J Cancer. 2011;2:107–15.
13. Wilt TJ, Harris RP, Qaseem A, High Value Care Task Force of the American College of Physicians. Screening for cancer: advice for high-value care from the American College of Physicians. Ann Intern Med. 2015;162(10):718–25.
14. Weitzel JN, Blazer KR, MacDonald DJ, Culver JO, Offit K. Genetics, genomics, and cancer risk assessment: state of the art and future directions in the era of personalized medicine. CA Cancer J Clin. 2011;61(5):327–59.
15. Baron JA. Screening for cancer with molecular markers: progress comes with potential problems. Nat Rev Cancer. 2012;12(5):368–71.
16. Shukla KK, Misra S, Pareek P, Mishra V, Singhal B, Sharma P. Recent scenario of microRNA as diagnostic and prognostic biomarkers of prostate cancer. Urol Oncol. 2017;35(3):92–101.
17. Saijo K, Ishioka C. Development of biomarkers for molecular target drugs. Nihon Rinsho. 2015;73(8):1308–12.
18. Leroy B, Anderson M, Soussi T. TP53 mutations in human cancer: database reassessment and prospects for the next decade. Hum Mutat. 2014;35(6):672–88.
19. Li D, Kumaraswamy E, Harlan-Williams LM, Jensen RA. The role of BRCA1 and BRCA2 in prostate cancer. Front Biosci (Landmark Ed). 2013;18:1445–59.
20. Foulkes WD. BRCA1 and BRCA2 - update and implications on the genetics of breast cancer: a clinical perspective. Clin Genet. 2014;85(1):1–4.
21. Poliseno L, Pandolfi PP. PTEN ceRNA networks in human cancer. Methods. 2015;77-78:41–50.
22. Krebs MG, Metcalf RL, Carter L, Brady G, Blackhall FH, Dive C. Molecular analysis of circulating tumour cells-biology and biomarkers. Nat Rev Clin Oncol. 2014;11(3):129–44.
23. Wang B, Yu L, Yang GZ, Luo X, Huang L. Application of multiplex nested methylated specific PCR in early diagnosis of epithelial ovarian cancer. Asian Pac J Cancer Prev. 2015;16(7):3003–7.
24. Zhao Y, Cao X, Tang J, Zhou L, Gao Y, Wang J, Zheng Y, Yin S, Wang Y. A novel multiplex real-time PCR assay for the detection and quantification of HPV16/18 and HSV1/2 in cervical cancer screening. Mol Cell Probes. 2012;26(2):66–72.
25. Mandhaniya S, Iqbal S, Sharawat SK, Xess I, Bakhshi S. Diagnosis of invasive fungal infections using real-time PCR assay in paediatric acute leukaemia induction. Mycoses. 2012 Jul;55(4):372–9.
26. Tipu HN, Shabbir A. Evolution of DNA sequencing. J Coll Physicians Surg Pak. 2015;25(3):210–5.
27. Boyd SD. Diagnostic applications of high-throughput DNA sequencing. Annu Rev Pathol. 2013;8:381–410.
28. Inaoka K, Inokawa Y, Nomoto S. Genomic-wide analysis with microarrays in human oncology. Microarrays (Basel). 2015;4(4):454–73.
29. Sekar D, Thirugnanasambantham K, Hairul Islam VI, Saravanan S. Sequencing approaches in cancer treatment. Cell Prolif. 2014;47(5):391–5.
30. Ferguson-Smith MA. History and evolution of cytogenetics. Mol Cytogenet. 2015;8:19.
31. Manola KN. Cytogenetic abnormalities in acute leukaemia of ambiguous lineage: an overview. Br J Haematol. 2013;163(1):24–39.
32. García-Peláez B, Trias I, Román R, Pubill C, Banús JM, Puig X. Fluorescent in situ hybridization as a predictor of relapse in urothelial carcinoma. Actas Urol Esp. 2013;37(7):395–400.

33. Van der Logt EM, Kuperus DA, van Setten JW, van den Heuvel MC, Boers JE, Schuuring E, Kibbelaar RE. Fully automated fluorescent in situ hybridization (FISH) staining and digital analysis of HER2 in breast cancer: a validation study. PLoS One. 2015;10(4):e0123201.
34. Ho DW, Yang ZF, Wong BY, Kwong DL, Sham JS, Wei WI, Yuen AP. Surface-enhanced laser desorption/ionization time-of-flight mass spectrometry serum protein profiling to identify nasopharyngeal carcinoma. Cancer. 2006;107(1):99–107.
35. Yang SY, Xiao XY, Zhang WG, Zhang LJ, Zhang W, Zhou B, Chen G, He DC. Application of serum SELDI proteomic patterns in diagnosis of lung cancer. BMC Cancer. 2005;5:83.
36. Zhang GQ, Du J, Pang D. Detection and clinical significance of serum proteomic patterns of breast cancers by surface enhanced laser desorption/ionization time of flight mass spectrometry. Zhonghua Zhong Liu Za Zhi. 2006;28(3):204–7.
37. Reubi JC. Regulatory peptide receptors as molecular targets for cancer diagnosis and therapy. Q J Nucl Med. 1997;41(2):63–70.
38. Wang W, Nag S, Zhang R. Pharmacokinetics and pharmacodynamics in breast cancer animal models. Methods Mol Biol. 2016;1406:271–87.
39. Lee W, Lockhart AC, Kim RB, Rothenberg ML. Cancer pharmacogenomics: powerful tools in cancer chemotherapy and drug development. Oncologist. 2005;10(2):104–11.

2 Molecular Diagnosis of Gall Bladder Cancer

Rajani Rai, Saumyak Gosai, Chinthalapally V. Rao, and Vishal Chandra

2.1 Gallbladder Cancer

Gallbladder Cancer (GBC), first described in 1771 by De Stoll, is a rare but an aggressive and highly fatal malignancy [1]. Worldwide, the incidence of GBC showed remarkable geographic variability that correlates with the prevalence of cholelithiasis (gallstone) with higher incidence being reported from developing nations like South American countries, Central and Northern Europe as well as some areas of India, Pakistan, Japan and Korea while it is infrequent in developed countries like USA [2]. According to The American Cancer Society's estimates, there will be approximately 12,190 new cases diagnosed (5450 in men and 6740 in women) with, and 3790 deaths (1530 in men and 2260 in women) due to, cancer of the gallbladder and nearby large bile ducts in the United States for 2018. The incidence rates of gallbladder cancer in Chile are more than 25 per 100,000 females and 9 per 100,000 males [3]. GBC is primarily classified as a disease of elderly females having 2–6 times higher incidence in female than males [4, 5]. Higher incidence and mortality rate of GBC is also reported in women from Delhi, Northern India (21.5/100,000) followed by South Karachi, Pakistan (13.8/100,000) and Quito, Ecuador (12.9/100,000) [2].

GBC is associated with poor prognosis due to its anatomic position (proximity to the major extrahepatic bile duct and liver) and feature (lack of a serosal layer) enabling early invasion of the liver and metastatic progression to the regional lymph nodes, the vagueness and nonspecificity of symptoms thereby contributing advanced stage at diagnosis and limited therapeutic options [6]. The overall 5-year survival for the GBC is less than 5% [7] with a median survival time of 4.8 months [8].

R. Rai
Department of Obstetrics and Gynecology, University of Oklahoma Health Sciences Center, Oklahoma City, OK, USA
e-mail: rajani-rai@ouhsc.edu

S. Gosai
Department of Obstetrics and Gynecology, University of Oklahoma Health Sciences Center, Oklahoma City, OK, USA

McAllen Family Medicine Residency Program, McAllen, TX, USA
e-mail: saumyakkumar.gosai@utrgv.edu

C. V. Rao
Hematology/Oncology Section, Department of Medicine, Center for Cancer Prevention and Drug Development, Stephenson Cancer Center (SCC), University of Oklahoma Health Sciences Center (OUHSC), Oklahoma City, OK, USA
e-mail: cv-rao@ouhsc.edu

V. Chandra (✉)
Department of Obstetrics and Gynecology, University of Oklahoma Health Sciences Center, Oklahoma City, OK, USA
e-mail: Vishal-chandra@ouhsc.edu

K. K. Shukla et al. (eds.), *Molecular Diagnostics in Cancer Patients*,
https://doi.org/10.1007/978-981-13-5877-7_2

2.2 Risk Factors GBC

The pathogenesis of the GBC is multifactorial comprising the combined effect of multiple genetic variations along with numerous dietary and environmental risk factors in addition to age, gender and race [9].

2.2.1 Age, Gender, Race and Socioeconomic Status

The incidence of GBC increases with age and most frequently diagnosed in the sixth and seventh decades of life with the mean age at diagnosis is 65 years [10]. GBC is mainly a female dominating disease affecting females 2–3 time more than males, which has been partly ascribed to increased incidence of gallstone in women. Worldwide, the highest female/male ratio (>3) was seen in Porto Alegre, Brazil (4.69), Israel (3.6), Pakistan (5.4), Colombia (6.1), Spain (5.5) and Denmark (5). In Northern India, GBC is considered the third most common malignancy of female with 1:3 male to female ratio [4] and in the United States, female to male ratio across all ethnic groups is 1.8. In the USA, white people have a 50% greater incidence than the black population [11]. A majority of GBC patients belong to low SES and hailed from rural background [4].

2.2.2 Gallstone and Other Pre-existing Diseases

Several pre-existed diseases (gallstone, anomalous pancreato-biliary ductal union, gallbladder polyps and Xanthogranulomatous cholecystitis etc.) are associated with increased risk of GBC. Gallstones are well-established cofactors in the causation of GBC [12] having 4–7 times increased risk of developing GBC [4, 13]. About 70–88% of GBC patients have a history or presence of stones, but the incidence of GBC among patients with stones is only 0.3–3.0% [14]. The risk of developing GBC increases directly with increasing duration and size or weight and volume of gallstone [15, 16]. Gallstones >3 cm in size confer a ten fold increased risk when compared with smaller stones [15]. Porcelain gallbladder, Gallbladder polyps, Xanthogranulomatous cholecystitis, Anomalous pancreato-biliary ductal union (APBDJ) and Gallbladder adenoma are also associated with increased risk of GBC [17].

2.2.3 Chronic Inflammation

Chronic inflammatory condition due to the repeated sequences of damage and repair in gallbladder epithelium stimulates progressive morphological deterioration through a metaplasia-dysplasia-carcinoma, and accumulative genome instability, and has been established as the most common causative factor for GBC [18]. Chronic inflammation of the gallbladder is suggested to encourage the loss of p53 gene heterozygosity and over-expression of p53 protein [19]. In addition, it may contribute to the survival and proliferation of mutated cells, apoptosis inhibition and stimulation of angiogenesis as well as metastasis [20].

2.2.4 Infections

Presence of pathogenic mixed bacteria in gallbladders and bile samples of GBC patients, and increased risk of GBC in Typhoid-endemic areas, such as Chile has evoked important role of bacterial infection in GBC [21, 22] S. *typhi* and H. *bilis* infection were associated with an increased risk of GBC [23, 24]. The risks of GBC are found 8.74 times greater in those positive for typhoid carriers than in non-carriers [25]. *S. typhi* produces a toxin named typhoid which causes DNA damage and cell cycle alterations thereby can exert its carcinogenic effect in intoxicated cells [26]. In addition, the bacterial colony may induce chronic inflammation and metabolize bile to produce carcinogenic compounds, and alteration in tumor suppressor genes or proto-oncogenes leading to malignant transformation [27].

2.2.5 Diet

Dietary factors may be either causative or protective for GBC [28]. High intakes of total energy, carbohydrate, red meat consumption, fats, and consumption of carcinogenic impurities in mustard oil are linked with the increased risk of GBC [28]. On the other hand adequate intake of fruits and vegetables, consumption of vitamin B6, vitamin E, Vitamin C and dietary fiber probably reduce the risk of GBC [28–30].

2.2.6 Obesity

Growing evidence have shown positively co-relation between obesity or BMI and the risk of GBC [31, 32]. Obesity promotes GBC risk by interrupting lipid and endogenous hormones, metabolism, and gallbladder motility thereby increasing the risk of gallstone formation [33]. Further, this association is found to be more prominent in women as compared to men [34]. A recent meta-analysis showed that obesity is associated with more than two fold GBC risk in the female, but reported no association between overweight and GBC in male [35].

2.2.7 Genetic Susceptibility and Family History

GBC patients have a significant association with previous family history [4] and gallstone. Subjects with both gallstone and positive family history were found to have a 57-fold increased risk as compared to the 21-fold risk for those with gallstone but without a family history of gallstone [36]. The relative risk for GBC was 13.9 in patients whose first-degree relatives had cancer of gallbladder [37]. The genetic mechanism underlying the development and progress of GBC is poorly understood and most of the research has been focused on K-ras, TP53, p16 gene abnormalities, loss of heterozygosity at tumor suppressor gene, microsatellite instability and loss of cell cycle regulation (Table 2.1).

Table 2.1 Genetic/epigenetic alterations in GBC

Genetic/ epigenetic alterations	Frequency in GBC
p53	p53 point mutation has been found in 30–70% of GBC malignancy. p53 deletion (LOH) is noted in an early stage of GBC [38]. Further, p53 expression was found to gradually increase from precancerous lesion to invasive carcinoma [39]
p16/ CDKN2	p16 abnormalities have been found in approximately 50% of all patients
K-ras	The frequency of K-ras mutation at codon 12 in the high-risk area, China, is reported to 2.7–5% [40, 41] while in India and Japan, it is reported to 38% and 10–67%, respectively [42, 43]
MSI	Low level of MSI (3–35%) is associated with GBC while higher frequency (80%) is found in those associated with APBDJ [43]
LOH	It is a common occurrence in cancer involving deletion of one of the two alleles or chromosomal region. In GBC LOH have been frequently reported on different regions of chromosome 1p, 3p, 8p, 9p, 9q, 13q, 16q, 18q and 22q

MSI microsatellite instability, *APBDJ* anomalous pancreatobiliary ductal union, *LOH* loss of heterozygosity

2.3 Pathogenesis of Gallbladder Cancer

GBC pathology is a multi-step process involving various genetic and epigenetic alterations. For gallbladder carcinogenesis, two models have been anticipated.

Dysplasia-Carcinoma Sequence: Dysplasia-carcinoma sequence of GBC pathogenesis has been described in more than 90% of GBC patients [1]. Roa et al. demonstrated the presence of metaplasia, dysplasia, and CIS in the mucosa adjacent to cancer in 66%, 81.3%, and 69%, respectively [44]. It is triggered by gallstones and chronic inflammation and involves a step-wise progression from normal epithelium into metaplasia that progresses to increasing grades of dysplasia followed by carcinoma in-situ (CIS) and invasive GBC over the years. It is well recognized that gallbladder dysplasia progresses to invasive most cancers normally over a path of 15–19 years [45].

It involves predominant p53 alteration with low K-ras mutation [46].

Adenoma-Carcinoma Sequence: This is the less common pathway for GBC pathogenesis which originates as mass-forming glandular proliferation, known as adenomas (pre-invasive neoplasia) which may progress to invasive carcinoma by an acquisition of increasing cytological and architectural dysplasia by this mass establishing lesion and subsequent invasive characteristics. The transition of benign adenoma into carcinoma was histologically traceable. In a study, the adenomatous residue was found in 19.0% of invasive carcinoma [47].

2.4 GBC Types

Histopathologically, more than 90% of GBC are adenocarcinoma originating in the fundus (60%), followed by body (30%), and neck (10%). Based on the degree of gland formation the adenocarcinomas are divided into four categories: well differentiated (grade 1, >95% gland formation), moderately differentiated (grade 2, 50–95% gland formation) and poorly differentiated (grade 3, 5–49% gland formation), and undifferentiated (grade 4, lack gland formation). The remaining 10% GBC cases include adenosquamous, squamous and anaplastic carcinomas and rare types of GBCs such as carcinosarcoma, small cell carcinoma, lymphoma, signet ring cell-type tumors, carcinoid tumors or embryonal rhabdomyosarcoma (Table 2.2). Adenocarcinomas originate in the mucus-producing gland cells in the gallbladder lining. These were further sub-classified into three types; non-papillary adenocarcinoma, papillary adenocarcinoma, and mucinous adenocarcinoma. Papillary adenocarcinoma develops in the connective tissues holding the gallbladder in place and less likely to spread to the liver and nearby lymph nodes and have the most favorable prognosis compared with other subtypes of GBC. Squamous cell cancers constitute only 2% of GBC and are treated in the same way as adenocarcinomas.

Table 2.2 GBC sub-types

PAC (5% of GBCs)	Characterized by the papillary proliferation of epithelial cells with delicate fibrovascular stalks. Noninvasive papillary tumors show intraluminal growth filling the gallbladder contributing to the early presentation of obstructive symptoms, delayed invasion, and thus associated with a better prognosis. While invasive papillary adenocarcinoma is associated with a 10-year relative survival rate of 52% for tumors confined to the gallbladder wall and of <10% with lymph node metastases [48]
MC (rare, 2.5% of GBCs)	Characterized by extracellular mucin comprising >50% of the tumor volume and when the mucinous component exceeds 90% the tumor is labeled as pure mucinous or colloid carcinoma. Mostly they are mixed-mucinous, not pure colloid, type. Large and advanced tumors at the time of diagnosis and more-aggressive. IHC profile is distinct: MUC2 (86%), MUC5AC (86%), loss of E-cadherin (86%), CDX2 and MUC6 negative and microsatellite stable [49, 50]
CCA (rarest)	Originates from gallbladder epithelium. The tumor cells were characterized by clear cytoplasm, large and well-defined cytoplasmic borders, hyperchromatic nuclei and little nuclear atypia. Cells were organized in nests, sheets, and trabeculae and positive for CK-7, CK-8, CK-18, CK-19, and negative for CK-20 and PAX8. Knowledge about its recurrence and overall survival is limited [51, 52]
ASC (5%)	It shows admixed malignant glandular and squamous component (>25%). Squamous component has a greater proliferative capacity compared with the glandular component. It grows more aggressively with frequent invasion to the liver and other organs. Diagnosed at an advanced stage with overall poor prognosis. Histologically, it may vary from well- to poorly-differentiated keratinizing squamous cell carcinoma [53, 54]
SRCC	An aggressive variant of mucinous adenocarcinoma associated with worse prognosis [23016488]. Characterized by the presence of rounded/ ring-shaped cells with a clear and mucinous cytoplasm and a peripheral nucleus [55]. Primary signet ring carcinoma shows surface dysplastic epithelium. IHC profile show CK7, CK20 positive and CDX2 negative [56]

Table 2.2 (continued)

Undifferentiated carcinomas (0.38%)	Characterized by little glandular or other specific epithelial differentiation [57] associated with worse prognosis. Classified into four types: 1. Spindle and giant cell type: the most common type also referred as sarcomatoid carcinoma. Consist of spindle, giant and polygonal cells 2. Osteoclast-like giant cells: consist of abundant multinucleated osteoclastic giant cells intermixed with pleomorphic malignant cells 3. Small cell type: consists of round undifferentiated cells with vesicular nuclei and prominent nucleoli 4. Nodular or lobular type: consists of well-defined nodules of neoplastic cells
NET (0.2% of all NETs)	Originate from multipotent stem cells or neuroendocrine cells in intestinal or gastric metaplasia of the gallbladder epithelium, and often coexists with gallstones with chronic cholecystitis. They are typically identified at an advanced stage, with a 5-year survival rate of ~36.9% [58–60]
SCC or oat cell carcinomas; (rare, 0.5% of GBCs)	Characterized by aggressive features and early metastasis, with a median survival time of 9 months and no survivors at 10 years Usually presents as a large mass comprising extensive necrosis with a prominent tendency for invasive submucosal growth. About 80% of cases are pure SCC and the remaining are combined SCC. Immunohistochemically, the tumor cells are positive for neuroendocrine markers, such as chromogranin A, synaptophysin, and/or CD56 [61–63]
Gallbladder Sarcoma (exceedingly rare)	Very aggressive, begins in the muscle layer of the gallbladder. Mainly occur in older female and have an overall poor prognosis. The mean survival after diagnosis is measured in months. Tumor types include leiomyosarcoma, rhabdomyosarcoma, angiosarcoma, kaposi's sarcoma, malignant fibrous histiocytoma (MFH), synovial sarcoma, malignant GIST, and liposarcoma. MFH is the predominant variant [64, 65]

PAC papillary adenocarcinoma, *MC* mucinous carcinoma, *CCA* clear cell adenocarcinoma, *ASC* adenosquamous carcinomas, *SRCC* signet-ring cell carcinoma, *NET* neuroendocrine tumors, *SCC* small cell carcinoma, *LSM* leiomyosarcomas, *GIST-like* gastrointestinal stromal tumor-like, *RSM* rhabdomyosarcomas

2.5 Clinical Presentation

Most GBC patients are very difficult to diagnose early and remain asymptomatic or have nonspecific symptoms until the disease progresses to an advanced stage. Most common clinical manifestation associated with GBC is gallstone and chronic inflammation. Patients with GBC present with following three different clinical scenarios; GBC diagnosed fortuitously on pathological examination after simple cholecystectomy, GBC diagnosed at the time of cholecystectomy for presumed non-malignant disease, and GBC suspected preoperatively. The first scenario (patients with acute cholecystitis) is the most common presentation of early-stage GBC leading to better prognosis and survival. Therefore, it is advised to inspect gallbladder mucosa for the presence of any suspicious lesions and its further evaluation following simple cholecystectomy. Patients with chronic cholecystitis present with vague upper GI pain and tenderness, food intolerance, and abdominal fullness. Patient having these symptoms with jaundice may have advanced disease and often is beyond the curable stage [66, 67]. Jaundice is an ominous sign of GBC suggesting obstruction of the distal common hepatic duct or proximal common bile duct and indicates poor prognosis and high postoperative morbidity [68, 69] (Table 2.3).

2.6 Diagnostic Methods

2.6.1 Blood test/Serum Markers

It involves liver function tests like; alkaline phosphatase (ALKP), albumin, aspartate aminotransferase (AST), alanine aminotransferase (ALT), total bilirubin (TBIL), direct bilirubin (DBIL), gamma glutamyl transpeptidase (GGT) and serum marker CA242, CA125, and CA199 and CEA which are found to be frequently elevated in GBC and associated with more advanced disease

Table 2.3 GBC diagnosis

Clinical diagnosis	
History/risk factors	• Age (>60 years) • Gender (female) • Presence of Gallstone or chronic cholecystitis, chronic inflammation • Infection (S. *typhi*, H. *pylori*) • Diet (higher intake of fat, carbohydrate, red meat, mustard oil etc.) • Disease (Obesity, APBDJ, gallbladder polyps, porcelain gallbladder, diabetes, XC) • Genetic factors and family history (having close relatives with GBC or other cancer) • Carcinogen Exposure (oil, heavy metal, free radical, oxidation products, Benzenes) • High parity, early age at first pregnancy, use of Oral contraceptives
Symptoms	• Asymptomatic or symptomatic (vague) • Vague upper GI pain and tenderness • Gastrointestinal bloating, indigestion, nausea or vomiting • Fever • Loss of appetite, weight loss • Itching • Jaundice (in advanced GBC)
Presumptive diagnosis	
Non-invasive diagnostic methods	Serum markers • Liver function tests (ALKP, AST, ALT, TBIL, DBIL, GGT) • Serum marker CA242, CA125, and CA199 CEA • LDH Imaging • USG • CT Scan • MRI • Elastography • PET and PET/CT
Invasive diagnostic methods	• ERCP/ERC • PTC
Definitive diagnosis	
Invasive diagnostic methods	Biopsy: FNAC

GBC gallbladder cancer, *APBDJ* anomalous pancreato-biliary ductal union, *XC* xanthogranulomatous cholecystitis, *ALKP* alkaline phosphatase, *AST* albumin aspartate aminotransferase, *ALT* alanine aminotransferase, *TBIL* total bilirubin, *DBIL* direct bilirubin, *GGT* gamma glutamyl-transpeptidase, *USG* ultrasonography, *CT* computerised tomography, *MRI* magnetic resonance imaging, *PET* positron emission tomography, *ERCP* endoscopic retrograde cholangiopancreatography, *PTC* percutaneous transhepatic cholangiography, *FNAC* fine-needle aspiration cytology, *GI* gastrointestinal

involving liver [70–74].The levels of LDH isoforms (3 and 4) are found to be significantly higher in GBC than cholelithiasis or chronic cholecystitis and total LDH and its isoforms alone or along with ALKP and TBIL is advocated to be potentially valuable biomarker for prognosis of gallbladder diseases like chronic cholecystitis, cholelithiasis and GBC [75, 76]. A study analyzing the serum level of CA242, CA125, and CA199 in GBC demonstrated the highest sensitivity of CA199 (71.7%) and highest specificity of in CA242 (98.7%) for GBC diagnosis with a single tumor marker while in combination of CA199, CA242, and CA125 diagnostic accuracy was 69.2% [70]. Another study showed CA 242 as a promising tumor marker for GBC with the sensitivity, specificity, positive predictive value, and negative predictive values of 64%, 83%, 88%, and 53%, respectively [71].

2.6.2 Imaging Techniques

Ultrasonography (USG): Abdominal ultrasound is the first-line standard diagnostic method in patients with right upper quadrant pain to confirm biliary duct dilatation, identify the obstruction, presence of GB mass and exclude stones. It shows hypo or iso-echogenic irregularly shaped lesion that appears as a subhepatic mass over the gallbladder and might reveal asymmetric gallbladder wall thickening, invasion of adjacent structures [67]. Dilatation of the intrahepatic bile ducts is the most frequent abnormality in patients with bile duct carcinoma [77]. USG is fast, real-time, non-invasive, and no ionizing radiation, cheap and easily available diagnostic method that provides information for disease staging, however, the overall accuracy is limited. In locally advanced disease, USG has a sensitivity of 85% and an overall accuracy of 80% in diagnosing GBC [66].

Color Doppler USG can be applied to identify the structures of the bile duct, compression, and thrombosis in the hepatic artery and portal vein due to the tumor. It is also helpful to assess the invasion into the portal vein and hepatic parenchyma.

Endoscopic ultrasound (EUS) is performed using high-frequency ultrasound (5–12 MHz) probes placed on the endoscope and is useful for the differential diagnosis of gallbladder tumors detected by mass screening, for estimating stage description with depth of tumor invasion and for distinguishing abnormal connections between pancreatobiliary ducts and local lymphadenopathy [78, 79]. EUS also offers safe and reliable sampling method via fine needle aspiration (FNA) biopsy [80]. It is considered more accurate than USG (76%) and useful in differential diagnosis to correctly detect histological neoplasia (97%).

Computerized tomography (CT) Scan: It is more advanced imaging study than USG that gives a 3-D picture of the organs and other structures including any tumors. CT scan can identify tumor invasion outside of the gallbladder and its metastases in the abdomen or pelvis. Combination of CT scan and US provides accurate details of disease extension and liver invasion which usually occurs in 60% of GBC cases. Dual-phase helical CT has an overall accuracy of 93.3% to evaluate GBC [81].

Magnetic resonance imaging (MRI): MRI offers superior soft tissue delineation of gallbladder lesions and biliary tree [82] and is useful in examining disease extension into other tissues or metastatic disease in the liver. MRI with cholangiography (MRCP) and 3D angiography (MR angiography) images may detect bile duct and vascular invasion with 100% sensitivity, but for hepatic invasion and lymph node metastases, sensitivity is less i.e., 67% and 56% respectively [83].

2.6.3 Elastography

Real-time elastography using acoustic radiation force impulse (ARFI) is a new developing method that can discriminate between benign and malignant nodules in various organs. It utilizes high-intensity focused ultrasound to estimate the tissue elasticity [84]. Elastography is a precise tool for discriminating benign gallbladder thickening with gallbladder carcinoma with an overall accuracy of 92.8%. For GBC diagnosing, its sensitivity is 100% and specificity is 91.3%, respectively [85]. It can be combined with sonography as the prime imaging tool for diagnosing gallbladder carcinoma at an early stage. It is also useful in obese (with BMI > 35 kg/m^2) or uncooperative patients and patients with acute cholecystitis [85].

2.6.4 PET and PET/CT

PET scans are especially useful in diagnosing vague primary lesions and identifying residual disease after cholecystectomy and metastases to other tissues and organs. PET and CT scans can be used in combination to locate the precise location of tumors. FDG PET/CT is a very sensitive investigation in predicting the malignant nature and recurrence of gallbladder lesions [86]. Overall diagnostic accuracy for the primary lesion, lymph node involvement, and metastatic disease was reported as 95.9%, 85.7% and 95.9%, respectively [87].

2.6.5 Endoscopic retrograde cholangiopancreatography (ERCP/ERC)

This method is used for diagnosis and treatment of liver, gallbladder, bile ducts, and pancreas related problems. It is best utilized for identifying tumor extension into the bile ducts. In this technique, a long, flexible endoscope is inserted into the first part of the small intestine via the esophagus and stomach and a small catheter is inserted into the common bile duct from the end of the endoscope. Then a contrast dye is injected through the tube followed by X-rays. The images can demonstrate narrowing or obstruction of these ducts and exclude ampullary pathology. This procedure is more invasive than MRCP but allow cells or fluid sample collection by brush cytology, biopsy, needle aspiration for further investigation, and can also be used to place a stent (a small tube) into a duct to help keep it open [88, 89].

2.6.6 Percutaneous Transhepatic Cholangiography (PTC)

It allows access to the proximal biliary tree that has become obstructed by extensive tumor growth from the gallbladder. In this procedure, a contrast dye is injected through a thin, hollow needle inserted into a bile duct via stomach and X-rays was performed. Similar to ERCP, this method is used to collect samples such as fluid or tissues or to place a stent into a duct to help keep it open. However, this method is more invasive and painful and usually used if ERCP failed due to some reason.

2.6.7 Biopsy

Biopsy is performed only after confirming the presence of GBC through other tests. It involves removing a sample of tissue from the gallbladder by laparoscopy or while ERCP and further histopathological evaluations. Ultrasound-guided fine-needle aspiration cytology is a safe method for GBC diagnosis.

2.7 Molecular Markers for GBC Diagnosis and Prognosis

With the rapid progress in molecular technology, the molecular pathogenesis GBC risk has been well established and various etiological factors have been identified. However, GBC is still a lethal disease and only a few valuable prognostic factors have been identified for GBC so far. The results, however, have been variable, and have not yielded clear clinical relevance. Since a subtle change at the molecular or genetic level may lead to the development of a new diagnostic as well as potential targets for personalized therapy, it is necessary to identify different biomarkers and molecular markers associated with GBC progression. Here we will discuss the recent development in GBC pathogenesis associated marker that can be used either alone or in combination to fulfill the gap between early diagnosis and therapy at advance stage GBC (Table 2.4).

p53: Alterations in p53, the tumor suppressor gene, is the most common event in the majority of human cancers. TP53 mutations leading to loss of function have been reported in approximately 27–70% of GBC. Missense mutations in exon 5,6,7,8 and 9 are the most common mutation type producing a nonfunctional protein that starts accu-

Table 2.4 Promising marker for GBC diagnosis and prognosis

Molecular markers	Alterations in GBC
P53	Mutation, over-expression (27–70%), LOH (50%)
K-ras	Mutation (10–67%)
P16	Mutation and loss of expression
Her-2/C-erB2	Overexpression (2–46.5%)
Rb	Mutation and loss of expression
Cyclin D1	Overexpression
Annexin A IV	Overexpression
Trx-1	Overexpression
ADAM-17	Overexpression
E-, N-, P-Cadherins	Altered expression
S100A4	Overexpression
Calpain-1	Overexpression
MicroRNA	Altered expression
NLR, PLR, CRP, GPS	Elevated level
ER PR	Altered expression

mulating in the cell. LOH is another commonest mechanism for loss of p53 function reported in more than 50% of GBC. p53 expression and its accumulation were found to increase in GBC from precancerous lesion to invasive carcinoma, while it has been found to be absent in normal mucosa adjacent to the tumor and normal gallbladder suggesting that p53 protein expression is an early event in the development of GBC. Further, increased expression of p53 was found to be correlated with disease progression in metaplasia-dysplasia-carcinoma sequence for GBC originating in the context of chronic cholecystitis [38]. However, the prognostic implication of p53 alteration in GBC is a subject of debate [90].

K-ras: KRAS mutations, particularly in codons 12, 13 have been reported 10–67% of GBC cases, however, a lower rate of K-ras mutation has been also reported [91]. GBC patients associated with an anomalous pancreaticobiliary duct junction (APBDJ) showed a higher rate of k-ras mutation (50–83%) suggesting it a promising diagnostic marker for these cases [42, 92].

Her-2/C-erB2: C-erbB2, a proto-oncogene, is a transmembrane glycoprotein with tyrosine kinase activity. It is a cell surface growth factor receptor frequently found to be upregulated in various cancers and has been established as a potential therapeutic target. Various studies have reported HER-2/neu (erbB-2) overexpression in 2–46.5% cases of GBC [93, 94]. Her-2 alterations have been proposed as a marker of metastatic disease as well as of poor prognosis [95].

Cell-cycle related proteins: The cyclin D1/p16/Rb pathway plays a critical role in cell cycle regulation and found to be dysregulation in various malignancies. GBC progression is associated with loss of p16 and Rb protein expression and upregulation of cyclin D1 expression [96]. P16 expression was reported in 12–48.8% of GBC and correlated with a low tumor stage and grade [96, 97]. p16/CDKN2A inactivation plays an important role in GBC pathogenesis suggesting it as a favorable prognostic marker [96, 98, 99]. RB protein expression was found in 24–58.5% of GBC [96, 97]. The expressions of Cyclin D1 increased along with the progression of GBC from gallbladder mucosa hyperplasia suggesting that Cyclin D1 may play a role in the early stage of gallbladder carcinoma. Cyclin D1 expression was seen in 40–68.3% of GBC patients [96, 97, 100].

Annexin A IV (ANX4): ANXA4, a member of the annexin family, has been shown to regulate membrane permeability and membrane trafficking. The ANXA4 overexpression has been reported in various epithelial tumors and it has been suggested as an indicator for tumor development, invasion, chemo-resistance, poor outcomes of cancer patients [101]. ANXA4 level is found to be significantly elevated in GBC tissue and has been reported as a significant diagnostic biomarker in GBC [102]. Further, a recent study showed that elevated ANXA4 expression is correlated with invasion depth in GBC patients and predicted a poor prognosis and ANXA4 knockdown demonstrated increased apoptosis and inhibited cell growth, migration, invasion and inhibited tumor growth, suggesting it as a potential therapeutic target [103].

Thioredoxin-1: Thioredoxin-1 (Trx-1) is a ubiquitous multifunctional redox protein having a conserved –Trp–Cys–Gly–Pro–Cys–Lys– redox catalytic site and is reduced by NADPH (nicotinamide adenine dinucleotide phosphate-oxidase) and Trx reductase (Trx-Red). Trx level was found elevated in many cancers. Aggressive tumors overexpress both Trx and Trx-Red. Increased Trx-1 leads to increased cell growth and resistance to apoptosis as well as chemotherapy [104]. TRX-1 protein levels were also found to be significantly high in GBC samples than in cholecystolithiasis samples, indicating a worse prognosis in the invasion front [105].

ADAM-17: The ADAM-17, also known as TACE (tumor necrosis factor-alpha converting enzyme), is a multi-functional gene family of membrane-anchored proteins having a disintegrin and metalloprotease domain. It has been implicated in a variety of biological processes involving cell-cell and cell-matrix interactions and tumor metastasis. Increased expression of ADAM-17 was significantly associated with high histological grade and pT stage and shorter overall survival of GBC patients. Therefore, it may be explored as a new therapeutic target for the GBC management [106].

Cadherins: Cadherins (-E, -N, -P), a class of type-1 transmembrane proteins, are a type of cell adhesion molecule (CAM) playing an important role in the formation of adherent junctions to bind cells with each other. Alterations in expression of these proteins were suggested to be involved in the loss of adhesive mechanisms leading carcinogenesis.

The function of the E-cadherin which is predominantly expressed in epithelial tissue is controlled by the β-catenin and alterations in the E-cadherin/β-catenin complex may contribute to metastasis of cancer cells due to loss of cell adhesion and cell polarity. In GBC, the expression of E-cadherin and β-catenin were found to be significantly differ between normal, inflamed and cancerous tissues; β-catenin expression was decreased between cholecystitis and malignant tissue, as well as between normal epithelium and carcinoma, while the E-cadherin membranous expression was reduced in normal gallbladder epithelia compared to carcinoma and also from inflammation to GBC. Further, the cytoplasmic E-cadherin was significantly different from normal gallbladders to carcinomas and between normal tissue and inflammation [107]. Priya et al., reported high LOH and loss of E-cadherin expression in GBC as compared to chronic cholecystitis, xanthogranulomatous cholecystitis and normal GB [108]. Recently Yi et al. demonstrated a close correlation between the expression of N- and P-cadherin and the clinicopathological as well as biological behaviors, and the poor-prognosis of GBC patients [109].

S100A4: The calcium-binding protein, S100A4, function in cell motility, invasion and tubulin polymerization. It has been established as a metastasis-inducing molecule. In a study, S100A4 staining was detected in 42% of resected GBC cases and 5-year survival rate of these cases is significantly less than that of S100A4 negative, indicating that S100A4 can be used as a GBC prognostic marker [110].

Calpain-1: Calpain-1 belonging to calpain protease family, regulate various physiological functions such as cell differentiation, transcriptional regulation, cell cycle, migration and apoptosis and has been shown to be involved in the cancer progression. In GBC patient's, calpain-1 expression was significantly upregulated as compared with those of cholecystitis patients, suggesting that calpain-1 expression may be associated with disease progression from cholecystitis to GBC [111].

Hormone Receptors: Female sex hormone receptors (ER and PR) expression have been shown in the majority of GBC suggesting an important role of sex hormones in GBC pathogenesis and their implications as anti-hormonal therapy. However, literature regarding their prognostic implication is inconclusive. Simultaneous expression of ER and PR was reported in 23.4% of GBC patients, which is correlated with metaplasia, dysplasia, and early/operable stage of the tumor [112]. Gupta et al. showed significantly high expression of ER in GBC as compared to chronic cholecystitis but no significant difference for PR expression in both groups [113], also their expression did not correlate with gender, age, menopausal status, the presence of gallstones, tumor differentiation, and tumor stage. However, Baskaran et al., showed higher expression of PR in GBC as compared to GSD, and was inversely correlated with tumor stage but positively associated longer overall survival suggesting PR as a prognostic marker [114]. Another study demonstrated the absence of both ER (alpha) and PR in GBC [115]. ERbeta expression was found to be significantly downregulated in GBC as compared to non-cancerous regions and was significantly associated with lymph node metastasis, advanced stage, lower grade, lymphatic invasion and a poor prognosis of the patients indicating the malignant property of GBC [116]. Another study reported ER-beta expression in 73.3% GBC which was associated with tumor differentiation and better 5-year survival rate [115].

MicroRNA: MicroRNAs (miRNAs) are small, non-coding RNA molecules that play a crucial role in carcinogenesis by acting like tumor suppressor- or onco-genes. Like other cancers, in GBC, miRNAs having a tumor suppressor function were found to be downregulated, while those with oncogenic property were upregulated (Table 2.5). The expression profile of miRNAs were significantly correlated with GBC prognosis and prediction. Forced overexpression/inhibition of these miRNAs was

Table 2.5 miRNA profile for GBC

Oncogenic/ up-regulated miRNA	Tumor suppressive/down-regulated miRNA				
miR-182	miR-335	miR-654-3p	miR-146b-5p	miR-379-5p	miR-145
mir-155	miR-34a	miR-411-5p	Mir-218-5p	miR-30e-3p	mir-130a
mir-29b	mir-122	miR-125a-5p	mir-143-3p, -5p	miR-299-5p	mir-99a-5p, -3p
mir-200a	mir-133a	miR-29b-3p	mir-125b-5p	miR-328	mir-29c-3p, -5p
mir-21	mir-195-5p	miR-29b-2-5p	miR-139-5p	miR-154-5p	miR-100-5p
mir-142-3p, -5p	miR-148a-3p	miR-495	miR-145-3p	miR-381-3p	miR-376c
mir-223	miR-187-3p	miR-101-5	miR-365a-3p	mir-133b**5p**	miR-101-3p
miR-182	miR-335	miR-654-3p	miR-146b-5p	miR-379-5p	miR-145

shown to affect tumor growth and development [117]. Further, let-7a, miR-21, miR-187, miR-143, miR-202 and miR-335 were found to be aberrantly expressed of in the blood samples of GBC patients as compared to healthy individuals and the expression of miR-187, miR-143 and miR-122, were correlated with lymph node metastasis and pathological TNM stage suggesting them as a promising noninvasive biomarker for early diagnosis of GBC [118].

Immune response-related index: Inflammation and inflammatory response has been well established as a critical player in the pathogenesis of various malignancies. Neutrophil to lymphocyte ratio (NLR), platelet to lymphocyte ratio (PLR), C-reactive protein (CRP) and Glasgow Prognostic Score (GPS) represents immune response-related index and elevated level of these inflammatory markers have been related to the poor prognosis and survival outcomes in patients of various cancers. In GBC patients, PLR was shown to be significantly associated with CA125 levels, TNM stage, and degree of differentiation [119]. Subsequently recent studies demonstrated that elevated NLR, GPS or CRP and PLR are associated with reduced survival in GBC patients and therefore are suggested as a straightforward, low-cost, valuable and potential prognostic marker for GBC [120–122].

2.8 Conclusion

Nonspecific symptoms, advanced stage of diagnosis and lack of well-defined therapeutic targets are the main factors contributing GBC lethality. Over the past few decades, there has been a remarkable improvement in diagnostic procedures and molecular technology. With the increased understanding of the molecular pathogenesis of GBC, significant effort has been made to identify a potential biomarker for GBC diagnosis at an early stage. Consequently, several potential candidates have been suggested that can be effectively used for diagnostic and prognostic purposes and can contribute to targeted therapy. Nevertheless, none of the biomarkers has shown consisting result predicting GBC prognosis and it is still an infrequent and puzzling malignancy with an overall poor outcome. Future studies need to focus on the combination of proteomics and genomics, including epigenetic alterations related to the molecular pathogenesis of GBC progression that could enhance the specificity and sensitivity of tumor prognosis and leads to the development of novel targeted therapies and contribute in personalized medicine.

References

1. Sharma A, et al. Gallbladder cancer epidemiology, pathogenesis and molecular genetics: recent update. World J Gastroenterol. 2017;23(22):3978–98.
2. Randi G, Franceschi S, La Vecchia C. Gallbladder cancer worldwide: geographical distribution and risk factors. Int J Cancer. 2006;118(7):1591–602.
3. Wernberg JA, Lucarelli DD. Gallbladder cancer. Surg Clin North Am. 2014;94(2):343–60.
4. Kumar JR, et al. An objective assessment of demography of gallbladder cancer. J Surg Oncol. 2006;93(8):610–4.
5. Gabbi C, et al. Estrogen-dependent gallbladder carcinogenesis in LXRbeta−/− female mice. Proc Natl Acad Sci U S A. 2010;107(33):14763–8.

6. Hundal R, Shaffer EA. Gallbladder cancer: epidemiology and outcome. Clin Epidemiol. 2014;6:99–109.
7. Lai CH, Lau WY. Gallbladder cancer—a comprehensive review. Surgeon. 2008;6(2):101–10.
8. Tomita K, et al. Long-term survival of a recurrent gallbladder carcinoma patient with lymph node and peritoneal metastases after multidisciplinary treatments: a case report. Surg Case Rep. 2016;2(1):12.
9. Rai R, et al. A multiple interaction analysis reveals ADRB3 as a potential candidate for gallbladder cancer predisposition via a complex interaction with other candidate gene variations. Int J Mol Sci. 2015;16(12):28038–49.
10. Dwivedi AN, Jain S, Dixit R. Gall bladder carcinoma: aggressive malignancy with protean loco-regional and distant spread. World J Clin Cases. 2015;3(3):231–44.
11. Misra S, et al. Carcinoma of the gallbladder. Lancet Oncol. 2003;4(3):167–76.
12. Shrikhande SV, et al. Cholelithiasis in gallbladder cancer: coincidence, cofactor, or cause! Eur J Surg Oncol. 2010;36(6):514–9.
13. Nervi F, Duarte I, Gómez G, Rodríguez G, Del Pino G, Ferrerio O, et al. Frequency of gallbladder cancer in Chile, a high-risk area. Int J Cancer. 1988;41:657–60.
14. Hamdani NH, et al. Clinicopathological study of gall bladder carcinoma with special reference to gallstones: our 8-year experience from eastern India. Asian Pac J Cancer Prev. 2012;13(11):5613–7.
15. Lowenfels AB, et al. Gallstone growth, size, and risk of gallbladder cancer: an interracial study. Int J Epidemiol. 1989;18(1):50–4.
16. Roa I, et al. Gallstones and gallbladder cancer-volume and weight of gallstones are associated with gallbladder cancer: a case-control study. J Surg Oncol. 2006;93(8):624–8.
17. Biswas PK. Carcinoma gallbladder. Mymensingh Med J. 2010;19(3):477–81.
18. Espinoza JA, et al. The inflammatory inception of gallbladder cancer. Biochim Biophys Acta. 2016;1865(2):245–54.
19. Tazuma S, Kajiyama G. Carcinogenesis of malignant lesions of the gall bladder. The impact of chronic inflammation and gallstones. Langenbeck's Arch Surg. 2001;386(3):224–9.
20. Li Y, Zhang J, Ma H. Chronic inflammation and gallbladder cancer. Cancer Lett. 2014;345(2):242–8.
21. Sharma V, et al. Role of bile bacteria in gallbladder carcinoma. Hepato-Gastroenterology. 2007;54(78):1622–5.
22. Andia ME, et al. Geographic variation of gallbladder cancer mortality and risk factors in Chile: a population-based ecologic study. Int J Cancer. 2008;123(6):1411–6.
23. Tewari M, Mishra RR, Shukla HS. Salmonella typhi and gallbladder cancer: report from an endemic region. Hepatobiliary Pancreat Dis Int. 2010;9(5):524–30.
24. Tyagi BB, Manoharan N, Raina V. Risk factors for gallbladder cancer: a population based case-control study in Delhi. Indian J Med Pediatr Oncol. 2008;29:16–26.
25. Shukla VK, et al. Carcinoma of the gallbladder—is it a sequel of typhoid? Dig Dis Sci. 2000;45(5):900–3.
26. Di Domenico EG, et al. Biofilm producing Salmonella typhi: chronic colonization and development of gallbladder cancer. Int J Mol Sci. 2017;18(9):1887.
27. Prieto AI, Ramos-Morales F, Casadesus J. Repair of DNA damage induced by bile salts in Salmonella enterica. Genetics. 2006;174(2):575–84.
28. Rai A, Mohapatra SC, Shukla HS. A review of association of dietary factors in gallbladder cancer. Indian J Cancer. 2004;41(4):147–51.
29. Makiuchi T, et al. The relationship between vegetable/fruit consumption and gallbladder/bile duct cancer: a population-based cohort study in Japan. Int J Cancer. 2017;140(5):1009–19.
30. Panda D, et al. Gall bladder cancer and the role of dietary and lifestyle factors: a case-control study in a North Indian population. Eur J Cancer Prev. 2013;22(5):431–7.
31. Li L, et al. Overweight, obesity and the risk of gallbladder and extrahepatic bile duct cancers: a meta-analysis of observational studies. Obesity (Silver Spring). 2016;24(8):1786–802.
32. Tan W, et al. Body mass index and risk of gallbladder cancer: systematic review and meta-analysis of observational studies. Nutrients. 2015;7(10):8321–34.
33. Wang F, Wang B, Qiao L. Association between obesity and gallbladder cancer. Front Biosci (Landmark Ed). 2012;17:2550–8.
34. Larsson SC, Wolk A. Obesity and the risk of gallbladder cancer: a meta-analysis. Br J Cancer. 2007;96(9):1457–61.
35. Liu H, et al. Body mass index can increase the risk of gallbladder cancer: a meta-analysis of 14 cohort studies. Med Sci Monit Basic Res. 2016;22:146–55.
36. Hsing AW, et al. Family history of gallstones and the risk of biliary tract cancer and gallstones: a population-based study in Shanghai, China. Int J Cancer. 2007;121(4):832–8.
37. Fernandez E, et al. Family history and the risk of liver, gallbladder, and pancreatic cancer. Cancer Epidemiol Biomark Prev. 1994;3(3):209–12.
38. Rai R, et al. p53: its alteration and gallbladder cancer. Eur J Cancer Prev. 2011;20(2):77–85.
39. Wistuba II, et al. p53 protein overexpression in gallbladder carcinoma and its precursor lesions: an immunohistochemical study. Hum Pathol. 1996;27(4):360–5.
40. Rashid A, et al. K-ras mutation, p53 overexpression, and microsatellite instability in biliary tract cancers: a population-based study in China. Clin Cancer Res. 2002;8(10):3156–63.
41. Wistuba II, et al. Allele-specific mutations involved in the pathogenesis of endemic gallbladder carcinoma in Chile. Cancer Res. 1995;55(12):2511–5.

42. Singh MK, et al. Mutational spectrum of K-ras oncogene among Indian patients with gallbladder cancer. J Gastroenterol Hepatol. 2004;19(8):916–21.
43. Saetta AA. K-ras, p53 mutations, and microsatellite instability (MSI) in gallbladder cancer. J Surg Oncol. 2006;93(8):644–9.
44. Roa I, et al. Preneoplastic lesions in gallbladder cancer. J Surg Oncol. 2006;93(8):615–23.
45. Segovia Lohse HA, Cuenca Torres OM. Prevalence and sequence of metaplasia-dysplasia-carcinoma of the gallbladder. A single centre retrospective study. Cir Esp. 2013;91(10):672–5.
46. Itoi T, et al. APC, K-ras codon 12 mutations and p53 gene expression in carcinoma and adenoma of the gallbladder suggest two genetic pathways in gall-bladder carcinogenesis. Pathol Int. 1996;46(5):333–40.
47. Kozuka S, et al. Relation of adenoma to carcinoma in the gallbladder. Cancer. 1982;50(10):2226–34.
48. Wan X, et al. Clinicopathological features of gallbladder papillary adenocarcinoma. Medicine (Baltimore). 2014;93(27):e131.
49. Dursun N, et al. Mucinous carcinomas of the gallbladder: clinicopathologic analysis of 15 cases identified in 606 carcinomas. Arch Pathol Lab Med. 2012;136(11):1347–58.
50. Singh SK, et al. Mucinous carcinoma of the gall bladder—an incidental diagnosis of a rare variant. J Cancer Res Ther. 2015;11(4):1045.
51. Maharaj R, et al. A case report of the clear cell variant of gallbladder carcinoma. Int J Surg Case Rep. 2017;32:36–9.
52. Zhang C, et al. A clear cell adenocarcinoma of the gallbladder with hepatoid differentiation: case report and review of literature. Onco Targets Ther. 2016;9:5797–802.
53. Oohashi Y, et al. Adenosquamous carcinoma of the gallbladder warrants resection only if curative resection is feasible. Cancer. 2002;94(11):3000–5.
54. Rustagi T, Rai M, Menon M. Ruptured adenosquamous cell carcinoma of the gallbladder: case report and review of literature. Gastrointest Cancer Res. 2011;4(1):29–32.
55. Bazan F, et al. Metastatic gallbladder adenocarcinoma with signet-ring cells: a case report. J Med Case Rep. 2011;5:458.
56. Ahmad Z, Qureshi A. Primary signet ring cell carcinoma of gall bladder: report of an extremely rare histological type of primary gall bladder carcinoma. BMJ Case Rep. 2010;2010:bcr0420091782.
57. Guo KJ, Yamaguchi K, Enjoji M. Undifferentiated carcinoma of the gallbladder. A clinicopathologic, histochemical, and immunohistochemical study of 21 patients with a poor prognosis. Cancer. 1988;61(9):1872–9.
58. Eltawil KM, et al. Neuroendocrine tumors of the gallbladder: an evaluation and reassessment of management strategy. J Clin Gastroenterol. 2010;44(10):687–95.
59. Monier A, et al. Neuroendocrine tumor of the gallbladder. Pol J Radiol. 2015;80:228–31.
60. Mezi S, et al. Neuroendocrine tumors of the gallbladder: a case report and review of the literature. J Med Case Rep. 2011;5:334.
61. Carrera C, Kunk P, Rahma O. Small cell carcinoma of the gallbladder: case report and comprehensive analysis of published cases. J Oncol. 2015;2015:304909.
62. Adachi T, et al. Gallbladder small cell carcinoma: a case report and literature review. Surg Case Rep. 2016;2(1):71.
63. Lee H, Choi HJ, Park IY. Small cell carcinoma of the gallbladder: a case report. Ann Hepatobiliary Pancreat Surg. 2017;21(3):168–71.
64. Al-Daraji WI, et al. Primary gallbladder sarcoma: a clinicopathologic study of 15 cases, heterogeneous sarcomas with poor outcome, except pediatric botryoid rhabdomyosarcoma. Am J Surg Pathol. 2009;33(6):826–34.
65. Husain EA, et al. Gallbladder sarcoma: a clinicopathological study of seven cases from the UK and Austria with emphasis on morphological subtypes. Dig Dis Sci. 2009;54(2):395–400.
66. Miller G, Jarnagin WR. Gallbladder carcinoma. Eur J Surg Oncol. 2008;34(3):306–12.
67. Gourgiotis S, et al. Gallbladder cancer. Am J Surg. 2008;196(2):252–64.
68. Yang XW, et al. The prognostic importance of jaundice in surgical resection with curative intent for gallbladder cancer. BMC Cancer. 2014;14:652.
69. Feng FL, et al. Role of radical resection in patients with gallbladder carcinoma and jaundice. Chin Med J. 2012;125(5):752–6.
70. Wang YF, et al. Combined detection tumor markers for diagnosis and prognosis of gallbladder cancer. World J Gastroenterol. 2014;20(14):4085–92.
71. Rana S, et al. Evaluation of CA 242 as a tumor marker in gallbladder cancer. J Gastrointest Cancer. 2012;43(2):267–71.
72. Chaube A, et al. CA 125: a potential tumor marker for gallbladder cancer. J Surg Oncol. 2006;93(8):665–9.
73. Xu XS, et al. Model based on alkaline phosphatase and gamma-glutamyltransferase for gallbladder cancer prognosis. Asian Pac J Cancer Prev. 2015;16(15):6255–9.
74. Ong SL, et al. Ten-year experience in the management of gallbladder cancer from a single hepatobiliary and pancreatic centre with review of the literature. HPB (Oxford). 2008;10(6):446–58.
75. Singh TD, et al. Quantitative assessment of expression of lactate dehydrogenase and its isoforms 3 and 4 may serve as useful indicators of progression of gallbladder cancer: a pilot study. Indian J Clin Biochem. 2011;26(2):146–53.
76. Singh TD, et al. The liver function test enzymes and glucose level are positively correlated in gallbladder cancer: a cancer registry data analysis from north central India. Indian J Cancer. 2012;49(1):125–36.
77. Oikarinen H. Diagnostic imaging of carcinomas of the gallbladder and the bile ducts. Acta Radiol. 2006;47(4):345–58.

78. Recio-Boiles A, Babiker HM. Cancer, gallbladder. Treasure Island: StatPearls; 2018.
79. Inui K, Yoshino J, Miyoshi H. Diagnosis of gallbladder tumors. Intern Med. 2011;50(11):1133–6.
80. Kim HJ, et al. Diagnostic role of endoscopic ultrasonography-guided fine needle aspiration of gallbladder lesions. Hepato-Gastroenterology. 2012;59(118):1691–5.
81. Kumaran V, et al. The role of dual-phase helical CT in assessing resectability of carcinoma of the gallbladder. Eur Radiol. 2002;12(8):1993–9.
82. Tan CH, Lim KS. MRI of gallbladder cancer. Diagn Interv Radiol. 2013;19(4):312–9.
83. Andren-Sandberg A. Diagnosis and management of gallbladder cancer. N Am J Med Sci. 2012;4(7):293–9.
84. Vijayakumar A, et al. Early diagnosis of gallbladder carcinoma: an algorithm approach. ISRN Radiol. 2013;2013:239424.
85. Kapoor A, Kapoor A, Mahajan G. Differentiating malignant from benign thickening of the gallbladder wall by the use of acoustic radiation force impulse elastography. J Ultrasound Med. 2011;30(11):1499–507.
86. Kumar R, et al. Role of 18F-FDG PET/CT in detecting recurrent gallbladder carcinoma. Clin Nucl Med. 2012;37(5):431–5.
87. Ramos-Font C, et al. Ability of FDG-PET/CT in the detection of gallbladder cancer. J Surg Oncol. 2014;109(3):218–24.
88. Hennedige TP, Neo WT, Venkatesh SK. Imaging of malignancies of the biliary tract–an update. Cancer Imaging. 2014;14:14.
89. De Moura DTH, et al. Endoscopic retrograde cholangiopancreatography versus endoscopic ultrasound for tissue diagnosis of malignant biliary stricture: systematic review and meta-analysis. Endosc Ultrasound. 2018;7(1):10–9.
90. Wang SN, et al. Aberrant p53 expression and the development of gallbladder carcinoma and adenoma. Kaohsiung J Med Sci. 2006;22(2):53–9.
91. Asai T, et al. High frequency of TP53 but not K-ras gene mutations in Bolivian patients with gallbladder cancer. Asian Pac J Cancer Prev. 2014;15(13):5449–54.
92. Maurya SK, et al. Genetic aberrations in gallbladder cancer. Surg Oncol. 2012;21(1):37–43.
93. Kumari N, et al. Role of C-erbB2 expression in gallbladder cancer. Indian J Pathol Microbiol. 2012;55(1):75–9.
94. Pujani M, et al. Expression of human epidermal growth factor receptor (Her 2/neu) and proliferative marker Ki-67: association with clinicopathological parameters in gallbladder carcinoma. Asian Pac J Cancer Prev. 2016;17(8):3903–9.
95. Kanthan R, et al. Gallbladder cancer in the 21st century. J Oncol. 2015;2015:967472.
96. Ma HB, et al. Association of cyclin D1, p16 and retinoblastoma protein expressions with prognosis and metastasis of gallbladder carcinoma. World J Gastroenterol. 2005;11(5):744–7.
97. Srivastava V, et al. Cyclin D1, retinoblastoma and p16 protein expression in carcinoma of the gallbladder. Asian Pac J Cancer Prev. 2013;14(5):2711–5.
98. Kim K, et al. Expression of cell cycle-related proteins, p16, p53 and p63 as important prognostic markers in gallbladder adenocarcinoma. Pathol Oncol Res. 2014;20(2):409–15.
99. Roa JC, et al. Inactivation of CDKN2A gene (p16) in gallbladder carcinoma. Rev Med Chil. 2004;132(11):1369–76.
100. Feng Z, et al. The risk factor of gallbladder cancer: hyperplasia of mucous epithelium caused by gallstones associates with p16/CyclinD1/CDK4 pathway. Exp Mol Pathol. 2011;91(2):569–77.
101. Yao H, et al. The role of annexin A4 in cancer. Front Biosci (Landmark Ed). 2016;21:949–57.
102. Huang HL, et al. Proteomic identification of tumor biomarkers associated with primary gallbladder cancer. World J Gastroenterol. 2014;20(18):5511–8.
103. Yao HS, et al. Annexin A4-nuclear factor-kappaB feedback circuit regulates cell malignant behavior and tumor growth in gallbladder cancer. Sci Rep. 2016;6:31056.
104. Jagannath P, Callery M. Molecular prognostic markers in gallbladder carcinoma. HPB (Oxford). 2012;14(9):571–2.
105. Nagano M, et al. Nuclear expression of thioredoxin-1 in the invasion front is associated with outcome in patients with gallbladder carcinoma. HPB (Oxford). 2012;14(9):573–82.
106. Wu K, et al. ADAM-17 over-expression in gallbladder carcinoma correlates with poor prognosis of patients. Med Oncol. 2011;28(2):475–80.
107. Puhalla H, et al. E-cadherin and beta-catenin expression in normal, inflamed and cancerous gallbladder tissue. Anticancer Res. 2005;25(6B):4249–54.
108. Priya TP, et al. Role of E-cadherin gene in gall bladder cancer and its precursor lesions. Virchows Arch. 2010;456(5):507–14.
109. Yi S, et al. N-cadherin and P-cadherin are biomarkers for invasion, metastasis, and poor prognosis of gallbladder carcinomas. Pathol Res Pract. 2014;210(6):363–8.
110. Nakamura T, et al. Prognostic significance of S100A4 expression in gallbladder cancer. Int J Oncol. 2002;20(5):937–41.
111. Luo W, et al. Clinical correlation of calpain-1 and glypican-3 expression with gallbladder carcinoma. Oncol Lett. 2016;11(2):1345–52.
112. Saranga Bharathi R, et al. Female sex hormone receptors in gallbladder cancer. J Gastrointest Cancer. 2015;46(2):143–8.
113. Gupta P, et al. Expression and clinicopathological significance of estrogen and progesterone receptors in gallbladder cancer. Gastrointest Cancer Res. 2012;5(2):41–7.

114. Baskaran V, et al. Do the progesterone receptors have a role to play in gallbladder cancer? Int J Gastrointest Cancer. 2005;35(1):61–8.
115. Park JS, et al. Estrogen receptor alpha, estrogen receptor beta, and progesterone receptor as possible prognostic factor in radically resected gallbladder carcinoma. J Surg Res. 2009;152(1):104–10.
116. Sumi K, et al. Loss of estrogen receptor beta expression at cancer front correlates with tumor progression and poor prognosis of gallbladder cancer. Oncol Rep. 2004;12(5):979–84.
117. Chandra V, et al. MicroRNA aberrations: an emerging field for gallbladder cancer management. World J Gastroenterol. 2016;22(5):1787–99.
118. Li G, Pu Y. MicroRNA signatures in total peripheral blood of gallbladder cancer patients. Tumour Biol. 2015;36(9):6985–90.
119. Pang Q, et al. Platelet to lymphocyte ratio as a novel prognostic tool for gallbladder carcinoma. World J Gastroenterol. 2015;21(21):6675–83.
120. Zhang L, et al. Prognostic significance of neutrophil to lymphocyte ratio in patients with gallbladder carcinoma. HPB (Oxford). 2016;18(7):600–7.
121. Zhang Y, et al. Prognostic significance of preoperative neutrophil/lymphocyte ratio and platelet/lymphocyte ratio in patients with gallbladder carcinoma. Clin Transl Oncol. 2015;17(10):810–8.
122. Saqib R, et al. Prognostic significance of preoperative inflammatory markers in resected gallbladder cancer: a systematic review. ANZ J Surg. 2018;88(6):554–9.

Molecular Diagnostics for Lung Cancer

3

Ashok Kumar and Ashwani Tandon

3.1 Introduction

Lung cancer is the leading cause of cancer-related deaths worldwide in both men and women [1]. Approximately 1.8 million new cases of lung cancer were diagnosed in 2012 and it accounts for 12.9% of all the cases [1]. It is broadly divided into two main histological groups: small cell lung carcinoma (SCLC) and non-small cell lung cancer (NSCLC). SCLC and NSCLC account for 13% and 87% of all lung cancers, respectively [2]. The main histological subtypes of NSCLC are adenocarcinoma, squamous cell carcinoma and large cell carcinoma [2]. Growing evidence suggests that lung cancer is a group of histologically and molecularly heterogeneous diseases even within the same histological subtype [2, 3]. Five year survival rate for stage I small and localized NSCLC varies from 70 to 90%. However, most of the patients with NSCLC are diagnosed in the advanced stages (III/IV) and have 1-year survival rate of just 15–19% [4]. SCLC is more aggressive than NSCLC and have overall 5-year survival rate of 5% [4]. In India as well as other south Asian countries, its diagnosis is compounded by the high incidence of pulmonary tuberculosis [5]. Therefore, the strategy for early and accurate diagnosis is of vital importance.

Identifying driver mutations in *EGFR, ALK* and other genes are central to management of lung cancer patients. International phase III randomized-controlled trials (RCT) have confirmed the superiority of tyrosine kinase inhibitors (TKIs) with improved progression-free survival (PFS) over systemic chemotherapy as first-line treatment for metastatic EGFR-mutated NSCLC [6]. A clinical trial showed that patients with an *EGFR* positive mutation had a longer progression free survival (PFS) treated with gefitinib versus carboplatin plus paclitaxel [6]. Conversely, patients negative for *EGFR* mutations had shorter PFS treated with gefitinib versus carboplatin plus paclitaxel [6].

3.2 Classification of Lung Cancer

For consistency in reporting, the revised histologic classification (Table 3.1) published by the World Health Organization (WHO) for tumors of the lung, including carcinoids, is practiced by pathologist [7]. In the era of molecular testing and targeted therapy accurate histologic typing of lung carcinoma is important. However, it may be limited in small biopsies, but in large resected

A. Kumar (✉)
Department of Biochemistry, All India Institute of Medical Sciences, Bhopal, Madhya Pradesh, India
e-mail: ashok.biochemistry@aiimsbhopal.edu.in

A. Tandon
Department of Pathology and Laboratory Medicine, All India Institute of Medical Sciences, Bhopal, Madhya Pradesh, India

K. K. Shukla et al. (eds.), *Molecular Diagnostics in Cancer Patients*,
https://doi.org/10.1007/978-981-13-5877-7_3

Table 3.1 WHO classification of tumors of the lung

Adenocarcinoma	Squamous cell carcinoma
Lepidic predominant	Keratinizing squamous cell carcinoma
Acinar predominant	Non-keratinizing squamous cell carcinoma
Papillary predominant	Basaloid squamous cell carcinoma
Solid predominant	Preinvasive lesions
Micropapillary predominant	Squamous cell carcinoma *in situ*
Invasive mucinous adenocarcinoma	Small cell carcinoma
Mixed invasive mucinous and nonmucinous	Combined small cell carcinoma (small cell carcinoma
adenocarcinoma	and non-small cell component)
Colloid adenocarcinoma	Large cell neuroendocrine carcinoma
Fetal adenocarcinoma	Typical carcinoid tumor
Enteric adenocarcinoma	Atypical carcinoid tumor
Minimally invasive adenocarcinoma	Large cell carcinoma
Nonmucinous	Adenosquamous carcinoma
Mixed nonmucinous and mucinous	Pleomorphic carcinoma
Mucinous	Spindle cell carcinoma
Preinvasive lesion	Giant cell carcinoma
Atypical adenomatous hyperplasia	Carcinosarcoma
Adenocarcinoma *in situ*	Pulmonary blastoma
Non mucinous/mucinous	Lymphoepithelioma-like carcinoma
	NUT carcinoma
	Mucoepidermoid carcinoma
	Adenoid cystic carcinoma
	Epithelial-myoepithelial carcinoma
	Carcinoma, type cannot be determined
	Non-small cell carcinoma, subtype cannot be determined
	Other histologic type not listed above

specimens, diagnosis of NSCLC is precise and accurate. Poorly differentiated carcinoma lacking microscopic evidence of glandular differentiation and positive for TTF-1 and Napsin A (Fig. 3.1a–c) by immunohistochemistry (IHC) is diagnosed as solid adenocarcinoma. If poorly differentiated carcinoma lacks microscopic evidence of squamous differentiation and shows the expression of p40 and CK5/6 and p63 (Fig. 3.1d–f), then it is diagnosed as non-keratinizing squamous cell carcinoma (SqCC) [3]. Sampling of lung carcinomas should be done and represented in the histological sections examined. A diagnosis of adenocarcinoma *in situ* (AIS) or minimally invasive adenocarcinoma (MIA) shall be made on entire specimen histological examination and lesion shall be solitary of ≤3 cm in diameter. The diagnosis of MIA is made in a lepidic predominant tumors with an invasive components measuring 0.5 cm or less in size [7].

Sub-classification of adenocarcinomas by predominant histologic pattern may be performed and can be useful for assessing pathologic grade. In poorly differentiated cases, immunohistochemistry can greatly aid in classification. This is particularly useful in making a diagnosis of solid-type adenocarcinoma or non-keratinizing SqCC.

Similarly, cytology specimens are also very informative and if material is adequate, pathologist may provide substantial information for patient management including broader classifier as adenocarcinoma, SqCC, small cell carcinoma or neuroendocrine tumors. Cytology specimens are very important as diagnostic material in effusion fluid cytology, aspirate material from metastatic tumor deposit in lymph nodes and even at distant sites. Immunocytochemistry on cytospin material or IHC on cell block material is important aid to further classify lung tumors [3].

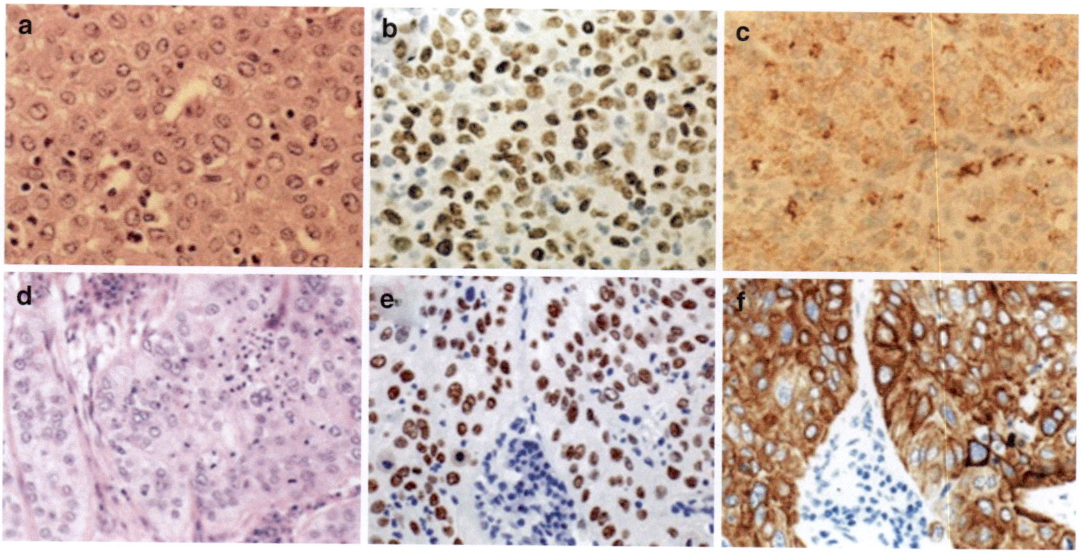

Fig. 3.1 Solid adenocarcinoma (**a–c**) and non-keratinizing squamous cell carcinoma (SqCC) (**d–f**). Solid adenocarcinoma [(**a**) HE staining] is immunohistochemically positive for TTF-1 (**b**) and Napsin A (**c**). Non-keratinizing SqCC [(**d**) HE staining] is immunohistochemically positive for p40 (**e**) and CK5/6 (**f**) (*Reprinted by permission from Frontiers Media S.A; Frontiers in Oncology* 2017; *7:193*)

3.3 Genetic Aberrations in Lung Cancer

While cancers are characterized by numerous genomic aberrations, some acquired mutation(s) may be sufficient to induce growth and impaired differentiation leading to cancer development. This powerful somatic effect has been commonly described as a driver mutation and the overall phenomenon as oncogene addiction [8]. Oncogene addiction becomes the rationale for targeted therapy of solid tumors enabling a model that delivers treatment with a higher probability of efficacy while at the same time lowers the risk for adverse events. A diversity of genomic and epigenetic abnormalities has been reported in NSCLC. Lung cancers develop through a multistep process involving development of multiple genetic and epigenetic alterations, particularly activation of growth promoting pathways and inhibition of tumour suppressor pathways. Activation of growth promoting oncogenes can occur by gene amplification or other genetic alterations including point mutations and structural rearrangements leading to uncontrolled signalling through oncogenic pathways. Improvements in our understanding of molecular alterations at multiple levels (genetic, epigenetic, protein expression) and their functional significance have the potential to impact lung cancer diagnosis and treatment [9]. Oncogenic driver mutations have been identified in over 50% of lung adenocarcinoma [9]. Oncogenic driver mutations refer to mutations that are responsible for both the initiation and maintenance of the cancer. These mutations are often found in genes that encode for signaling proteins that are critical for maintaining normal cellular proliferation and survival [10]. NSCLC, especially lung adenocarcinomas, can be further subclassified by their genetic mutation profiles, making personalized treatment strategies based on the identification of oncogenic driver mutations feasible. Clinically relevant genetic aberrations in common genes involved in lung cancer are described below.

3.3.1 Epidermal Growth Factor Receptor (EGFR)

The human *EGFR* gene is a member of the ErbB family of receptor tyrosine kinases (RTK). Binding of the receptor with epidermal growth factor (EGF) or other cognate ligands induces receptor dimerization and auto-phosphorylation. Crosslinking of EGFR to its ligand activates downstream signaling cascade, resulting in the stimulation of cell proliferation [11]. Mutations in EGFR gene in lung cancer are mostly detected in the first four exons of the RTK domain (exon 18–21) (Fig. 3.2). The most frequent mutations are missense mutations in exon 21 (41% of all mutations) and in-frame deletions in exon 19 (44% of all mutations) [12]. These mutations are frequently detected in lung adenocarcinoma (20–48%) and are also frequently detected in females (40–60%), never smokers (50–60%) and East Asian patients (30–50%) [12]. Two most common genetic alterations in *EGFR* gene are; a point mutation in exon 21 L858R and an in-frame deletion in

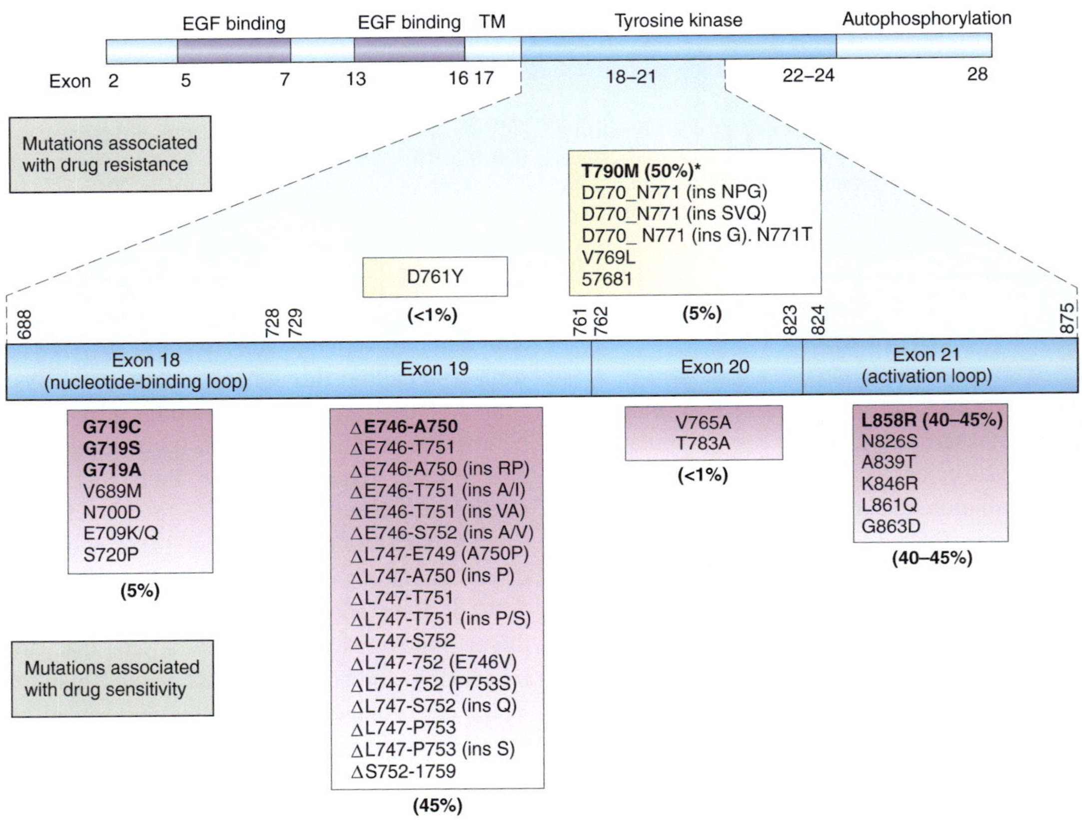

Fig. 3.2 Different domains of EGFR and various mutations in *EGFR* gene. Exons 18–21 in the tyrosine kinase region where the relevant mutations are located are expanded (represented by the cyan bar), and a detailed list of EGFR mutations in these exons that are associated with sensitivity (magenta boxes) or resistance (yellow boxes) to gefitinib or erlotinib is shown. Occurrence of various EGFR mutations in NSCLC is shown as percentage (%). The most prevalent of EGFR kinase domain mutations, accounting for 45% of EGFR mutations in NSCLC, are in-frame deletions of exon 19. Another recurrent mutation is the L858R substitution in exon 21, which comprises approximately 40–45% of EGFR mutations. Nucleotide substitutions in exon 18 (for example, G719C or G719S) account for another 5% of EGFR mutations. The most noteworthy, clinically relevant mutation in exon 20 is T790M, which is detected in 50% of the cases (denoted by asterisk) as a second site mutation associated with acquired gefitinib and erlotinib resistance. D761Y, a T790M-like secondary mutation in exon 19 of EGFR, has also reported to be associated with resistance to gefitinib and erlotinib in NSCLC cells (*Reprinted by permission from Macmillan Publishers Ltd Nature Reviews Cancer 7(3):169–181*; Copyright 2007)

exon 19 (del E746_A750); together these account for 90–95% of all mutations in *EGFR*. Most of these mutations in the RTK domain are activating mutations resulting into constitutive activation of EGFR. Detection of these EGFR mutations is clinically important because they have been associated with enhanced sensitivity to small molecule tyrosine kinase inhibitors (TKIs) (gefitinib, erlotinib and afatinib) [13, 14]. In contrast, several EGFR mutations produce resistance to targeted therapy. These include the missense mutation p.T790M, small insertions/duplications of exon 20 and missense mutations at p.S768 and p.V769p [15].

Furthermore, approximately in 30–75% of samples from NSCLCs, overexpression of EGFR protein is detected which may be due to epigenetic causes (transcriptional hyper-activation), gene amplification or oncogenic viruses [12].

3.3.2 Anaplastic Lymphoma Kinase (ALK)

Aberrant ALK expression is detected in a subset of NSCLC, mostly adenocarcinomas. Most prevalent ALK alterations are chromosomal rearrangements resulting in fusion genes. ALK fusions arise from fusion of the 3′ half of ALK, derived from Chromosome 2 that retains its kinase catalytic domain, and the 5′ portion of a different gene that provides its promoter [16]. Multiple different 5′ partners have been identified in variety of cancers. In lung cancer, the most common fusion partner for ALK is EML4 (echinoderm microtubule associated protein like-4), EML4-ALK rearrangements have multiple distinct isoforms with demonstrated transforming activity (Fig. 3.3). The three major variants (v1:E13;A20; v2:E20;A20, and v3; E6;A20)

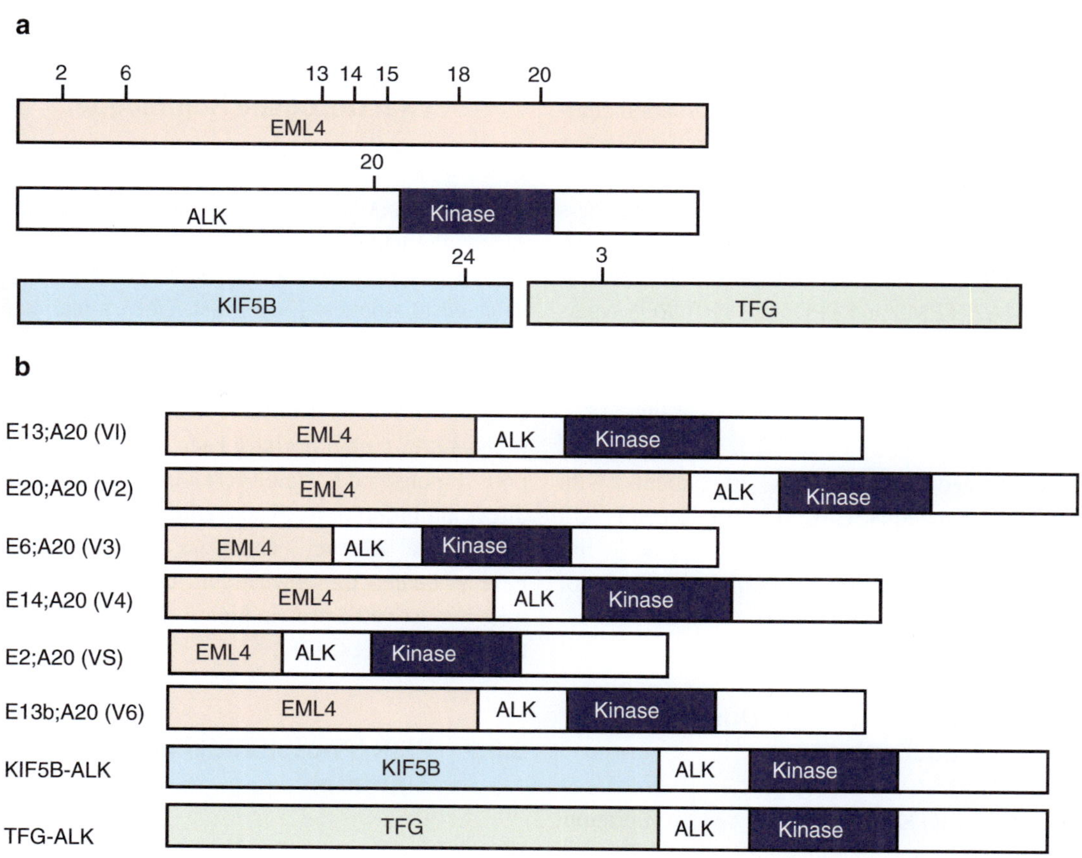

Fig. 3.3 (**a**) Exons of ALK, EML4 KIF5B and TFG are shown that are involved in chromosomal rearrangement, (**b**) Different variants of *EML4-ALK* and fusion partners with other genes are depicted

account for more than 90% of all ALK rearrangement in lung cancers. EML4-ALK fusion protein is detected in 2–7% NSCLC. The frequency of this genomic alteration is even higher (17–20%) in the non-smokers [17]. In lung cancers, other fusion partners of ALK4 such as *TFG, KIF5B, HIP1* and *KLC1* have been reported [16]. Tumors with EML4-ALK rearrangement usually lack mutations in *EGFR* and *KRAS* genes. ALK inhibitors, crizotinib, ceritinib, and alectinib are effective in advanced NSCLC with EML4-ALK translocation [12, 16].

3.3.3 ROS1 (c-Ros Oncogene 1)

ROS1 gene is located at chromosome 6q22 and encodes for a RTK of the insulin receptor family [18]. It is closely related to ALK and LTK and it has 80% sequence identity with ALK in their ATP binding domain. *ROS1* gene rearrangement leads to a constitutively activated downstream signaling leading to oncogenesis [19]. Its gene rearrangement has been reported in several tumors including NSCLC [19]. All rearrangements involve the 3′ region of the kinase domain of ROS1 and 5′ region of the partner gene. Several fusion partners of ROS1 has been reported, these include CD74, EZR, Fig. 3.1, CCD6, KDELR2, LRI3, SDC4, SLC34A2, TPM3 and TPD52L1 [19]. *ROS1* rearrangements have been identified in about 0.5–2% of NSCLC, and more frequently in younger, non-smoking patients with adenocarcinoma [12]. Crizotinib, an inhibitor of ALK and ROS1 has demonstrated high efficacy in patients with ROS1-rearranged NSCLC [12, 19]. Recently, US Food and Drug Administration (FDA) has approved the use of crizotimib in the treatment of *ROS1* rearranged NSCLC [19].

3.3.4 RET (Rearranged During Transfection)

The *RET*, a RTK is involved in cell proliferation, differentiation and migration [20]. The RET fusion protein has been detected as a driver mutation in 1–2% of NSCLC, mostly young never smokers with adenocarcinoma. The presence of RET rearrangement in NSCLC is mutually exclusive to mutation or rearrangement in commonly altered genes such as *EGFR, KRAS, ROS1* and *ALK*. The most common fusion partner of RET is *KIF5B* (Kinesin family member 5B) [21]. Alectinib is an approved ALK inhibitor that is also effective for *RET* fusion-positive NSCLC [21].

3.3.5 MET

MET encodes for a RTK that activates multiple signaling pathways involved in cell survival, proliferation, migration and invasion [22]. *MET* occurs in 2–7% of NSCLC patients [23] and these patients show rapid and durable response to crizotinib [24]. *MET* amplification has also identified as one of the acquired secondary resistance mechanisms in patients treated with TKIs [25].

3.3.6 KRAS (Kirsten Rat Sarcoma Viral Oncogene Homologue)

KRAS gene is a member of *RAS* family and it is one of the most commonly activated genes in lung cancer. Point mutations in *KRAS* gene are detected in 20% of lung adenocarcinoma, more frequently detected in smokers [26]. Most *KRAS* mutations are single base substitutions affecting codon 12, 13 and 61. In lung adenocarcinoma, *KRAS* mutations are mutually exclusive with *EGFR* mutations. *KRAS* mutations have been associated with poor response rates to EGFR-TKIs [27], however, direct inhibition of RAS activation failed to show any clinical efficacy. Therefore, recent studies have evaluated the downstream target of *KRAS*, mitogen-activated protein kinase (MAPK) for the therapy of NSCLC [28].

3.3.7 PI3K (Phosphatidylinositol-3-Kinase)

PI3K signaling cascade plays a critical role in the initiation and/or progression of NSCLC [29]. Mutations in the *PIK3CA* gene encoding the class I PI3K p110α, are commonly found in a variety of cancers including lung cancers. In NSCLC, mutations within *PIK3CA* usually occur in exon 9 (E545K and E542K) or exon 20 (H1047R and H1047L), are considered oncogenic and targetable [30]. *PIK3CA* mutations occur in approximately 1–4% of NSCLC, with higher frequency in squamous cell carcinoma (8.9%) compared to adenocarcinoma (2.9%) [30]. Majority of patients with *PIK3CA* mutations, have additional oncogenic driver mutations [30]. *PIK3CA* copy number gain is also a common abnormality in NSCLC, mostly in squamous cell carcinoma [12].

3.4 Various Techniques Used in Molecular Diagnostics

A variety of methods can be used to genetic aberrations including immunohistochemistry, fluorescent *in situ* hybridization (FISH), allele-specific polymerase chain reaction (PCR), quantitative real-time PCR (qRT-PCR), sanger sequencing and next generation sequencing (NGS). Each method has its merits and demerits thus molecular pathologists should consider the available approaches and the advantages and disadvantages of each method including turnaround time and analytical sensitivity [31].

3.4.1 Fluorescent *In Situ* Hybridization (FISH)

The first widely adopted test to detect ALK rearrangement was FISH, which has been approved by the FDA in 2001. FISH using a dual color "break-apart" probes approach is considered the gold standard in detecting *ALK* (Fig. 3.4) and *ROS1* gene rearrangement. The probes label the 5′ (telomeric) part with red fluorochrome and the 3′ (centromeric) part of the fusion breakpoint with green fluorochrome or vice versa [19]. Several probes can be used to visualize the gene arrangement, however, regardless of the probe,

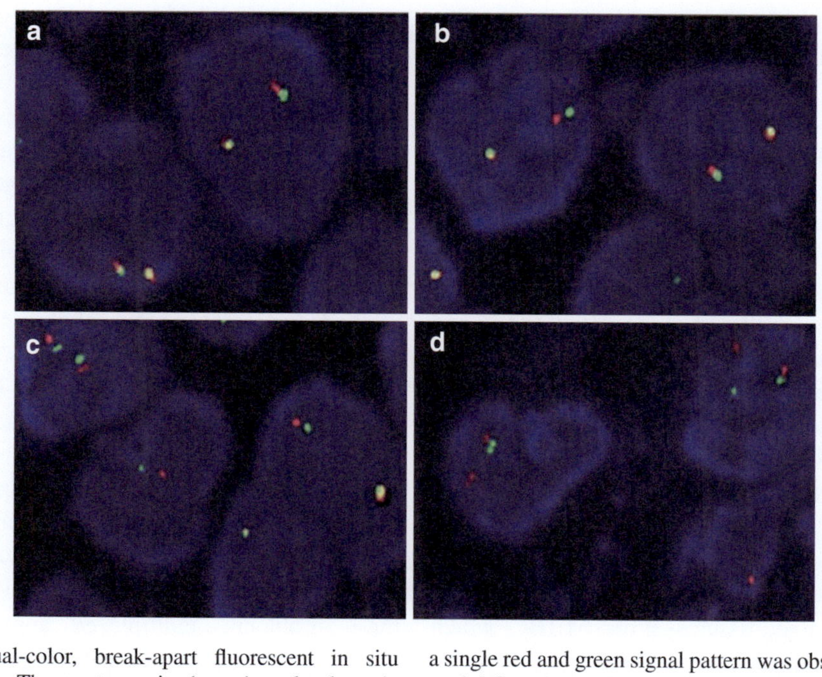

Fig. 3.4 Dual-color, break-apart fluorescent in situ hybridization. The centromeric (green) and telomeric (red) flank the ALK locus. Splitting of the red and green signals indicates ALK rearrangement. (**a**) No EML4-ALK rearrangement. (**b**–**d**) EML4-ALK rearrangements. A break-apart signal pattern, where one fusion signal and a single red and green signal pattern was observed in most nuclei (**b** and **c**). A few nuclei showed a predominant signal pattern of deletion of the 5′ region (**d**) (*Reprinted by permission from Biomed Central; Journal of Experimental & Clinical Cancer Research* 2014; *33:109*)

the cutoff for a positive result is 50 tumor cells with the arrangement. Tissue sections or cytology specimens are subjected to a protocol that labels either side of *ALK*/*ROS1* breakpoint locus with two different fluorochromes (red/green). In cell nuclei that are negative for gene rearrangement, colored dots overlap and appear yellow, whereas cell nuclei positive for gene arrangement isolated red and/or green signals are observed [32]. Break-apart FISH detects a break in the chromosomal region encoding tyrosine kinase domain of *ALK* or *ASK1* and it does not identify specific fusion partners. FISH is a technically demanding method, which requires specialized equipment and experienced pathologist [32]. Until the commercialization of anti-ALK antibodies, FISH was the most frequently used and most laboratories continue to use FISH either as first line test or to validate the results of IHC [12]. There are few limitations with FISH. Sometimes, the observed signal is difficult to interpret or ambiguous and requires more than 100 tumor cells to get the reliable results. Thus, this can be more challenging with small biopsy samples which may not contain few tumor cells [17].

3.4.2 Immunohistochemistry (IHC)

IHC is a widely used method in all pathology laboratories. Identifying the tumor histological subtype has shown to be predictive of response to certain types of therapy [33]. Both *ROS1* and *ALK* gene rearrangements are present in a low percentage of cases and can occur with multiple fusion partners. FISH can detect multiple rearrangements by a split signal but is a cumbersome and expensive method. RT-PCR is also possible but requires multiple primer sets, and rare rearrangements can be missed. Thus, it is possible to rapidly evaluate ALK and ROS1 rearrangement on formalin-fixed tissue sections by IHC, which is cheaper and easier than FISH. Two clones of ALK1 antibodies D5F3 (Cell Signaling Technology, Danvers, MA, USA); 54A (Novocastra, Leica Biosystems) have been widely used and are reliable [34]. In case of ROS1 expression D4D6 clone shows better correlation between IHC and FISH data [19, 35]. Furthermore, expression of ALK and ROS1 is low in normal lung tissue, and gene rearrangements are associated with constitutive high protein expression of ALK and ROS1. Thus, IHC is an ideal method to screen for lung cancer cases with *ROS1* gene rearrangements [28]. ROS1 expression at IHC typically shows finely granular cytoplasmic and/or membranous staining. Four tiered scoring system is used to evaluate ALK and ROS1 IHC data. IHC is less specific than FISH, thus, to obtain a reliable interpretation certain pitfalls must be avoided such as false positive results close to necrotic zones. For quality assurance, validation of the method and inter-laboratory controls are important considerations.

3.4.3 Sanger Sequencing

Sanger sequencing or chain terminating sequencing is considered the gold standard for mutation analysis. Sanger sequencing is performed on PCR products and requires sequencing primers spanning the region of interest, DNA polymerase, nucleotides bases and a low concentration of modified nucleotide (also known as dideoxyNTP). All four dideoxy nucleotides (cytosine, guanine, adenosine and thymine) are labelled with a different flourophore. In Sanger sequencing, DNA fragments of different lengths are generated, which are then separated out with capillary gel electrophoresis [36]. It is one of the preferred methods to detect mutations of clinically relevant genes, such as the EGFR hot-spot mutations. Sanger sequencing can detect all known and novel base substitutions, small insertions and deletions. However, direct DNA sequencing requires a high ratio of tumor cells to normal cells (more than 50%) for reliable results. Furthermore, it is unable to analyze multiple gene hot-spots simultaneously. To overcome these problems, multiplexed approaches for molecular testing, particularly for gene mutation analysis have been developed [12, 36]. The limited sensitivity of Sanger sequencing has created a need for alternative techniques to detect common mutations, such as well RT- PCR based assays, pyrosequencing and NGS [37].

3.4.4 Allele-Specific PCR and Real-Time PCR

Allele-specific PCR is also known as an amplification-refractory mutation system. Allele-specific PCR has the advantage of mutant enrichment, resulting in high sensitivity, which is essential for mutation detection in samples with a low tumor cell percentage. It is based on the principle that extension is efficient when the 3′ terminal base of a primer matches its target, whereas extension is inefficient or nonexistent when the terminal base is mismatched [38]. Furthermore, combining allele-specific PCR with qRT-PCR techniques allows monitoring template amplification, resulting into improved interpretation of PCR results [39]. Based on this technology, several commercial kits have been developed to detect mutations in *EGFR*, *BRAF* and *KRAS* genes. Cobas® EGFR Mutation test (Roche Molecular Systems) is a FDA approved kit, which is based on allele-specific qRT-PCR assay. This kit detects 42 mutations in *EGFR* gene in exons 18–21 in DNA extracted from formalin-fixed paraffin-embedded tissue samples. These mutations include exon 19 deletions and L858R, T790M, G719X, exon 20 insertions, S768I and L861Q. Cobas EGFR mutation test kit is based on Taqman chemistry, where two target specific primers flanking the region of interest and a third sequence specific probe, which hybridizes within the area of interest. The probe is labelled with a reporter fluorophore on 5′ end and a quencher on the 3′ end. When the reporter dye and quencher are in close proximity, quencher prevents the fluorescence signal of reporter dye. The exonuclease activity of Taq DNA polymerase, cleaves the probe resulting in the separation of reporter dye and quencher, allowing reporter dye to emit fluorescence signal. Algorithm for the detection of EGFR mutation in adenocarcinoma is described in Fig. 3.5 [40].

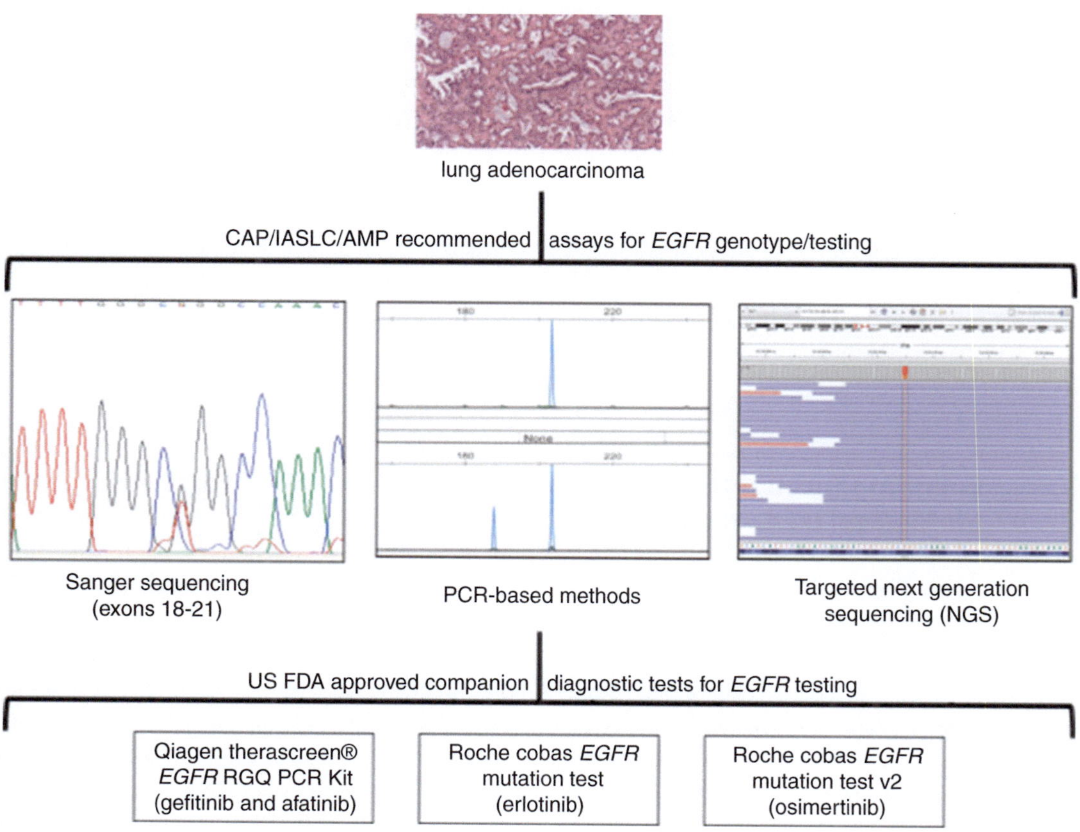

Fig. 3.5 Algorithm for detection of *EGFR* mutations in clinical practice (*Reprinted by permission from Elsevier; Clinical Lung Cancer* 2016;17:483–92)

The therascreen EGFR kit (Qiagen, Hilden, Germany) is another allele specific qRT-PCR assay. This kit detects 29 mutations in *EGFR* gene cover 4 exons 18–21. The mutation detected by this kit include G719X (X = S, A or C) in exon 18, deletions in exon 19, 3 insertions in exon 20, T790M andS7681 in exon 20, L858R and L861Q in exon 21. This kit utilizes ARMS method and Scorpions chemistry for the detection of these mutations. Scorpions are molecules that contain a PCR primer linked to a probe (labelled with reporter dye and quencher). When the Scorpion primer bind to the ARMS amplicon, it starts primer extension resulting separation of reporter dye from the quencher resulting into release of fluorescence [36]. Several other CE approved kits such as PNAClamp™ EGFR Mutation Detection Kit (Panagen Corp, Daejeon, Korea), RealLine EGFR-7R (Bioron Diagnostics, Ludwigshafen, Germany) have also been developed for *EGFR* mutation detection. Targeted assays are also available for *KRAS* and *BRAF* from Qiagen and Roche.

Reverse Transcription PCR (RT-PCR) method is also used to detect rearrangement in *ALK* and *ROS1* gene [17, 19]. Several factors affect the sensitivity and specificity of RT-PCR for gene rearrangement, but mainly by the quantity and quality of the extracted RNA. RT-PCR is a sensitive technique for detection of some EML4-ALK variants but it is not currently advocated for routine use as it may not detect ALK fusions with rarer fusion partners [33]. It has an advantage over IHC and FISH that it is free from subjectivity of the analysis.

3.5 Emerging Technologies for Molecular Diagnostics

3.5.1 High-Throughput Multiplexing Assays

High-throughput targeted assays have been developed to screen mutations in *EGFR*, *KRAS*, *NRAS* and *BRAF* genes. These include MassARRAY iPLEX HS (Agena Bioscience, San Diego, CA, USA) and SNaPShot (Applied Biosystems). Agena MassARRAY system is based on PCR and allele specific single base primer extension. Each nucleotide having a defined molecular mass is added to the primer and the primer extension products are analyzed using the principle of matrix-assisted laser desorption/ionization time-of-flight (MALDI-TOF). The TOF is proportional to the mass/charge ratio which is translated into a specific genotype call [36, 41]. MassARRAY iPLEX HS facilitates mutation detection as low as 1% allele frequency even from poor quality and degraded samples such as FFPE tissue, FNA, and cytology blocks and it requires only 10 ng of DNA. iPLEX HS Lung Panel covers 70 mutations in five genes including *EGFR, BRAF, KRAS, ERB2* and *PIK3CA*. The MassARRAY LungFUSION Panel offers a rapid screening method for detecting an oncogenic fusion partner in *ALK*, *RET* and *ROS1 genes*.

The SNapShot platform is based on multiplex PCR and single base primer extension using fluorescent labelled probes. Primer extension products are then detected by capillary electrophoresis. The SNapShot panel analyzes smaller panel of mutations and genes (~10 mutations) compared to the Agena MassARRAY system. The workflow of SNapShot platform is simpler than Agena MassARRAY system, however the main disadvantage of SNapShot platform is the limit to the number of assays that can be multiplexed. Furthermore, it is not designed to detect deletions, insertions and amplifications [30].

3.5.2 Next Generation Sequencing (NGS)

NGS is high-throughput method, which allows massive parallel sequencing that affords maximal tumor genomic assessment. NGS approach is utilizes to sequence both DNA and RNA. DNA sequencing includes whole genome, whole exome, epigenome and targeted sequencing. RNA sequencing allows whole transcriptome analysis which provide information of alternative spliced transcripts, gene fusion, mutations, SNPs, small and long non-coding RNAs and changes in gene expression [42]. NGS is rapidly changing the paradigm of lung cancer research and patient care. Presently, several NGS platforms are available these include Ion Torrent systems (ThermoFisher Scientific, Waltham, MA, USA) and Illumina HiSeq 2500 (Illumina Inc., San Diego, CA). A variety of genomic aberrations such as point mutations, small and large insertions/deletions, copy number variations, fusion transcripts can be detected with high accuracy and sensitivity. Each of the available platforms uses different sequencing chemistry for signal detection; irrespective of the method used, the sensitivity of NGS is much higher than Sanger sequencing. Currently, clinical application of NGS is hampered by computational bioinformatics challenges to analyze the large amount of data generated [12, 42]. The Oncomine™ Dx Target Test is a FDA-approved [43] NGS test that uses targeted high throughput, parallel-sequencing technology to detect single nucleotide variants (SNVs) and deletions in 23 genes from DNA and fusions in ROS1 from RNA isolated from FFPE tumor tissue samples from patients with NSCLC using the Ion PGM™ Dx System (ThermoFisher).

3.5.3 Liquid Biopsy

In order to create a molecular profile of a tumor, a biopsy or several biopsies may be required. Recurrent biopsies are invasive and may miss parts of the tumor that are developing resistance to the treatment or have acquired new driver mutations. Studies have revealed that tumors have significant molecular heterogeneity, with cells from portion of a tumor having different mutations than other areas [44]. Therefore, minimally invasive modalities that could guide early detection, follow patients regularly, allow early emerging treatment assessment and identify new driver mutations would be useful in the management of lung cancer [45]. Analysis of blood-based biomarkers including circulating cell-free tumor DNA (cfDNA), circulating tumor cells (CTCs) and tumor-educated platelets (TEPs) suggest that these biomarkers may facilitate early detection of lung cancer with frequent monitoring. cfDNA gives ladder-like appearance on electrophoresis due to presence of multimers of 180 base pairs (bps) DNA ladder, possibly arising from apoptotic cells [46]. However, other studies have shown that a significant portion of tumor-derived cfDNA is smaller than 145 bps, which suggest non-apoptotic origin of cfDNA [47]. Though, tumor cfDNA is present in blood, lymph, milk, spinal fluid, urine and saliva. However, sample for cfDNA is collected by phlebotomy in EDTA vials and cfDNA is extracted from plasma. Tumor cfDNA is analyzed by variety of techniques including droplet digital PCR (ddPCR), qRT-PCR, peptide nucleic acid-locked clamp PCR (PNA-LNA) and NGS. Analysis of cfDNA could be challenging as it can make up as little as 0.01% of the total cfDNA pool [44].

Analysis of cfDNA has several applications in the management of lung cancer including analyzing tumor molecular heterogeneity, monitoring disease burden and prognosis [44]. A study used ddPCR to analyze EGFR mutations in cfDNA and compared it with conventional tissue biopsies [48]. Interestingly, ddPCR cfDNA analysis could detect EGFR mutation in 34% additional patients that were otherwise negative by tumor biopsy analysis [48]. However, recent studies have shown variable sensitivity and specificity for different EGFR mutations by cfDNA ddPCR [49, 50]. Further, a study showed that plasma cfDNA levels were higher in NSCLC patients (prior to tumor resection) compared to healthy individuals [51], plasma cfDNA levels were decreased in NSCLC patients after tumor resection [51]. The EGFR mutation detection rate in pleural fluid by ddPCR is better than both the direct sequencing and ARMS PCR [52]. Liquid biopsy by qRT-PCR showed a reduction in the sensitizing EGFR mutations (L858R or ex19Del) and concomitant increase in T790M (EGFR resistant mutation) in THI-treated patients. With liquid biopsy, T790M mutations could be detected as early as 344 days before clinical lung cancer progression was evident. Therefore, persistent monitoring for T790M may allow the earlier detection of TKI-resistant-related lung cancer progression [53]. The cobas® EGFR Mutation Test v2 CE-IVD (Roche) is the first FDA approved test which identifies 42 mutations in exons 18, 19, 20 and 21 of the EGFR gene using plasma as a sample [43].

Liquid biopsy approaches hold great potential in lung cancer diagnostics. Currently, several challenges must be resolved before the liquid biopsy can enter clinical practice. These challenges include (a) optimizing and standardizing sample collection (b) implementing uniform analytical procedures (c) identifying the analytes in the various body fluids to yield clinical information (d) performing the large multicentre clinical trials necessary for validating specific analysis protocol [44].

3.6 Challenges

Molecular testing in lung cancer patients is of undeniable benefit; however, it is not without its pitfalls. Obtaining adequate tissue for diagnosis and molecular testing is a key for management of lung cancer patients. Usually, the large tissue samples obtained via open thoracotomy are of sufficient quantity and quality. However, the tumor is not always easily accessible in patients presenting with a probable lung cancer. Thus, in patients with advanced diseases sample is collected by CT guided or US guided endoscopic biopsy or with fine needle aspiration. The sample quality and quantity from needle biopsy is the most limiting for histological and molecular testing [32]. Earlier, only two molecular markers, EGFR mutation testing and ALK rearrangement by FISH were the FDA approved standard of care tests for NSCLC [33]. Whether molecular analysis is successfully performed depends on the proportion of tumor cells compared to total nucleated cells, absolute number of tumor cells and the method used for molecular testing [32]. Macro- or microdissection may be performed to increase the tumor cells in the sample. Each type of molecular test has its advantages and disadvantages. Thus, mentioning the limitations of an assay along with the result is useful for clinical interpretation. Sanger sequencing without any enrichment procedure has lower limit of mutation detection of 10–25% of total DNA. Samples with low tumor number can result in false negative mutation calls. On the other hand, highly sensitive methods which can detect mutations in low tumor cellularity samples (<10%) can give false positive results [32]. Resistance to EGFR TKIs is due to acquisitions of secondary mutations in *EGFR* or other driver genes. Due to inherent heterogeneity in lung cancer, multiple resistance mechanism may exist in the same person in different lesions. Thus, single sample may not be sufficient to determine the cause of TKI resistance and it may require multiple sample collections [32].

Several factors affect the sensitivity of assays for hot-spot mutation detection is a key issue in molecular diagnostics due to several limitations of tumor samples: the poor quality of the DNA extracted from formalin fixed paraffin embedded (FFPE) tissues, the low quantity of DNA available, and the contamination of tumor sample by non-neoplastic cells carrying wild type alleles. Laboratories must incorporate molecular testing methods into their overall laboratory quality improvement program. In particular, laboratories should participate in a formal proficiency testing program [31].

The Cancer Genome Atlas (TCGA) data for squamous cell carcinoma [54] and adenocarcinoma are likely to increase the number of mutations being tested in clinical trials. Large multicenter trials need to be carried out to evaluate the clinical benefit of new novel mutations.

3.7 Quality Control for Molecular Pathology Testing for Lung Cancer

These guidelines are adopted from the College of American Pathologists, International Association for the Study of Lung Cancer, and Association for Molecular Pathology which were published in 2013 and under revision [55, 56].

3.7.1 Pre-analytical

Recommendation Pathologists should select and utilize tissue sparing techniques to preserve tumor tissue for diagnosis and to enable subsequent lung cancer biomarker testing. It should use FFPE, fresh, frozen specimen, cell block and cytology preparation for lung cancer biomarker molecular testing. Other tissue treatments, such as acidic or heavy metal fixatives, or acid decalcifying solutions, should be avoided.

Expert Consensus Opinion Pathologists should select and assess the tumor content adequacy of each specimen for biomarker testing. If tumor content is inadequate then pathologist should perform, microdissection for tumor cell enrichment and assess nucleic acid quality and quantity. Specimens should be received within 3 working days from histopathology lab and recommended turnaround time should be 2 weeks. In patients with multiple, apparently separate, primary lung adenocarcinomas, laboratories may test each tumor, but testing of multiple different areas within a single tumor is not necessary.

3.7.2 Analytical

Strong Recommendation Laboratories should not use total EGFR expression by IHC testing for copy number analysis to select patients for EGFR-targeted tyrosine kinase inhibitor therapy.

Recommendation Laboratories testing for EGFR T790M mutation in patients with acquired resistance to EGFR-targeted kinase inhibitors should deploy assays capable of detecting EGFR T790M mutations in as little as 4% of viable cells (2% of EGFR alleles). When performing ALK testing, physicians can utilize IHC as an equivalent alternative to FISH. In some clinical settings in which tissue is limited and/or insufficient for molecular testing, physicians may use a cell-free plasma DNA (cfDNA) assay for EGFR.

Expert Consensus Opinion Clinical EGFR mutation testing should be able to detect all individual mutations that have been reported with a frequency of at least 1% of EGFR-mutated lung adenocarcinomas. In some clinical settings in which tissue is limited and/or insufficient for molecular testing, physicians may utilize a mutation-specific IHC assay for EGFR testing. Laboratories should employ, or have available at an external reference laboratory, clinical lung cancer biomarker molecular testing assays that are able to detect molecular alterations in specimens with as little as 20% cancer cells. Physicians may use ROS1 IHC as a screening test in lung adenocarcinoma patients; however, positive ROS1 IHC results should be confirmed by a molecular or cytogenetic method. Pathologists should participate in the interpretation of FISH, either by performing the analysis directly or by reviewing the interpretations of cytogeneticists or technologists with specialized training in solid tumor FISH analysis. Physicians may use cell-free plasma DNA (cfDNA) methods to identify EGFR T790M mutations in lung adenocarcinoma patients with progression or acquired resistance to EGFR-targeted tyrosine kinase inhibitors; testing of the tumor sample is recommended if the plasma result is negative. Multiplexed genetic sequencing panels are preferred over multiple single-gene tests to identify other treatment options beyond EGFR, ALK, and ROS1.

No Recommendation There is currently insufficient evidence to support the use of circulating cell-free plasma DNA (cfDNA) molecular methods for the diagnosis of primary lung adenocarcinoma. There is currently insufficient evidence to recommend IHC or FISH testing for ERBB2 (HER2) amplification or expression status to guide selection of therapy in lung adenocarcinoma patients. There is currently insufficient evidence to support the use of circulating tumor cell (CTC) molecular methods for the diagnosis of primary lung adenocarcinoma.

References

1. Ferlay J, Soerjomataram I, Dikshit R, Eser S, Mathers C, Rebelo M, et al. Cancer incidence and mortality worldwide: sources, methods and major patterns in GLOBOCAN 2012. Int J Cancer. 2015;136(5):E359–86. Epub 2014/09/16.
2. Herbst RS, Heymach JV, Lippman SM. Lung cancer. N Engl J Med. 2008;359(13):1367–80. Epub 2008/09/26.
3. Inamura K. Lung cancer: understanding its molecular pathology and the 2015 WHO classification. Front Oncol. 2017;7:193. Epub 2017/09/13.
4. Blandin Knight S, Crosbie PA, Balata H, Chudziak J, Hussell T, Dive C. Progress and prospects of early detection in lung cancer. Open Biol. 2017;7(9). Epub 2017/09/08.

5. Bhatt M, Kant S, Bhaskar R. Pulmonary tuberculosis as differential diagnosis of lung cancer. South Asian J Cancer. 2012;1(1):36–42. Epub 2012/07/01.
6. Mok TS, Wu YL, Thongprasert S, Yang CH, Chu DT, Saijo N, et al. Gefitinib or carboplatin-paclitaxel in pulmonary adenocarcinoma. N Engl J Med. 2009;361(10):947–57. Epub 2009/08/21.
7. Travis WD, Brambilla E, Nicholson AG, Yatabe Y, Austin JHM, Beasley MB, et al. The 2015 World Health Organization classification of lung tumors: impact of genetic, clinical and radiologic advances since the 2004 classification. J Thorac Oncol. 2015;10(9):1243–60. Epub 2015/08/21.
8. Sharma SV, Bell DW, Settleman J, Haber DA. Epidermal growth factor receptor mutations in lung cancer. Nat Rev Cancer. 2007;7(3):169–81. Epub 2007/02/24.
9. Cooper WA, Lam DC, O'Toole SA, Minna JD. Molecular biology of lung cancer. J Thorac Dis. 2013;5(Suppl 5):S479–90. Epub 2013/10/29.
10. Stratton MR, Campbell PJ, Futreal PA. The cancer genome. Nature. 2009;458(7239):719–24. Epub 2009/04/11.
11. Yarden Y. The EGFR family and its ligands in human cancer. Signalling mechanisms and therapeutic opportunities. Eur J Cancer. 2001;37(Suppl 4):S3–8. Epub 2001/10/13.
12. Fujimoto J, Wistuba II. Current concepts on the molecular pathology of non-small cell lung carcinoma. Semin Diagn Pathol. 2014;31(4):306–13. Epub 2014/09/23.
13. Rosell R, Carcereny E, Gervais R, Vergnenegre A, Massuti B, Felip E, et al. Erlotinib versus standard chemotherapy as first-line treatment for European patients with advanced EGFR mutation-positive non-small-cell lung cancer (EURTAC): a multicentre, open-label, randomised phase 3 trial. Lancet Oncol. 2012;13(3):239–46. Epub 2012/01/31.
14. Lynch TJ, Bell DW, Sordella R, Gurubhagavatula S, Okimoto RA, Brannigan BW, et al. Activating mutations in the epidermal growth factor receptor underlying responsiveness of non-small-cell lung cancer to gefitinib. N Engl J Med. 2004;350(21):2129–39. Epub 2004/05/01.
15. Wang S, Song Y, Yan F, Liu D. Mechanisms of resistance to third-generation EGFR tyrosine kinase inhibitors. Front Med. 2016;10(4):383–8. Epub 2016/10/23.
16. Holla VR, Elamin YY, Bailey AM, Johnson AM, Litzenburger BC, Khotskaya YB, et al. ALK: a tyrosine kinase target for cancer therapy. Cold Spring Harb Mol Case Stud. 2017;3(1):a001115. Epub 2017/01/05.
17. Hofman P. ALK in non-small cell lung cancer (NSCLC) pathobiology, epidemiology, detection from tumor tissue and algorithm diagnosis in a daily practice. Cancers. 2017;9(8). Epub 2017/08/15.
18. Davies KD, Doebele RC. Molecular pathways: ROS1 fusion proteins in cancer. Clin Cancer Res. 2013;19(15):4040–5. Epub 2013/05/31.
19. Rossi G, Jocolle G, Conti A, Tiseo M, Zito Marino F, Donati G, et al. Detection of ROS1 rearrangement in non-small cell lung cancer: current and future perspectives. Lung Cancer (Auckl). 2017;8:45–55. Epub 2017/07/26.
20. Mulligan LM. RET revisited: expanding the oncogenic portfolio. Nat Rev Cancer. 2014;14(3):173–86. Epub 2014/02/25.
21. Takeuchi S, Murayama T, Yoshimura K, Kawakami T, Takahara S, Imai Y, et al. Phase I/II study of alectinib in lung cancer with RET fusion gene: study protocol. J Med Invest. 2017;64(3.4):317–20. Epub 2017/09/29.
22. Birchmeier C, Birchmeier W, Gherardi E, Vande Woude GF. Met, metastasis, motility and more. Nat Rev Mol Cell Biol. 2003;4(12):915–25. Epub 2003/12/20.
23. Cappuzzo F, Marchetti A, Skokan M, Rossi E, Gajapathy S, Felicioni L, et al. Increased MET gene copy number negatively affects survival of surgically resected non-small-cell lung cancer patients. J Clin Oncol Off J Am Soc Clin Oncol. 2009;27(10):1667–74. Epub 2009/03/04.
24. Zhang Y, Wang W, Wang Y, Xu Y, Tian Y, Huang M, et al. Response to crizotinib observed in lung adenocarcinoma with MET copy number gain but without a high-level MET/CEP7 ratio, MET overexpression, or exon 14 splicing mutations. J Thorac Oncol. 2016;11(5):e59–62. Epub 2016/01/03.
25. Yu HA, Arcila ME, Rekhtman N, Sima CS, Zakowski MF, Pao W, et al. Analysis of tumor specimens at the time of acquired resistance to EGFR-TKI therapy in 155 patients with EGFR-mutant lung cancers. Clin Cancer Res. 2013;19(8):2240–7. Epub 2013/03/09.
26. Kranenburg O. The KRAS oncogene: past, present, and future. Biochim Biophys Acta. 2005;1756(2):81–2. Epub 2005/11/05.
27. Roberts PJ, Stinchcombe TE, Der CJ, Socinski MA. Personalized medicine in non-small-cell lung cancer: is KRAS a useful marker in selecting patients for epidermal growth factor receptor-targeted therapy? J Clin Oncol Off J Am Soc Clin Oncol. 2010;28(31):4769–77. Epub 2010/10/06.
28. Kempf E, Rousseau B, Besse B, Paz-Ares L. KRAS oncogene in lung cancer: focus on molecularly driven clinical trials. Eur Respir Rev. 2016;25(139):71–6. Epub 2016/03/02.
29. Xu CX, Jin H, Shin JY, Kim JE, Cho MH. Roles of protein kinase B/Akt in lung cancer. Front Biosci (Elite Ed). 2010;2:1472–84. Epub 2010/06/03.
30. Scheffler M, Bos M, Gardizi M, Konig K, Michels S, Fassunke J, et al. PIK3CA mutations in non-small cell lung cancer (NSCLC): genetic heterogeneity, prognostic impact and incidence of prior malignancies. Oncotarget. 2015;6(2):1315–26. Epub 2014/12/05.
31. Shim HS, Choi YL, Kim L, Chang S, Kim WS, Roh MS, et al. Molecular testing of lung cancers. J Pathol Transl Med. 2017;51(3):242–54. Epub 2017/04/22.
32. Hiley CT, Le Quesne J, Santis G, Sharpe R, de Castro DG, Middleton G, et al. Challenges in molecular testing in non-small-cell lung cancer patients with advanced disease. Lancet. 2016;388(10048):1002–11. Epub 2016/09/07.
33. O'Brien CP, Taylor SE, O'Leary JJ, Finn SP. Molecular testing in oncology: problems, pitfalls

and progress. Lung Cancer. 2014;83(3):309–15. Epub 2014/01/30.
34. Conklin CM, Craddock KJ, Have C, Laskin J, Couture C, Ionescu DN. Immunohistochemistry is a reliable screening tool for identification of ALK rearrangement in non-small-cell lung carcinoma and is antibody dependent. J Thorac Oncol. 2013;8(1):45–51. Epub 2012/12/01.
35. Boyle TA, Masago K, Ellison KE, Yatabe Y, Hirsch FR. ROS1 immunohistochemistry among major genotypes of non-small-cell lung cancer. Clin Lung Cancer. 2015;16(2):106–11. Epub 2014/12/04.
36. Khoo C, Rogers TM, Fellowes A, Bell A, Fox S. Molecular methods for somatic mutation testing in lung adenocarcinoma: EGFR and beyond. Transl Lung Cancer Res. 2015;4(2):126–41. Epub 2015/04/15.
37. Roma C, Esposito C, Rachiglio AM, Pasquale R, Iannaccone A, Chicchinelli N, et al. Detection of EGFR mutations by TaqMan mutation detection assays powered by competitive allele-specific TaqMan PCR technology. Biomed Res Int. 2013;2013:385087. Epub 2013/12/24.
38. Weber B, Meldgaard P, Hager H, Wu L, Wei W, Tsai J, et al. Detection of EGFR mutations in plasma and biopsies from non-small cell lung cancer patients by allele-specific PCR assays. BMC Cancer. 2014;14:294. Epub 2014/04/30.
39. Lang AH, Drexel H, Geller-Rhomberg S, Stark N, Winder T, Geiger K, et al. Optimized allele-specific real-time PCR assays for the detection of common mutations in KRAS and BRAF. J Mol Diagn. 2011;13(1):23–8. Epub 2011/01/14.
40. Sheikine Y, Rangachari D, McDonald DC, Huberman MS, Folch ES, VanderLaan PA, et al. EGFR testing in advanced non-small-cell lung cancer, a mini-review. Clin Lung Cancer. 2016;17(6):483–92. Epub 2016/10/23.
41. Storm N, Darnhofer-Patel B, van den Boom D, Rodi CP. MALDI-TOF mass spectrometry-based SNP genotyping. Methods Mol Biol. 2003;212:241–62. Epub 2002/12/21.
42. Serrati S, De Summa S, Pilato B, Petriella D, Lacalamita R, Tommasi S, et al. Next-generation sequencing: advances and applications in cancer diagnosis. OncoTargets Ther. 2016;9:7355–65. Epub 2016/12/17.
43. In Vitro Diagnostics [database on the Internet]. US Food and Drug Administration. 2017 [cited 26 Oct 2017]. https://www.fda.gov/MedicalDevices/ProductsandMedicalProcedures/InVitroDiagnostics/ucm301431.htm.
44. Ansari J, Yun JW, Kompelli AR, Moufarrej YE, Alexander JS, Herrera GA, et al. The liquid biopsy in lung cancer. Genes Cancer. 2016;7(11–12):355–67. Epub 2017/02/14.
45. Zhang Z, Ramnath N, Nagrath S. Current status of CTCs as liquid biopsy in lung cancer and future directions. Front Oncol. 2015;5:209. Epub 2015/10/21.
46. Stroun M, Lyautey J, Lederrey C, Olson-Sand A, Anker P. About the possible origin and mechanism of circulating DNA apoptosis and active DNA release. Clin Chim Acta. 2001;313(1–2):139–42. Epub 2001/11/06.
47. Mouliere F, Robert B, Arnau Peyrotte E, Del Rio M, Ychou M, Molina F, et al. High fragmentation characterizes tumour-derived circulating DNA. PLoS One. 2011;6(9):e23418. Epub 2011/09/13.
48. Alegre E, Fusco JP, Restituto P, Salas-Benito D, Rodriguez-Ruiz ME, Andueza MP, et al. Total and mutated EGFR quantification in cell-free DNA from non-small cell lung cancer patients detects tumor heterogeneity and presents prognostic value. Tumour Biol. 2016;37(10):13687–94. Epub 2016/07/31.
49. Mohrmann L, Huang H, Hong DS, Tsimberidou AM, Fu S, Piha-Paul S, et al. Liquid biopsies using plasma exosomal nucleic acids and plasma cell-free DNA compared with clinical outcomes of patients with advanced cancers. Clin Cancer Res. 2018;24(1):181–8. Epub 2017/10/21.
50. Zhu YJ, Zhang HB, Liu YH, Zhu YZ, Chen J, Li Y, et al. Association of mutant EGFR L858R and exon 19 concentration in circulating cell-free DNA using droplet digital PCR with response to EGFR-TKIs in NSCLC. Oncol Lett. 2017;14(2):2573–9. Epub 2017/08/10.
51. Sozzi G, Roz L, Conte D, Mariani L, Andriani F, Lo Vullo S, et al. Plasma DNA quantification in lung cancer computed tomography screening: five-year results of a prospective study. Am J Respir Crit Care Med. 2009;179(1):69–74. Epub 2008/09/13.
52. Li X, Liu Y, Shi W, Xu H, Hu H, Dong Z, et al. Droplet digital PCR improved the EGFR mutation diagnosis with pleural fluid samples in non-small-cell lung cancer patients. Clin Chim Acta. 2017;471:177–84. Epub 2017/06/13.
53. Sorensen BS, Wu L, Wei W, Tsai J, Weber B, Nexo E, et al. Monitoring of epidermal growth factor receptor tyrosine kinase inhibitor-sensitizing and resistance mutations in the plasma DNA of patients with advanced non-small cell lung cancer during treatment with erlotinib. Cancer. 2014;120(24):3896–901. Epub 2014/08/12.
54. Cancer Genome Atlas Research Network. Comprehensive genomic characterization of squamous cell lung cancers. Nature. 2012;489(7417):519–25. Epub 2012/09/11.
55. Lindeman NI, Cagle PT, Beasley MB, Chitale DA, Dacic S, Giaccone G, et al. Molecular testing guideline for selection of lung cancer patients for EGFR and ALK tyrosine kinase inhibitors: guideline from the College of American Pathologists, International Association for the Study of Lung Cancer, and Association for Molecular Pathology. J Thorac Oncol. 2013;8(7):823–59. Epub 2013/04/05.
56. Molecular Testing guideline for selection of lung cancer patients – revision 2016 draft recommendations. IASLC; 2016 [cited 2017 30 Nov 2017]. https://www.iaslc.org/sites/default/files/wysiwyg-assets/5-20160616capiaslcamplungguideline-2016draftrecommendations_ocpfinal.pdf.

Predicting E3 Ubiquitin Ligases as Possible Promising Biomarkers for Brain Tumors

4

Vibhuti Joshi, Arun Upadhyay, Ayeman Amanullah, Ribhav Mishra, and Amit Mishra

Abbreviations

AIP4	Atrophin-1 interacting protein 4
APC/C	Anaphase promoting complex/ cyclosome;
BCA2	Breast cancer associated protein 2
BMP	Bone morphogenic protein
BRCA 1	Breast cancer gene 1
c-Cbl	Casitas B- lineage lymphoma
Cdc4	Cell division control protein 4
CHIP	Carboxy terminus of Hsp70-interacting protein
CRLs	Cullin-RING ubiquitin ligases
E6-AP	E6-associated protein
GC	Gas chromatography
Gp78	Glycoprotein 78
HCC	Hepatocellular carcinoma
HECT	Homologous to E6-associated protein C-terminus
HPV	Human papilloma virus
IAPs	Inhibitors of apoptosis protein
IHC	Immunohistochemistry
KRAS	Kirsten rat sarcoma viral oncogene homolog
LATS1	Large tumor suppressor kinase 1
LC3	Light chain 3
MALDI	Matrix assisted laser desorption/ ionization
MDM2	Mouse double minute 2
MIC-1	Macrophage inhibitory cytokine-1
NCT	Neoadjuvant chemotherapy
NEDD4	Neural precursor cell expressed developmentally downregulated 4
PEP	Protein elution plate
PHD	Plant homeodomain
PQC	Protein quality control
PTK	Protein tyrosine kinase
RBR	RING-in-between-RING
RING	Really interesting new gene
RT-PCR	Reverse transcriptase-polymerase chain reaction
SCF	Skp1, Cullins and F-box complex
Siah2	Seven in absentia homolog 2
Smad4	S-Mothers against decapentaplegic homolog 4
Smurf 1/2	Smad ubiquitin regulatory factors
TGF-β	Transforming growth factor-β
TNF-α	Tumor necrosis factor-α
TRIM2	Tripartite motif containing 2
TRIM25	Tripartite motif containing 25
UBE2C	Ubiquitin conjugating enzyme 2C
ULK1	Unc-51 like autophagy activating kinase 1
UPS	Ubiquitin proteasome system
XIAP	X-chromosome-linked IAP

V. Joshi · A. Upadhyay · A. Amanullah · R. Mishra
A. Mishra (✉)
Cellular and Molecular Neurobiology Unit,
Indian Institute of Technology Jodhpur,
Jodhpur, Rajasthan, India
e-mail: pg201384014@iitj.ac.in;
pg201384004@iitj.ac.in; pg201384005@iitj.ac.in;
mishra.1@iitj.ac.in; amit@iitj.ac.in

K. K. Shukla et al. (eds.), *Molecular Diagnostics in Cancer Patients*,
https://doi.org/10.1007/978-981-13-5877-7_4

4.1 Introduction

In the last few decades, despite all the progress in basic and advanced research, cancer still remains the major challenge of medical science. However, understanding of its initiation and progression has grown tremendously, still more efforts are needed to reach up to the application level. The onset of the disease marks a plethora of molecular alterations, including several genetic mutations, loss-of-function of many crucial proteins, dysregulated cellular pathways and abnormal metabolism [1]. In fact, cancer is a very broad term, which encompasses a number of diseases occurring in different tissue types with some common underlying features. Advancement in research and diagnostic tools led us to describe this disease as an outcome of several genetic alterations, which provide cells with advantageous gain-of-survival factors and mechanisms giving them with uninterrupted division capacity even under stress conditions [2]. Failure in the maintenance of normal homeostatic conditions due to poor cellular quality control adds up to the severity of the disease condition, whereas the immune system of the organisms supports the growth and metastasis of cancer cells and tissues. For a long time, surgery and radiotherapy were two widely used methods for patients with various grades and stages of cancer [3]. But, the last few decades have provided us with multiple classes of chemotherapeutic molecules to target affected molecular pathways and kill the cancer cells [4].

Charles Huggins first time attempted molecular targeting of cancer by inventing, designing and applying several translational approaches in the oncotherapy [5]. Advances in biochemical, computational and imaging techniques facilitate us to understand the underlying causes and affected molecular pathways in most of the cancers in a better and more elaborative manner [6]. Experts from different backgrounds have started looking onto the etiology and progression of the disease with their own viewpoints. A summarized overview of the causes and mechanism of cancer onset and several associated cellular changes during the progression of the disease and crucial brain tumor causing factors has been represented in Fig. 4.1. After so many years of research, several therapeutic approaches have been devised for cancer treatment, e.g. radiotherapy, chemotherapy, hormonal therapy, immunotherapy, combination therapy, and many more [7]. Owing to the progress in genomics and proteomics, various new molecular targets are continuously added in the category of probable druggable molecules. But, unfortunately, none of the approaches and therapeutic models for the prevention of disease initiation and progression has got enough success [8]. Those, which are already in trials and practice, are reported with a number of toxic side effects on normal cells and tissues, and this is one of the major challenges for scientists and clinicians working in the area of cancer therapeutics and drug development [9].

To identify and diagnose the disease at an early stage, classify and grade them according to their stage, and target the tumor in a more specific and accurate manner are other areas of concern where the current status of medical science falls short of understanding and combating this biological problem [10]. Therefore, clinical scientists need to develop effective tools and efficient techniques to address the aforementioned obstacles in cancer detection and treatment. In last one decade, identification of biomarkers and their prospective applications in current models of disease therapeutics has been welcomed with significant success in early detection and diagnosis of the disease, followed by personalized medical treatment and follow up of patients with different types and grades of cancer [11]. Further, several contemporary cutting-edge molecular advancements have added more productivity and precision in the development of future therapeutic tools. For example, integration of genomic and proteomic knowledge in pinpointing the specific genetic mutations has accelerated the process of identification of the respective biomarkers of several types of cancer. In pursuit of identifying prospective biomarkers for cancer, multiple cellular systems and pathways have been targeted so far and several genes have been investigated in detail for their perspective roles as putative diagnostic tools in upcoming years of research.

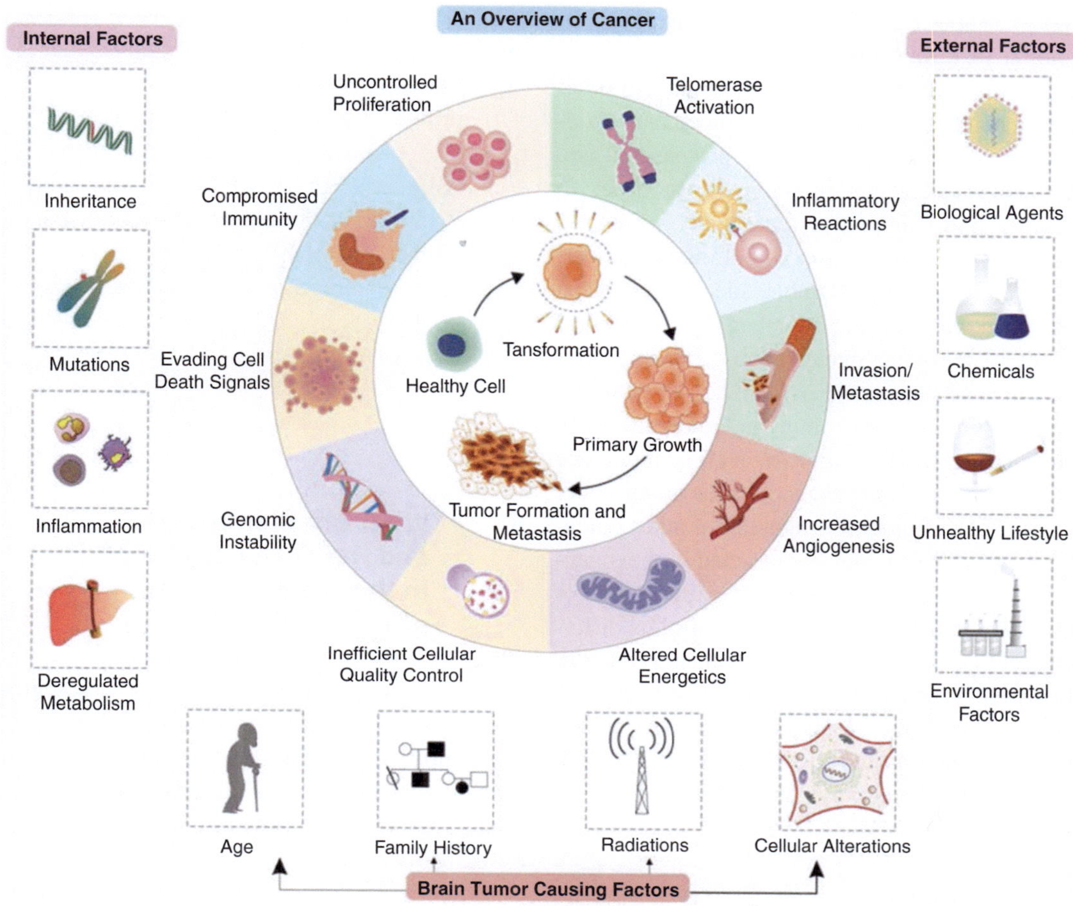

Fig. 4.1 Concise description of cancer causing factors and alterations during tumor formation: Various external and internal factors, causing cancer are represented in square boxes. The alterations generated by these cancer-causing factors are shown in the outer circle; whereas common pathway of tumor formation is represented in the inner circle

In furtherance, cellular protein quality control (PQC) systems are crucial components to maintain the overall homeostasis of the cells and any irregularity or imbalance in the functioning of the components of these pathways may result in significant loss of cellular and organism health [12]. The dysregulated ubiquitin proteasome system (UPS) and autophagy have been acknowledged for their contribution in initiation and progression of cancer and several other diseases. Components of these systems have been found to be significantly upregulated or downregulated in patients diagnosed with different cancers [13, 14]. Identification and characterization of these molecules and pathways would benefit us in developing and expanding a new area of research with a huge potential of modulating several cellular and molecular pathways [15].

In brain tumors like medulloblastoma and glial cell tumors, oncoproteins stabilization in absence of UPS regulation is often reported in adults and children [16]. UPS components, including few E3 ubiquitin ligases, are key regulators of glioma cell cycle and may help to prevent cancer progression via regulating various target proteins [17]. Expression levels of few E3 ubiquitin ligases including SKP2, Huwe1, FBW7, and β-TrCP were found to be altered in medulloblastoma, which signifies the importance of UPS pathway and its components in cell cycle regulation and tumor suppression in brain cells [18]. Similarly, autophagy pathway and its indispensable roles have also been explored in glioma to utilize this pathway of bulk protein degradation in therapeutics of glioma and other associated brain cancers [19]. Hence, many studies have been done to exploit proteasome and autophagy pathways in the past, in order to achieve the cumulative target of preventing uncontrolled cell division and eliminate cancerous cells [14, 20]. Notable success has been observed when certain autophagy inhibitors had been given to mice models with different malignancies and cancer types [21, 22]. Proteasome inhibitors (e.g. bortezomib) have already been approved by the FDA and are in clinical practice with many other similar molecules being under trials [23]. E3 ubiquitin ligases are other potential targets, which could be targeted for next generation molecular therapy for exploitation of their large variety of functional control on different cellular pathways and mechanisms [24, 25]. In recent years, many of them have been proposed as probable biomarker candidates, which we are discussing in further sections of the text; summary has been provided in Box 4.1.

Box 4.1 Summary

- Biomarkers are the crucial early diagnosis tools for brain tumors and various other types of cancers.
- Biomolecules and chemicals produced by cancer cells generally function as biomarkers. On the basis of applications, three broad categories of biomarkers are: prognostic, predictive and pharmacodynamic.
- Multiple advanced methods and tools were developed with time to identify biomarkers at different levels including gene, protein and metabolite analysis.
- Failure or improper functioning of Protein Quality Control pathways: UPS and autophagy were found to be associated with multiple cancer types, along with brain tumors.
- E3 ubiquitin ligases, the key component of Ubiquitin Proteasome System plays critical roles as biomarkers in the detection of tumor by their altered expression or regulation of substrate proteins.
- The potential of E3 ubiquitin ligase families (HECT, RING, U-box, and PHD) and their member E3s as probable biomarkers for different cancer types is still unexplored and needed to be a thoroughly investigated.

4.2 What Are Biomarkers and How Are They Helpful in the Early Diagnosis of Tumors?

Cancer is a categorical term for the representation of an array of diseases that are developed due to simultaneous modifications in several genes of a particular cell type, providing them an advantageous survival capacity with uncontrolled cellular division [1, 26].

Etiology of cancer consists of a cluster of internal and external factors, making it hard to detect the transformational changes in normal cells at earlier stages and if detected, it is difficult to efficiently pinpoint the actual stage of the disease progression [27, 28]. Therefore, clinical oncology needs the development of techniques that can selectively recognize and target transformed cells, preferably by identifying the altered molecular signatures [29–31]. Biomarkers are a similar translational medicinal tool, used widely for the detection and localization of cancers with high selectivity. They also assist in the prognosis and individualization of the treatment with increased specificity and affordability [10, 11]. Malignant tissues are unique in the way of molecules and chemicals they produce i.e. proteins, metabolites, carbohydrates etc. either in secretary or accumulated form in the response of microenvironment, which indicates the progression of the disease. These can be detected qualitatively or quantitatively in different body fluids through various molecular and biochemical techniques

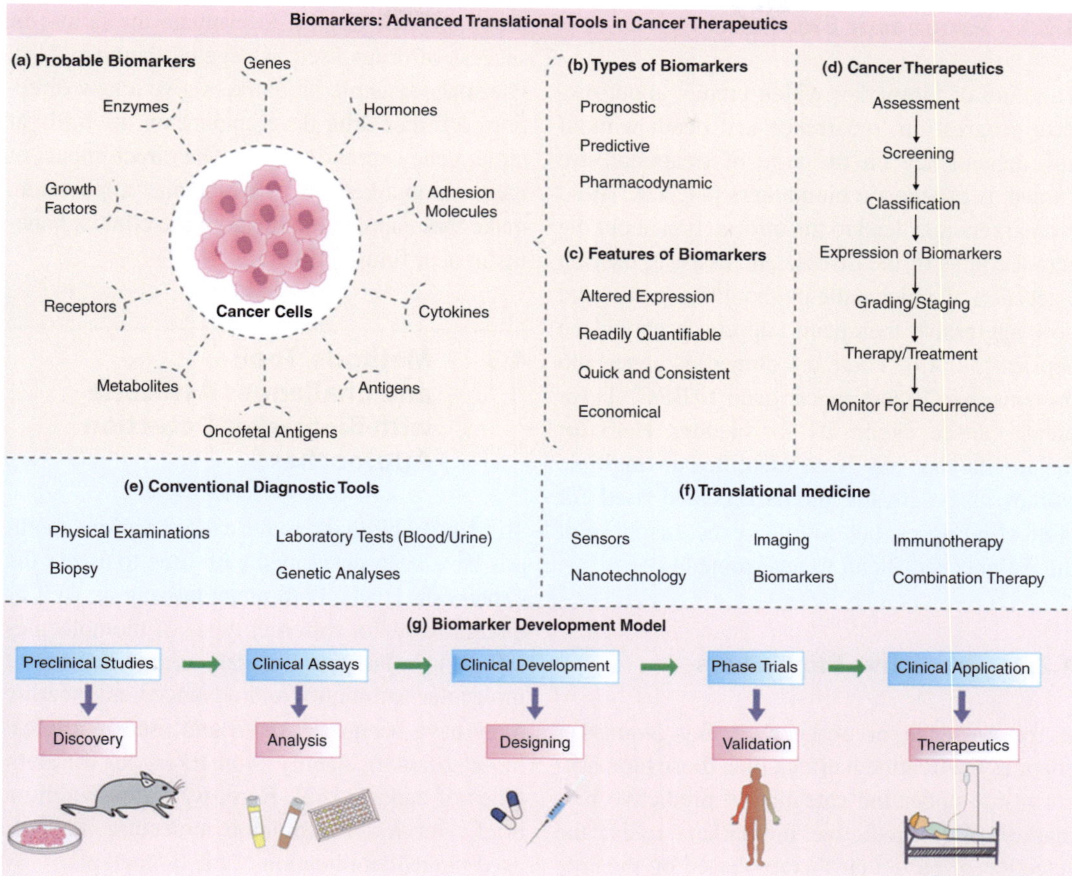

Fig. 4.2 Cancer biomarkers, as an advanced translational tool in cancer therapeutics: A brief overview of cancer biomarkers and advancements in cancer therapeutics. (**a**) Different types of cellular proteins and components that could be used as potential biomarker candidates. (**b**) Currently, available biomarkers could be categorized into different classes based on their potential applications. (**c**) Desirable characteristic features of suitable biomarkers. (**d**) The flow chart presented here shows a stepwise plan of assessment and treatment of cancer. (**e**) Conventional diagnostic tools for cancer. (**f**) Advanced translational medicinal approaches against cancer. (**g**) Schematic overview of the steps involved in identification, assessment, and validation of a biomarker

[32–34]. Figure 4.2 summarizes various categories, characteristic features and possible applications of biomarkers. It also depicts the multi- stage process of how a biomarker is identified, characterized, designed and validated before reaching up to a stage of clinical trial.

Several genes, proteins, enzymes, hormones, carbohydrate moieties and a few oncofetal antigens have been recognized by date as potential biomarkers [35, 36]. Despite progress in molecular methods of cancer biomarker identification, finding a universal biomarker, in place of individual cancer specific marker is still a big challenge, which needs more efforts in near future. Recent advancements in the genomic, proteomic and molecular imaging tools have led to the development of a better molecular understanding of the disease progression. These techniques have also assisted in developing many non-invasive tools for early-stage molecular profiling of cancer patients [37, 38]. But, selection of specific diagnosis tools, and the prediction of which preventive therapeutics should be applied in a particular case, still remains a challenge for scientists [32, 39]. Tumor biomarkers have provided an edge to the oncologists in making these decisions. Based on applications, tumor biomarkers could be classified into three broader categories, which are briefly mentioned below [37, 40].

4.2.1 Prognostic Biomarkers

The kind of biomarker which predict about disease progression, recurrence and death without any dependency on the type of treatment, are known as prognostic biomarkers [41, 42]. These biomarkers may lead to the information about the actual course of the disease and assist in making a decision of which patients should be treated and how aggressive therapeutic approach should be applied [32, 43]. There are numerous genes and proteins, like Breast cancer gene 1 (BRCA1) for breast cancer, cyclin D1 for bladder, Her3 for melanoma that has been identified in multiple studies as prognostic biomarkers and used for clinical purposes, but still, the exact response of the patients is difficult to determine [44].

4.2.2 Predictive Biomarkers

If the presence or absence of any biomarker changes the treatment effect, then those biomarkers reside under the category of predictive biomarker [41]. Predictive biomarkers assist the selection of particular therapy based on the specific mutation or polymorphism in a specific cancer type and predict the scope and success of the treatment [43]. The alternative nomenclature of predictive biomarkers is response biomarkers as they help in identifying the type of treatment and also assess the effect of any particular treatment method [42, 45]. The genes, like p53, PTEN, Her2/neu etc., come under the class of predictive biomarkers for their crucial roles in the prediction of the therapy required [44].

4.2.3 Pharmacodynamic Biomarkers

Biomarkers specifically facilitating the selection of chemotherapeutic drug doses are known as pharmacodynamic biomarkers [42]. Assessment or evaluation of the drug potency, as well as selection and measurement of that drug dose for drugs in the trail, is the major advantage of pharmacodynamic biomarkers [46]. Biomarkers of this class provide information about the effect of drugs on their targets, to evaluate the failure or success of drugs used in targeted therapies [47]. Pharmacodynamic biomarkers give a new direction to tumor drug development on the basis of target gene expression [48]. The direct impact of these biomarkers in therapeutic application, make them applicable for multiple clinical benefits in near future [49].

4.3 Methods, Tools and Challenges Associate with Biomarker Detection Approaches

To identify biomarkers for cancer, various methods have been developed with time to assess the expression levels, both quantitatively as well as qualitatively, for different types of biomolecules [50, 51]. In last two decades, a large number of molecular techniques and advanced engineering tools have been discovered and used in clinical laboratories to identify biomarkers for different types of cancers [52]. Here, we are providing a brief overview of common molecular methods used in the identification of the biomarkers.

4.3.1 Gene Analysis

Quick and commonly used method of biomarker identification is microarray based genome analysis of specific tissue samples or whole proteome analysis to give information of the possible biomarkers [53, 54]. Microarray analysis also gives gene expression profiling of particular cancer type to distinguish highly expressed genes, which may function as prognostic biomarkers [55, 56]. Traditional microarray technique has been modified in multiple ways over the years to develop protein biomarker detection methods [57, 58]. As microarray analysis is used for whole genome analysis, various other methods were developed for the individual sequence analysis, such as PCR (polymerase chain reaction) and its variations like real-time RT-PCR (reverse transcriptase-PCR), competitive RT-PCR and gradient PCR etc. to obtain accurate detection of various types of cancers [59, 60].

4.3.2 Proteome Analysis

Proteins either in normal functional or in mutated forms are recognized as the second level of cancer biomarker, which could be identified and validated by multiple advanced techniques [61, 62]. Earlier, the basic techniques, like western blotting and 2D gel electrophoresis that separate the proteins according to charge and molecular weight, were commonly used for biomarker detection [63, 64]. Advancements in 2D gel electrophoresis and mass spectrometry methods have given a new direction to proteomics-based biomarker identification in various types of cancers [65]. Other methods like isotope tagging, magnetic beads, free flow electrophoresis are also used for cancer biomarker detection [66]. Other widely used methods in clinical practice for detection of biomarker proteins are immunohistochemistry (IHC) and immunocytochemistry, which is now combined with computer- assisted quantification methods for better analysis [67, 68]. Different versions of mass spectrometry, like Matrix Assisted Laser Desorption/Ionization (MALDI) and electron transfer dissociation are advanced methods for cancer biomarker discovery [69]. Fluorescence in situ hybridization is one of the recent techniques, which is playing important roles in the detection of specific biomarkers for neoplasms; and hence are participating in the development of personalized medicines [70, 71].

4.3.3 Metabolite Analysis

In last few years, extended research on various metabolic pathways suggests plasma metabolites as possible biomarkers for pancreatic cancer [72]. Serum and plasma are commonly used for the study of metabolites in developing metabolomic technologies, which help in biomarker detection for multiple cancer types [73]. Gas chromatography (GC)-MS, GC to time-of-flight (TOF) mass analyzers and mass spectrometry based kits are in frequent use currently to detect metabolite cancer biomarkers [52]. Another latest technology prepared to identify lung cancer patients is metabolic biomarker identification using Protein Elution Plate (PEP) [74]. Monitoring the presence of circulating tumor cells or T regulatory cells in the bloodstream could be a possible strategy in understanding and detecting cancer progression. Similarly, the occurrence of cancer antigens in the bloodstream and urine, e.g., prostate-specific antigen, cancer antigen 19-9, and human chorionic gonadotropin could have potential applications as cancer biomarkers [32].

Biopsy is another important detection strategy that provides a definitive diagnosis of cancer in a suspicious area. In this method, a tissue sample is removed from the area to be diagnosed and is assessed in the laboratory through techniques like microscopic imaging. Depending on the tissue or region to be analyzed, various procedures have been developed to collect tissues; for example, needle biopsy, endoscopic biopsy and bone marrow biopsy [75–77]. Besides these conventional techniques, tremendous advancements have been made in the area of biosensors for early detection of cancers, such as, molecularly imprinted polymer based sensors, which give low cost stable method to detect target molecule with high affinity. Biosensors made by proteins, DNA and RNA for accurate assessment of effective therapeutic methods against cancer progression, and metastasis [78, 79]. Designing detection techniques based on multiplexing, i.e. use of more than a single biomarker will overcome few shortcomings of traditional methods, e.g. specificity and accuracy issues of sensors that are generated due to the complexity of the biological system [80]. Apart from these technologies used for biomarker detection, techniques like fluorescence tagging, molecular imaging, nanoparticle development, bioinformatics predictions also have prominent roles in the identification, detection and therapeutic applications of various biomolecules [52].

4.4 The Protein Quality Control Mechanism and Its Association with Cancers

Genetic information encoded in the genes is translated into proteins via mRNA at ribosomes with utmost accuracy. The cellular QC systems start their functions at mRNA level to achieve the healthy set of cellular molecules in the cytoplasmic *milieu* [81]. Failure in this procedure due to any internal or external factor may cause accumulation of aberrant or misfolded proteins inside the cells; therefore, to prevent this, cells have evolved various strategies against protein aggregation [82]. The quality control machinery makes crucial decisions on the refolding or elimination of these aberrant proteins and maintains the homeostatic condition inside the cell [83–85]. The two major pathways of cellular PQC system are UPS and autophagy [86]. PQC systems do have a significant contribution in the carcinogenesis and they also play a significant role in the regulation of cancer cell metabolism [87]. Figure 4.3 represents how cellular PQC components effectively maintain the proteostatic

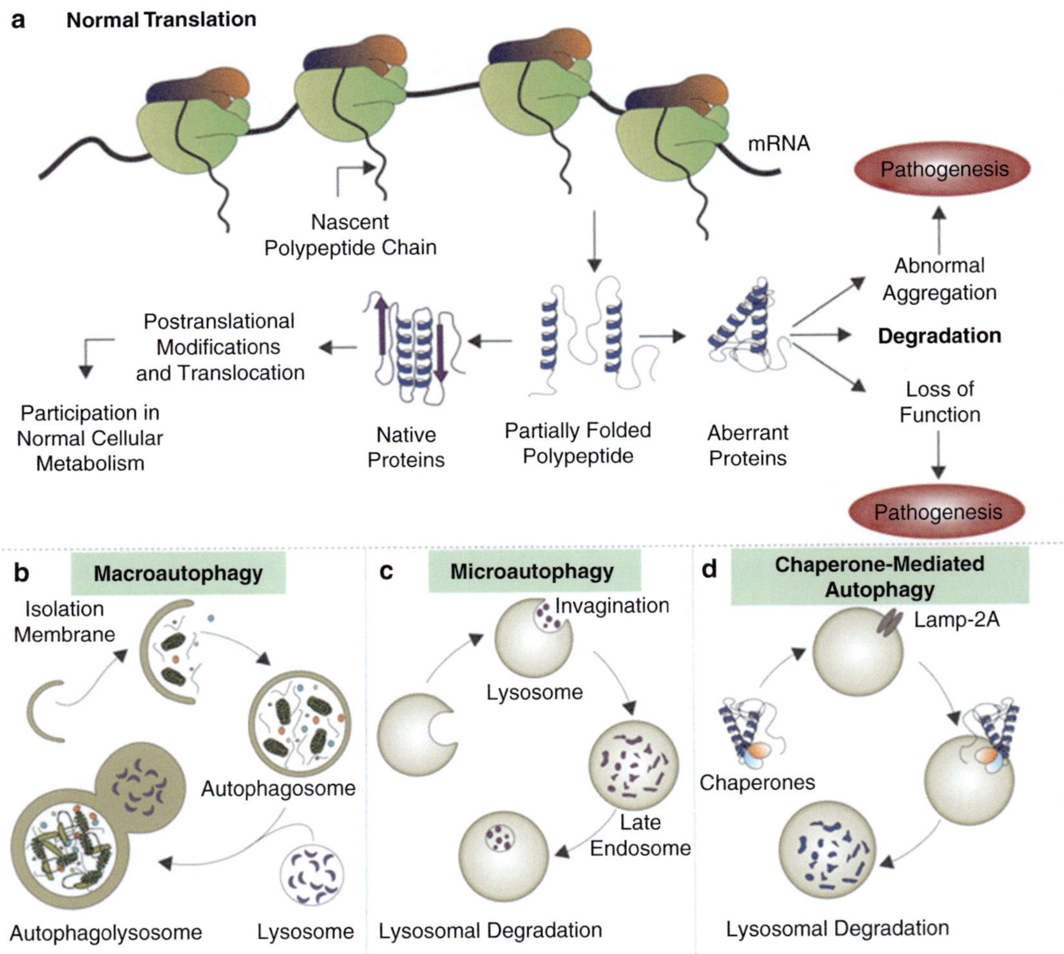

Fig. 4.3 Protein quality control system: From synthesis to degradation: A diagrammatic representation of cellular protein quality control system, taking care of aberrant cellular proteins and their accumulation. (**a**) A normal cellular translation process synthesizing proteins. Cellular stresses or lack-of-function of the quality control pathways result in misfolding of cellular proteins leading to their accumulation that may result in several types of pathological conditions. (**b**) An illustration of ubiquitin proteasome system showing different components, ubiquitinating the substrate proteins in a well coordinated manner to target it for proteasomal degradation. (**c–e**) Autophagy is the bulk degradation process of the cell, which could target the bulk of cellular debris and cellular aggregates of proteins in three different ways. (**c**) Macroautophagy is unique because of isolation membrane and formation of autophagolysosome. (**d**) In microautophagy, invagination of accumulated proteins occurs, and proteins are targeted for lysosomal degradation. (**e**) Chaperone mediated autophagy identifies substrate proteins for degradation with the help of molecular chaperones and degrades them via lysosomal degradation pathways

balance inside the cell, under various proteotoxic stress conditions. In further subsections, we are describing how these two crucial pathways are linked with maintenance of cellular homeostasis and their slight abnormality may lead to improper cellular health.

4.4.1 Autophagy

The complex role of autophagy in cancer has made it difficult to be utilized in cancer therapeutics and diagnosis. Autophagy is a cellular catabolic process having the ability of self-destruction, which enables cells to get rid of cellular waste, such as, toxic proteinaceous inclusions and defective cellular organelles [14]. Autophagy is an important process that plays a crucial role in organism development and cellular protection from environmental and other stresses. It also plays critical roles in developmental processes and diseases, like neurodegeneration and immunological disorders etc. [88, 89]. Initially, the mechanism of autophagy involves sequestration of cytoplasmic material or organelles through double membrane structures, termed as autophagosomes. In the next step, the autophagosome vesicle further fuses with a lysosome containing digestive enzymes; which help in the degradation of sequestered material into basic units, such as amino acids or nucleotides that can be further reused by the cell for its maintenance [90, 91]. In normal tissues, the basal level of autophagy aids in cellular homeostasis maintenance and disturbances in autophagic pathways may have cancer-promoting effects.

It has been reported that disruption of the autophagy gene beclin-1 resulted in the promotion of tumorigenesis in a mice models [92, 93]. Similarly, other studies have also shown the roles of autophagic degradation pathways in tumor suppression [93–95]. Although so many possible links between autophagy and cancer have been identified, still a clear and definitive picture of direct methodological linkage is missing. Autophagy helps cancer cells to survive under nutrient-deprived conditions; contrary to that a mutation in autophagy genes may result in the development of cancer [96]. The role of autophagy genes in cancer prevention gives a new direction to studies, where inducing autophagy by chemotherapeutic agents, such as, sodium butyrate and suberoylanilide hydroxamic acid etc., and naturally derived molecules like resveratrol and saponins have shown potential in reducing the growth of cancer. Surprisingly, different autophagy inhibitors, such as chloroquine, hydroxychloroquine, bafilomycin A1 etc. are also found to be effective in suppressing the growth of breast cancer cells [97]. Recently, it was reported that inhibition of autophagy may overcome the resistance developed due to BRAFV600E inhibition in pediatric brain tumors [98, 99]. Autophagy modulation also regulates chemosensitivity in this type of brain cancer [100].

A recent study has provided prognostic relevance of autophagy proteins light chain 3 (LC3), p62, beclin-1 and Unc-51 like autophagy activating kinase 1 (ULK1) by immunoexpression analysis in Kirsten Rat Sarcoma Viral Oncogene Homolog (KRAS) mutated colorectal cancer patients, where the correlation between expression of these proteins was studied with overall survival of patients [101]. Similarly, it has been proposed that LC3 can be used to identify autophagy status in residual breast cancer cells after neoadjuvant chemotherapy (NCT), which may help in determining the risk of disease relapse or death [102]. Single nucleotide polymorphism study on seven core autophagy genes like ULK1, beclin 1, Atg12 etc. in prostate cancer patients signifies role of autophagy pathway in cancer biomarker development and detection of recurrence after therapy [103, 104]. Autophagy proteins LC3A, p62 were also studied in different types of thyroid cancers by microarray and immunohistochemical analysis, which showed variation in expression of these proteins in different types of thyroid cancers, hence, these are possible biomarker with a specific cancer type [105]. Analysis of LC3 and beclin1 in breast cancer cells reported higher immunoreactivity in cancer cells; whereas baseline level of beclin1 was found to be associated with poor pathological and clinical responses [106]. These studies provide considerable evidence of the utility of the autophagy mechanism in designing cancer treatment strategies. However, to translate these into clinical tools, further work is required. Analysis of autophagy proteins in detail will help in exploring more links between autophagy proteins and cancer types. This may provide basic aid in designing novel biomarkers and treatment methods for cancer therapy.

4.4.2 Ubiquitin Proteasome System

Ubiquitin proteasome system is another protein quality control mechanism, which works independently or synergistically with autophagy to prevent the occurrence of several complex diseases, including cancer and neurodegeneration [87, 107, 108]. Critical control of UPS over the degradation of various cell cycle regulatory proteins like cyclin-dependent kinase inhibitor p27, p53, and cyclin E points towards the possible roles of the pathway in cancer and possibility for future therapeutic implications [13, 109]. UPS got recognition for its wide involvement in various cancers, via its multiple components like E1 ubiquitin activating enzyme, E2 ubiquitin conjugating enzyme and E3 ubiquitin ligases as well as deubiquitinating enzymes and proteasome [110, 111]. The whole cascade of E1, E2 and E3 enzymes of UPS functions in a coordinated manner to transfer the small ubiquitin molecule on target substrate protein, which is eventually degraded in to smaller oligopeptides by the catalytic activity of proteasome [112, 113]. Several components of this protein homeostasis maintaining system have been proposed as the drug targets for multiple cancers and many other severe diseases [114, 115]. In Fig. 4.4, we briefly describe the ubiquitin proteasome system, its enzymes, and their types, for a proper understanding of further sections of this chapter. The UPS as a whole is less explored for cancer

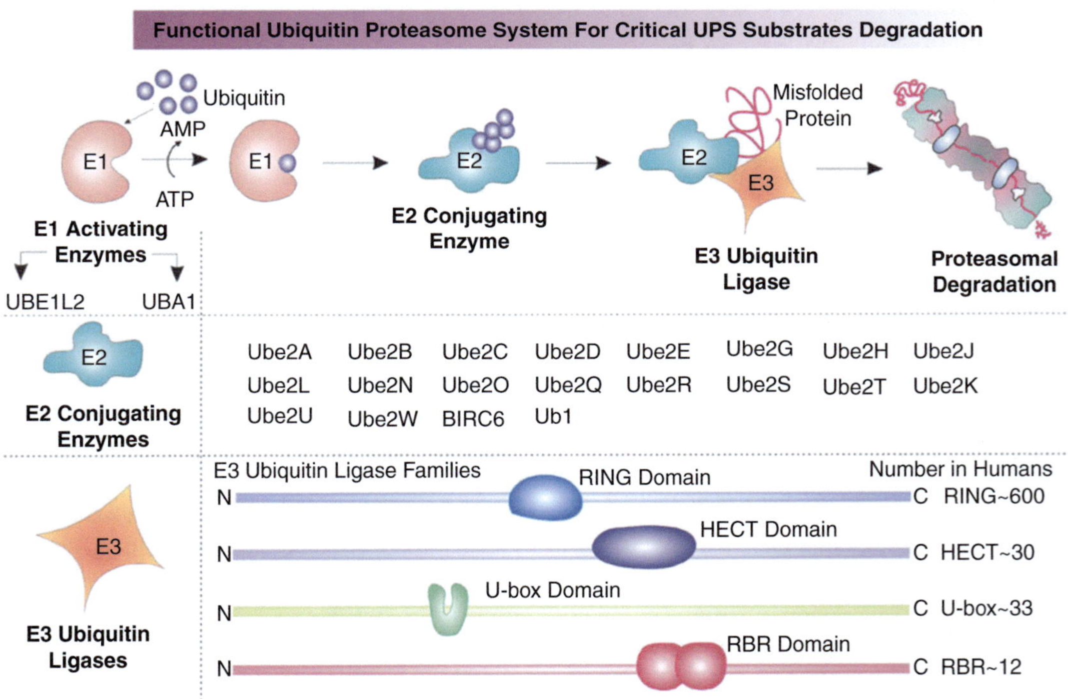

Fig. 4.4 Ubiquitin Proteasome Systems and its enzymes for critical substrate degradation: Schematic brief introduction of UPS mediated substrates protein degradation by enzyme cascade has been described to understand its functional aspects. Just below UPS pathway, various types of E1 activating, E2 conjugating enzymes and E3 ubiquitin ligase families are represented with an approximate number of E3 ubiquitin ligases in each family along with their functional domains

biomarker development, whereas E3 ubiquitin ligases have been studied in detail for biomarker development [25].

The increased proteasome activity and high expression levels of different subunits of proteasome were observed in breast cancer patients by immunoblot and immunofluorescence analysis, proposing possibilities of various UPS components to serve as biomarkers for cancers [116]. These proteasome complexes and their increased catalytic activities were commonly targeted by synthetic and natural compounds, which may suppress angiogenesis and induce apoptosis in cancer cells [117]. Bortezomib is a well-explored proteasome inhibitor, implicated for therapeutic intervention of cancer, but still, leaves the question of broader applicability as it is effective against few cancer types [118]. Not only proteasome, but other components of UPS, e.g. E1 ubiquitin activating enzymes were also studied for cancer treatment [119]. Firstly, a chemical inhibitor 4[4-(5-nitro-furan-2-ylmethylene)-3,5-dioxo-pyrazolidin- 1-yl]-benzoic acid ethyl ester (PYR-41) was reported to block E1 ubiquitin activating enzyme and cause an increase in sumoylation in cells, hence proposed for cancer therapeutics [120]. Inhibitors of E2 conjugating enzymes have also been explored in further research; and MLN4924, an AMP analog inhibits the Nedd8-activating enzyme and trigger autophagy in liver cancer cells [121]. Apart from treatment, PQC system and its components are also investigated for their potential applications as cancer biomarkers.

Microarray analysis of genes associated with hepatocellular carcinoma (HCC) revealed the elevated expression of ubiquitin conjugating enzyme E2C (UBE2C), which was further confirmed by RT-PCR and hence reported as an indicator or biomarker of HCC [122]. E2 ubiquitin conjugating enzymes UbcH10 and UBE2C were found to be highly expressed in primary tumors of uterus, bladder, lung, stomach and thyroid malignant tissues with poor clinical outcomes, which signifies their importance as potential biomarkers for a number of cancer types [123–125]. The most studied component of UPS in association with cancer are E3 ubiquitin ligases, which provide specificity of substrate identification [126]. Mutations and abnormal regulation by the E3 ubiquitin ligases lead to cancer development; moreover, the high-level expression of some E3 ubiquitin ligases in cancer makes them prognostic biomarker and the critical target for multiple types of cancers [25, 127, 128]. Variation in the expressions and functions of the E3 ubiquitin ligases, e.g. overexpression of Hdm2 and Skp2, or functional loss of BRCA1 and Fbw7 like enzymes, are commonly reported in some cancer types [115, 129]. Recently, other UPS components have also been proposed as possible therapeutic targets for glioblastoma. For example, increased expression of ubiquitin-specific protease (USP1) has been reported in patient-derived primary glioblastoma tumor cells, which was further established by the importance of USP1 in GBM growth and maintenance [130]. Several efforts have also been made to develop therapy targeting deubiquitinating enzymes and ubiquitin-specific proteases [131–133].

4.5 How E3 Ubiquitin Ligase Families Are Linked with Deregulated Cell-Cycle Progression and Cancer?

The specific substrate recognizing ability of E3 ubiquitin ligases make them a crucial component of UPS that work towards maintaining homeostatic conditions inside the cells [134, 135]. E3 ubiquitin ligases facilitate the covalent bond formation between the ubiquitin molecules and a lysine residue of substrate protein either in a direct or indirect manner [136]. There are four classes of E3 ubiquitin ligases identified so far, varying with respect to the presence of domains; they are: homologous to E6-associated protein C-terminus (HECT) domain, U-box domain, really interesting new gene (RING) finger domain and plant homeodomain (PHD) [126, 137]. Recently, a new hybrid class of E3 ubiquitin ligases was also reported and named as RING-in-between-RING (RBR) ubiquitin ligases, which are multidomain complex proteins, e.g. parkin [138, 139]. The difference in domains present in these classes of E3 ubiquitin ligases brings divergence in their mode of transferring ubiquitin molecules to the substrate proteins for proteasomal degradation and hence are divided into various classes [140–142].

4.5.1 HECT E3 Ubiquitin Ligases

The HECT domain containing E3 ubiquitin ligases first bind themselves with the ubiquitin molecule via thioester bond and then transfer it to substrate protein [141, 143, 144]. E3 ubiquitin ligases of HECT family are implicated in degrading the substrates involved in various pathways that are associated with cancer development. Moreover, overexpression of E3 ubiquitin ligases like Huwe1, EDD, Nedd4-1, WWP1, and Smurf1/2 may serve as prognostic biomarkers for various cancer types, including breast, prostate, pancreatic and esophageal cancer [145]. Other members of this class of E3 ubiquitin ligases, such as ITCH and NEDD4-2 do not directly function as biomarker, but by regulating transcription factors, like p73 and Smad4 (S-Mothers against decapentaplegic homolog 4), they have regulatory control on the overall development of cancer; and hence they could be targeted for therapeutic developments [146]. HECT domain E3 ubiquitin ligase Huwe1 has a critical regulatory role in neural differentiation and proliferation by ubiquitin-mediated degradation of oncoprotein N-Myc [147].

4.5.2 RING E3 Ubiquitin Ligases

The second class of E3 ubiquitin ligases directly transfer the ubiquitin molecule from E2 conjugating enzymes to a lysine residue of substrate protein for either monoubiquitination or polyubiquitination by forming an E2- E3 complex [148]. RING E3 ubiquitin ligases show variations in E2 conjugating enzymes binding, as their E2 binding site is different from RING domain [149]. Many of the RING E3 ubiquitin ligases are involved in the cellular processes like signaling, transcription, apoptosis, cell cycle regulation and DNA repair mechanism which have direct linkage with cancer cell metabolism, suggesting a possible role of these E3s as cancer biomarkers [150]. Mdm2 is one of the most explored E3 ubiquitin ligases in cancer biology because of its ability to regulate tumor suppressor p53 protein [151]. Its inhibition may result in altered expression of macrophage inhibitory cytokine-1 (MIC-1), a p53 target gene that may serve as biomarkers [152]. Similarly, overexpression of other RING domain E3 ubiquitin ligases, e.g. COP1 and Pirh2 were also reported in breast and lung cancers, respectively that signifies the probability of using these two as cancer biomarkers [153, 154]. High expression levels of novel RING E3 ubiquitin ligases breast cancer associated protein 2 (BCA2) and RING finger protein 11 (RNF11) were also observed in invasive breast cancer cells [155–157].

4.5.3 U-box, PHD and RBR E3 Ubiquitin Ligases

U-box domain containing E3 ubiquitin ligases are a small family of these enzymes with special function as the E4 enzyme, i.e. adding ubiquitin molecules to already ubiquitinated substrate protein. U-box domain is generally considered as modified RING E3 ubiquitin ligase because of structural similarity with RING domain [158]. CHIP is the widely studied U-box E3 ubiquitin ligase involved in the degradation of various substrates associated with the occurrence of multiple cancer types [159, 160]. Another class of proteins, with a zinc finger containing PHD domains, also has E3 ubiquitin ligase activities [161, 162]. Although less explored, but these proteins have shown to have regulation over the trafficking of several proteins [163]. These proteins can also help viruses evading host immunity by downregulating the surface expression of CD4 and MHC class I molecules [164, 165]. The RBR, a hybrid family of HECT and RING E3 ubiquitin ligases, is less studied in the field of complex diseases like cancer, but their ability of auto-inhibition, which causes posttranslational modifications and protein-protein interaction, need to be explored more in the future [166]. The above described different families of E3 ubiquitin ligases and association of member ligases with cancer affirm their involvement in cell cycle regulation and cancer [24]. For a better understanding of their implication and possible therapeutic advantages over other class of molecular targets, in the next section of this chapter, we are describing crucial E3 ubiquitin ligases, which retain a huge potential to work as a biomarker for various cancers.

4.6 Major E3 Ubiquitin Ligases Promising Possible Candidates as Cancer Biomarkers

In the maintenance of cellular physiological processes, protein degradation may sometimes become more crucial regulatory mechanism than the others, like transcription and translation [167]. Regulation of cell cycle is one of the most tightly regulated cellular processes and the preciseness and timing of cell division are dominantly regulated by ubiquitin-dependent proteasomal degradation of cell cycle regulatory proteins [24]. Cyclins and their inhibitors are very crucial proteins for the fine- tuning of the cell cycle progression, which is regulated by two basic mechanisms, i.e., ubiquitination and phosphorylation [168, 169]. A number of E3 ubiquitin ligases coordinate various phases of the cell cycle by regulating differential expression and activity of several crucial proteins during different stages of the cell cycle progression [109]. Alterations in the activities and modulations in the functions of these E3 ubiquitin ligases and their substrates have shown considerable promises in the diagnostics and therapeutics of different types of cancers [110, 170]. In Table 4.1 we have summarized major E3 ubiquitin ligases, which are involved in the regulation of cell cycle progression and tumor formation. Here, in this section, we are providing a brief description of major E3 ubiquitin ligases and their associated mechanisms of action in the cell cycle regulatory processes.

Table 4.1 Involvement of few crucial E3 ubiquitin ligases in cancer and cell proliferation: Table represents crucial E3 ubiquitin ligases with their associated substrate proteins and pathways known to be involved in various types of cancers

S.N.	E3 Ubiquitin Ligases	Target Molecule	Affected Cellular Process	References
1.	Mdm2	p53	Cell cycle	(Haupt et al., 1997)
2.	SCF-Skp2	p27	Cell cycle	(Tsvetkov et al., 1999)
3.	β-TrCP	IkB-α	Transcriptional regulation	(Winston et al., 1999)
4.	CHIP	ErbB2	Tyrosine kinase activity	(Zhou et al., 2003)
5.	ITCH	LATS1	Hippo pathway	(Ho et al., 2011)
6.	E6-AP	p53	Proteasomal degradation	(Scheffner et al., 1993)
7.	Gp78	KAI1	Tumour Metastasis	(Tsai et al., 2007)
8.	Cullin4B	Cyclin E	Cell cycle	(Zou et al., 2009)
9.	NEDD4A	LATS1	Hippo pathway	(Salah et al., 2013)
10.	XIAP	Caspase 3 and 7	Apoptosis	(Deveraux et al., 1997)
11.	c-IAP-1	Caspase 3 and 7	Apoptosis	(Roy et al., 1997)
12	c-IAP-2	Caspase 3 and 7	Apoptosis	(Roy et al., 1997)
13.	Cdc4	Cyclin E	Cell cycle	(Koh et al., 2006)
14.	APC	Cyclin A	Cell cycle	(Amador et al., 2007)
15.	Smurf1/2	TGF-β	TGF-β signaling	(Derynck et al., 2001)
16.	Cbl-b	Tyrosine kinases	Cell signaling	(Paolino et al., 2014)
17.	Siah1	β-catenin	Cell cycle	(Liu et al., 2001)
18.	BRCA1	Rb protein	Transcriptional regulation	(Aprelikova et al., 1999)

4.6.1 Gp78 (Glycoprotein 78)

Initially discovered in melanoma cells, this glycoprotein is well explored in the field of cancer as a possible biomarker, mainly in metastatic tissues [171]. High-level expression of autocrine motility factor receptor or Gp78 (RING E3 ubiquitin ligase) has been observed in various cancers including esophageal, cutaneous malignant melanoma, lung, liver, colon, rectum and stomach, where it is associated with tumor stage and lower survival rate [172]. In breast cancer, comparative analysis of non-neoplastic normal tissues and breast cancer tissues by immunohistochemistry and RT-PCR revealed its inverse correlation with patient's survival [173]. Studies on the expression of Gp78 in cancers, like hepatocellular carcinoma and tongue squamous cell carcinoma suggested a positive correlation between higher expression and invasion of a cancer cells with a low survival rate of patients [174, 175]. Elevated expression of Gp78 in metastatic tissues was explained by degradation of metastasis suppressor protein KAI1 through its E3 ubiquitin ligase activity [176, 177]. Gp78 was proposed as a prostate cancer biomarker, as it is specifically expressed in cancer tissues, while no or very low level is detected in normal prostate tissues [178]. In high-grade astrocytomas, *in situ* hybridization analysis reported high expression level of Gp78 and its ligand autocrine motility factor, which proposes this protein as a bad prognostic factor for glioblastoma and anaplastic astrocytomas [179].

4.6.2 CHIP (Carboxy Terminus of Hsp70-Interacting Protein)

A multifaceted E3 ubiquitin ligase CHIP is well explored in various diseases, like neurodegeneration, heart disease and cancer [160]. Histology sections of breast cancer tissues were analyzed by IHC and a computer-aided image analysis system for CHIP expression and proposed it as a prognostic biomarker for breast cancer [180, 181]. Similarly, expression analysis of CHIP in esophageal squamous cell carcinoma patients by IHC and microarray signifies the importance of CHIP as a predictor of metastatic tumors [182]. Further, the study of CHIP expression in gastric cancer reported its decreased expression in the correlation with increased angiogenesis and a poor prognosis, which suggests CHIP as a prognostic marker of gastric cancer [183]. Same results were also observed in Gall bladder cancer and hence CHIP is proposed as a putative biomarker for these cancers as well [184]. Considering a wide range of functions affected by this E3 ubiquitin ligase, it remains a great challenge for scientists and clinicians to devise a successful therapeutics based on CHIP, although there remains a notable potential in this molecule to be considered as a putative biomarker for multiple cancer types [185]. Downregulated mRNA level of CHIP was observed in glioblastoma as compared to the normal brain tissues, which provides possible clues for possible roles of CHIP as a glioblastoma biomarker [186].

4.6.3 BRCA1 (Breast Cancer Gene 1)

Breast and ovarian cancer associated RING figure protein 53 or BRCA1 acts as a tumor suppressor by regulating DNA repair mechanisms and hence studied for its therapeutic importance [157, 187]. BRCA1 was reported as a potential biomarker for the prediction of breast cancer and beneficial in DNA damage based chemotherapy for this cancer [188]. Similar to breast cancer, the mRNA expression analysis of BRCA1 in ovarian cancer helps in the prediction of patient survival after chemotherapy [189]. The study observed a correlation between BRCA1 and BRCA2 germline or somatic mutations with abnormalities in TP53 gene, which resulted in increased filtrates of immune cells [190]. Predictive biomarker analysis of drugs olaparib and carboplatin is under phase I/Ib trials for ovarian and breast cancers [191]. Recently, IHC results of epithelial ovarian carcinoma for BRCA1 expression provide the significant prognostic importance and support for clinical trials [192]. However, the risk of brain cancer in BRCA1 mutation is very low, but detailed studies in future may explore the possible relationship between this E3 ubiquitin ligase and brain cells cancer [193]. Recently it has been observed that BRAC1 play a tumor-promoting role for glioblastoma by preventing replication stress [194, 195].

4.6.4 SCF (Skp, Cullin, F-box Containing Complex)

The proteins Skp1, Cullins, F-box and ROC/Rbx/SAG forms the SCF complex, which is mainly involved in the degradation of the cell cycle regulatory proteins that are directly associated with multiple cancers [196]. The component of the complex, such as F-box proteins provide substrate specificity and may work as an ideal biomarker in cancers like prostate and squamous cell carcinomas, with possible applications in targeted therapy [197, 198]. Other than cell cycle regulation, this complex is also involved in glycolysis, serine–threonine kinase ubiquitination and tumorigenesis [199]. The significance of Skp2 in human gastric carcinoma could be shown by its high expression and thus it could be proposed as a prognostic biomarker for this cancer [200]. Other components of this complex RING box proteins, RBX1 and RBX2 also have regulatory roles in multiple cancers and might be used as a biomarker in near future [201]. A small molecule MLN4924 was identified as an inhibitor of a SCF complex, and its use in trials has given new hopes for the targeting of SCF complex in anticancer therapy [202]. The components of SCF complex ROC/Rbx were also identified as a biomarker in melanoma with Skp2, SCF-FBW7 and other E3 ubiquitin ligases [127, 203]. Small interfering RNA mediated downregulation of Skp2 in T98G glioblastoma type causes induction of p27 and growth arrest that finally leads to apoptosis [204].

4.6.5 ITCH

ITCH or atrophin-1 interacting protein 4 (AIP4) was first studied for its role in coat color alterations in mouse skin [205]. It was observed that a 18H mutation, which produces this coat colored variations, arises from the chromosomal inversions with deletion of 18–20 bases, hampering expression of *agouti* and ITCH genes [146, 205]. ITCH is basically involved in regulating the inflammatory [206] and immune responses [207] of the cell, but it also controls ubiquitination and thus the degradation of different proteins, which have functions in regulation of cell death, such as tumor necrosis factor-α (TNF-α) [208]; and apoptosis via regulating proteins such as p73 [209] and p63 [210]. The functions of ITCH in modulating cell cycle and uncontrolled cellular growth, as observed in tumor cells, is also provided by a study, where this E3 ubiquitin ligase was found to degrade protein such as RASSF5, which is necessary for causing apoptosis in cells [211]. Other studies also link ITCH with tumorigenicity, as ITCH induces the degradation of LATS1 (large tumor suppressor kinase 1) in cells, resulting in uncontrolled cellular proliferation and growth [212]. Recently, ITCH is proposed as a prognostic biomarker in pancreatic cancer, as loss-of- function in this gene is responsible for metastasis [213]. All these above mentioned different studies indicate that ITCH is a prominent candidate, with substrate proteins, having roles in cellular proliferation. Thus, observing changes in ITCH functions and levels can help in monitoring and modulating cellular proliferation and uncontrolled growth.

4.6.6 NEDD4 (Neural Precursor Cell Expressed Developmentally Down-Regulated 4)

NEDD4, a HECT family E3 ubiquitin ligase mediates its cellular effects by regulating ubiquitination and degradation of its substrates in ER, proteasome, and autophagy [214]. NEDD4 is a multifunctional E3 ubiquitin ligase regulating a range of protein substrates (e.g. ENac, AMPA receptors, etc.) with important functions in different biological processes. It also affects signaling pathways, linked with uncontrolled cellular growth and proliferation [215]. NEDD4 regulates the levels of LATS1 protein by ubiquitination and its proteasomal degradation, thus can influence tumorigenesis directly [216]. NEDD4 can also suppress the oncogenic pathway of Notch signaling and reduce the levels of important proteins of the pathway, such as Notch and Deltex [217]. NEDD4-1 has a direct role in regulating pancreatic cancer cells growth, as it controls the level of PTEN, a cancer inhibitor protein, by its polyubiquitination and degradation; its levels were drastically increased when monitored in mouse model of cancer [218]. Thus, these findings indicate that NEDD4 is a critical regulator of tumor growth and its increased level in pancreatic cancer cells suggests that it could be considered as prognostic marker for these cancers. NEDD4 is associated with glioblastoma also by regulating invasion and migration of glioma cells via ubiquitinating cyclic nucleotide Ras guanine nucleotide exchange factor and RAS-related protein 2A [219, 220].

4.6.7 CUL Family (Cullin-RING Ubiquitin Ligases)

Cullin basically acts as a scaffold protein and with its C-terminal region binds to a RING-finger containing protein known as ROC1/ROC2 that makes the family of cullin RING finger ligases (CRLs). Neddylation is a process by which protein such as NEDD8, may regulate the activity of CRLs proteins [221]. Human cullin family of E3 ubiquitin ligases consists of eight members (CUL1, CUL2, CUL3, CUL4A, CUL4B, CUL5, CUL7, and CUL9). Each cullin works as a scaffold protein to recruit adaptor and other interacting proteins. Cullin proteins may have a specific role in cancer, as their expression pattern (CUL4A) was found to alter under these conditions, such as in the breast and hepatocellular carcinoma [222, 223]. Furthermore, in different processes, which are linked with tumorigenicity, such as cell cycle regulation, DNA damage, signaling and tumor suppression, this E3 ubiquitin ligase complex plays indispensable roles [224]. Another member of this family, CUL4B modulates cell cycle proteins, such as cyclin E and a knockdown of CUL4B is associated with an increase in cyclin E [225]. Since cyclin E controls cell cycle transition from G1 to S phase, a decrease in cyclin E is associated with an increase in cellular proliferation, as is observed in tumor cells [226]. Similarly, CUL4A is also found to regulate another cell cycle protein p21, which is degraded by a highly expressed CUL4A, resulting in a loss of control on cell cycle and an increase in proliferation, as observed in different cancerous cells [227, 228]. The role of Cullin 1 was also explored in glioma cells proliferation, invasion, and migration [229]. It has been reported that decrease in the expression of CUL4B, under both *in vitro* and *in vivo* condition, inhibits proliferation of glioma cells in brain tumor [230].

4.6.8 Cdc4 (Cell Division Control Protein 4)

Cdc4 is an F-box protein and is a vital component in the big complex of SCF. It acts as one of the substrate binding proteins in the SCF complex and thus can regulate important proteins, which have critical roles in cell cycle progression, e.g. cyclin E [197]. This has been observed in cells of pancreatic cancer, where different isoforms of this protein are found in higher stage cancer [231]. Similarly, in other pathological conditions, such as in colorectal cancer, Cdc 4 is found to be present in a mutated form, which highlights the possible implication of this protein in cell cycle control and tumorigenesis [232]. There is also a report that establishes the involvement of the Cdc4 gene in chromosomal stability [233], which could probably be in p53 dependent manner; however loss of this protein may result in genomic instability [232]. These reports clearly establish the importance of this E3 ubiquitin ligase in controlling the growth rate of cells. hCdc4 was proposed as a prognostic biomarker for glioblastoma as it controls the cell proliferation in glioma under *in vitro* conditions [234].

4.6.9 MDM2 (Mouse Double Minute 2)

MDM2, a 90 kDa protein, is designated to be the major regulator of tumor suppressor protein TP53, which lies at the center of many oncogenic pathways [235, 236]. A feedback loop formed of MDM2 and p53 forms a regulatory control over the maintenance of genomic integrity and cellular transformation [237]. MDM2 overexpression is one among the many reported genetic alterations in several types of cancers. It has also been reported to retain p53-independent oncogenic potential, which could be related to few other cell fate regulatory proteins, e.g., retinoblastoma, Numb, E2F1 etc. [238–240]. MDM2-p53 complex inhibition has been exploited for therapeutic purposes in multiple cancer types, but toxicity generated by used inhibitors also cause damage to healthy tissues [151].

Multiple discoveries have led to the identification of MDM2 as one of the promising prognostic biomarker, which helps us to detect early stage tumors like gastric cancer development and post-therapy recurrences [241–243]. MDM2 has been proposed as a negative biomarker in breast carcinoma as no remarkable relation was observed in the MDM2 expression levels and patient survival [244]. In non-small-cell lung cancer, IHC analysis of MDM2 expression reported the protein as a probable prognostic biomarker, especially in patients without accumulation of p53 protein [245]. Development of small peptide antagonists and identification of many inhibitors in the past have gained significant success in cancer therapeutics [246]. Expression levels of MDM2 in primary and secondary glioblastoma lacking p53 mutations were analyzed and were reportedly high in primary glioblastoma only [247].

4.6.10 E6-AP (Human Papilloma Virus E6-Associated Protein)

E6-AP is another major E3 ubiquitin ligase that is directly associated with regulation of p53 expression, stability, and function [248]. Human papilloma virus (HPV) is sexually transmitted DNA tumor viruses that underlie the majority of the worldwide cases of cervical cancer [249]. E6 viral oncoprotein, after binding to E6-AP, alters its cellular functions and causes E6-AP mediated polyubiquitination of p53, followed by degradation [250]. E6/E6-AP complex can also target NFX1-91, a putative repressor of hTERT, causing its induction, which leads to the activation of telomerase enzyme [251]. Similarly, in several knockdowns and transgenic mouse model based studies, E6-AP has been shown to mediate most of the oncogenic effects imparted by HPV via its interaction with viral E6 protein [252, 253]. However, E6-AP is also crucial for the stability of intracellularly expressed E6 oncoprotein itself [254]. Apart from regulating the turnover of p53 [255], E6-AP also ubiquitylates and degrades other cell cycle regulatory proteins, e.g., p27 [256]. Considering these prominent functions of E6-AP, either in complex with E6, or in an independent manner, E6-AP could be considered to be a major therapeutic target for various types of cancers [135, 255, 257].

4.6.11 APC/C (Anaphase-Promoting Complex/Cyclosome)

APC/C, E3 ubiquitin ligase is known for its cell cycle regulatory functions over the S-phase and early mitosis *via* its substrate proteins, such as cyclin A, Skp2, securin etc [258]. The activities of APC/C are regulated by two effector proteins, i.e., Cdc20 and Cdh1 [259]. Loss of control over the regulatory pathway of APC/C complex results in the formation of malignant tumors; and thus suggests the importance of this crucial protein in the pathogenesis of cancer [260]. High concentration of various APC/C substrate proteins, including Cdc20, polo-like kinase 1, Aurora kinase A and Skp2 are observed in multiple types of human cancers, proposes them as potential biomarkers and APC/C as a crucial target for cancer therapy [261]. Regulatory pathway of Skp2 was analyzed in colon cancer patients by biochemical analysis and reported APC/C-Cdh1 complex as a potential biomarker for colorectal tumor formation [262]. APC/C-Cdh1 also regulates another E3 ubiquitin ligase, *viz* NEDD4-like ubiquitin ligase 2, which is involved in the progression of cervix or colon cancer [263]. Recently, a research suggests that functional inactivation of APC/C reduces chromosomal instability in cancer cells [264]. As APC/C is involved in regulation of cell cycle as well as cell death pathways, it is considered as a crucial drug target for cancer treatment [265]. APC/C-Cdh1 also targets inhibitor of DNA binding 2 protein which is involved in tumor progression and cell proliferation [266]. Recently, it has been reported that self-renewal and invasiveness of stem-like cells of glioblastoma are controlled by the Cdc20-APC complex in glioblastoma patients [267].

4.6.12 Smurf 1/2 (Smad Ubiquitin Regulatory Factors)

Smurf 1 and 2 are putative regulators of the transforming growth factor-β (TGF-β) and bone morphogenic protein (BMP) signaling cascades; and are associated with multiple cellular functions, like cell proliferation, cell cycle regulation, DNA damage response, metastasis and maintenance of genomic stability [268]. They modulate pathways by mediating the proteasomal degradation of Smads, and few crucial receptors involved in various signaling pathways [269–271]. A very delicate regulation is required for TGF-β signaling pathways at various life stages as well as tissue types; so targeting of TGF-β signaling pathways for cancer therapeutics through Smurf1/2 still remains a challenge as the pathway may cause both suppression and induction of tumor development and metastasis [272, 273]. Smurf2 overexpression was found to be linked with poor prognosis in certain breast cancer tissues and esophageal squamous cell carcinoma patients [274, 275]. Similarly, in renal cell carcinoma, Smurf1 significantly expressed in high amount and found to be associated with stages of metastasis, tumor size and vascular invasion; thus might be proposed as a prognostic biomarker [276]. Although, the roles of Smurf 1/2 as a biomarker is well explored in several cancer types, but their involvement in brain tumors is still unexplored, which could be established in future by conducting detailed research in glioma patients.

4.6.13 IAPs (Inhibitors of Apoptosis Proteins)

IAP family of proteins consists of various members, some of which contains RING domain, like XIAP, c-IAP1, and c-IAP2. The effect of expression levels of various IAPs in different types of cancer has been checked in various studies in order to understand their prognostic significance [277]. In patients of malignant pleural mesothelioma, IAP1 and survivin were found to be linked with a short lifespan, whereas X- chromosome-linked IAP (XIAP) and livin had positive effects on patient survival [278]. Interestingly, in another study involving acute myeloid leukemia patients, low levels of XIAP was associated with patient's longer survival [279]. However, the presence of higher XIAP and survivin expression level in childhood acute myeloid leukemia samples were correlated with decrease in survival [280]. Similarly, the prognostic significance of XIAP and survivin were also observed in another study, where high expression of these two E3 ubiquitin ligases was observed in advanced tumor stages of breast cancer patients [281].

Recently, another study provided evidence of the potential of IAPs level in identifying the risk of cancer progression [282]. Furthermore, IAPs have also been found to be involved in establishing resistance in cancer cells to drugs like paclitaxel, 5-FU, and doxorubicin [283]. It was also found in this study that ectopic expression of c-IAP2 resulted in reduced cytotoxicity of cisplatin [284]. Altogether, these studies provide useful information about IAPs, which can be utilized to develop biomarkers for cancer detection. However, there are some studies that provide different results, such as in the case of XIAP that have been shown to have no or opposite effects in acute myeloid leukemia and resected non- small cell lung cancer patients respectively, making their applicability limited [285, 286]. IAP family gene Apollon was found to be expressed in brain cancer cells, where it protects cells from apoptosis [287]. However, amplification of cIAP1/2 was also explored in glioblastoma, where IAPs are related with the negative progression of cancer [288]. Thus careful further investigation is needed to understand the potential of these proteins to be used as biomarkers for cancer.

4.6.14 CBL (Casitas B-Lineage Lymphoma)

c-Cbl is a RING type E3 ubiquitin ligase, which is involved in attenuation of protein tyrosine kinase (PTK) signaling. Studies have identified CBL gene mutations in patients with myeloid malignancies [289, 290]. In gastric carcinoma and primary colorectal cancer tissues the expression of Cbl protein has been reported to be elevated, hence it may function as a biomarker for these two cancers [291, 292]. Increased Cbl level in prostate cancer tissues has also been associated with reduced patient survival [293]. Cbl has also been found to be mutated in lung cancers [294]. Recently, the role of Cbl in gliomas was also elucidated, when in glioma tissues patients had a high level of Cbl E3 ubiquitin ligase [295]. The altered levels and mutations of Cbl in various cancer tissues give an idea of the crucial roles played by them in cellular homeostasis and their ability to serve as biomarkers for cancer detection. Expression analysis for tyrosine phosphorylated c-Cbl was performed in different cancer patients and it has been observed that an equal number of negative and positive patients were present for brain cancer [296]. Later, c-Cbl exon skipping was reported to be a possible mutation contributing to growth and malignancy of glioma [297]. Further, another study proposed expression of c-Cbl with poor prognosis and tumor progression in high grade glioma [295].

4.6.15 Siah2 (Seven In Absentia Homolog 2)

Siah2 is another RING type E3 ubiquitin ligase involved in mechanisms such as in apoptosis, DNA damage response, cellular proliferation and response to hypoxia condition [298, 299]. Siah2 high level has also been associated with drug resistance and inhibition of it resulted in sensitivity to anti- cancer drug [300]. Siah2 has been shown to have possible roles in tumor development and progression in epithelial ovarian carcinoma [301]. The expression of Siah2 has also been found to be elevated in human lung cancer [302]. Increased level of Siah2 has been reported in breast cancer with probable roles in progression and metastasis [303]. Recently, another study provided evidence in support of Siah2 as a promoter of invasion capacity of breast cancer cell line [304]. Under hypoxia condition ubiquitin ligase Siah2 regulates HIF-1α facilitating the migration and invasion of glioma cells [305]. The metastatic role of Siah2 can be further analyzed, as it can serve as a promising tool in identifying and detecting progressive cancers.

4.6.16 TRIM25 (Tripartite Motif Containing Protein 25)

TRIM25 is another E3 ubiquitin ligase and a member of the vast family of TRIM proteins having RING, B box, and coiled coil motif. Like above E3 ubiquitin ligases, TRIM25 role in cancer has also been studied [306]. Abnormal expression of TRIM25 has been observed in cancers of breast and ovary [307, 308]. Also, TRIM25 has been shown to be linked with poor prognosis of gastric cancer patients [309]. Recently, the proliferative and migratory role of TRIM25 in lung and colorectal cancer has also been elucidated [310, 311]. These recent identifications of the roles of TRIM25 in multiple cancers show that more studies are needed to unravel its involvement in other cancers like brain cancer, glioblastoma. In depth analysis of this RING type E3 ubiquitin ligase may add significantly in the field of early stage detection of cancer and may also prove to be a novel therapeutic target for inhibition of cancer proliferation and migration.

4.7 Key Questions and Future Perspectives

In spite of several translational approaches being developed for the treatment of cancer, not much success has been received in transforming the research outcomes into clinical tools. The most challenging task for oncologists still remains the early diagnosis and targeted drug delivery to specific sites with least side effects on other cells and tissues. The advent of biomarkers has minimized both, the costs of the diagnosis and the treatment of the disease. Despite the increase in the use of 'omics' and other analytical techniques in research, which enabled us to identify new proteins as possible markers for future therapeutics; these techniques do not get enough success in clinical practices. Applicability of most of these biomarkers is limited to only few cancer types. The urgent need of present scenario is to identify and develop universal or broad-spectrum biomarkers relevant for several cancer types including brain cancer [312, 313]. In this direction, integration of biomarkers with other translational medicine tools like nanoparticles will increase the success rate in upcoming years [314]. E3 ubiquitin ligases, like many other protein misfolding associated diseases, also play crucial roles in regulating cell division and proliferation. Past many years have seen increasing literature presenting these molecules as future therapeutic targets in many biological diseases like neurodegeneration and ageing [24]. But their remedial exploration and successful applications are yet to be tested and verified in diseases like brain cancer.

Finding out solutions to the problem of cancer lies in its early stage diagnosis, as this helps in predetermining and designing a rational therapy against this dreadful disease. Utilizing E3 ubiquitin ligases as a prognostic biomarker for cancer can be a useful option which remains to be tested at clinical and laboratory level to understand its full potential. Researchers have hypothesized that, as many members of E3 ubiquitin ligases family are involved in different regulatory processes in cancer, they may serve as possible candidates in early stage cancer diagnosis [25]. This hypothesis has been supported by various studies as mentioned earlier in the text, where the altered level of many E3 ubiquitin ligases have been found in cancer cells and tissues. Interestingly, E3 ubiquitin ligase-based anti-cancer drugs, such as nutlin have been identified, giving an idea of their crucial importance in cancer mechanism [315]. However, developing E3 ubiquitin ligases as a potential biomarker for brain cancer will require further studies. Altogether, to translate E3 ubiquitin ligases as a biomarker for brain cancer at the clinical level, future studies should be aimed at identifying the roles of these enzymes in different types of cancers along with cost effectiveness, production at industrial level and their clinical usefulness in terms of specificity and accuracy.

Acknowledgement In this work, VJ and AU were supported by a research fellowship from University Grants Commission, Council for Scientific and Industrial Research, Government of India. The authors would like to thank Mr. Bharat Pareek for his technical assistance and entire lab management during the manuscript preparation. We apologize to various authors whose work could not be included due to space limitations.

Conflict of interest: The authors do not have any actual or potential conflicts of interests to disclose.

References

1. Hanahan D, Weinberg RA. Hallmarks of cancer: the next generation. Cell. 2011;144:646–74.
2. Vogelstein B, Papadopoulos N, Velculescu VE, Zhou S, Diaz LA Jr, Kinzler KW. Cancer genome landscapes. Science. 2013;339:1546–58.
3. Sudhakar A. History of cancer, ancient and modern treatment methods. J Cancer Sci Ther. 2009;1:1–4.
4. Meyskens FL Jr, Mukhtar H, Rock CL, Cuzick J, Kensler TW, et al. Cancer prevention: obstacles, challenges and the road ahead. J Natl Cancer Inst. 2016;108.
5. Huggins C, Hodges CV. Studies on prostatic cancer. I. The effect of castration, of estrogen and of androgen injection on serum phosphatases in metastatic carcinoma of the prostate. Cancer Res. 1941;1:293–7.

6. Weissleder R, Ntziachristos V. Shedding light onto live molecular targets. Nat Med. 2003;9:123–8.
7. Drake CG. Combination immunotherapy approaches. Ann Oncol. 2012;23:viii41–6.
8. Dang CV, Reddy EP, Shokat KM, Soucek L. Drugging the 'undruggable' cancer targets. Nat Rev Cancer. 2017;17(8):502–8.
9. Hedigan K. Cancer: herbal medicine reduces chemotherapy toxicity. Nat Rev Drug Discov. 2010;9:765.
10. Henry NL, Hayes DF. Cancer biomarkers. Mol Oncol. 2012;6:140–6.
11. Liotta LA, Petricoin E. Cancer biomarkers: closer to delivering on their promise. Cancer Cell. 2011;20:279–80.
12. Chhangani D, Mishra A. Protein quality control system in neurodegeneration: a healing company hard to beat but failure is fatal. Mol Neurobiol. 2013;48:141–56.
13. Mani A, Gelmann EP. The ubiquitin-proteasome pathway and its role in cancer. J Clin Oncol. 2005;23:4776–89.
14. Mathew R, Karantza-Wadsworth V, White E. Role of autophagy in cancer. Nat Rev Cancer. 2007;7:961–7.
15. Upadhyay A, Joshi V, Amanullah A, Mishra R, Arora N, et al. E3 ubiquitin ligases neurobiological mechanisms: development to degeneration. Front Mol Neurosci. 2017;10:151.
16. Hede SM, Savov V, Weishaupt H, Sangfelt O, Swartling FJ. Oncoprotein stabilization in brain tumors. Oncogene. 2014;33:4709–21.
17. Vlachostergios PJ, Voutsadakis IA, Papandreou CN. The ubiquitin-proteasome system in glioma cell cycle control. Cell Div. 2012;7:18.
18. Vriend J, Ghavami S, Marzban H. The role of the ubiquitin proteasome system in cerebellar development and medulloblastoma. Mol Brain. 2015;8:64.
19. Kaza N, Kohli L, Roth KA. Autophagy in brain tumors: a new target for therapeutic intervention. Brain Pathol. 2012;22:89–98.
20. Adams J, Palombella VJ, Sausville EA, Johnson J, Destree A, et al. Proteasome inhibitors: a novel class of potent and effective antitumor agents. Cancer Res. 1999;59:2615–22.
21. McAfee Q, Zhang Z, Samanta A, Levi SM, Ma X-H, et al. Autophagy inhibitor Lys05 has single-agent antitumor activity and reproduces the phenotype of a genetic autophagy deficiency. Proc Natl Acad Sci. 2012;109:8253–8.
22. Yuan N, Song L, Zhang S, Lin W, Cao Y, et al. Bafilomycin A1 targets both autophagy and apoptosis pathways in pediatric B-cell acute lymphoblastic leukemia. Haematologica. 2015;100:345–56.
23. Adams J. The development of proteasome inhibitors as anticancer drugs. Cancer Cell. 2004;5:417–21.
24. Nakayama KI, Nakayama K. Ubiquitin ligases: cell-cycle control and cancer. Nat Rev Cancer. 2006;6:369–81.
25. Sun Y. E3 ubiquitin ligases as cancer targets and biomarkers. Neoplasia. 2006;8:645–54.
26. Vogelstein B, Kinzler KW. Cancer genes and the pathways they control. Nat Med. 2004;10:789–99.
27. Danaei G, Vander Hoorn S, Lopez AD, Murray CJ, Ezzati M, Group CRAc. Causes of cancer in the world: comparative risk assessment of nine behavioural and environmental risk factors. Lancet. 2005;366:1784–93.
28. Ferrari M. Cancer nanotechnology: opportunities and challenges. Nat Rev Cancer. 2005;5:161–71.
29. Gelmon KA, Eisenhauer EA, Harris AL, Ratain MJ, Workman P. Anticancer agents targeting signaling molecules and cancer cell environment: challenges for drug development? J Natl Cancer Inst. 1999;91:1281–7.
30. Hait WN. Anticancer drug development: the grand challenges. Nat Rev Drug Discov. 2010;9:253–4.
31. Hollingsworth SJ, Biankin AV. The challenges of precision oncology drug development and implementation. Public Health Genomics. 2015;18:338–48.
32. Bhatt AN, Mathur R, Farooque A, Verma A, Dwarakanath BS. Cancer biomarkers—current perspectives. Indian J Med Res. 2010;132:129–49.
33. Kawakami Y, Fujita T, Matsuzaki Y, Sakurai T, Tsukamoto M, et al. Identification of human tumor antigens and its implications for diagnosis and treatment of cancer. Cancer Sci. 2004;95:784–91.
34. Rusling JF, Kumar CV, Gutkind JS, Patel V. Measurement of biomarker proteins for point-of-care early detection and monitoring of cancer. Analyst. 2010;135:2496–511.
35. Ludwig JA, Weinstein JN. Biomarkers in cancer staging, prognosis and treatment selection. Nat Rev Cancer. 2005;5:845–56.
36. Sell S, Wahren B. Human cancer markers. Berlin: Springer Science & Business Media; 2012.
37. Sawyers CL. The cancer biomarker problem. Nature. 2008;452:548–52.
38. Sorio C, Mauri P, Pederzoli P, Scarpa A. Non-invasive cancer detection: strategies for the identification of novel cancer markers. IUBMB Life. 2006;58:193–8.
39. Gonzalez de Castro D, Clarke PA, Al-Lazikani B, Workman P. Personalized cancer medicine: molecular diagnostics, predictive biomarkers, and drug resistance. Clin Pharmacol Ther. 2013;93:252–9.
40. Ulaner GA, Riedl CC, Dickler MN, Jhaveri K, Pandit-Taskar N, Weber W. Molecular imaging of biomarkers in breast cancer. J Nucl Med. 2016;57(Suppl 1):53S–9S.
41. Ballman KV. Biomarker: predictive or Prognostic? J Clin Oncol. 2015;33:3968–71.
42. Mishra A, Verma M. Cancer biomarkers: are we ready for the prime time? Cancer. 2010;2:190.
43. Nalejska E, Maczynska E, Lewandowska MA. Prognostic and predictive biomarkers: tools in personalized oncology. Mol Diagn Ther. 2014;18:273–84.
44. Mehta S, Shelling A, Muthukaruppan A, Lasham A, Blenkiron C, et al. Predictive and prognostic

molecular markers for cancer medicine. Ther Adv Med Oncol. 2010;2:125–48.
45. Shaw A, Bradley MD, Elyan S, Kurian KM. Tumour biomarkers: diagnostic, prognostic, and predictive. BMJ. 2015;351:h3449.
46. Sarker D, Workman P. Pharmacodynamic biomarkers for molecular cancer therapeutics. Adv Cancer Res. 2007;96:213–68.
47. Gainor JF, Longo DL, Chabner BA. Pharmacodynamic biomarkers: falling short of the mark? Clin Cancer Res. 2014;20:2587–94.
48. Mizuarai S, Irie H, Kotani H. Gene expression-based pharmacodynamic biomarkers: the beginning of a new era in biomarker-driven anti-tumor drug development. Curr Mol Med. 2010;10:596–607.
49. Mito S, Sakai M, Suzuki M. Pharmacodynamics biomarkers: application and considerations in clinical development. Nihon Yakurigaku Zasshi. 2016;148:302–4.
50. Kulasingam V, Diamandis EP. Strategies for discovering novel cancer biomarkers through utilization of emerging technologies. Nat Clin Pract Oncol. 2008;5:588–99.
51. Sahab ZJ, Semaan SM, Sang QX. Methodology and applications of disease biomarker identification in human serum. Biomark Insights. 2007;2:21–43.
52. Jain KK. Technologies for discovery of biomarkers. In: The handbook of biomarkers. Berlin: Springer; 2010. p. 23–72.
53. Camp RL, Neumeister V, Rimm DL. A decade of tissue microarrays: progress in the discovery and validation of cancer biomarkers. J Clin Oncol. 2008;26:5630–7.
54. Hanash SM, Pitteri SJ, Faca VM. Mining the plasma proteome for cancer biomarkers. Nature. 2008;452:571.
55. Chai JC, Park S, Seo H, Cho SY, Lee YS. Identification of cancer-specific biomarkers by using microarray gene expression profiling. Biochip J. 2013;7:57–62.
56. Ramaswamy S, Tamayo P, Rifkin R, Mukherjee S, Yeang C-H, et al. Multiclass cancer diagnosis using tumor gene expression signatures. Proc Natl Acad Sci. 2001;98:15149–54.
57. Lee HJ, Wark AW, Corn RM. Microarray methods for protein biomarker detection. Analyst. 2008;133:975–83.
58. Perez-Diez A, Morgun A, Shulzhenko N. Microarrays for cancer diagnosis and classification. In: Microarray technology and cancer gene profiling. 2007. p. 74–85.
59. Kang K, Peng X, Luo J, Gou D. Identification of circulating miRNA biomarkers based on global quantitative real-time PCR profiling. J Anim Sci Biotechnol. 2012;3:4.
60. Scott A, Ambannavar R, Jeong J, Liu ML, Cronin MT. RT-PCR-based gene expression profiling for cancer biomarker discovery from fixed, paraffin-embedded tissues. Methods Mol Biol. 2011;724:239–57.
61. Rifai N, Gillette MA, Carr SA. Protein biomarker discovery and validation: the long and uncertain path to clinical utility. Nat Biotechnol. 2006;24:971–83.
62. Wang Q, Chaerkady R, Wu J, Hwang HJ, Papadopoulos N, et al. Mutant proteins as cancer-specific biomarkers. Proc Natl Acad Sci. 2011;108:2444–9.
63. Issaq HJ, Veenstra TD. The role of electrophoresis in disease biomarker discovery. Electrophoresis. 2007;28:1980–8.
64. Wulfkuhle JD, Liotta LA, Petricoin EF. Proteomic applications for the early detection of cancer. Nat Rev Cancer. 2003;3:267.
65. Wong SC, Chan CM, Ma BB, Lam MY, Choi GC, et al. Advanced proteomic technologies for cancer biomarker discovery. Expert Rev Proteomics. 2009;6:123–34.
66. Jain KK. Cancer biomarkers: current issues and future directions. Curr Opin Mol Ther. 2007;9:563–71.
67. Dunstan RW, Keith A, Wharton J, Quigley C, Lowe A. The use of immunohistochemistry for biomarker assessment—can it compete with other technologies? Toxicol Pathol. 2011;39:988–1002.
68. Matos LL, Trufelli DC, de Matos MG, da Silva Pinhal MA. Immunohistochemistry as an important tool in biomarkers detection and clinical practice. Biomark Insights. 2010;5:9–20.
69. Crutchfield CA, Thomas SN, Sokoll LJ, Chan DW. Advances in mass spectrometry-based clinical biomarker discovery. Clin Proteomics. 2016;13:1.
70. Hu L, Ru K, Zhang L, Huang Y, Zhu X, et al. Fluorescence in situ hybridization (FISH): an increasingly demanded tool for biomarker research and personalized medicine. Biomark Res. 2014;2:3.
71. Min L, Shou C. In situ hybridization of breast cancer markers. In: Cao J, editor. Breast cancer: methods and protocols. New York: Springer; 2016. p. 53–9.
72. Xie G, Lu L, Qiu Y, Ni Q, Zhang W, et al. Plasma metabolite biomarkers for the detection of pancreatic cancer. J Proteome Res. 2015;14:1195–202.
73. Zhang A, Sun H, Yan G, Wang P, Wang X. Metabolomics for biomarker discovery: moving to the clinic. Biomed Res Int. 2015;2015:354671.
74. Sun Z, Chen X, Wang G, Li L, Fu G, et al. Identification of functional metabolic biomarkers from lung cancer patient serum using PEP technology. Biomark Res. 2016b;4:11.
75. Porro G, Ménard S, Tagliabue E, Orefice S, Salvadori B, et al. Monoclonal antibody detection of carcinoma cells in bone marrow biopsy specimens from breast cancer patients. Cancer. 1988;61:2407–11.
76. Reid BJ, Blount PL, Feng Z, Levine DS. Optimizing endoscopic biopsy detection of early cancers in Barrett's high-grade dysplasia. Am J Gastroenterol. 2000;95:3089–96.
77. Stewart CS, Leibovich BC, Weaver AL, Lieber MM. Prostate cancer diagnosis using a saturation needle biopsy technique after previous negative sextant biopsies. J Urol. 2001;166:86–91. Discussion 91–2.

78. Bohunicky B, Mousa SA. Biosensors: the new wave in cancer diagnosis. Nanotechnol Sci Appl. 2010;4:1–10.
79. Selvolini G, Marrazza G. MIP-based sensors: promising new tools for cancer biomarker determination. Sensors. 2017;17:E718.
80. Wei F, Patel P, Liao W, Chaudhry K, Zhang L, et al. Electrochemical sensor for multiplex biomarkers detection. Clin Cancer Res. 2009;15:4446–52.
81. Shoemaker CJ, Green R. Translation drives mRNA quality control. Nat Struct Mol Biol. 2012;19:594–601.
82. Tyedmers J, Mogk A, Bukau B. Cellular strategies for controlling protein aggregation. Nat Rev Mol Cell Biol. 2010;11:777–88.
83. Maurizi MR. Love it or cleave it: tough choices in protein quality control. Nat Struct Biol. 2002;9:410–2.
84. Sandefur CI, Schnell S. Effects of protein quality control machinery on protein homeostasis. In: Dubitzky W, Southgate J, Fuß H, editors. Understanding the dynamics of biological systems: lessons learned from integrative systems biology. New York: Springer; 2011. p. 1–17.
85. Swaminathan S. Protein quality control: knowing when to fold. Nat Cell Biol. 2005;7:647.
86. Cohen-Kaplan V, Livneh I, Avni N, Cohen-Rosenzweig C, Ciechanover A. The ubiquitin-proteasome system and autophagy: coordinated and independent activities. Int J Biochem Cell Biol. 2016;79:403–18.
87. Trcka F, Vojtesek B, Muller P. Protein quality control and cancerogenesis. Klin Onkol. 2012;25(Suppl 2):2S38–44.
88. Amaravadi RK. Cancer. Autophagy in tumor immunity. Science. 2011;334:1501–2.
89. Chhangani D, Chinchwadkar S, Mishra A. Autophagy coupling interplay: can improve cellular repair and aging? Mol Neurobiol. 2014;49:1270–81.
90. Glick D, Barth S, Macleod KF. Autophagy: cellular and molecular mechanisms. J Pathol. 2010;221: 3–12.
91. Levine B. Cell biology: autophagy and cancer. Nature. 2007;446:745–7.
92. Qu X, Yu J, Bhagat G, Furuya N, Hibshoosh H, et al. Promotion of tumorigenesis by heterozygous disruption of the beclin 1 autophagy gene. J Clin Invest. 2003;112:1809–20.
93. Yue Z, Jin S, Yang C, Levine AJ, Heintz N. Beclin 1, an autophagy gene essential for early embryonic development, is a haploinsufficient tumor suppressor. Proc Natl Acad Sci U S A. 2003;100:15077–82.
94. Rohatgi RA, Janusis J, Leonard D, Bellve KD, Fogarty KE, et al. Beclin 1 regulates growth factor receptor signaling in breast cancer. Oncogene. 2015;34:5352–62.
95. Takamura A, Komatsu M, Hara T, Sakamoto A, Kishi C, et al. Autophagy-deficient mice develop multiple liver tumors. Genes Dev. 2011;25: 795–800.
96. White E. Deconvoluting the context-dependent role for autophagy in cancer. Nat Rev Cancer. 2012;12:401–10.
97. Yang YP, Hu LF, Zheng HF, Mao CJ, Hu WD, et al. Application and interpretation of current autophagy inhibitors and activators. Acta Pharmacol Sin. 2013;34:625–35.
98. Levy JMM, Thompson JC, Griesinger AM, Amani V, Donson AM, et al. Autophagy inhibition improves chemosensitivity in BRAF V600E brain tumors. Cancer Discov. 2014;4:773–80.
99. Mulcahy Levy JM, Zahedi S, Griesinger AM, Morin A, Davies KD, et al. Autophagy inhibition overcomes multiple mechanisms of resistance to BRAF inhibition in brain tumors. Elife. 2017;6:e19671.
100. Levy JM, Thorburn A. Modulation of pediatric brain tumor autophagy and chemosensitivity. J Neurooncol. 2012;106:281–90.
101. Schmitz KJ, Ademi C, Bertram S, Schmid KW, Baba HA. Prognostic relevance of autophagy-related markers LC3, p62/sequestosome 1, Beclin-1 and ULK1 in colorectal cancer patients with respect to KRAS mutational status. World J Surg Oncol. 2016;14:189.
102. Chen S, Jiang YZ, Huang L, Zhou RJ, Yu KD, et al. The residual tumor autophagy marker LC3B serves as a prognostic marker in local advanced breast cancer after neoadjuvant chemotherapy. Clin Cancer Res. 2013;19:6853–62.
103. Huang C-Y, Huang S-P, Lin VC, Yu C-C, Chang T-Y, et al. Genetic variants of the autophagy pathway as prognostic indicators for prostate cancer. Sci Rep. 2015;5:14045.
104. Liu B, Miyake H, Nishikawa M, Tei H, Fujisawa M. Expression profile of autophagy-related markers in localized prostate cancer: correlation with biochemical recurrence after radical prostatectomy. Urology. 2015;85:1424–30.
105. Kim HM, Kim ES, Koo JS. Expression of autophagy-related proteins in different types of thyroid cancer. Int J Mol Sci. 2017;18:E540.
106. Ueno T, Saji S, Sugimoto M, Masuda N, Kuroi K, et al. Clinical significance of the expression of autophagy-associated marker, beclin 1, in breast cancer patients who received neoadjuvant endocrine therapy. BMC Cancer. 2016;16:230.
107. Korolchuk VI, Menzies FM, Rubinsztein DC. Mechanisms of cross-talk between the ubiquitin- proteasome and autophagy-lysosome systems. FEBS Lett. 2010;584:1393–8.
108. Wojcik S. Crosstalk between autophagy and proteasome protein degradation systems: possible implications for cancer therapy. Folia Histochem Cytobiol. 2013;51:249–64.
109. Bassermann F, Eichner R, Pagano M. The ubiquitin proteasome system—implications for cell cycle control and the targeted treatment of cancer. Biochim Biophys Acta. 2014;1843:150–62.
110. Hoeller D, Dikic I. Targeting the ubiquitin system in cancer therapy. Nature. 2009;458:438–44.

111. Weathington NM, Mallampalli RK. Emerging therapies targeting the ubiquitin proteasome system in cancer. J Clin Invest. 2014;124:6–12.
112. Ciechanover A, Iwai K. The ubiquitin system: from basic mechanisms to the patient bed. IUBMB Life. 2004;56:193–201.
113. Nandi D, Tahiliani P, Kumar A, Chandu D. The ubiquitin-proteasome system. J Biosci. 2006;31:137–55.
114. Bedford L, Lowe J, Dick LR, Mayer RJ, Brownell JE. Ubiquitin-like protein conjugation and the ubiquitin-proteasome system as drug targets. Nat Rev Drug Discov. 2011;10:29–46.
115. Shen M, Schmitt S, Buac D, Dou QP. Targeting the ubiquitin-proteasome system for cancer therapy. Expert Opin Ther Targets. 2013;17:1091–108.
116. Chen L, Madura K. Increased proteasome activity, ubiquitin-conjugating enzymes, and eEF1A translation factor detected in breast cancer tissue. Cancer Res. 2005;65:5599–606.
117. Chen D, Dou QP. The ubiquitin-proteasome system as a prospective molecular target for cancer treatment and prevention. Curr Protein Pept Sci. 2010;11:459–70.
118. Buac D, Shen M, Schmitt S, Rani Kona F, Deshmukh R, et al. From bortezomib to other inhibitors of the proteasome and beyond. Curr Pharm Des. 2013;19:4025–38.
119. Xu GW, Ali M, Wood TE, Wong D, Maclean N, et al. The ubiquitin-activating enzyme E1 as a therapeutic target for the treatment of leukemia and multiple myeloma. Blood. 2010;115:2251–9.
120. Yang Y, Kitagaki J, Dai RM, Tsai YC, Lorick KL, et al. Inhibitors of ubiquitin-activating enzyme (E1), a new class of potential cancer therapeutics. Cancer Res. 2007;67:9472–81.
121. Luo Z, Yu G, Lee HW, Li L, Wang L, et al. The Nedd8-activating enzyme inhibitor MLN4924 induces autophagy and apoptosis to suppress liver cancer cell growth. Cancer Res. 2012;72:3360–71.
122. Ieta K, Ojima E, Tanaka F, Nakamura Y, Haraguchi N, et al. Identification of overexpressed genes in hepatocellular carcinoma, with special reference to ubiquitin-conjugating enzyme E2C gene expression. Int J Cancer. 2007;121:33–8.
123. Hao Z, Zhang H, Cowell J. Ubiquitin-conjugating enzyme UBE2C: molecular biology, role in tumorigenesis, and potential as a biomarker. Tumor Biol. 2012;33:723–30.
124. Okamoto Y, Ozaki T, Miyazaki K, Aoyama M, Miyazaki M, Nakagawara A. UbcH10 is the cancer-related E2 ubiquitin-conjugating enzyme. Cancer Res. 2003;63:4167–73.
125. Xie C, Powell C, Yao M, Wu J, Dong Q. Ubiquitin-conjugating enzyme E2C: a potential cancer biomarker. Int J Biochem Cell Biol. 2014;47:113–7.
126. Ardley HC, Robinson PA. E3 ubiquitin ligases. Essays Biochem. 2005;41:15–30.
127. Bielskienė K, Bagdonienė L, Mozūraitienė J, Kazbarienė B, Janulionis E. E3 ubiquitin ligases as drug targets and prognostic biomarkers in melanoma. Medicina. 2015;51:1–9.
128. Lub S, Maes K, Menu E, De Bruyne E, Vanderkerken K, Van Valckenborgh E. Novel strategies to target the ubiquitin proteasome system in multiple myeloma. Oncotarget. 2016;7:6521–37.
129. Yang Y, Kitagaki J, Wang H, Hou DX, Perantoni AO. Targeting the ubiquitin-proteasome system for cancer therapy. Cancer Sci. 2009;100:24–8.
130. Lee JK, Chang N, Yoon Y, Yang H, Cho H, et al. USP1 targeting impedes GBM growth by inhibiting stem cell maintenance and radioresistance. Neuro Oncol. 2016;18:37–47.
131. Cheng C, Niu C, Yang Y, Wang Y, Lu M. Expression of HAUSP in gliomas correlates with disease progression and survival of patients. Oncol Rep. 2013;29:1730–6.
132. Summers MK, Venere M. Targeting the ubiquitin proteasome system in glioblastoma. Transl Cancer Res. 2016;S920–22.
133. Zhang L, Wang H, Tian L, Li H. Expression of USP7 and MARCH7 is correlated with poor prognosis in epithelial ovarian cancer. Tohoku J Exp Med. 2016;239:165–75.
134. Chhangani D, Jana NR, Mishra A. Misfolded proteins recognition strategies of E3 ubiquitin ligases and neurodegenerative diseases. Mol Neurobiol. 2013;47:302–12.
135. Upadhyay A, Amanullah A, Chhangani D, Mishra R, Mishra A. Selective multifaceted E3 ubiquitin ligases barricade extreme defense: potential therapeutic targets for neurodegeneration and ageing. Ageing Res Rev. 2015;24:138–59.
136. Glickman MH, Ciechanover A. The ubiquitin-proteasome proteolytic pathway: destruction for the sake of construction. Physiol Rev. 2002;82:373–428.
137. Berndsen CE, Wolberger C. New insights into ubiquitin E3 ligase mechanism. Nat Struct Mol Biol. 2014;21:301–7.
138. Dove KK, Stieglitz B, Duncan ED, Rittinger K, Klevit RE. Molecular insights into RBR E3 ligase ubiquitin transfer mechanisms. EMBO Rep. 2016;17:1221–35.
139. Spratt DE, Walden H, Shaw GS. RBR E3 ubiquitin ligases: new structures, new insights, new questions. Biochem J. 2014;458:421–37.
140. Cyr DM, Höhfeld J, Patterson C. Protein quality control: U-box-containing E3 ubiquitin ligases join the fold. Trends Biochem Sci. 2002;27:368–75.
141. Huibregtse JM, Scheffner M, Beaudenon S, Howley PM. A family of proteins structurally and functionally related to the E6-AP ubiquitin-protein ligase. Proc Natl Acad Sci U S A. 1995;92:5249.
142. Morreale FE, Walden H. Types of ubiquitin ligases. Cell. 2016;165(248-48):e1.
143. Rotin D, Kumar S. Physiological functions of the HECT family of ubiquitin ligases. Nat Rev Mol Cell Biol. 2009;10:398–409.

144. Scheffner M, Kumar S. Mammalian HECT ubiquitin-protein ligases: biological and pathophysiological aspects. Biochim Biophys Acta. 2014;1843:61–74.
145. Bernassola F, Karin M, Ciechanover A, Melino G. The HECT family of E3 ubiquitin ligases: multiple players in cancer development. Cancer Cell. 2008;14:10–21.
146. Melino G, Gallagher E, Aqeilan RI, Knight R, Peschiaroli A, et al. Itch: a HECT-type E3 ligase regulating immunity, skin and cancer. Cell Death Differ. 2008;15:1103–12.
147. Zhao X, Heng JI, Guardavaccaro D, Jiang R, Pagano M, et al. The HECT-domain ubiquitin ligase Huwe1 controls neural differentiation and proliferation by destabilizing the N-Myc oncoprotein. Nat Cell Biol. 2008;10:643–53.
148. Deshaies RJ, Joazeiro CA. RING domain E3 ubiquitin ligases. Annu Rev Biochem. 2009;78:399–434.
149. Metzger MB, Pruneda JN, Klevit RE, Weissman AM. RING-type E3 ligases: master manipulators of E2 ubiquitin-conjugating enzymes and ubiquitination. Biochim Biophys Acta. 2014;1843:47–60.
150. Joazeiro CAP, Weissman AM. RING finger proteins. Cell. 2000;102:549–52.
151. Chene P. Inhibiting the p53-MDM2 interaction: an important target for cancer therapy. Nat Rev Cancer. 2003;3:102–9.
152. Shangary S, Wang S. Targeting the MDM2-p53 interaction for cancer therapy. Clin Cancer Res. 2008;14:5318–24.
153. Dornan D, Bheddah S, Newton K, Ince W, Frantz GD, et al. COP1, the negative regulator of p53, is overexpressed in breast and ovarian adenocarcinomas. Cancer Res. 2004;64:7226–30.
154. Duan W, Gao L, Druhan LJ, Zhu WG, Morrison C, et al. Expression of Pirh2, a newly identified ubiquitin protein ligase, in lung cancer. J Natl Cancer Inst. 2004;96:1718–21.
155. Azmi P, Seth A. RNF11 is a multifunctional modulator of growth factor receptor signalling and transcriptional regulation. Eur J Cancer. 2005;41:2549–60.
156. Brahemi G, Kona FR, Fiasella A, Buac D, Soukupová J, et al. Exploring the structural requirements for inhibition of the ubiquitin E3 ligase breast cancer associated protein 2 (BCA2) as a treatment for breast cancer. J Med Chem. 2010;53:2757–65.
157. Burger A, Amemiya Y, Kitching R, Seth AK. Novel RING E3 ubiquitin ligases in breast cancer. Neoplasia. 2006;8:689–95.
158. Hatakeyama S, Yada M, Matsumoto M, Ishida N, Nakayama KI. U box proteins as a new family of ubiquitin-protein ligases. J Biol Chem. 2001;276:33111–20.
159. Cao Z, Li G, Shao Q, Yang G, Zheng L, et al. CHIP: a new modulator of human malignant disorders. Oncotarget. 2016;7:29864–74.
160. Joshi V, Amanullah A, Upadhyay A, Mishra R, Kumar A, Mishra A. A decade of boon or burden: what has the CHIP ever done for cellular protein quality control mechanism implicated in neurodegeneration and aging? Front Mol Neurosci. 2016;9:93.
161. Bienz M. The PHD finger, a nuclear protein-interaction domain. Trends Biochem Sci. 2006;31:35–40.
162. Coscoy L, Ganem D. PHD domains and E3 ubiquitin ligases: viruses make the connection. Trends Cell Biol. 2003;13:7–12.
163. Coscoy L, Sanchez DJ, Ganem D. A novel class of herpesvirus-encoded membrane-bound E3 ubiquitin ligases regulates endocytosis of proteins involved in immune recognition. J Cell Biol. 2001;155:1265–74.
164. Hewitt EW, Duncan L, Mufti D, Baker J, Stevenson PG, Lehner PJ. Ubiquitylation of MHC class I by the K3 viral protein signals internalization and TSG101-dependent degradation. EMBO J. 2002;21:2418–29.
165. Mansouri M, Bartee E, Gouveia K, Hovey Nerenberg BT, Barrett J, et al. The PHD/LAP-domain protein M153R of myxomavirus is a ubiquitin ligase that induces the rapid internalization and lysosomal destruction of CD4. J Virol. 2003;77:1427–40.
166. Smit JJ, Sixma TK. RBR E3-ligases at work. EMBO Rep. 2014;15:142–54.
167. Varshavsky A. Discovery of cellular regulation by protein degradation. J Biol Chem. 2008;283:34469–89.
168. Hershko A. Roles of ubiquitin-mediated proteolysis in cell cycle control. Curr Opin Cell Biol. 1997;9:788–99.
169. Lu Z, Hunter T. Ubiquitylation and proteasomal degradation of the p21Cip1, p27Kip1 and p57Kip2 CDK inhibitors. Cell Cycle. 2010;9:2342–52.
170. Craney A, Rape M. Dynamic regulation of ubiquitin-dependent cell cycle control. Curr Opin Cell Biol. 2013;25:704–10.
171. Nabi IR, Raz A. Cell shape modulation alters glycosylation of a metastatic melanoma cell-surface antigen. Int J Cancer. 1987;40:396–402.
172. Chiu CG, St-Pierre P, Nabi IR, Wiseman SM. Autocrine motility factor receptor: a clinical review. Expert Rev Anticancer Ther. 2008;8:207–17.
173. Jiang WG, Raz A, Douglas-Jones A, Mansel RE. Expression of autocrine motility factor (AMF) and its receptor, AMFR, in human breast cancer. J Histochem Cytochem. 2006;54:231–41.
174. Endo K, Shirai A, Furukawa M, Yoshizaki T. Prognostic value of cell motility activation factors in patients with tongue squamous cell carcinoma. Hum Pathol. 2006;37:1111–6.
175. Wang W, Yang LY, Yang ZL, Peng JX, Yang JQ. Elevated expression of autocrine motility factor receptor correlates with overexpression of RhoC and indicates poor prognosis in hepatocellular carcinoma. Dig Dis Sci. 2007a;52:770–5.
176. Joshi B, Li L, Nabi IR. A role for KAI1 in promotion of cell proliferation and mammary gland hyperplasia by the gp78 ubiquitin ligase. J Biol Chem. 2010;285:8830–9.
177. Tsai YC, Mendoza A, Mariano JM, Zhou M, Kostova Z, et al. The ubiquitin ligase gp78 promotes

sarcoma metastasis by targeting KAI1 for degradation. Nat Med. 2007;13:1504–9.
178. Shang Y, Zhu Z. gp78 is specifically expressed in human prostate cancer rather than normal prostate tissue. J Mol Histol. 2013;44:653–9.
179. Tanizaki Y, Sato Y, Oka H, Utsuki S, Kondo K, et al. Expression of autocrine motility factor mRNA is a poor prognostic factor in high-grade astrocytoma. Pathol Int. 2006;56:510–5.
180. Jan CI, Yu CC, Hung MC, Harn HJ, Nieh S, et al. Tid1, CHIP and ErbB2 interactions and their prognostic implications for breast cancer patients. J Pathol. 2011;225:424–37.
181. Jang KW, Lee KH, Kim SH, Jin T, Choi EY, et al. Ubiquitin ligase CHIP induces TRAF2 proteasomal degradation and NF-κB inactivation to regulate breast cancer cell invasion. J Cell Biochem. 2011;112:3612–20.
182. Wen J, Luo KJ, Hu Y, Yang H, Fu JH. Metastatic lymph node CHIP expression is a potential prognostic marker for resected esophageal squamous cell carcinoma patients. Ann Surg Oncol. 2013;20:1668–75.
183. Wang S, Wu X, Zhang J, Chen Y, Xu J, et al. CHIP functions as a novel suppressor of tumour angiogenesis with prognostic significance in human gastric cancer. Gut. 2013;62:496–508.
184. Liang ZL, Kim M, Huang SM, Lee HJ, Kim JM. Expression of carboxyl terminus of Hsp70-interacting protein (CHIP) indicates poor prognosis in human gallbladder carcinoma. Oncol Lett. 2013;5:813–8.
185. Sun C, Li HL, Shi ML, Liu QH, Bai J, Zheng JN. Diverse roles of C-terminal Hsp70-interacting protein (CHIP) in tumorigenesis. J Cancer Res Clin Oncol. 2014;140:189–97.
186. Paul I, Ahmed SF, Bhowmik A, Deb S, Ghosh MK. The ubiquitin ligase CHIP regulates c-Myc stability and transcriptional activity. Oncogene. 2013;32:1284–95.
187. Wu W, Koike A, Takeshita T, Ohta T. The ubiquitin E3 ligase activity of BRCA1 and its biological functions. Cell Div. 2008;3:1.
188. James CR, Quinn JE, Mullan PB, Johnston PG, Harkin DP. BRCA1, a potential predictive biomarker in the treatment of breast cancer. Oncologist. 2007;12:142–50.
189. Quinn JE, James CR, Stewart GE, Mulligan JM, White P, et al. BRCA1 mRNA expression levels predict for overall survival in ovarian cancer after chemotherapy. Clin Cancer Res. 2007;13:7413–20.
190. McAlpine JN, Porter H, Kobel M, Nelson BH, Prentice LM, et al. BRCA1 and BRCA2 mutations correlate with TP53 abnormalities and presence of immune cell infiltrates in ovarian high-grade serous carcinoma. Mod Pathol. 2012;25:740–50.
191. Lee JM, Hays JL, Annunziata CM, Noonan AM, Minasian L, et al. Phase I/Ib study of olaparib and carboplatin in BRCA1 or BRCA2 mutation-associated breast or ovarian cancer with biomarker analyses. J Natl Cancer Inst. 2014;106:dju089.
192. Hjortkjaer M, Waldstrom M, Jakobsen A, Kanstrup H, Sogaard-Andersen E, Dahl SK. The prognostic value of BRCA1 and PARP expression in epithelial ovarian carcinoma: immunohistochemical detection. Int J Gynecol Pathol. 2017;36:180–9.
193. Thompson D, Easton DF. Cancer incidence in BRCA1 mutation carriers. J Natl Cancer Inst. 2002;94:1358–65.
194. Chen C, Sun C, Tang D, Yang G, Zhou X, Wang D. Identification of key genes in glioblastoma-associated stromal cells using bioinformatics analysis. Oncol Lett. 2016;11:3999–4007.
195. Rasmussen RD, Gajjar MK, Tuckova L, Jensen KE, Maya-Mendoza A, et al. BRCA1-regulated RRM2 expression protects glioblastoma cells from endogenous replication stress and promotes tumorigenicity. Nat Commun. 2016;7:13398.
196. Nakayama KI, Nakayama K. Regulation of the cell cycle by SCF-type ubiquitin ligases. Semin Cell Dev Biol. 2005;16:323–33.
197. Koh MS, Ittmann M, Kadmon D, Thompson TC, Leach FS. CDC4 gene expression as potential biomarker for targeted therapy in prostate cancer. Cancer Biol Ther. 2006;5:78–83.
198. Kudo Y, Kitajima S, Sato S, Miyauchi M, Ogawa I, Takata T. High expression of S-phase kinase- interacting protein 2, human F-box protein, correlates with poor prognosis in oral squamous cell carcinomas. Cancer Res. 2001;61:7044–7.
199. Chan CH, Li CF, Yang WL, Gao Y, Lee SW, et al. The Skp2-SCF E3 ligase regulates Akt ubiquitination, glycolysis, herceptin sensitivity, and tumorigenesis. Cell. 2012;149:1098–111.
200. Masuda TA, Inoue H, Sonoda H, Mine S, Yoshikawa Y, et al. Clinical and biological significance of S- phase kinase-associated protein 2 (Skp2) gene expression in gastric carcinoma. Cancer Res. 2002;62:3819–25.
201. Wei D, Sun Y. Small RING finger proteins RBX1 and RBX2 of SCF E3 ubiquitin ligases: the role in cancer and as cancer targets. Genes Cancer. 2010;1: 700–7.
202. Jia L, Sun Y. SCF E3 ubiquitin ligases as anticancer targets. Curr Cancer Drug Targets. 2011;11:347–56.
203. Xie CM, Wei W, Sun Y. Role of SKP1-CUL1-F-box-protein (SCF) E3 ubiquitin ligases in skin cancer. J Genet Genomics. 2013;40:97–106.
204. Lee SH, McCormick F. Downregulation of Skp2 and p27/Kip1 synergistically induces apoptosis in T98G glioblastoma cells. J Mol Med. 2005;83:296–307.
205. Perry WL, Hustad CM, Swing DA, O'Sullivan TN, Jenkins NA, Copeland NG. The itchy locus encodes a novel ubiquitin protein ligase that is disrupted in a18H mice. Nat Genet. 1998;18:143–6.
206. Parravicini V, Field AC, Tomlinson PD, Basson MA, Zamoyska R. Itch-/- alphabeta and gammadelta T cells independently contribute to autoimmunity in Itchy mice. Blood. 2008;111:4273–7282.
207. Fang D, Elly C, Gao B, Fang N, Altman Y, et al. Dysregulation of T lymphocyte function in itchy

mice: a role for Itch in TH2 differentiation. Nat Immunol. 2002;3:281–7.
208. Chang L, Kamata H, Solinas G, Luo JL, Maeda S, et al. The E3 ubiquitin ligase itch couples JNK activation to TNFalpha-induced cell death by inducing c-FLIP(L) turnover. Cell. 2006;124:601–13.
209. Rossi M, De Laurenzi V, Munarriz E, Green DR, Liu YC, et al. The ubiquitin-protein ligase Itch regulates p73 stability. EMBO J. 2005;24:836–48.
210. Rossi M, Aqeilan RI, Neale M, Candi E, Salomoni P, et al. The E3 ubiquitin ligase Itch controls the protein stability of p63. Proc Natl Acad Sci U S A. 2006;103:12753–8.
211. Suryaraja R, Anitha M, Anbarasu K, Kumari G, Mahalingam S. The E3 ubiquitin ligase Itch regulates tumor suppressor protein RASSF5/NORE1 stability in an acetylation-dependent manner. Cell Death Dis. 2013;4:e565.
212. Salah Z, Melino G, Aqeilan RI. Negative regulation of the Hippo pathway by E3 ubiquitin ligase ITCH is sufficient to promote tumorigenicity. Cancer Res. 2011;71:2010–20.
213. Luo ZL, Luo HJ, Fang C, Cheng L, Huang Z, et al. Negative correlation of ITCH E3 ubiquitin ligase and miRNA-106b dictates metastatic progression in pancreatic cancer. Oncotarget. 2016;7: 1477–85.
214. Shearwin-Whyatt L, Dalton HE, Foot N, Kumar S. Regulation of functional diversity within the Nedd4 family by accessory and adaptor proteins. Bioessays. 2006;28:617–28.
215. Ye X, Wang L, Shang B, Wang Z, Wei W. NEDD4: a promising target for cancer therapy. Curr Cancer Drug Targets. 2014;14:549–56.
216. Salah Z, Cohen S, Itzhaki E, Aqeilan RI. NEDD4 E3 ligase inhibits the activity of the Hippo pathway by targeting LATS1 for degradation. Cell Cycle. 2013;12:3817–23.
217. Sakata T, Sakaguchi H, Tsuda L, Higashitani A, Aigaki T, et al. Drosophila Nedd4 regulates endocytosis of notch and suppresses its ligand-independent activation. Curr Biol. 2004;14:2228–36.
218. Wang X, Trotman LC, Koppie T, Alimonti A, Chen Z, et al. NEDD4-1 is a proto-oncogenic ubiquitin ligase for PTEN. Cell. 2007b;128:129–39.
219. Wang L, Zhu B, Wang S, Wu Y, Zhan W, et al. Regulation of glioma migration and invasion via modification of Rap2a activity by the ubiquitin ligase Nedd4-1. Oncol Rep. 2017;37:2565–74.
220. Zhang H, Nie W, Zhang X, Zhang G, Li Z, et al. NEDD4-1 regulates migration and invasion of glioma cells through CNrasGEF ubiquitination in vitro. PLoS One. 2013;8:e82789.
221. Jackson S, Xiong Y. CRL4s: the CUL4-RING E3 ubiquitin ligases. Trends Biochem Sci. 2009;34:562–70.
222. Melchor L, Saucedo-Cuevas LP, Munoz-Repeto I, Rodriguez-Pinilla SM, Honrado E, et al. Comprehensive characterization of the DNA amplification at 13q34 in human breast cancer reveals TFDP1 and CUL4A as likely candidate target genes. Breast Cancer Res. 2009;11:R86.
223. Yasui K, Arii S, Zhao C, Imoto I, Ueda M, et al. TFDP1, CUL4A, and CDC16 identified as targets for amplification at 13q34 in hepatocellular carcinomas. Hepatology. 2002;35:1476–84.
224. Petroski MD, Deshaies RJ. Function and regulation of cullin-RING ubiquitin ligases. Nat Rev Mol Cell Biol. 2005;6:9–20.
225. Zou Y, Mi J, Cui J, Lu D, Zhang X, et al. Characterization of nuclear localization signal in the N terminus of CUL4B and its essential role in cyclin E degradation and cell cycle progression. J Biol Chem. 2009;284:33320–32.
226. Lopez-Beltran A, MacLennan GT, Montironi R. Cyclin E as molecular marker in the management of breast cancer: a review. Anal Quant Cytol Histol. 2006;28:111–4.
227. Higa LA, Yang X, Zheng J, Banks D, Wu M, et al. Involvement of CUL4 ubiquitin E3 ligases in regulating CDK inhibitors Dacapo/p27Kip1 and cyclin E degradation. Cell Cycle. 2006;5:71–7.
228. Li B, Jia N, Kapur R, Chun KT. Cul4A targets p27 for degradation and regulates proliferation, cell cycle exit, and differentiation during erythropoiesis. Blood. 2006;107:4291–9.
229. Fan Y-C, Zhu Y-S, Mei P-J, Sun S-G, Zhang H, et al. Cullin1 regulates proliferation, migration and invasion of glioma cells. Med Oncol. 2014;31:227.
230. Dong J, Wang XQ, Yao JJ, Li G, Li XG. Decreased CUL4B expression inhibits malignant proliferation of glioma in vitro and in vivo. Eur Rev Med Pharmacol Sci. 2015;19:1013–21.
231. Kemp Z, Rowan A, Chambers W, Wortham N, Halford S, et al. CDC4 mutations occur in a subset of colorectal cancers but are not predicted to cause loss of function and are not associated with chromosomal instability. Cancer Res. 2005;65:11361–6.
232. Mao JH, Perez-Losada J, Wu D, Delrosario R, Tsunematsu R, et al. Fbxw7/Cdc4 is a p53-dependent, haploinsufficient tumour suppressor gene. Nature. 2004;432:775–9.
233. Rajagopalan H, Jallepalli PV, Rago C, Velculescu VE, Kinzler KW, et al. Inactivation of hCDC4 can cause chromosomal instability. Nature. 2004;428:77–81.
234. Hagedorn M, Delugin M, Abraldes I, Allain N, Belaud-Rotureau MA, et al. FBXW7/hCDC4 controls glioma cell proliferation in vitro and is a prognostic marker for survival in glioblastoma patients. Cell Div. 2007;2:9.
235. Kubbutat MH, Jones SN, Vousden KH. Regulation of p53 stability by Mdm2. Nature. 1997;387:299.
236. Moll UM, Petrenko O. The MDM2-p53 Interaction. Mol Cancer Res. 2003;1:1001–8.
237. Vousden KH, Lu X. Live or let die: the cell's response to p53. Nat Rev Cancer. 2002;2:594–604.
238. Blattner C, Sparks A, Lane D. Transcription factor E2F-1 is upregulated in response to DNA damage in a manner analogous to that of p53. Mol Cell Biol. 1999;19:3704–13.

239. Juven-Gershon T, Shifman O, Unger T, Elkeles A, Haupt Y, Oren M. The Mdm2 oncoprotein interacts with the cell fate regulator Numb. Mol Cell Biol. 1998;18:3974–82.
240. Xiao ZX, Chen J, Levine AJ, Modjtahedi N, Xing J, et al. Interaction between the retinoblastoma protein and the oncoprotein MDM2. Nature. 1995;375:694–8.
241. Chen H, Xie L, Liu B. Clinical significance of MDM2 as a tumor biomarker. Chin German J Clin Oncol. 2012;11:356–60.
242. Onel K, Cordon-Cardo C. MDM2 and prognosis. Mol Cancer Res. 2004;2:1–8.
243. Ye Y, Li X, Yang J, Miao S, Wang S, et al. MDM2 is a useful prognostic biomarker for resectable gastric cancer. Cancer Sci. 2013;104:590–8.
244. Turbin DA, Cheang MC, Bajdik CD, Gelmon KA, Yorida E, et al. MDM2 protein expression is a negative prognostic marker in breast carcinoma. Mod Pathol. 2006;19:69–74.
245. Higashiyama M, Doi O, Kodama K, Yokouchi H, Kasugai T, et al. MDM2 gene amplification and expression in non-small-cell lung cancer: immunohistochemical expression of its protein is a favourable prognostic marker in patients without p53 protein accumulation. Br J Cancer. 1997;75:1302–8.
246. Fischer PM. Peptide, peptidomimetic, and small-molecule antagonists of the p53-HDM2 protein-protein interaction. Int J Pept Res Ther. 2006;12:3–19.
247. Biernat W, Kleihues P, Yonekawa Y, Ohgaki H. Amplification and overexpression of MDM2 in primary (de novo) glioblastomas. J Neuropathol Exp Neurol. 1997;56:180–5.
248. Scheffner M, Huibregtse JM, Vierstra RD, Howley PM. The HPV-16 E6 and E6-AP complex functions as a ubiquitin-protein ligase in the ubiquitination of p53. Cell. 1993;75:495–505.
249. Beaudenon S, Huibregtse JM. HPV E6, E6AP and cervical cancer. BMC Biochem. 2008;9(Suppl 1):S4.
250. Huibregtse JM, Scheffner M, Howley PM. A cellular protein mediates association of p53 with the E6 oncoprotein of human papillomavirus types 16 or 18. EMBO J. 1991;10:4129–35.
251. Gewin L, Myers H, Kiyono T, Galloway DA. Identification of a novel telomerase repressor that interacts with the human papillomavirus type-16 E6/E6-AP complex. Genes Dev. 2004;18:2269–82.
252. Kelley ML, Keiger KE, Lee CJ, Huibregtse JM. The global transcriptional effects of the human papillomavirus E6 protein in cervical carcinoma cell lines are mediated by the E6AP ubiquitin ligase. J Virol. 2005;79:3737–47.
253. Nguyen M, Song S, Liem A, Androphy E, Liu Y, Lambert PF. A mutant of human papillomavirus type 16 E6 deficient in binding alpha-helix partners displays reduced oncogenic potential in vivo. J Virol. 2002;76:13039–48.
254. Tomaic V, Pim D, Banks L. The stability of the human papillomavirus E6 oncoprotein is E6AP dependent. Virology. 2009;393:7–10.
255. Mishra A, Jana NR. Regulation of turnover of tumor suppressor p53 and cell growth by E6-AP, a ubiquitin protein ligase mutated in Angelman mental retardation syndrome. Cell Mol Life Sci. 2008;65: 656–66.
256. Mishra A, Godavarthi SK, Jana NR. UBE3A/E6-AP regulates cell proliferation by promoting proteasomal degradation of p27. Neurobiol Dis. 2009;36:26–34.
257. Matentzoglu K, Scheffner M. Ubiquitin ligase E6-AP and its role in human disease. Biochem Soc Trans. 2008;36:797–801.
258. Acquaviva C, Pines J. The anaphase-promoting complex/cyclosome: APC/C. J Cell Sci. 2006;119:2401–4.
259. Manchado E, Eguren M, Malumbres M. The anaphase-promoting complex/cyclosome (APC/C): cell- cycle-dependent and -independent functions. Biochem Soc Trans. 2010;38:65–71.
260. Lehman NL, Tibshirani R, Hsu JY, Natkunam Y, Harris BT, et al. Oncogenic regulators and substrates of the anaphase promoting complex/cyclosome are frequently overexpressed in malignant tumors. Am J Pathol. 2007;170:1793–805.
261. Penas C, Ramachandran V, Ayad NG. The APC/C ubiquitin ligase: from cell biology to tumorigenesis. Front Oncol. 2011;1:60.
262. Fujita T, Liu W, Doihara H, Wan Y. Regulation of Skp2-p27 axis by the Cdh1/anaphase-promoting complex pathway in colorectal tumorigenesis. Am J Pathol. 2008;173:217–28.
263. Lu L, Hu S, Wei R, Qiu X, Lu K, et al. The HECT type ubiquitin ligase NEDL2 is degraded by anaphase-promoting complex/cyclosome (APC/C)-Cdh1, and its tight regulation maintains the metaphase to anaphase transition. J Biol Chem. 2013;288:35637–50.
264. Sansregret L, Patterson JO, Dewhurst S, Lopez-Garcia C, Koch A, et al. APC/C dysfunction limits excessive cancer chromosomal instability. Cancer Discov. 2017;7:218–33.
265. Lee SJ, Langhans SA. Anaphase-promoting complex/cyclosome protein Cdc27 is a target for curcumin- induced cell cycle arrest and apoptosis. BMC Cancer. 2012;12:44.
266. Lasorella A, Stegmuller J, Guardavaccaro D, Liu G, Carro MS, et al. Degradation of Id2 by the anaphase-promoting complex couples cell cycle exit and axonal growth. Nature. 2006;442:471–4.
267. Mao DD, Gujar AD, Mahlokozera T, Chen I, Pan Y, et al. A CDC20-APC/SOX2 signaling axis regulates human glioblastoma stem-like cells. Cell Rep. 2015;11:1809–21.
268. David D, Nair SA, Pillai MR. Smurf E3 ubiquitin ligases at the cross roads of oncogenesis and tumor suppression. Biochim Biophys Acta Rev Cancer. 2013;1835:119–28.
269. Ebisawa T, Fukuchi M, Murakami G, Chiba T, Tanaka K, et al. Smurf1 interacts with transforming growth factor-β type I receptor through Smad7 and induces receptor degradation. J Biol Chem. 2001;276:12477–80.

270. Kavsak P, Rasmussen RK, Causing CG, Bonni S, Zhu H, et al. Smad7 binds to Smurf2 to form an E3 ubiquitin ligase that targets the TGFβ receptor for degradation. Mol Cell. 2000;6:1365–75.
271. Murakami G, Watabe T, Takaoka K, Miyazono K, Imamura T. Cooperative inhibition of bone morphogenetic protein signaling by Smurf1 and inhibitory Smads. Mol Biol Cell. 2003;14:2809–17.
272. Derynck R, Akhurst RJ, Balmain A. TGF-β signaling in tumor suppression and cancer progression. Nat Genet. 2001;29:117–29.
273. Massague J. TGFbeta in cancer. Cell. 2008;134:215–30.
274. Fukuchi M, Fukai Y, Masuda N, Miyazaki T, Nakajima M, et al. High-level expression of the Smad ubiquitin ligase Smurf2 correlates with poor prognosis in patients with esophageal squamous cell carcinoma. Cancer Res. 2002;62:7162–5.
275. Jin C, Yang Y-a, Anver MR, Morris N, Wang X, Zhang YE. Smad ubiquitination regulatory factor 2 promotes metastasis of breast cancer cells by enhancing migration and invasiveness. Cancer Res. 2009;69:735–40.
276. Ke M, Mo L, Li W, Zhang X, Li F, Yu H. Ubiquitin ligase SMURF1 functions as a prognostic marker and promotes growth and metastasis of clear cell renal cell carcinoma. FEBS Open Bio. 2017;7:577–86.
277. Deveraux QL, Reed JC. IAP family proteins—suppressors of apoptosis. Genes Dev. 1999;13:239–52.
278. Gordon GJ, Mani M, Mukhopadhyay L, Dong L, Edenfield HR, et al. Expression patterns of inhibitor of apoptosis proteins in malignant pleural mesothelioma. J Pathol. 2007;211:447–54.
279. Tamm I, Kornblau SM, Segall H, Krajewski S, Welsh K, et al. Expression and prognostic significance of IAP-family genes in human cancers and myeloid leukemias. Clin Cancer Res. 2000;6:1796–803.
280. Tamm I, Richter S, Oltersdorf D, Creutzig U, Harbott J, et al. High expression levels of x-linked inhibitor of apoptosis protein and survivin correlate with poor overall survival in childhood de novo acute myeloid leukemia. Clin Cancer Res. 2004;10:3737–44.
281. Pluta P, Jeziorski A, Cebula-Obrzut AP, Wierzbowska A, Piekarski J, Smolewski P. Expression of IAP family proteins and its clinical importance in breast cancer patients. Neoplasma. 2015;62:666–73.
282. Rodriguez-Berriguete G, Torrealba N, Ortega MA, Martinez-Onsurbe P, Olmedilla G, et al. Prognostic value of inhibitors of apoptosis proteins (IAPs) and caspases in prostate cancer: caspase-3 forms and XIAP predict biochemical progression after radical prostatectomy. BMC Cancer. 2015;15:809.
283. Lopes RB, Gangeswaran R, McNeish IA, Wang Y, Lemoine NR. Expression of the IAP protein family is dysregulated in pancreatic cancer cells and is important for resistance to chemotherapy. Int J Cancer. 2007;120:2344–52.
284. Wu HH, Wu JY, Cheng YW, Chen CY, Lee MC, et al. cIAP2 upregulated by E6 oncoprotein via epidermal growth factor receptor/phosphatidylinositol 3-kinase/AKT pathway confers resistance to cisplatin in human papillomavirus 16/18-infected lung cancer. Clin Cancer Res. 2010;16:5200–10.
285. Carter BZ, Kornblau SM, Tsao T, Wang RY, Schober WD, et al. Caspase-independent cell death in AML: caspase inhibition in vitro with pan-caspase inhibitors or in vivo by XIAP or Survivin does not affect cell survival or prognosis. Blood. 2003;102:4179–86.
286. Ferreira CG, van der Valk P, Span SW, Ludwig I, Smit EF, et al. Expression of X-linked inhibitor of apoptosis as a novel prognostic marker in radically resected non-small cell lung cancer patients. Clin Cancer Res. 2001;7:2468–74.
287. Chen Z, Naito M, Hori S, Mashima T, Yamori T, Tsuruo T. A human IAP-family gene, apollon, expressed in human brain cancer cells. Biochem Biophys Res Commun. 1999;264:847–54.
288. Oberoi-Khanuja TK, Murali A, Rajalingam K. IAPs on the move: role of inhibitors of apoptosis proteins in cell migration. Cell Death Dis. 2013;4:e784.
289. Naramura M, Nadeau S, Mohapatra B, Ahmad G, Mukhopadhyay C, et al. Mutant Cbl proteins as oncogenic drivers in myeloproliferative disorders. Oncotarget. 2011;2:245–50.
290. Thien CB, Langdon WY. Cbl: many adaptations to regulate protein tyrosine kinases. Nat Rev Mol Cell Biol. 2001;2:294.
291. Cristobal I, Manso R, Rincon R, Carames C, Madoz-Gurpide J, et al. Up-regulation of c-Cbl suggests its potential role as oncogene in primary colorectal cancer. Int J Colorectal Dis. 2014;29:641.
292. Ito R, Nakayama H, Yoshida K, Matsumura S, Oda N, Yasui W. Expression of Cbl linking with the epidermal growth factor receptor system is associated with tumor progression and poor prognosis of human gastric carcinoma. Virchows Arch. 2004;444:324–31.
293. Knight JF, Shepherd CJ, Rizzo S, Brewer D, Jhavar S, et al. TEAD1 and c-Cbl are novel prostate basal cell markers that correlate with poor clinical outcome in prostate cancer. Br J Cancer. 2008;99:1849–58.
294. Tan YH, Krishnaswamy S, Nandi S, Kanteti R, Vora S, et al. CBL is frequently altered in lung cancers: its relationship to mutations in MET and EGFR tyrosine kinases. PLoS One. 2010;5:e8972.
295. Jing Z, Li L, Wang X, Wang M, Cai Y, et al. High c-Cbl expression in gliomas is associated with tumor progression and poor prognosis. Oncol Lett. 2016;11:2787–91.
296. Kamei T, Machida K, Nimura Y, Senga T, Yamada I, et al. C-Cbl protein in human cancer tissues is frequently tyrosine phosphorylated in a tumor-specific manner. Int J Oncol. 2000;17:335–9.
297. Seong MW, Ka SH, Park JH, Park JH, Yoo HM, et al. Deleterious c-Cbl exon skipping contributes to human glioma. Neoplasia. 2015;17:518–24.
298. Nakayama K, Qi J, Ronai ZE. The ubiquitin ligase Siah2 and the hypoxia response. Mol Cancer Res. 2009;7:443–51.
299. Qi J, Nakayama K, Gaitonde S, Goydos JS, Krajewski S, et al. The ubiquitin ligase Siah2 regulates tumorigenesis and metastasis by HIF-dependent

and-independent pathways. Proc Natl Acad Sci. 2008;105:16713–8.

300. Kim Y, Kim H, Park D, Jeoung D. miR-335 targets SIAH2 and confers sensitivity to anti-cancer drugs by increasing the expression of HDAC3. Mol Cells. 2015;38:562–72.
301. Gao Y, Liu Y, Meng F, Shang P, Wang S, et al. Overexpression of Siah2 is associated with poor prognosis in patients with epithelial ovarian carcinoma. Int J Gynecol Cancer. 2016;6:114–9.
302. Moreno P, Lara-Chica M, Soler-Torronteras R, Caro T, Medina M, et al. The Expression of the Ubiquitin Ligase SIAH2 (Seven In Absentia Homolog 2) Is Increased in Human Lung Cancer. PLoS One. 2015;10:e0143376.
303. Adam MG, Matt S, Christian S, Hess-Stumpp H, Haegebarth A, et al. SIAH ubiquitin ligases regulate breast cancer cell migration and invasion independent of the oxygen status. Cell Cycle. 2015;14:3734–47.
304. Sun J, Zhang X, Han Y, Zhen J, Meng Y, Song M. Overexpression of seven in absentia homolog 2 protein in human breast cancer tissues is associated with the promotion of tumor cell malignant behavior in in vitro. Oncol Rep. 2016a;36:1301–12.
305. Shi H, Zheng B, Wu Y, Tang Y, Wang L, et al. Ubiquitin ligase Siah1 promotes the migration and invasion of human glioma cells by regulating HIF-1α signaling under hypoxia. Oncol Rep. 2015;33:1185–90.
306. Hatakeyama S. TRIM proteins and cancer. Nat Rev Cancer. 2011;11:792.
307. Sakuma M, Akahira J, Suzuki T, Inoue S, Ito K, et al. Expression of estrogen-responsive finger protein (Efp) is associated with advanced disease in human epithelial ovarian cancer. Gynecol Oncol. 2005;99:664–70.
308. Suzuki T, Urano T, Tsukui T, Horie-Inoue K, Moriya T, et al. Estrogen-responsive finger protein as a new potential biomarker for breast cancer. Clin Cancer Res. 2005;11:6148–54.
309. Zhu Z, Wang Y, Zhang C, Yu S, Zhu Q, et al. TRIM25 blockade by RNA interference inhibited migration and invasion of gastric cancer cells through TGF-beta signaling. Sci Rep. 2016;6:19070.
310. Qin Y, Cui H, Zhang H. Overexpression of TRIM25 in lung cancer regulates tumor cell progression. Technol Cancer Res Treat. 2016;15:707–15.
311. Sun N, Xue Y, Dai T, Li X, Zheng N. Tripartite motif containing 25 promotes proliferation and invasion of colorectal cancer cells through TGF-beta signaling. Biosci Rep. 2017.
312. Abu-Asab MS, Chaouchi M, Alesci S, Galli S, Laassri M, et al. Biomarkers in the age of omics: time for a systems biology approach. Omics. 2011;15:105–12.
313. Srivastava S. Biomarkers in cancer screening and early detection. New York: Wiley; 2017.
314. Phan JH, Moffitt RA, Stokes TH, Liu J, Young AN, et al. Convergence of biomarkers, bioinformatics and nanotechnology for individualized cancer treatment. Trends Biotechnol. 2009;27:350–8.
315. Vassilev LT, Vu BT, Graves B, Carvajal D, Podlaski F, et al. In vivo activation of the p53 pathway by small-molecule antagonists of MDM2. Science. 2004;303:844–8.

5 Molecular Diagnostics in Melanoma: An Update

A. Srivastava, P. Srivastava, and A. B. Pant

5.1 Introduction

The malignant tumor of the melanocytes present primarily in skin is called melanoma. So far there have been no or negligible reports of a benign melanoma [1–6]. Amongst all the major health disorders gripping the society globally today melanoma remains one of the most alarming conditions. It has been declared as the fastest growing cancer in the US affecting the fair-skinned people the most. It is also known as the black cancer. Unlike other forms of cancers melanoma can develop anywhere on skin and not necessarily on the sun-exposed portions. Its occurrence is not limited to skin only. It can also target the eye (especially conjunctiva, uvea and ciliary body), and several mucosal surfaces along with the meninges. While the melanomas are predominantly severely pigmented there are reports of their amelanotic form as well. They tend to metastasize and therefore make the prognosis a grueling task. Melanomas contribute to approximately 90% of the mortality reported in cutaneous tumours [7]. Melanomas are usually cutaneous in nature and most of their cases turn lethal for the patients. The geriatric populations report the greatest incidence of melanoma, and it is also the most common type of cancers occurring in adolescents and young adults [8]. Upon early diagnosis melanoma can be treated successfully through surgical procedures. However, at advanced stages it demonstrates poor prognosis. Due to its property of targeting the young population it has a substantial societal impact. Once it becomes metastatic none of the therapies actually work to curb it. The treatment to be meted out to the patients depends upon the histopathological features of the primary tumor [9].

A. Srivastava · P. Srivastava · A. B. Pant (✉)
System Toxicology and Health Risk Assessment Group, CSIR-Indian Institute of Toxicology Research (CSIR-IITR), MG Marg, Lucknow, Uttar Pradesh, India
e-mail: abpant@iitr.res.in

5.2 Historical Background

Melanoma, derived from *melas* ("dark") and *oma* ("tumor") first came into light in fifth century in the writings of Hippocrates of Cos, and subsequently of Rufus of Eupheses, a Greek physician. The earliest evidence of melanoma can be traced back to the 2400 years old fossil remains or mummies of the Pre Columbian era. The skeletons of these mummies showed diffused melanotic metastases [10]. It were the efforts of John Hunter, a Scottish surgeon, who worked at St George's Hospital Medical School in London that the surgical removal of melanoma became possible as mentioned in the Western medical literature. Dr. William Norris from Stourbridge, UK was the first one to report the complete etiology and disease progression of melanoma in

K. K. Shukla et al. (eds.), *Molecular Diagnostics in Cancer Patients*,
https://doi.org/10.1007/978-981-13-5877-7_5

1820 who termed it as "fungoid disease" [11]. He further elaborated his observations and classified melanoma in 8 more cases. He laid down certain principles or norms governing epidemiology and management of melanoma by linking its incidence with environmental stressors. He also reported that most of the patients who came to him were pale looking with light colored hair. As per his reports melanoma had a pigmented or an amelanotic form and could reach to visceral organs following which none of the medical treatment or surgery really worked. The most effective treatment regime that he suggested was removal of tumor along with the adjoining unaffected skin [12]. The word 'melanoma' was coined by Robert Carswell in 1838 who described it in his piece of work called the "Illustrations of the Elementary Forms of Disease" [13]. The untreatable and incurable nature of melanoma at its advanced stages came into light in 1840. It was Cooper who stated that the only way to treat melanoma is to excise it during the initial stages [14]. Earlier studies during nineteenth century somehow failed to shed light on the basic mechanistic aspect of the disease. It was later in twentieth century that a proper prognosis and therapy of melanoma was deciphered after careful observation and quantitative estimations. Wallace Clark in 1966 developed a standard scale and through histological details analyzed the prognosis of melanoma. The fact that cutaneous melanoma prognosis depends upon the size of tumor as well as the invasion level in respect of tumor thickness was discovered by Alexander Breslow in 1970. This concept of Breslow thickness is defined as the complete vertical depth of melanoma beginning from the granular layer of the epidermis till the point it penetrates most deeply in the skin. This path breaking concept of Clark and Breslow gave tumor thickness the significance of being one of the most important and vital prognostic factors for identifying localized melanoma as mentioned in the present version of the AJCC Melanoma Staging System [15]. Another method developed for treating melanoma was the sentinel lymph node biopsy by Donald Morton. It is a lesser invasive method of staging the regional nodes thereby limiting dissection of node in people exhibiting proven metastases [16, 17]. A histological examination of status of mitosis in the primary melanoma is another important method of prognosis [18], primarily for thin lesions that helps in identifying thin melanomas that may have a higher risk of nodal metastasis for sentinel node biopsy [19]. Presently the histopathological observations of Breslow and Clark are being amalgamated with the available genetic data for a more comprehensive insight into the mechanistic details of melanoma progression and its influence on distinct pathological behavior [20].

5.3 Epidemiology and Etiology

There has been a constant increase in the incidence of melanoma globally and the worst affected are the fair-skinned people receiving too much of sun exposure [21–24]. This incidence rate amounts to 10–14 per 100,000 population in Central Europe while in Southern Europe it is 6–10 per 100,000 population. USA stands at a higher rate of 20–30 per 100,000 population and Australia has the highest incidence rate of 50–60 per 100,000 population [25]. Although it forms a very small proportion of the total classes of skin cancer (only 1%) its menace is continuously rising. In US alone, last year in 2017 there emerged about 87, 110 new reporting of melanoma and 9730 melanoma caused deaths [26, 27]. Melanoma exhibits polygenic inheritance. Approximately 5–10% of it occurs in families genetically predisposed towards it [28, 29]. However, the key factor responsible for melanoma incidence is UV exposure, especially the intermittent one [30–33].

Malignant melanoma is a rapidly emerging health scare in the US and in the entire world. Its incidence rate has been found to be increasing with time. Early in 1930s, the probability of an American contracting malignant melanoma was around 1 in 1500. As per reports mortality rate due to malignant melanoma has soared to nearly 2% per year since 1960. If the melanoma is restricted to the epidermis (*in-situ*) it does not carry any risk of mortality while a thin melanoma lesion is associated with a minute risk of becoming metastatic. The most vital parameter governing the survival in melanoma patients is the tumor thickness.

Malignant melanoma comes under the category of potentially fatal melanocytic neoplasm that has a tendency to metastasize. Lesions may be a result of a de novo process, or they may occur within congenital, dysplastic or banal nevi. The best way to reduce the risk of metastasis is an early detection and precise therapy. Some basic behavioral alterations might virtually prevent melanoma. Therefore the focus is being centered on to find ways of prevention or early diagnosis of melanoma and its subsequent treatment with the progress in scientific and medical techniques. As such identifying people with a higher predisposition towards melanoma becomes necessary for developing effective prevention strategies. Besides acute sun exposure that leads to sunburn various other factors are involved in melanoma etiology. These include atypical mole syndrome/dysplastic nevus syndrome, prior psoralen based therapy with ultraviolet (UV) A light, blistering sunburns, UV exposure at salons providing tanning services, immunosuppression, history of melanoma in an immediate family member or relative and higher socioeconomic status [34]. Some phenotypic characteristics also influence melanoma incidence. These include eye color (blue/green), fair skin, hair color (blond or red), freckles, sensitivity to sun, etc. Blacks and Caucasians demonstrate same probability of plantar surface melanoma incidence [35].

5.3.1 Melanoma-Associated Risk Factors

Through extensive studies it was concluded that the most prominent risk factors that independently influence development of malignant melanoma are:

- A known family history of malignant melanoma
- Hair coloration (blond or red hair)
- Presence of freckles on the upper back
- Exposure to three or more sunburns that had led to blisters before attaining 20 years of age
- Nature of outdoor job in summers for three or more years
- Evidence of actinic keratosis

People who possess even one or two of the above mentioned risk factors are more prone to developing malignant melanoma in comparison to the general unexposed population. If the risk factors involved are three or more an increase of approximately 20-fold has been witnessed. Several studies have established a correlation between germline and somatic mutations of tumor suppressor p16 and melanoma development [36]. A deeper insight into such mutations and identification of other possible risk factors might help in devising better targeting approach for affected individuals for preventing disease onset and enabling early diagnosis.

5.3.2 Classification Based on Clinical Features and Histology

Although there are no evidences directly correlating the histological subtypes with behavioral prediction in malignant melanoma patients an in-depth analysis of these subtypes does help in recognizing several other factors. Based on clinical and histological variations there are four main subtypes of melanomas:

5.3.2.1 Superficial Spreading Melanoma (SSM)

It is the most commonly occurring histological pattern in melanoma. It has an intra-epidermal, radial or horizontal growth phase in the initial stage, similar to a macule that gradually becomes a plaque, having different colors as well as pale areas of regression. At times there could be a development of secondary nodular areas. Its most distinct feature is an epidermal lateral component possessing malignant melanocytes spread in a pagetoid fashion all along the epidermis [37, 38]. They account for almost 75% of the total cases of melanomas. It is the best example for defining the characteristic histologic findings of melanoma. SSM exhibits poorly circumscribed melanocytes with isolated melanocytes overshadowing the melanocyte nests in a haphazard manner above the basal layer and termed as Pagetoid spread. Some discontinuous nests of melanocytes also exist. The malignant melanocytes extend out laterally within the epidermis. Stretches of single cells run adjacent to bigger nests. These nests lie alongside rete ridges, or within suprapapillary plates. The most distinct feature of SSM is the pagetoid migration of melanin cells but it does not form a pathogenic hallmark of the disease. Another key feature of SSM is the loose or detached arrangement of cells within the nests. The intraepidermal melanocytes in melanoma are the large cells whose cytoplasm and nucleoli are eosinophil rich with large vesicular multiple nuclei. The cells are of pleomorphic nature with frequently occurring mitosis. At times there may also be small hyperchromatic malignant cells that have very scanty cytoplasm and are called small nevoid melanoma. As the melanocytes penetrate inside the papillary dermis, their size reduces, and the cytoplasm, nuclei and nucleoli become inconspicuous [39].

5.3.2.2 Nodular Melanoma

Another subtype of melanoma known as nodular melanoma is a brown-black outward growing tumor that appears eroded and lacks a horizontal growth phase. That's why this kind of melanoma is hardly diagnosed in the intraepidermal stage [40]. These tumors commonly affect the middle-aged adults and have an affinity for the trunk. Histologically these melanomas are quiet similar to SSM with an exception in circumscription pattern that is far improved in nodular melanoma. Further, there is no lateral extension of the epidermal component in to the dermal component. Instead there is a sharp boundary along the two regions of the tumor. This justifies their nodular clinical appearance and difficult prognosis. The epidermal component of nodular melanomas harbors epithelioid melanocytes with a dense cytoplasm, vesicular nuclei and distinct nucleoli. Ulceration is also a characteristic feature of these neoplasms [41]. There is hardly any histological disparity in the dermal component of nodular melanoma and superficial spreading melanoma in the vertical growth phase.

5.3.2.3 Lentigo Maligna Melanoma

This kind of melanoma usually arises from lentigo maligna post several years in a majority of aged people with sun-damaged skin. It demonstrates lentiginous proliferation of atypical melanocytes located at the dermo-epidermal junction and also has histological similarity with cases of chronic sun exposure (solar elastosis) [42, 43]. Its intraepidermal features vary from the other subtypes. Its epidermis is atrophic found solely in extremely sun-damaged skin. The Pagetoid spread appears during later stages of disease progression probably on the initiation of dermal invasion. Another distinct feature is the occurrence of melanocytes at the convergence of dermis and epidermis that may sometimes extend into appendageal epithelium. The cells are small and hyperchromatic with dense nuclear chromatin and unapparent nucleoli and melanoma cells with multiple nuclei may also be present in some cases.

5.3.2.4 Acral Lentiginous Melanoma

It is classified as palmoplantar or subungual melanoma. Initially it shows a circumscribed pigmentation followed by appearance of a nodular region having an invasive growth pattern [44]. It is a rarely reported melanoma present in acral surfaces. Their sites of appearance are the nail beds and nail plates. The melanocytes exist as nests and single cells at the point of convergence of dermis and epidermis. There's an extensive and elaborate Pagetoid migration in the lesions. The intraepidermal melanocytes are similar to those of lentigo maligna and are hyperchromatic and spindled. The nucleoli are usually unapparent. Dermal invasion features proliferating spindle, hyperchromatic melanocytes travelling in fascicles, nests and often as single cells along the dermis. There can be some accumulation around blood vessels too [45].

Based on histological features melanoma can also be broken down into several stages (namely,

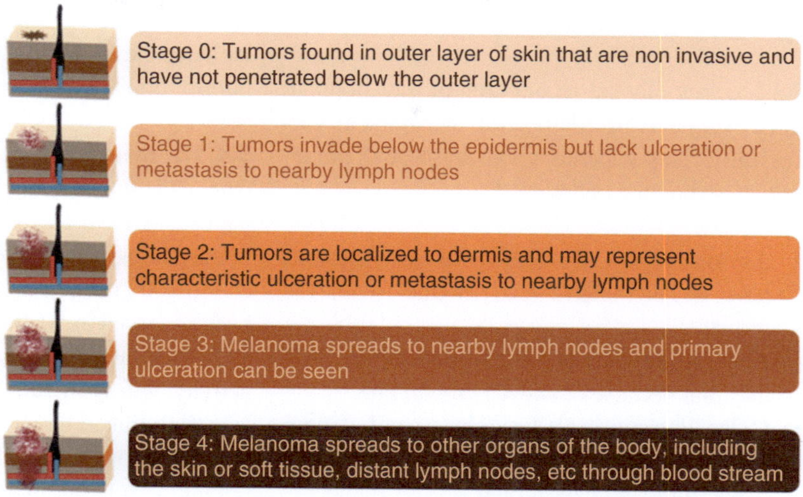

Fig. 5.1 Schematic representation of various stages of melanoma

0, I, II, III and IV). This classification is based upon the thickness level of tumor, depth of penetration and how far it spreads (Fig. 5.1).

5.3.3 Prognosis and Staging

During diagnosis almost 90% melanomas come across as primary tumors with no proven metastasis. The 10-year survival rule specific for these kinds of tumors is 75–85%. Some of the vital parameters that influence prognosis for primary melanoma not exhibiting metastases are as follows [15, 46, 47]:

- **Breslow's depth**, defined as the vertical tumor thickness, as measured using an optical micrometer on histological specimen.
- **Ulceration** that forms a key feature. Melanoma ulceration is a combination of features like the defect of full-thickness in epidermis (lacking stratum corneum as well as basement membrane), presence of host response (i.e. activity of neutrophils and fibrin deposition), and dissipation, reactive hyperplasia in adjacent epidermal region and effacement [16].
- Another independent and influential prognostic factor in certain affected population is the **mitotic activity**.
- **Invasion level** (or the Clark's level) is applicable only in case of thin tumors having less than 1 mm thickness.

There are two routes of melanoma metastasis, namely, lymphatic route or haematogenous route. Approximately two-thirds of total cases of metastases remain confined solely till the lymph nodes and their drainage areas [48]. The cardinal features of occurrence of regional metastasis are:

- **Micro-metastases** exhibited in the regional lymph nodes that is identified using sentinel lymph node biopsy. It is otherwise clinically unrecognizable by other existing techniques [49].
- **Satellite metastases** (exists up to 2 cm from the site of primary tumour).
- **In-transit metastases** (occurs in skin between the site of satellite metastases and the primary draining lymph node) [50].
- **Regional lymph node metastases** that is clinically recognizable [51].

The 10-year survival rule stands at 30–70% for micrometastases suffering patients, 30–50% for patients suffering from satellite and in-transit metastases and 20–40% for patients with clinically proven regional lymph node metastases. The chances of a successful prognosis are bleak in distant metastases with a median survival rate of 6–9 months in untreated patients. However variation exists on the basis of involvement of internal organ and levels of lactate dehydrogenase in serum.

5.4 Clinical Features

An accurate clinical recognition of melanoma at initial stages is mandatory for managing it successfully. This depends upon the ABCD guideline as elaborated below [52]:

- **Asymmetry** – A majority of early lesions have an asymmetric pattern due to uneven growth.
- **Border Irregularity** - The borders also become irregular because of uneven growth rate.
- **Color Variegation** - Irregular growth pattern gives rise to a patchy appearance of colors black, light and dark brown.
- **Diameter** - Lesions expressing above stated ABC features along with a diameter greater than 6 mm fall under suspicious category.

5.4.1 Genetics of Melanoma

Genetic mutations and genomic aberrations primarily underlie melanoma pathogenesis [53]. These genetic mutations further affect the signaling cascades involved in cell proliferation, especially the PI3K/MAP kinase pathway [54]. A thorough analysis of the modifications occurring in pathways in response to mutations helps in identifying the erring target molecules for therapy development too. Some of the vital genes and their mutated forms responsible for triggering melanoma pathogenesis and etiology have been elaborated below:

5.4.1.1 Neuroblastoma RAS (NRAS)

Mutations in MAP kinase pathway, one of the key pathways involved in melanoma, are known to play a role in its incidence. Around 15–20% of melanoma cases have been found to be associated with *NRAS* mutations. Substitution of glutamine by leucine at codon 61 is the most commonly occurring *NRAS* mutation. It leads to an over activation of protein NRAS resulting in uncontrolled proliferation of cells [55]. It was recently observed that NRAS mutations are correlated with nodular melanomas and those present in case of chronically sun-damaged skin. Moreover, the characteristic features of *NRAS* mutations included elevated mitosis, thick tumor and highly inferior clinical outcome [56].

5.4.1.2 B-Raf (BRAF)

One of the downstream molecules of MAP kinase pathway known as BRAF also influences melanoma pathogenesis. Its mutant form, especially at codon 600 (Valine substitutes glutamic acid), has been observed in 40–60% instances of melanoma [57]. It results in activation of its innate kinase activity which in turn triggers the downstream signaling linked to MAP kinase pathway [58]. A few mutations were also reported in the loop domain (exon 11) of BRAF. BRAF mutation is reportedly a key event during the early stages of melanoma. Although both NRAS and BRAF mutations are associated with MAPK signaling pathway, they themselves generally remain mutually exclusive. The Food and Drug Administration (FDA) approved Vemurafenib, a targeted drug developed against V600-mutant form of BRAF, for combating advanced stage symptoms of melanoma, with proven positive clinical outcomes [59]. The FDA also approved a test kit for identifying BRAF V600E mutation that was called the cobas® 4800 BRAF V600 Mutation Test. It was based on real-time PCR assay using TaqMan probes conjugated with fluorescent tags that bind with wild-type and mutant forms of BRAF [60].

5.4.1.3 KIT

KIT belongs to receptor tyrosine kinase family present on cell surface and plays a role in normal development of melanocyte, along with the pathogenesis of lentiginous, acral and mucosal melanoma. It triggers several intracellular signaling pathways, like the PI3K and MAPK pathways [61]. Analysis of various types of melanoma samples revealed increased copy number accompanied with somatic mutations in KIT in approximately 30% of tumors that led to enhanced expression of KIT. These mutations exist in exons 9, 11, 13, and 17 [62].

5.4.1.4 PTEN

Present on chromosome 10q23 *PTEN* functions as a tumor suppressor gene and also modulates the PI3K pathway that drives melanoma pathogenesis. Mutations in *PTEN* have been implicated in melanoma tumors as well and they mostly co-exist with mutant forms of BRAF [63]. These mutations usually involve missense mutations, insertions, deletions, and epigenetic silencing.

5.4.1.5 GNAQ/GNA11

Uveal melanomas affecting the eyes in adults are another category of melanomas [64]. BRAF and NRAS mutations are found to be absent in them. The causative factors of uveal melanoma are the mutant forms of GNAQ and GNA11 [65]. They encode the alpha subunits of G-protein-coupled receptors. Mice injected with GNAQ Q209 carrying melanocytes exhibited increased tumorigenicty and increased activity of MAP kinases [66]. These mutations can be targeted for devising a therapeutic mechanism against uveal melanoma.

5.4.1.6 CDK4 and CDKN2A

Approximately 3–15% of melanoma cases are familial that indicates their hereditary nature. However, the familial cases exhibit genetic heterogeneity. CDK4 and CDKN2A, 2 genes susceptible to high penetrance, are found to be mutated in around 30–40% cases of familial melanoma [67]. Another oncogene called CDK4 is expressed in a mutant form in a few cases of familial melanoma (~2%). The most abundant and prominent mutations present in about 20–40% of familial cases of melanoma are the germline mutations of CDKN2A. The tumor suppressor proteins p14ARF and p16INK4 are encoded by CDKN2A. Its penetrance reaches to 0.67 when the patient reaches 80 years of age. It has been reported that melanoma patients carrying a CDKN2A mutation experience an early disease onset with high risk of developing multiple primary melanomas (MPM) [68].

5.4.1.7 Melanocortin-1 Receptor Gene (MC1R)

Since human pigmentation is a complex process a possible involvement of some more genetic factors in melanoma etiology is assumed. One such gene known as melanocortin-1 receptor gene (MC1R), present as chromosomal locus 16q24.3 and encoding a G-protein-coupled receptor carrying 7 membrane-spanning domains, regulates the process of human pigmentation. It stimulates the transduction process of tyrosinase thus boosting eumelanin synthesis. Being a vital part of melanin production pathway MC1R determines the risk of developing melanoma [33]. Alterations in *MC1R* gene lead to the risk of developing malignant melanoma. Subjects from nine different geographical regions were selected and monitored for MC1R changes. Although there wasn't any hint of a possible association between MC1R related changes and development of tumor characteristics it was still linked with melanoma anatomy [69]. Due to its polymorphic nature the white-skinned people harbor over 70 variants of MC1R gene. Several studies brought forth the functional outcomes of these variations. They led to amino acid substitutions that could impair the eumelanin synthesis and predispose an individual towards UV burns and development of skin tumors. The study results differ with the difference in phenotype of the human subjects selected based on region they dwell in. The variants observed in a Spanish population were different and novel in comparison to other populations studied earlier [33].

Genetic mutations are largely responsible for causing both familial and spontaneous melanoma. The upcoming molecular techniques ensure retrieval of precise and specific data regarding melanoma tumors that further sheds light on the exact melanoma pathogenesis. As a result advancement in developing new target based therapy became possible that was way ahead than the conventional therapeutic approaches in terms of clinical benefits. Using the genetic and genomic information derived from patients personalized medicine against melanoma could be developed as an ideal treatment strategy [70].

5.4.2 Molecular Diagnostics in Melanoma

The incessant technological advancements in the area of molecular pathology have simplified identification of disease prone individuals and clinical sub-types of diseases, error-free diagnosis for developing effective therapeutic measures and achieving improved results. The histological parameters largely govern discerning and prognosis of primary cutaneous melanoma. These are the depth of tumor and ulceration. Besides that certain clinical factors like number of lymph nodes or distant metastases also act as an influence over disease prognosis. However, in a few cases sentinel lymph node biopsy fails to identify highly prone individuals suffering from thin melanomas and their chances of developing distant metastasis. The discovery of certain new markers has also aided in melanoma identification, treatment and possibility of recurrence and correlated these factors with disease progression [71, 72]. However, none of the treatment methods existing today guarantee survival for longer periods.

The identification of nucleic acid (DNA, RNA) or protein related pathogenic mutations for an effective diagnosis, identification of subtypes, prognosis, chosen therapy and monitoring of outcome can be achieved via molecular diagnosis. Over the last 50 years a substantial advancement and knowledge gathered in the field of medicine related to detection of human cancer has led to development of high throughput techniques of molecular diagnosis. For example, by decoding the signaling pathways governing the cell cycle, proliferation, growth and differentiation, and cell death (apoptosis) of cancer cells, suitable candidates for anticancer drugs were identified and developed which were found to be effective for some patients. The concept of personalized medicine signifies specificity of disease progression and the response towards therapy for a given individual [73]. In context to melanoma, the personalized medicine concept includes estimation of an individual's predisposition towards the disease, screening followed by an early diagnosis of the disease, analysis of its prognosis and identification of the associated minimal residual disease if any, determination of pharmacogenomic characteristics of drug efficacy and the related toxic effects due to the adopted treatment of metastatic melanoma, and finally its possible recurrence [74].

It is comparatively tougher to predict the clinical outcome in melanoma of intermediate thickness (2.0 to 4.0 mm in Breslow depth). Therefore it's extremely essential to identify patient derived molecular biomarkers of tumor for an improved disease prognosis [75]. To achieve this establishing an elaborate and detailed tumor bank along with its morphological characteristics and clinical follow-up becomes mandatory. Evidence obtained from several studies in the past suggest that this kind of molecular data can be drawn from formalin-fixed, paraffin-embedded (FFPE) material, thus bypassing the requirement of freshly obtained primary melanoma samples [76]. This approach offers several advantages: (a) provides a vast repository of biopsy specimens analyzed for histologic diagnosis that are held valid worldwide, (b) these specimens create a disease signature in terms of morphology, and (c) in a few cases, these samples were preserved for up to 20 years, which facilitated back tracing the current studies with the previous clinical outcomes [77].

There are however certain issues that need to be focused upon while pursuing molecular testing in metastatic melanoma to achieve targeted therapy [78]. These are as follows:

1. There needs to be a close alliance between the clinician handling the case, the pathologist conducting the tests and the molecular biologist analyzing the data. Testing is necessary only when targeted therapy is deemed as the only treatment option. The final call towards this lies with the clinician.
2. All the tests must be conducted in a molecular laboratory holding a valid accreditation. This ensures the process is performed under standard conditions and has followed the required guidelines yielding reliable results.
3. The pathologist should take care of the diagnostic procedures checking the affected tissue and selecting the area to be dissected for DNA analysis.
4. The molecular biologists should conclude the test results and report them after their adequate interpretation. The report should highlight important areas like the block of tissue

that was tested, test sensitivity, genes under study, the mutations observed along with their complete description.
5. The molecular test should preferentially be conducted using a recent metastasis case.
6. The test should minutely pinpoint every single relevant and targetable gene mutation.
7. The test should ideally take less turnaround time because this therapy is adopted in cases of rapidly advancing melanoma (highly metastatic).

5.5 Testing for Genetic Mutations

Genetic mutations and aberrations are predominant factors underlying cancer pathogenesis in different types of cancers, like *KRAS* in colon cancer, *EGFR* in lung cancer and *BRAF* in melanoma. In case of melanoma the most consistently occurring mutations are the point mutations while the genomic aberrations encountered are heterozygosity loss at specific locus points of genes or amplification, and the epigenetic silencing. The somatic, genomic and genetic alterations arising in genes like *BRAF, NRAS, KIT, GNAQ/GNA11, PTEN,* and *MAP 2 K1/2 (MEK1/2)* are crucial events of melanoma pathogenesis [79]. An assimilation of these genetic facts behind melanoma incidence facilitated the designing of target therapeutic compounds/drugs directed against the erring forms of genes like KIT, MEK 1/2, and BRAF that resulted in numerous mutation-based clinical trials, including the most recent approval of vemurafenib by the FDA. A successful identification of the involved genetic aberrations in the formalin-fixed paraffin embedded as well as fresh samples is the key factor responsible for developing an effective therapeutic measure in any form of genetic mutation based cancer. Additionally knowledge of the existing genetic mutations in a given patient also aids in determining the efficacy of the developed therapy as well as its inclusion or exclusion in a clinical trial based on observed mutations. Somatic mutations can

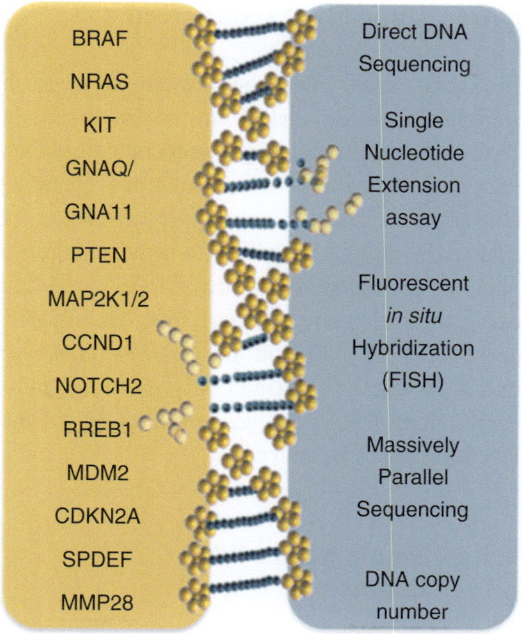

Fig. 5.2 Schematic representation of major genes and techniques involved in pathogenic mutations and molecular diagnosis of melanoma respectively

be evaluated using direct sequencing techniques, single nucleotide extension techniques, high density sequencing and copy number analysis. The type of technique selected for analysis further depends upon the kind of mutation and the number of samples under study (Fig. 5.2).

The USFDA approved 2 drugs against metastatic melanoma in 2011. These were ipilimumab, a CTLA-4 inhibitor and vemurafenib, a BRAF inhibitor. The fact that activating BRAF mutations are a major underlying reason behind melanoma pathogenesis led the scientists to develop Vemurafenib [80]. To identify this mutation **Fine-needle aspiration (FNA) method** came into light through the study of Bernacki et al. (2012). It is a minimally invasive and inexpensive process designed for melanoma diagnosis that can do away with the painful invasive procedures like surgical excisions. In cases of deep seated lesions during the advanced stages FNA technique is the only technique with the potential to extract out the sample for diagnosis [81].

5.5.1 Direct DNA sequencing

Each and every mutation present in a given stretch of DNA obtained from the tumor sample can be identified using direct sequencing of DNA [82]. In case where some mutations occur as clusters over a small area, pyrosequencing (a trademark of Qiagen), proves to be advantageous than single nucleotide extension [83, 84]. It can carry out sequencing of short stretches of DNA comprising of 300–500 nucleotides. However mutations can be identified only when the damaged/mutant DNA occupies a total of 5% of the DNA sample to be analyzed.

5.5.2 Single Nucleotide Extension assay

Single nucleotide extension assays facilitate identification of known point mutation. These assays are confined to the interrogated base and evaluate the mutations strictly within it [85]. Two forms of this technique that are commonly employed are iPlex (Sequenom Inc) and SNaPshot (Applied Biosystems, Inc). These techniques can multiplex to interrogate several varying point mutations at a time [86]. However multiple base changes occurring within a small stretch of nucleotides cannot be investigated using Single nucleotide extension tests efficiently. These techniques are usually taken into use in clinical molecular pathology for diagnostic purposes. They especially recognize genes with mutation hotspots like *GNAQ/GNA11, NRAS* and *BRAF*.

5.5.3 Fluorescent In Situ Hybridization (FISH)

Fluorescent in situ Hybridization (FISH) also came into picture for melanoma diagnosis while analyzing ambiguous samples. Senetta et al. used specific probes against *GNAQ/GNA11, RREB1* and *CCND1* genes, along with the centromere control probe in benign nevi and malignant melanoma [87]. Hossain et al. focused on FISH probes specific for chromosomes for distinguishing between benign lesions and malignant melanoma. A whopping 94% of the total melanoma samples exhibited chromosomal abnormalities while those of compound nevi and normal skin had 6% and 0% abnormality respectively. The most commonly occurring abnormality was the chromosome 11 gain, followed by chromosomes 7, 20, and 6 [88]. Although FISH cannot solely be relied upon as an interrogative tool for melanoma it can still be employed as a supplementary or an add-on test when dealing with ambiguous samples and tricky diagnosis [89].

5.5.4 Estimation of DNA Copy Number Changes

Variations in DNA copy number are reportedly associated with cancer pathogenesis and may influence disease progression and clinical outcome in several types of tumor. Copy number profiling helps in analysis of multiple genomic aberrations and the subsequent genomic alterations occurring in melanoma [90]. Gene amplifications in *MITF, BRAF, NRAS, CCNE1, CCND1, MDM2* and *NOTCH2* and homozygous deletions in *CDKN2A* and *PTEN* are reportedly involved in melanoma pathogenesis. Analysis of DNA copy number also helps in identifying novel genes and the associated pathways in melanoma. This turns out to be useful in cases of ambiguous samples with difficult diagnosis by providing extra details about their expression profiles. There has been an enhancement in technologies used for genome wide copy number over the last few years. These include **Single Nucleotide Polymorphism (SNP) arrays** that carry 25 nucleotide long probes while the oligonucleotide platforms employed in a CGH carry 60-mer probes [91]. Studies also concluded that probes with more oligonucleotides give an improved output while investigating low-amplitude genomic alterations in tumor cells of melanoma whereas SNP arrays were preferred for copy number changes in noncoding DNA elements. This technique helps in producing a signature genomic sequence for each melanoma tumor which further eases the process of target identification. Another technique for targeted analysis is **multiplex probe ligation amplification** (MLPA; MRC-Holland). It determines genomic deletions and amplifications [92]. It is more advantageous in comparison to aCGH since the starting tumor DNA used for this is lesser in amount.

5.5.5 Massively Parallel Sequencing

Outdoing the traditional sequencing methods is the fast emerging massively parallel sequencing approach. It enables the exome sequencing as well as the sequencing of the complete genomes of tumor samples. Through this technique sequencing of multiple genes at a time and rapid estimation of genetic mutations and variations in copy number has become feasible [93]. **Next generation sequencing** works by constructing libraries using genomic DNA or even from exons accompanied by their flanking DNA sequence. It is executed on a flow cell surface, with short adaptor ligated DNA fragments, their subsequent capture, amplification, and recurring rotations of sequencing and sequence detection [94]. Additionally these methods are regularly improved so as to increase the level of multiplexing in every single flow cell. Another sequencing technique known as the **Whole genome sequencing** evaluates the genomes of malignant melanoma [95]. In the beginning studies conducted analyzed a metastasized malignant melanoma derived cell line based on the comparison with a matching lymphoblastoid cell line. The alterations and mutations identified were as follows: 33,345 somatic mutations, 303 small insertions, 680 small deletions and 51 somatic rearrangements. Mutations consistent with UV exposure and significantly involved in melanoma were also noted. These included BRAF V600E (corresponding to a noticeable genomic deletion of PTEN) and deletion of two base pairs in CDKN2A. Novel mutations in SPDEF encoding an ETS transcription factor family member were also reported. Mutations also occurred in MMP28, a matrix metalloproteinase gene and autophagy associated gene UVRAG which is also supposedly a tumor suppressor gene [96, 97]. A further extensive sequencing of melanoma genome will shed light on additional novel mutations underlying melanoma pathogenesis [98]. Whole genome sequencing revealed several new and frequently occurring somatic mutations in about 14 cases of metastatic melanoma. Wei et al. in a study reported a repetitive TRRAP mutation at locus p.S722F, in approximately 4% (6/167) of the total melanoma samples. Its further functional analysis suggested its role as an oncogene. Another gene GRIN2A also had mutations in about 33% (17/52) of the total samples. Reinstating the findings of previous studies BRAF was again found to be mutated in as high as 50% of samples. Although reported to occur in 15–20% of melanomas there was no evidence of NRAS mutations in this study. MAP 2K1 and MAP 2K2 were also present in their recurrent mutant form in melanoma [99]. Hence massively parallel sequencing method promises to provide an elaborate data based on genes and genome of melanoma. This could further aid in molecular profiling of melanoma and the resulting stratification of the patients [100]. This can predict an individual's response towards a chosen therapy and likewise conduct the treatment [101]. Its ability to discover novel mutations has led to identification of novel drug targets. Whole genome and whole exome sequencing are usually not the first choice for diagnosing tumor due to their high cost and available alternative therapeutics [102]. Next generation sequencing also facilitates identification of unknown mutations. Moreover, it also offers advantage in cases where patients develop resistance towards existing therapy, thereby promoting identification of new targets and therapeutic approaches.

The technological advancements in the area of disease diagnosis have thus helped a great deal in unearthing the molecular basis of various severe health disorders. The advent of genetic testing methods altogether modified the diagnostic processes world over. These methods can clearly identify even the minutest of deletions, duplication and insertions of DNA unlike the conventional microscopic methods. Analysis of multiple genes in one go during the same instant has been made possible by massively parallel next-generation sequencing technique. The influence of a patient's genetic factors on his/her response towards the selected therapeutic measure can also be ascertained by DNA testing. This further enables customizing the most suitable method of treatment and drug dosage for each patient based on his/her genetic profile. Gauging the genetic alterations using exome and genome sequencing has helped the clinicians to identify the degree of susceptibility of a person towards developing cancer in the long run and likewise choose the most optimum therapy against the same. If abiding by the ethics and stringently following the legal and social norms the genetic testing methods can satisfactorily improve the clinical diagnostic procedures as well as the interpretation of the final outcomes [103].

5.6 The Need for Regulatory Approval in Molecular Diagnosis

The molecular diagnostic procedures required to estimate cancer (here melanoma) progression do not require an approval from the USFDA unlike the medical devices. It is the laboratory engaged in performing these diagnostic tests that needs a certificate of Clinical Laboratory Improvement Amendments (CLIA) bestowed by the Centers for Medicare and Medicaid Services (CMS) [104]. It governs all the clinical diagnostic procedures being conducted on human subjects in that laboratory. Once a laboratory receives a CLIA certification for a given diagnostic test it signifies its ability to carry out that test reproducibly under the standard conditions [105]. However, this certification procedure does not consider the resulting clinical implications associated with the test, its influence on the decision-making in terms of disease remedy by physicians, or the probable side-effects associated with the test that can adversely affect the patient as interpreted by the physician. Before conducting any such test it is highly recommended that the clinicians go through the published peer-reviewed records and studies on these tests as well as the CLIA-certification of the laboratory performing these tests [106].

5.7 Conclusion

A robust and reproducible detection method in melanoma involves identification of an array of factors that must be screened for effective and fast diagnosis. However, the key challenges remain in the form of translation traits that must travel from bench to bedside in clinical settings. In addition, the incessantly expanding incidence and complex etiology of melanoma have triggered an alarming health concern the world over. The abundance of melanoma-associated environmental risk factors around us, with the UV rays of sun being the most common out of them, has significantly magnified the susceptibility of developing the disease in exposed people, especially the fair-skinned ones. As opposed to sporadic melanoma caused by external factors the familial melanoma is a case of genetic inheritance from the family. Furthermore, an attempt has also been made in the present chapter to highlight the pathological state of melanoma by citing information on genetic and epigenetics markers including genetic mutations and genomic aberrations that might aid towards better diagnosis of the disease in individuals who are genetically predisposed towards melanoma. Additionally, sections focusing on current methods for early detection of melanoma containing pertinent genes involved in genetic mutations along with radical scientific detection methods to outline molecular diagnostics have also been mentioned. Keeping in view the highly versatile nature of the disease, we conclude that a rational approach equipped with logistical consideration must be explored to answer highly specific diagnostic strategy against this disease. In order to achieve this milestone, an explorative technique focusing on each gene should be developed that should be cost effective for the patient as well.

References

1. Dummer R, Hauschild A, Jost L. Cutaneous malignant melanoma: ESMO clinical recommendations for diagnosis, treatment and follow-up. Ann Oncol. 2008;19(2):ii86–8.
2. Dummer R, Panizzon R, Bloch P, Burg G. Updated Swiss guidelines for the treatment and follow-up of cutaneous melanoma. Dermatology. 2005;210(1):39–44.
3. Garbe C, Hauschild A, Volkenandt M, Schadendorf D, Stolz W, Reinhold U, et al. Evidence and interdisciplinary consense-based German guidelines: diagnosis and surveillance of melanoma. Melanoma Res. 2007;17(6):393–9.
4. Garbe C, Hauschild A, Volkenandt M, Schadendorf D, Stolz W, Reinhold U, et al. Evidence and interdisciplinary consensus-based German guidelines: surgical treatment and radiotherapy of melanoma. Melanoma Res. 2008;18(1):61–7.
5. Roberts D, Anstey A, Barlow R, Cox N, Bishop J, Corrie P, et al. UK guidelines for the management of cutaneous melanoma. Br J Dermatol. 2002;146(1):7–17.
6. Saiag P, Bosquet L, Guillot B, Verola O, Avril M-F, Bailly C, et al. Management of adult patients with cutaneous melanoma without distant metastasis. 2005 update of the French Standards, Options and Recommendations guidelines. Summary report. Eur J Dermatol. 2007;17(4):325–31.
7. Garbe C, Peris K, Hauschild A, Saiag P, Middleton M, Spatz A, et al. Diagnosis and treatment of melanoma: European consensus-based interdisciplinary guideline. Eur J Cancer. 2010;46(2):270–83.
8. Matthews N, Li W, Qureshi A, Weinstock M, Cho E. Epidemiology of melanoma. In: Ward WH, Farma JM, editors. Cutaneous Melanoma: Etiology and Therapy [Internet]. Brisbane: Codon Publications; 2017.
9. Goyal A, Duncan LM. Pathology and molecular pathology of melanoma. Pathology and epidemiology of cancer. Berlin: Springer; 2017. p. 613–53.
10. Urteaga B, Pack GT. On the antiquity of melanoma. Cancer. 1966;19(5):607–10.
11. Norris W. Case of fungoid disease. Edinb Med Surg J. 1820;16:562–5.
12. Norris W. Eight cases of melanosis: with pathological and therapeutical remarks on that disease. London: Longman, Brown, Green, Longmans, and Roberts; 1857.
13. Carswell R. Illustrations of the elementary forms of disease. London: Longman; 1838.
14. Cooper S. The first lines of the theory and practice of surgery: including the principle operations. SS and W. Wood; 1844.
15. Balch CM, Gershenwald JE, S-j S, Thompson JF, Atkins MB, Byrd DR, et al. Final version of 2009 AJCC melanoma staging and classification. J Clin Oncol. 2009;27(36):6199–206.
16. Morton DL, Wen D-R, Wong JH, Economou JS, Cagle LA, Storm FK, et al. Technical details of intraoperative lymphatic mapping for early stage melanoma. Arch Surg. 1992;127(4):392–9.
17. Morton DL, Thompson JF, Cochran AJ, Mozzillo N, Elashoff R, Essner R, et al. Sentinel-node biopsy or nodal observation in melanoma. N Engl J Med. 2006;355(13):1307–17.
18. Azzola MF, Shaw HM, Thompson JF, Sj S, Scolyer RA, Watson GF, et al. Tumor mitotic rate is a more powerful prognostic indicator than ulceration in patients with primary cutaneous melanoma. Cancer. 2003;97(6):1488–98.
19. Sondak VK, Taylor JM, Sabel MS, Wang Y, Lowe L, Grover AC, et al. Mitotic rate and younger age are predictors of sentinel lymph node positivity: lessons learned from the generation of a probabilistic model. Ann Surg Oncol. 2004;11(3):247–58.
20. Viros A, Fridlyand J, Bauer J, Lasithiotakis K, Garbe C, Pinkel D, et al. Improving melanoma classification by integrating genetic and morphologic features. PLoS Med. 2008;5(6):e120.
21. de Vries E, Bray FI, Coebergh JWW, Parkin DM. Changing epidemiology of malignant cutaneous melanoma in Europe 1953–1997: rising trends in incidence and mortality but recent stabilizations in western Europe and decreases in Scandinavia. Int J Cancer. 2003;107(1):119–26.
22. Garbe C, Blum A. Epidemiology of cutaneous melanoma in Germany and worldwide. Skin Pharmacol Physiol. 2001;14(5):280–90.
23. MacKie RM, Bray CA, Hole DJ, Morris A, Nicolson M, Evans A, et al. Incidence of and survival from malignant melanoma in Scotland: an epidemiological study. Lancet. 2002;360(9333):587–91.
24. Månsson-Brahme E, Johansson H, Larsson O, Rutqvist LE, Ringborg U. Trends in incidence of cutaneous malignant melanoma in a Swedish population 1976-1994. Acta Oncol. 2002;41(2):138–46.
25. Garbe C, Peris K, Hauschild A, Saiag P, Middleton M, Bastholt L, et al. Diagnosis and treatment of melanoma. European consensus-based interdisciplinary guideline–Update 2016. Eur J Cancer. 2016;63:201–17.
26. Cheng L, Lopez-Beltran A, Massari F, MacLennan GT, Montironi R. Molecular testing for BRAF mutations to inform melanoma treatment decisions: a move toward precision medicine. Mod Pathol. 2018;31(1):24.
27. Siegel RL, Miller KD, Fedewa SA, Ahnen DJ, Meester RG, Barzi A, et al. Colorectal cancer statistics, 2017. CA Cancer J Clin. 2017;67(3):177–93.
28. Bishop JN, Harland M, Randerson-Moor J, Bishop DT. Management of familial melanoma. Lancet Oncol. 2007;8(1):46–54.
29. de Snoo FA, Kroon MW, Bergman W, ter Huurne JA, Houwing-Duistermaat JJ, van Mourik L, et al. From sporadic atypical nevi to familial melanoma: risk analysis for melanoma in sporadic atypical nevus patients. J Am Acad Dermatol. 2007;56(5):748–52.

30. Tsao H, Atkins MB, Sober AJ. Management of cutaneous melanoma. N Engl J Med. 2004;351(10):998–1012.
31. Curtin JA, Busam K, Pinkel D, Bastian BC. Somatic activation of KIT in distinct subtypes of melanoma. J Clin Oncol. 2006;24(26):4340–6.
32. Curtin JA, Fridlyand J, Kageshita T, Patel HN, Busam KJ, Kutzner H, et al. Distinct sets of genetic alterations in melanoma. N Engl J Med. 2005;353(20):2135–47.
33. Avilés J, Lázaro P, Fernández L, Benítez J, Ibarrola-Villava M, Ribas G. Phenotypic and histologic characteristics of cutaneous melanoma in patients with melanocortin-1 receptor polymorphisms. Actas Dermosifiliogr. 2012;103(1):44–50.
34. Berwick M, Buller DB, Cust A, Gallagher R, Lee TK, Meyskens F, et al. Melanoma epidemiology and prevention. Cancer Treat Res. 2016;167:17–49.
35. Potrony M, Badenas C, Aguilera P, Puig-Butille JA, Carrera C, Malvehy J, et al. Update in genetic susceptibility in melanoma. Ann Transl Med. 2015;3(15):210.
36. Diseati L, Scheinfeldt LB, Kasper RS, Zhaoyang R, Gharani N, Schmidlen TJ, et al. Common genetic risk for melanoma encourages preventive behavior change. J Pers Med. 2015;5(1):36–49.
37. D'Ath P, Thomson P. Superficial spreading melanoma. BMJ. 2012;344:e2319.
38. Longo C, Casari A, Pellacani G. Superficial spreading melanoma. Reflectance confocal microscopy for skin diseases. Berlin: Springer; 2012. p. 151–78.
39. Vu M, Adler N, Wee E, Wolfe R, McLean C, Kelly J, et al. Impact of naevus association on survival for nodular and superficial spreading melanomas. Br J Dermatol. 2018;172(3):761–2.
40. Pizzichetta M, Kittler H, Stanganelli I, Bono R, Cavicchini S, De Giorgi V, et al. Pigmented nodular melanoma: the predictive value of dermoscopic features using multivariate analysis. Br J Dermatol. 2015;173(1):106–14.
41. Skala SL, Arps DP, Zhao L, Cha KB, Wang M, Harms PW, et al. Comprehensive histopathological comparison of epidermotropic/dermal metastatic melanoma and primary nodular melanoma. Histopathology. 2018;72(3):472–80.
42. Greveling K, Wakkee M, Nijsten T, van den Bos RR, Hollestein LM. Epidemiology of lentigo maligna and lentigo maligna melanoma in the Netherlands, 1989–2013. J Investig Dermatol. 2016;136(10):1955–60.
43. Charifa A, Chen C. Cancer, melanoma, Lentigo maligna. In: StatPearls [Internet]. Treasure Island: StatPearls Publishing; 2018.
44. Goydos JS, Shoen SL. Acral lentiginous melanoma. Melanoma. Berlin: Springer; 2016. p. 321–9.
45. Smoller BR. Histologic criteria for diagnosing primary cutaneous malignant melanoma. Mod Pathol. 2006;19(S2):S34.
46. Breslow A, Macht S. Optimal size of resection margin for thin cutaneous melanoma. Surg Gynecol Obstet. 1977;145(5):691–2.
47. Boland GM, Gershenwald JE. Principles of melanoma staging. Melanoma. Berlin: Springer; 2016. p. 131–48.
48. Adler NR, Haydon A, McLean CA, Kelly JW, Mar VJ. Metastatic pathways in patients with cutaneous melanoma. Pigment Cell Melanoma Res. 2017;30(1):13–27.
49. Caulley L, Balch CM, Ross MI, Robert C. Management of sentinel-node metastasis in melanoma. N Engl J Med. 2018;378(1):85–8.
50. Neuschmelting V, Lockau H, Ntziachristos V, Grimm J, Kircher MF. Lymph node micrometastases and in-transit metastases from melanoma: in vivo detection with multispectral optoacoustic imaging in a mouse model. Radiology. 2016;280(1):137–50.
51. Amit M, Tam S, Abdelmeguid AS, Roberts DB, Raza SM, Su SY, et al. Approaches to regional lymph node metastasis in patients with head and neck mucosal melanoma. Cancer. 2018;124(3):514–20.
52. Mar VJ, Chamberlain AJ, Kelly JW, Murray WK, Thompson JF. Clinical practice guidelines for the diagnosis and management of melanoma: melanomas that lack classical clinical features. Med J Aust. 2017;207(8):348–50.
53. Kwong LN, Zou L, Chagani S, Pedamallu CS, Liu M, Jiang S, et al. Modeling genomic instability and selection pressure in a mouse model of melanoma. Cell Rep. 2017;19(7):1304–12.
54. Rosenberg SA, Niglio SA, Salehomoum N, Chan JL-K, Jeong B-S, Wen Y, et al. Targeting glutamatergic signaling and the PI3 kinase pathway to halt melanoma progression. Transl Oncol. 2015;8(1):1–9.
55. Vu HL, Aplin AE. Targeting mutant NRAS signaling pathways in melanoma. Pharmacol Res. 2016;107:111–6.
56. Cicenas J, Tamosaitis L, Kvederaviciute K, Tarvydas R, Staniute G, Kalyan K, et al. KRAS, NRAS and BRAF mutations in colorectal cancer and melanoma. Med Oncol. 2017;34(2):26.
57. Heppt MV, Siepmann T, Engel J, Schubert-Fritschle G, Eckel R, Mirlach L, et al. Prognostic significance of BRAF and NRAS mutations in melanoma: a German study from routine care. BMC Cancer. 2017;17(1):536.
58. Amaral T, Sinnberg T, Meier F, Krepler C, Levesque M, Niessner H, et al. MAPK pathway in melanoma part II—secondary and adaptive resistance mechanisms to BRAF inhibition. Eur J Cancer. 2017;73:93–101.
59. Eroglu Z, Ribas A. Combination therapy with BRAF and MEK inhibitors for melanoma: latest evidence and place in therapy. Ther Adv Med Oncology. 2016;8(1):48–56.
60. Ascierto PA, McArthur GA, Dréno B, Atkinson V, Liszkay G, Di Giacomo AM, et al. Cobimetinib combined with vemurafenib in advanced BRAFV600-mutant melanoma (coBRIM): updated efficacy results from a randomised, double-blind, phase 3 trial. Lancet Oncol. 2016;17(9):1248–60.

61. Manzano JL, Layos L, Bugés C, de los Llanos Gil M, Vila L, Martínez-Balibrea E, et al. Resistant mechanisms to BRAF inhibitors in melanoma. Ann Transl Med. 2016;4(12).
62. Carvajal RD, Antonescu CR, Wolchok JD, Chapman PB, Roman R-A, Teitcher J, et al. KIT as a therapeutic target in metastatic melanoma. JAMA. 2011;305(22):2327–34.
63. Brown K, Yang P, Salvador D, Kulikauskas R, Ruohola-Baker H, Robitaille A, et al. WNT/β-catenin signaling regulates mitochondrial activity to alter the oncogenic potential of melanoma in a PTEN-dependent manner. Oncogene. 2017;36(22):3119.
64. Decatur CL, Ong E, Garg N, Anbunathan H, Bowcock AM, Field MG, et al. Driver mutations in uveal melanoma: associations with gene expression profile and patient outcomes. JAMA Ophthalmol. 2016;134(7):728–33.
65. Staby KM, Gravdal K, Mørk SJ, Heegaard S, Vintermyr OK, Krohn J. Prognostic impact of chromosomal aberrations and GNAQ, GNA11 and BAP1 mutations in uveal melanoma. Acta Ophthalmol. 2018;96(1):31–8.
66. Chen X, Wu Q, Depeille P, Chen P, Thornton S, Kalirai H, et al. RasGRP3 mediates MAPK pathway activation in GNAQ mutant uveal melanoma. Cancer Cell. 2017;31(5):685–696. e6.
67. Marzuka-Alcalá A, Gabree MJ, Tsao H. Melanoma susceptibility genes and risk assessment. Molecular diagnostics for melanoma. Berlin: Springer; 2014. p. 381–93.
68. van der Rhee JI, Krijnen P, Gruis NA, de Snoo FA, Vasen HF, Putter H, et al. Clinical and histologic characteristics of malignant melanoma in families with a germline mutation in CDKN2A. J Am Acad Dermatol. 2011;65(2):281–8.
69. Taylor NJ, Busam KJ, From L, Groben PA, Anton-Culver H, Cust AE, et al. Inherited variation at MC1R and histological characteristics of primary melanoma. PLoS One. 2015;10(3):e0119920.
70. Wilson MA, Nathanson KL. Molecular testing in melanoma. Cancer J. 2012;18(2):117.
71. Harbour JW, Chao DL. A molecular revolution in uveal melanoma: implications for patient care and targeted therapy. Ophthalmology. 2014;121(6):1281–8.
72. Janku F, Claes B, Huang HJ, Falchook GS, Devogelaere B, Kockx M, et al. BRAF mutation testing with a rapid, fully integrated molecular diagnostics system. Oncotarget. 2015;6(29):26886.
73. Dancey JE, Bedard PL, Onetto N, Hudson TJ. The genetic basis for cancer treatment decisions. Cell. 2012;148(3):409–20.
74. Carlson JA, Ross JS, Slominski A, Linette G, Mysliborski J, Hill J, et al. Molecular diagnostics in melanoma. J Am Acad Dermatol. 2005;52(5):743–75.
75. Axelrod ML, Johnson DB, Balko JM, editors. Emerging biomarkers for cancer immunotherapy in melanoma. Seminars in cancer biology. Amsterdam: Elsevier; 2017.
76. Van Allen EM, Wagle N, Stojanov P, Perrin DL, Cibulskis K, Marlow S, et al. Whole-exome sequencing and clinical interpretation of formalin-fixed, paraffin-embedded tumor samples to guide precision cancer medicine. Nat Med. 2014;20(6):682.
77. Dadras SS. Molecular diagnostics in melanoma: current status and perspectives. Arch Pathol Lab Med. 2011;135(7):860–9.
78. van Engen-van Grunsven AC, Kusters-Vandevelde H, Groenen PJ, Blokx WA. Update on molecular pathology of cutaneous melanocytic lesions: what is new in diagnosis and molecular testing for treatment? Front Med. 2014;1:39.
79. Ribas A. Novel insights/translational implication from the emerging biology of melanoma. Molecular diagnostics for melanoma. Berlin: Springer; 2014. p. 3–9.
80. Gedye C, Hogg D, Butler M, Joshua AM. New treatments for metastatic melanoma. Can Med Assoc J. 2014;186(10):754–60.
81. Bernacki KD, Betz BL, Weigelin HC, Lao CD, Redman BG, Knoepp SM, et al. Molecular diagnostics of melanoma fine-needle aspirates: a cytology-histology correlation study. Am J Clin Pathol. 2012;138(5):670–7.
82. Lyu J, Wu Y, Li C, Wang R, Song H, Ren G, et al. Mutation scanning of BRAF, NRAS, KIT, and GNAQ/GNA11 in oral mucosal melanoma: a study of 57 cases. J Oral Pathol Med. 2016;45(4):295–301.
83. McEvoy AC, Wood BA, Ardakani NM, Pereira M, Pearce R, Cowell L, et al. Droplet digital PCR for mutation detection in formalin-fixed, paraffin-embedded melanoma tissues: a comparison with Sanger sequencing and pyrosequencing. J Mol Diagn. 2018;20(2):240–52.
84. de Araújo ÉS, Pramio DT, Kashiwabara AY, Pennacchi PC, Maria-Engler SS, Achatz MI, et al. DNA methylation levels of melanoma risk genes are associated with clinical characteristics of melanoma patients. Biomed Res Int. 2015;Article ID 376423.
85. Stence A, Gailey M, Robinson R, Jensen C, Ma D. Simultaneously detection of 50 mutations at 20 Sites in the BRAF and RAS genes by multiplexed single-nucleotide primer extension assay using fine-needle aspirates of thyroid nodules. Yale J Biol Med. 2015;88(4):351–8.
86. Wilson MA, Nathanson KL. Molecular diagnostics and tumor mutational analysis. BRAF targets in melanoma. Berlin: Springer; 2015. p. 47–65.
87. Senetta R, Paglierani M, Massi D. Fluorescence in-situ hybridization analysis for melanoma diagnosis. Histopathology. 2012;60(5):706–14.
88. Hossain D, Qian J, Adupe J, Drewnowska K, Bostwick DG. Differentiation of melanoma and benign nevi by fluorescence in-situ hybridization. Melanoma Res. 2011;21(5):426–30.
89. Gerami P, Jewell SS, Morrison LE, Blondin B, Schulz J, Ruffalo T, et al. Fluorescence in situ hybridization (FISH) as an ancillary diagnostic tool

in the diagnosis of melanoma. Am J Surg Pathol. 2009;33(8):1146–56.

90. Pfarr N, Penzel R, Klauschen F, Heim D, Brandt R, Kazdal D, et al. Copy number changes of clinically actionable genes in melanoma, non-small cell lung cancer and colorectal cancer—a survey across 822 routine diagnostic cases. Genes Chromosom Cancer. 2016;55(11):821–33.
91. North JP, Vemula SS, Bastian BC. Chromosomal copy number analysis in melanoma diagnostics. Molecular diagnostics for melanoma. Berlin: Springer; 2014. p. 199–226.
92. Bunyan D, Eccles D, Sillibourne J, Wilkins E, Thomas NS, Shea-Simonds J, et al. Dosage analysis of cancer predisposition genes by multiplex ligation-dependent probe amplification. Br J Cancer. 2004;91(6):1155.
93. Akabane H, Sullivan RJ. The future of molecular analysis in melanoma: diagnostics to direct molecularly targeted therapy. Am J Clin Dermatol. 2016;17(1):1–10.
94. Serratì S, De Summa S, Pilato B, Petriella D, Lacalamita R, Tommasi S, et al. Next-generation sequencing: advances and applications in cancer diagnosis. Onco Targets Ther. 2016;9:7355.
95. Hayward NK, Wilmott JS, Waddell N, Johansson PA, Field MA, Nones K, et al. Whole-genome landscapes of major melanoma subtypes. Nature. 2017;545(7653):175.
96. Palavalli LH, Prickett TD, Wunderlich JR, Wei X, Burrell AS, Porter-Gill P, et al. Analysis of the matrix metalloproteinase family reveals that MMP8 is often mutated in melanoma. Nat Genet. 2009;41(5):518.
97. Liang C, Feng P, Ku B, Dotan I, Canaani D, Oh B-H, et al. Autophagic and tumour suppressor activity of a novel Beclin1-binding protein UVRAG. Nat Cell Biol. 2006;8(7):688.
98. De Paoli-Iseppi R, Johansson PA, Menzies AM, Dias K-R, Pupo GM, Kakavand H, et al. Comparison of whole-exome sequencing of matched fresh and formalin fixed paraffin embedded melanoma tumours: implications for clinical decision making. Pathology. 2016;48(3):261–6.
99. Wei X, Walia V, Lin JC, Teer JK, Prickett TD, Gartner J, et al. Exome sequencing identifies GRIN2A as frequently mutated in melanoma. Nat Genet. 2011;43(5):442.
100. Lang UE, Yeh I, McCalmont TH. Molecular melanoma diagnosis update: gene fusion, genomic hybridization, and massively parallel short-read sequencing. Clin Lab Med. 2017;37(3):473–84.
101. Kalia M. Biomarkers for personalized oncology: recent advances and future challenges. Metabolism. 2015;64(3):S16–21.
102. Krauthammer M, Kong Y, Bacchiocchi A, Evans P, Pornputtapong N, Wu C, et al. Exome sequencing identifies recurrent mutations in NF1 and RASopathy genes in sun-exposed melanomas. Nat Genet. 2015;47(9):996.
103. Korf BR, Rehm HL. New approaches to molecular diagnosis. JAMA. 2013;309(14):1511–21.
104. Katsanis SH, Katsanis N. Molecular genetic testing and the future of clinical genomics. Nat Rev Genet. 2013;14(6):415.
105. Singh RR, Patel KP, Routbort MJ, Reddy NG, Barkoh BA, Handal B, et al. Clinical validation of a next-generation sequencing screen for mutational hotspots in 46 cancer-related genes. J Mol Diagn. 2013;15(5):607–22.
106. March J, Hand M, Truong A, Grossman D. Practical application of new technologies for melanoma diagnosis: Part II. Molecular approaches. J Am Acad Dermatol. 2015;72(6):943–58.

6 Molecular Diagnostics in Breast Cancer

Rajeshwari Sinha and Sanghamitra Pati

6.1 Introduction

Cancer, in the simplest of terms, could be defined as "cells gone wrong" [1]. It refers to the continuous and unregulated proliferation of cells, accompanied by metabolic and behavioral changes. These changes occur through alterations in cellular mechanisms that control cell proliferation, as a result of which cancer cells can spread and also invade other tissues. One of the leading causes of morbidity and mortality worldwide, cancer has resulted in approximately 14 million new cases in 2012 and this number is projected to rise to over 21 million by 2030 [2]. It is also the second leading cause of death globally, and has been responsible for 8.8 million deaths in 2015. The most frequently diagnosed cancer among men in the United States is prostrate, lung and colorectal cancer, while those in women are breast, lung and colorectal cancer [3]. The developing world is said to face a larger burden of cancer incidence, morbidity, and mortality. More than 50% cases and 65% cancer deaths have been attributed to less developed regions [4].

Breast cancer is the most common cause of cancer among women. In the United States, it is expected to account for 30% of all new cancer diagnoses in women [3]. The precise causes that lead to cancer of the breast are yet to be fully understood, however some of the key risk factors include increasing age, previous family history, previous history of breast cancer, role of hormones (for example, increased exposure to hormone estrogen can trigger breast cancer cells), role of genes (for example, BRCA1 and BRCA2 gene mutations in women are more likely to induce breast cancer), lifestyle factors such as obesity or alcohol consumption, exposure to radiation, early menstruation or late menopause etc. [5]. The GLOBOCAN project under the International Agency for Research on Cancer (IARC) of the World Health Organization (WHO) estimates the possible incidence, mortality and prevalence of major cancers across different countries. As per GLOBOCAN estimates for 2012, globally, there have been an estimated 1.67 million new cancer cases diagnosed and over 5 lakh deaths in 2012 [6]. The number of deaths due to breast cancer in less developed regions is about 1.6 times higher than those in more developed regions. The higher mortality and gradually increasing prevalence of breast cancer in developing countries has largely been attributed to increased urbanization, increased life expectancy and westernized lifestyles coupled with limited resources and weak health

R. Sinha
Independent Researcher, New Delhi, India

S. Pati (✉)
ICMR-Regional Medical Research Centre
Department of Health Research, Govt. of India
Bhubaneswar, Odisha, India

K. K. Shukla et al. (eds.), *Molecular Diagnostics in Cancer Patients*,
https://doi.org/10.1007/978-981-13-5877-7_6

systems [7]. Furthermore, the low survival rates owing to breast cancer in such less developed countries are also a result of late-stage disease detection, lack of early detection programmes, and inadequate access to appropriate diagnosis and treatment facilities [8].

Breast cancer incidences in Asia are rising rapidly. According to the Cancer Atlas, it is one of the top three cancers and also one of the top three causes of cancer death in women belonging to Southern, Eastern, and Southeastern Asia [9]. In India, there were 145,000 new cases and 70,000 deaths reported as on 2012 [6]. Another recent review on the breast cancer epidemiology in Indian women in 2017 by Malvia et al. [10] projects that number of people in India with breast cancer is set to cross 1.7 million by 2020. The authors also observe that breast cancer mortality and morbidity in females is the highest in metropolitan cities as compared to other cities in India [10].

Diagnosis and treatment of breast cancer has come a long way, transitioning from clinical to genomic approaches. Furthermore, with the introduction of new biomarkers and molecular diagnostics tools, breast cancer diagnosis has also recently undergone a paradigm shift. The present chapter focuses on the understanding of how molecular tools and technologies have revolutionized diagnosis and treatment of breast cancer. The chapter also simultaneously reflects on the existing traditional as well as newer screening and diagnosis approaches for breast cancer. The increasing importance of newer "omics' based approaches such as proteomics in breast cancer biomarker discovery has also been highlighted.

6.2 Early Detection of Breast Cancer

Early detection of disease is the cornerstone of not just breast cancer, but for any cancer control. It is deemed to be an essential component for improved breast cancer outcome and survival. When identified early, there is a greater possibility of treatments being more effective and less expensive, higher chances of survival and lesser morbidity.

The WHO's latest guide to early diagnosis of cancer [11] outlines that improved chances of survival for people living with cancer can be achieved by ensuring that health services focus on early diagnosis and treatment. The guidance outlines the need for improved public awareness of cancer symptoms, strengthened and well equipped health services and access to safe and effective treatment as key elements to early detection of cancer.

Challenges associated with the early detection of breast cancer are reportedly greater in low- and middle-income countries (LMICs). A review by Unger-Saldaña [12] identifies different possible factors associated with delay in provision of breast cancer care which may ultimately lead to delay in early stage detection, particularly in developing countries. These factors include low socioeconomic status, lack of health insurance, longer travel time or distance to hospital, longer waiting times, multiple consultations at different health services before arrival to a cancer center, awareness levels of healthcare professional or errors in screening, diagnosis, interpretation of results. The rate of individuals diagnosed with early-stage tumors in developing countries was relatively low and ranged from 5 to 14% across countries such as India, Pakistan and Iran [13].

6.3 Routine Breast Cancer Screening and Detection Methods

There are two early detection methods-early diagnosis and screening. **Early diagnosis** entails creation of awareness on early signs and symptoms while **screening** involves the use of a screening test to identify individuals with any abnormality that is indicative of cancer. This section discusses some of the commonly used breast cancer screening and detection methods. Some of these are also used for diagnosis of the cancer (Fig. 6.1).

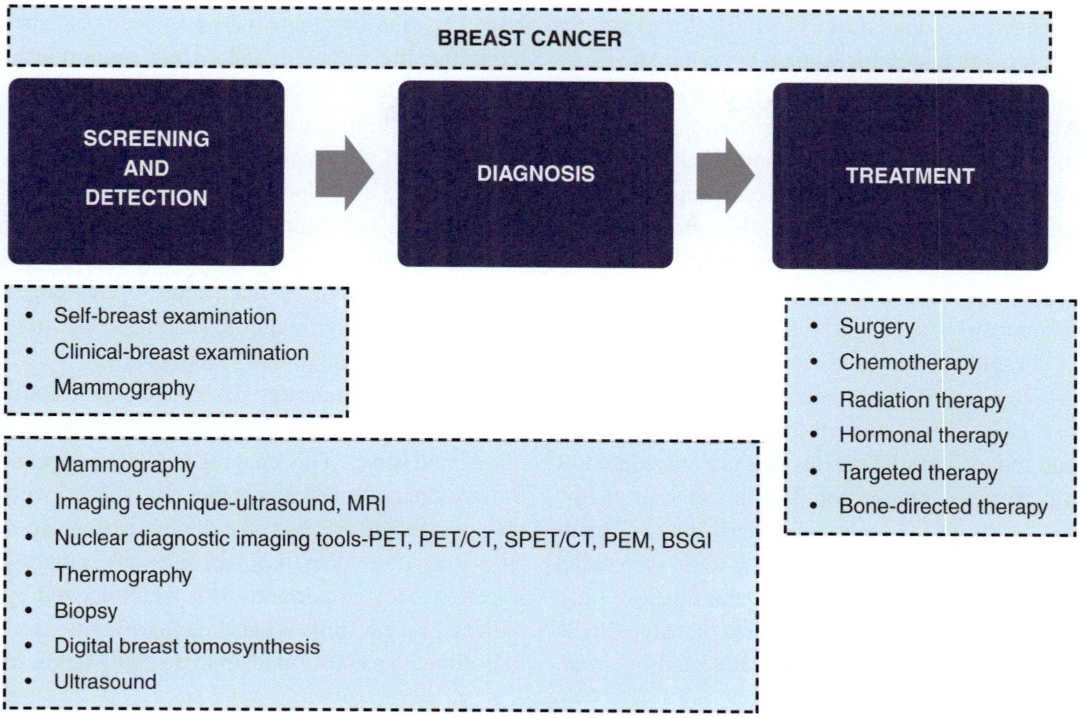

Fig. 6.1 Commonly used screening and diagnostic approaches for breast cancer

The most common and widely used approaches for breast cancer screening are **Breast Self-Examination** (BSE; examination of breast by own self) and **Clinical Breast Examination** (CBE; examination of breasts by a trained health professional). Although there have been several awareness campaigns to educate women on the need for regular and periodic breast examinations through the use of BSE or CBE approaches, there has been very limited scientific evidence to validate the success of these approaches in reducing chances of breast cancer or mortality linked to it. BSE is in fact no longer recommended by most guidelines. In Nigeria, 75.6% of studied women had never performed a BSE [14] and in Bangladesh, 71% and 96% did not know what screening and BSE is respectively [15]. Contrarily, a cross-sectional study on awareness and screening behavior of breast cancer among 100 urban women without history of breast cancer in Mysuru, India showed that 99% of women under study were aware of breast cancer, 63% were aware of BSE and 66% had practiced BSE once [16].

Mammography or **Screen Film Mammography (SFM)** is one of the most widely accepted screening approaches for breast cancer. In fact, it is often referred to as the "gold standard" of screening. Mammography uses X-rays to identify breast related abnormalities and is by far, the only screening method that has reportedly been proven to be effective in reducing breast cancer. In high-resource settings, mammography has reportedly helped reduce mortality by approximately 20% [7]. In case of LMICs, it is difficult to implement screening strategies such as mammography owing to high cost, lack of health care infrastructure, higher incidence in younger women wherein mammography screening may not be as effective [17–19].

Digital Mammography or **Full-Field Digital Mammography (FFDM)**, as the name suggests, involves digital display of mammographic images on a computer monitor for faster interpretation of results. It also enables the use of computer-aided detection (CAD) software to aid in cancer detection. FFDM has higher contrast, lower noise, greater accuracy, better ease of data storage as compared to SFM [20]. It is generally not recommended for women over age 50.

Contrast Enhanced (CE) Digital Mammography is another mammography technique which requires injection of an iodinated contrast agent. Tumor detection using CE digital mammography has shown high sensitivity [21]. It is however, not useful as a screening tool for breast cancer in isolation but used as an adjunct to standard mammographic techniques.

Despite evidence that mammography is an efficient method for screening large populations, has successfully detected early breast cancers and reduced mortality, it is still not considered as a perfect screening tool. This is because of low sensitivity of the technique. Sensitivity of mammography gradually decreases with increasing density of the breast under examination [22]. FFDM has been found to be more sensitive in the detection of tumors in dense breast tissue than FSM [21]. Further, there have also been concerns regarding the radiation risks from mammography, high rate of false positives, increased cost, unnecessary biopsies and patient anxiety.

In view of the fact that successful breast cancer screening aims for maximum sensitivity and specificity at minimum cost, a large number of other screening or detection methods are also available. While these may address challenges faced in mammographic screening, they may have their own limitations (Table 6.1).

Ultrasound imaging, also called sonography, creates image from reflected high-frequency ultrasound waves. This imaging technique appears much more advantageous in that it is widely available, less expensive, has no risk of radiation exposure and also does not require any contrast injection. Most importantly, it is well tolerated by patients, owing to its widespread use across several ailments. Ultrasound imaging also helps in

Table 6.1 Screening or detection approaches for breast cancer

Screening/detection methods	Advantages	Gaps	Supplementary role
Physical examination			
Self Breast Examination	– Preliminary or basic screening – Examination by self	– No scientific evidence for reduction in mortality – Chances of increased false positives and more testing	No
Clinical Breast Examination	– Preliminary or basic screening	– No scientific evidence for reduction in mortality	No
Mammography			
Mammography	– Detects early breast cancers – Recommended for screening large populations – Evidences of reduction in mortality	– Reduced sensitivity – Chances of radiation exposure – False positives – High cost – Overdiagnosis – Pain and discomfort, mental anxiety	No
Digital mammography	– Detect tumors in dense breast tissue – Higher contrast, reduced noise, greater accuracy and sensitivity compared to regular mammography	– Not much recommended for women over age of 50	No
Contrast Enhanced Mammography	– High sensitivity of tumor detection	– Need for contrast injection	Used as adjunct to mammography

Table 6.1 (continued)

Screening/detection methods	Advantages	Gaps	Supplementary role
Imaging techniques			
Ultrasound imaging	– Differentiation of solid tumors from fluid-filled cysts – Wide availability and use – Low cost involved – No risk of exposure to radiation – Well received among patients	– Not recommended for screening of general population	Used as supplement to mammography
Magnetic resonance imaging	– Effective in detecting invasive breast cancer – Higher sensitivity to mammography and ultrasound	– Reduced specificity – False identification of benign lesions as malignant – Expensive – Need for contrast injection – Limited data to show a reduction in mortality	Used as an adjunct to mammography in select high-risk patients
Nuclear medicine imaging techniques			
Positron Emission Tomography (PET) or FDG-PET	– High resolution – High sensitivity – High accuracy	– Chances of radiation exposure – False positives – False negatives – Low sensitivity/specificity in very small lesions (<0.5 cm)	Used as supplement to mammography
Positron Emission Mammography	– Higher sensitivity than PET/CT – High positive predictive values	– Chances of radiation exposure – Not recommended for general or regular screening	Used as supplement to mammography
Breast-Specific Gamma Imaging	– High positive predictive values	– Chances of radiation exposure – Not recommended for general or regular screening	Used as supplement to mammography
Others			
Biopsy	– Helps detect/confirm presence of cancer after initial screening by mammography, MRI or ultrasound	– Surgical biopsy: painful procedure – FNAB:no histological data – CNB: larger needle used	Used after primary detection by mammography, ultrasound or MRI
Digital Breast Tomosynthesis	– Three dimensional view – Lower recall rates on screening mammography – Reduced false negatives – Less expensive and easier to use than other supplemental breast imaging tests	– Decreased sensitivity for detection of micro-calcifications	Used as supplement to mammography

differentiating solid tumors from fluid-filled cysts. However, it is not used as an isolated screening tool by itself, but often used along with mammography. Studies have reported that Automated Whole-Breast Ultrasound System (AWBUS) devices have aided significant improvement in detection of cancer in women with dense breasts, as compared to mammography alone.

Magnetic Resonance Imaging (MRI) is another widely used imaging tool for breast cancer detection. MRI uses an intravenous contrast injection, a powerful magnetic field and radio frequency to create images of organs and tissues. While MRI has been reported to have higher sensitivity and is quite effective in detecting invasive breast cancer, but it may also lead to false identification of benign lesions as malignant. It is recommended for use as a supplemental screening approach for high risk patients.

Nuclear diagnostic imaging tools, such as **Positron emission tomography (PET)** have been used in the early detection of breast cancer in women. A scan uses a radioactive substance (tracer) to track breast cancer. Along with fluorodeoxyglucose (FDG; a radiopharmaceutical), PET forms a powerful imaging technique FDG-PET, which has significantly improved diagnostic opportunities. It has also enabled detection of small sized lesions. Studies have shown FDG-PET to be highly sensitive and specific towards the detection of primary large and palpable breast tumors [23]. The sensitivity is however low in case of lesions which are small and non-palpable.

Sometimes, PET is used in combination with a computed tomography (CT) to form **PET/CT**, which enables image formation from both devices at the same time which are superimposed. A study that compares PET, CT, and PET/CT in breast cancer patients found that in more than 50% of the patients under study, PET/CT was more effective than with PET or CT alone [24]. Some of the limitations of PET or PET/CT include high false negative rates in the detection of small sized or low grade tumors, high rate of false positives and low sensitivity towards detection of axillary nodal metastasis [25].

Single photon emission tomography-computed tomography (SPET/CT) is another nuclear medicine imaging technique that uses gamma rays. Simanek and Koranda [26] have reviewed the current status and challenges with SPET/CT. This technique has the advantage of increased diagnostic accuracy and has been known to offer advantages in detection of sentinel lymph nodes in breast cancer [26].

Positron emission mammography (PEM) uses gamma rays to detect hot-spots of rapidly growing cells. Similar to PET, PEM involves intravenous administration of a contrast agent, FDG. PEM is considered to have significantly higher sensitivity than PET/CT in detection small-sized tumours less than 2 cm. It is used in addition to mammography**. Breast-Specific Gamma Imaging (BSGI)**, employs a radioactive tracer to identify cancer cells. BSGI has been found to have high diagnostic performance as an effective supplementary imaging modality along with mammography [27]. Rechtman et al. [28] evaluated the sensitivity of BSGI for detection of breast cancer and found overall high sensitivity of 95.4%. Despite high positive predictive values associated with PEM and BSGI, both approaches involve the risk of radiation exposure to the patient, owing to use of radioactive tracer.

Thermography detects breast cancer by identifying skin areas with higher local temperature. The higher temperature is due to increased vascularization and inflammation caused by a developing malignancy. There is however limited evidence that supports the use of thermography as a breast cancer screening or diagnostic tool.

Biopsy generally refers to the removal of breast tissue from a suspicious area, which may have been found after mammography, ultrasound or MRI. Three major kinds of biopsy techniques are commonly used, namely **Surgical biopsy**, **Fine needle Aspiration biopsy** (FNAB) and **Core Needle biopsy**. FNAB is inexpensive and simple, but does not show histological architecture. There is also a possibility of higher rates of tissue sampling error. Core needle biopsy involves used of larger needle than FNAB but provides more specific diagnostic information as compared to FNAB. Surgical biopsy is definitely the "gold standard" for breast cancer diagnosis and shows tissue architecture, however the process is painful.

To overcome the problem of false positives in standard mammography due to overlapping breast tissues, **Digital Breast Tomosynthesis (DBT)** is generally used. A rotating gantry captures images of the breast from various angles in order to produce three-dimensional image, thus diminishing the overlapping effect. DBT is approved for use as an adjunct along with mammography. Tomosynthesis is also limited by its decreased sensitivity for detection of microcalcifications, which are small deposits of calcium within the soft breast tissue. Studies on breast cancer screening using DBT have often been carried out using a combination with digital mammography and have shown improved cancer detection rates and lower recall rates [29].

6.4 Role of Molecular Diagnostics and Biomarkers in Breast Cancer Detection

It is known that during cancer development and progression, various genetic changes occur. This may include genetic mutations, deletions, amplifications, rearrangements etc. Such changes are manifested in the form of release of biochemical substances called tumor biomarkers. Any biological material (for example, nucleic acids, proteins etc.) provided by cancer cells that can be detected and used as an indicator of tumor status therefore qualifies as a tumor biomarker. Biomarkers are otherwise referred to as the "molecular signposts" reflecting the state of a cell at any point of time [30]. In addition to biomarkers, molecular level diagnostics for cancer have also evolved and now play a key role in cancer management. Molecular diagnostics refer to a set of analytical tools that can detect or analyze such biomarkers and provide an assessment of the individual's health. New molecular diagnostic tools or assays developed for testing of biomarkers for breast cancer have been successful not only because of their prognostic and predictive value but also because it has enabled simplified and early breast cancer detection, along with accurate and tailored treatment.

As seen in Table 6.1, available standard and traditional breast cancer screening and diagnostic methods are associated with own limitations. Hence, the need to develop new biomarkers or molecular diagnostics becomes pertinent. Moving on from imaging techniques, "omics" based approaches such as genomics, proteomics and transcriptomics have been explored for discovery of potential biomarkers of breast cancer detection and diagnosis. This has enabled better characterization and improved understanding of tumor cells and associated new biomarkers. Several researchers have reviewed the available standard biomarkers or molecular diagnostic approaches for breast cancer diagnosis (Fig. 6.2) [31–34].

The following section of this chapter revisits key such molecular entities and techniques and provide updates on recent novel approaches in the field.

6.4.1 Hormone Based Receptors as Biomarkers

Hormone receptors, namely **estrogen receptor** (ER), **progesterone receptor** (PR), **and human epidermal growth factor receptor 2** (HER2) are used routinely for breast cancer prognosis and therapeutic purposes.

6.4.1.1 Estrogen Receptor and Progesterone Receptor

The presence of estrogen receptors (ER) and/or progesterone receptors (PR) are considered as one of the most important biomarkers. Excessive secretion of estrogen and/or progesterone from the tumor cells is indicative of the presence of breast cancer. The cell expression is analyzed and the results are indicated as ER+/PR− or ER−/PR+ or ER+/PR+ or ER−/PR− depending on whether any one or both receptors are present. Diagnosis for this test is carried out by ligand binding assay (LBA) or immuno-histochemical (IHC) assays. While IHC assay is the more widely accepted standard protocol, there is a lack of standardization in the use and interpretation of

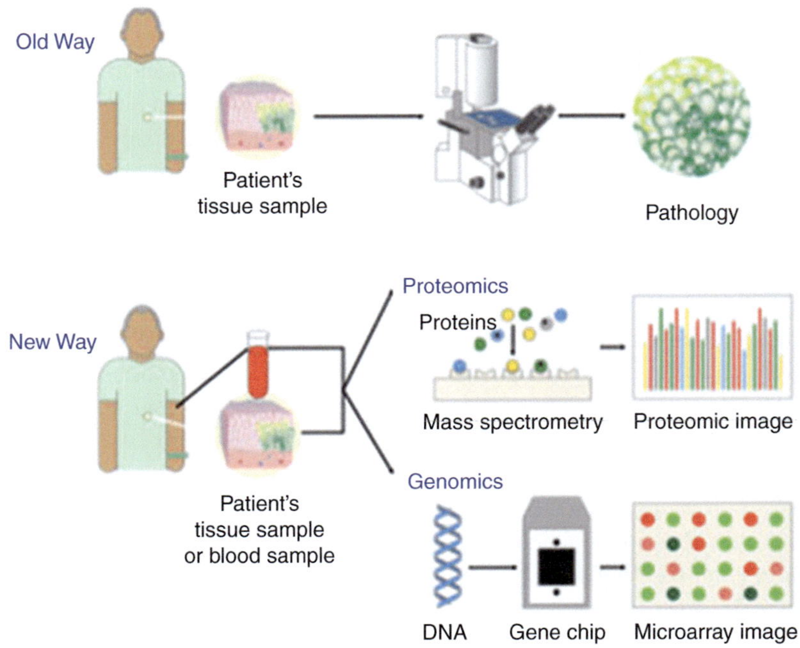

Fig. 6.2 Role of molecular diagnostics in disease diagnosis and management (Image courtesy: National Cancer Institute)

this assay. Several retrospective studies have shown that patients with ER or PR-containing tumours tend to have a better outcome than those lacking the receptors [35].

6.4.1.2 HER2/neu Analysis

Human Epidermal growth factor Receptor 2 (HER2) is the second important biomarker of prognostic value, widely used for diagnosis of invasive breast cancer. HER2 is a protein found on some breast cancer cells. Overexpression of the HER2 gene which codes for HER2 protein is predictive of the presence of cancer. HER2 protein overexpression is found in almost 25% of breast cancers [36]. Breast cancer patients with HER2 positive status are treated with trastuzumab, a monoclonal antibody that blocks activation of the HER2 receptor. HER2 is detected using IHC and Fluorescence in situ Hybridization (FISH).

Another assay that measures the total HER2 protein and functional HER2 homodimer (H2D) levels on the cell surface of breast cancer tissue is the HERmark™ assay. The assay reports whether a patient is HER2 negative, positive or equivocal (wherein no useful information is obtained). HER2 expression measured by routine HER2 testing as well as by HERmark assay showed that the assay method was much more sensitive and accurately identified HER2 expression, the results of which correlated well with results of the routine testing method [37].

6.4.1.3 KI-67 Proliferation Index

The Ki-67 proliferation index has been studied as a prognostic and predictive biomarker for breast cancer [38, 39]. It has also been used as a predictor of recurrence in breast cancer. Ki-67 antigen is expressed in the nuclei of all proliferating cells and therefore often also considered as a key proliferation biomarker. Ki-67 can be measured by immune-histochemistry. High levels of Ki67 have been linked to adverse outcome in patients with breast cancer [35].

6.4.2 Gene Expression Based Assays

Interpretation and analysis of the expression pattern of specific tumor-related genes offers another approach for identifying tumors and predicting a patient's prognosis. Several RNA-based molecular diagnostic tools are currently available commercially. A few of the more common gene expression tests are discussed here.

6.4.2.1 MammaPrint™

The MammaPrint test is a molecular diagnostic tool that assesses chances of tumor recurrence in a breast cancer patient. It measures a 70-gene expression profile signature. The clinical utility of Mammaprint has been studied in a prospective, randomized, phase three controlled clinical trial, MINDACT. Results from this trial showed that Mammaprint test can decrease the frequency of administering adjunct chemotherapy to patients who are at a high risk [35]. The assay is however only recommended for patients with stage 1 or 2 invasive breast cancer. One of the limitations with the MammaPrint assay is that it is currently only performed in the Agendia laboratory in Amsterdam, the Netherlands; therefore, the test is not available across a variety of laboratories. Moreover, the test utilizes up quite a large amount of sample, therefore there may not be enough sample remaining for routine histological assessments.

6.4.2.2 Oncotype DX®

This is a 21-gene expression assay that uses quantitative real time polymerase chain reaction (qRT-PCR) and microarray technology. Oncotype DX® assay helps to estimate the likelihood of recurrence of invasive breast cancer in patients who have been successfully treated with chemotherapy. Also known as the 21-gene Recurrence Score (RS) assay, it is the standard screening test for women with early-stage (Stage I or II), node-negative, ER+ invasive breast cancer [40]. A recent study assessing the National Cancer Database data, a database that contains information on cancer patients diagnosed and treated across the USA, reported immense impact in reducing chemotherapy recommendation among those who had RS assay in comparison to those who did not [41].

6.4.2.3 Theros H/I℠ and MGI℠ or Breast Cancer Index (BCI)

Theros H/I℠ is a molecular diagnostic test that measures the ratio of expression of two genes HOXB13 and IL17BR. The ratio serves as an indicator of clinical outcome in breast cancer patients who have been treated with tamoxifen, a hormone therapy drug used to treat breast cancer [42]. A high level of expression of the two-gene ratio reflects a failure with respect to response to tamoxifen treatment [43]. Similarly, an additional test that uses a five-gene expression index instead of two is the Theros MGI℠. It is used to stratify ER+ breast cancer patients into high or low risk of recurrence [44].

6.4.2.4 Prosigna Breast Cancer Assay

Another assay based on tumor gene expression is the Prosigna Breast Cancer Assay. The assay measures the expression of the fifty PAM50 genes and 8 housekeeping genes. As compared to other gene expression based assays, Prosigna test has the advantage of having a simplified approach. The assay is currently validated for postmenopausal women with hormone receptor-positive (HR+), node-negative (stage I or II) or node-positive (stage II) disease. A prospective multicentre French study evaluating the clinical impact of Prosigna Test in management of breast cancer at early stage showed that availability of the test increased the confidence of the physicians and also simultaneously decreased anxiety and improved health related quality of life in patients [45]. The clinical utility of Prosigna in a real world setting was established by testing a comprehensive population-based cohort of patients that included all Danish Women diagnosed with breast cancer between 2000 to 2003 [46].

6.4.2.5 Genomic Grade Index (GGI)

The GGI signature is a gene-expression signature which was developed to reclassify patients with histological grade 2 tumors. It is a 97 gene expression assay, in which the genes are associated with cell cycle regulation and proliferation. Differential expression of genes is observed in case of high- and low-grade breast tumors. The GGI test is said to help improve treatment decisions and also increase the accuracy of tumor grading [31].

6.4.2.6 EndoPredict Test

EndoPredict Test is a multi-gene assay that analyses the activity of 12 genes in breast cancer cells which include eight target genes, three housekeeper genes and one control gene. These genes are linked to the likelihood that the cancer will recur in another part of the body within 10 years after diagnosis. Several prospective-retrospective trials have validated the prognostic value of EndoPredict test [35]. A study comparing the 21-gene Oncotype DX Recurrence Score and EndoPredict score with respect to a 10 year breast cancer recurrence risk showed that EndoPredict test provided more prognostic information than Oncotype DX Recurrence Score [47].

6.4.2.7 Urokinase Plasminogen Activator and PAI-1

Urokinase plasminogen activator (uPA) and its inhibitor, PAI-1 are also among the best validated prognostic biomarkers for lymph node–negative breast cancer. High levels of these biomarkers in the tumor tissue imply faster growth of the tumor. These are however not used very widely. Several retrospective and prospective studies have shown the linkages between high concentrations of uPA and PAI-1 with poor outcomes in breast cancer patients [48].

A summary of key molecular tools for breast cancer detection and diagnosis is provided in Table 6.2.

Apart from the molecular diagnostic tools discussed above, **Next Generation Sequencing (NGS)** is another emerging area [49]. NGS allows for the sequencing of large numbers of genes in the tumor cells at the same platform and

Table 6.2 Key molecular tools for breast cancer detection and diagnosis

	Biomarker/assay	Component measured	Diagnosis method	Applicability
Hormone receptor based	Estrogen receptor and Progesterone receptor	Over-expression of estrogen receptor and progesterone receptor from tumor cells	Ligand binding assay (LBA) or immunohistochemical (IHC) assay	All stages
	HER2	HER2 gene over-expression to produce HER2	IHC and Fluorescence in situ Hybridization (FISH)	All stages
	HERmark™ assay	Total HER2 protein and functional HER2 homodimer levels		All stages
	Ki-67	Over-expression of Ki-67 antigen	Immunohistochemistry	
Gene expression based	Mammaprint™	70-gene expression profile	Microarray platform	Stage 1 or 2 invasive breast cancer
	Oncotype DX®	21-gene expression profile	qRT-PCR and microarray technologies	ER+, HER2-, node-negative and node-positive cancer, stage I and II, ductal carcinoma in situ
	Theros H/I℠ and MGI℠	Two-gene ratio and five-gene expression index	qRT-PCR	Stage 1, 2 and 3
	Prosigna breast cancer assay	Expression of fifty PAM50 genes and 8 housekeeping genes	Nucleic acid profiling platform	Postmenopausal women with HR+, node-negative (stage I or II) or node-positive (stage II) disease
	Genomic Grade Index	97-gene expression profile	Microarray platform	Grade 2 tumors
	EndoPredict	Analyses activity of 8 disease-relevant genes, 3 housekeeper genes and one control gene	PCR based	Patients newly diagnosed with early-stage, ER+, HER2-negative breast cancer

also in a single test to detect all possible genetic variations and mutations [32]. NGS allows for increased chances of discovery of new genes as biomarkers since numerous genes are being tested. Often referred to in cases where breast cancer is hereditary, NGS is cost effective and requires less time in comparison to single gene testing. NGS also provide systemic results with all tissue samples irrespective of ER/PR status. Similarly, **microRNA (miRNA) analysis** is another emerging molecular field that has also been reported to play a key role in providing prognostic and/or predictive information in breast cancer [50]. MicroRNAs are small noncoding RNAs which can act as tumor suppressor genes when they are dysregulated. Many miRNAs have been identified as potential biomarkers for breast cancer such as miR-21, miR-9, miR-10b, miR-335, miR-206 etc. [51]. Over recent years, nanoparticles are also being explored for their potential use in development of molecular-level diagnostics for breast cancer [52–54].

6.5 Exploring Proteomics Approach in Breast Cancer Diagnostics

The field of proteomics holds promise for the discovery of new biomarkers for early detection and diagnosis of disease. This is primarily because the cellular proteome is a complex and dynamic entity, which reflects the in vivo status of the cell. Moreover, proteomic technologies have enabled improved understanding of cellular proteins which may help infer trends in cell behaviors. Protein profiling is deemed to provide more information over those obtained by gene profiling. Analysis of protein profiles and deciphering the alterations of cellular proteins have been found to be useful in discovery of new biomarker entities, development of novel therapeutics approaches and assessment of protein level changes within the cell in response to drugs/treatment etc.

A variety of proteomic approaches such as 2D Polyacrylamide Gel Electrophoresis (PAGE), mass spectrometry; matrix assisted laser desorption ionization time of flight (MALDI-TOF), surface enhanced laser desorption ionization time of flight (SELDI-TOF), laser capture microdissection (LCM), etc. have been used in biomarker discovery [55–57].

Samples used for proteomic analysis in case of breast cancer patients range from body-tissue samples to biological fluids such as serum, plasma, saliva, nipple aspirate fluid (NAF) etc. Proteomic studies in samples from tumor and non-tumor sources have reported identification of biomarkers [58], but these have remained limited to research and have not been are yet not used commercially. It has been said that such studies often suffer from a low proteome coverage and low cohort size. Body fluids have also been explored as sources of biomarkers using the proteomic approach. Hudler et al. [59], in their review enlists several potential biomarkers for breast cancer that have been isolated from serum such as transferrins, epidermal growth factor receptor, fibronectins, apolipoproteins etc. In a recent study, functional proteomics was applied for identification of serum based biomarkers for breast cancer [60]. Two prospective clinical trials which were conducted to test and validate Videssa® Breast, a blood based combinatorial proteomic biomarker assay, showed that the assay was effective in detecting breast cancer for women under age of 50 [61]. Salivary biomarkers have also been examined as potential biomarkers for breast cancer using proteomic approaches [62]. NAF-based biomarkers offer great potential for developing newer screening strategies. Based on the differential levels of testosterone in NAF samples, these have been found to be a suitable biomarker to predict breast cancer risk [63]. Likewise proteomic analysis of urine as well as tear fluid have yielded evidences of proteins which could be identified as biomarkers for breast cancer [64, 65].

Protein-profiling studies using proteomics could eventually play important role in improving cancer patient outcome. Yet, there are limitations associated with proteomic analysis of samples such as heterogeneous composition of the tissue type which may have multiple cell types masking cancerous cells of interest, huge protein abundance in body fluid samples, protein denaturation during sample processing, low coverage etc., all of which may lead to false discovery. While these challenges can be addressed using experimental optimizations, it is worth mentioning that despite diagnostic, predictive or prognostic value of many proteins identified by proteomics, only very few have so far successfully entered into clinical stages for being considered for commercial use. This is primarily because biomarkers identified across such studies need to be further validated appropriately before being put to clinical use or patient care. Moreover, protein biomarkers identified by proteomic approaches do not provide any information pertaining to its cellular localization, leaving scope for further analysis.

6.6 Conclusion

The role of personalized and precise approaches for management of cancer to improve patient outcomes is gradually becoming increasingly more evident. New molecular diagnostic tools or assays for breast cancer have demonstrated some success not only because of their prognostic and predictive value but also for their simplified treatment protocols, thus enabling early breast cancer detection. Such tools are therefore likely to become the cornerstone of much envisaged personalized treatment models in the future. Newer "omics" based approaches, particularly proteomics, are also paving way for discovery of novel potential biomarkers in the field of breast cancer. It is however imperative that each molecular test or tool undergoes extensive clinical and analytical validations, so as to catalyze design of effective breast cancer treatments, and improved public health.

References

1. O'Connor CM, Adams JU. Essentials of cell biology. 2010. https://www.nature.com/scitable/ebooks/essentials-of-cell-biology-14749010/122997842. Accessed 2 Jan 2018.
2. World Health Organization. Cancer Factsheet. 2018. http://www.who.int/mediacentre/factsheets/fs297/en/. Accessed 2 Jan 2018.
3. Siegel RL, Miller KD, Jemal A. Cancer statistics, 2018. CA Cancer J Clin. 2018;68(1):7–30.
4. Torre LA, Bray F, Siegel RL, Ferlay J, Lortet-Tieulent J, Jemal A. Global cancer statistics, 2012. CA Cancer J Clin. 2015;65(2):87–108.
5. McPherson K, Steel C, Dixon JM. Breast cancer—epidemiology, risk factors, and genetics. BMJ. 2000;321(7261):624–8.
6. World Health Organization-International Agency for Research on Cancer. GLOBOCAN 2012: estimated cancer incidence, mortality and prevalence worldwide in 2012. 2012. http://globocan.iarc.fr/Pages/fact_sheets_cancer.aspx. Accessed 2 Jan 2018.
7. World Health Organization. Breast cancer. n.d. http://www.who.int/cancer/prevention/diagnosis-screening/breast-cancer/en/. Accessed 2 Jan 2018.
8. World Health Organization. Breast cancer: prevention and control. n.d. http://www.who.int/cancer/detection/breastcancer/en/. Accessed 2 Jan 2018.
9. Cancer Atlas. n.d. http://canceratlas.cancer.org/the-burden/cancer-in-southern-eastern-and-southeastern-asia/. Accessed 2 Jan 2018.
10. Malvia S, Bagadi SA, Dubey US, Saxena S. Epidemiology of breast cancer in Indian women. Asia Pac J Clin Oncol. 2017;13(4):289–95.
11. World Health Organization. Guide to cancer early diagnosis. 2017. http://apps.who.int/iris/bitstream/10665/254500/1/9789241511940-eng.pdf?ua=1. Accessed 2 Jan 2018.
12. Unger-Saldaña K. Challenges to the early diagnosis and treatment of breast cancer in developing countries. World J Clin Oncol. 2014;5(3):465–77.
13. da Costa Vieira RA, Biller G, Uemura G, Ruiz CA, Curado MP. Breast cancer screening in developing countries. Clinics. 2017;72(4):244–53.
14. Amoran OE, Toyobo OO. Predictors of breast self-examination as cancer prevention practice among women of reproductive age-group in a rural town in Nigeria. Niger Med J. 2015;56(3):185–9.
15. Hossain MS, Ferdous S, Karim-Kos HE. Breast cancer in South Asia: a Bangladeshi perspective. Cancer Epidemiol. 2014;38(5):465–70.
16. Madhu B, Shankar P. Awareness and screening behaviors of breast cancer among urban women in Mysuru, India-need for breast health education program. Int J Commun Med Publ Health. 2017;4(8):2967–72.
17. Arslan AA, Formenti SC. Mammography in developing countries: the risks associated with globalizing the experiences of the Western world. Nat Rev Clin Oncol. 2009;6(3):136–7.
18. Breast Cancer in Developing Countries. Lancet. 2009;374(9701):1567–2131.
19. Rizwan MM, Saadullah M. Lack of awareness about breast cancer and its screening in developing countries. Indian J Cancer. 2009;46(3):252–3.
20. Shtern F. Digital mammography and related technologies: a perspective from the National Cancer Institute. Radiology. 1992;183(3):629–30.
21. Drukteinis JS, Mooney BP, Flowers CI, Gatenby RA. Beyond mammography: new frontiers in breast cancer screening. Am J Med. 2013;126(6):472–9.

22. Carney PA, Miglioretti DL, Yankaskas BC, et al. Individual and combined effects of age, breast density, and hormone replacement therapy use on the accuracy of screening mammography. Ann Intern Med. 2003;138(3):168–75.
23. Vercher-Conejero JL, Pelegrí-Martinez L, Lopez-Aznar D, Cózar-Santiago MD. Positron emission tomography in breast cancer. Diagnostics. 2015;5(1):61–83.
24. Tatsumi M, Cohade C, Mourtzikos KA, Fishman EK, Wahl RL. Initial experience with FDG-PET/CT in the evaluation of breast cancer. Eur J Nucl Med Mol Imaging. 2006;33(3):254–62.
25. Evangelista L, Rita Cervino A. Nuclear imaging and early breast cancer detection. Curr Radiopharm. 2014;7(1):29–35.
26. Simanek M, Koranda P. SPECT/CT imaging in breast cancer-current status and challenges. Biomed Papers. 2016;160(4):474–83.
27. Sun Y, Wei W, Yang HW, Liu JL. Clinical usefulness of breast-specific gamma imaging as an adjunct modality to mammography for diagnosis of breast cancer: a systemic review and meta-analysis. Eur J Nucl Med Mol Imaging. 2013;40(3):450–63.
28. Rechtman LR, Lenihan MJ, Lieberman JH, Teal CB, Torrente J, Rapelyea JA, Brem RF. Breast-specific gamma imaging for the detection of breast cancer in dense versus nondense breasts. Am J Roentgenol. 2014;202(2):293–8.
29. Skaane P. Breast cancer screening with digital breast tomosynthesis. Breast Cancer. 2017;24(1):32–41.
30. Schwab M, editor. Encyclopedia of cancer. Berlin: Springer Science & Business Media; 2008.
31. De Abreu FB, Wells WA, Tsongalis GJ. The emerging role of the molecular diagnostics laboratory in breast cancer personalized medicine. Am J Pathol. 2013;183(4):1075–83.
32. Hagemann IS. Molecular testing in breast cancer: a guide to current practices. Arch Pathol Lab Med. 2016;140(8):815–24.
33. Zoon CK, Starker EQ, Wilson AM, Emmert-Buck MR, Libutti SK, Tangrea MA. Current molecular diagnostics of breast cancer and the potential incorporation of microRNA. Expert Rev Mol Diagn. 2009;9(5):455–66.
34. von Wahlde MK, Kurita T, Sanft T, Hofstatter E, Pusztai L. Clinical utility of emerging molecular diagnostics in breast cancer. Am J Hematol Oncol. 2016;12(2). http://www.gotoper.com/publications/ajho/2016/2016Feb/Clinical-Utility-of-Emerging-Molecular-Diagnostics-in-Breast-Cancer. Accessed 21 Jan 2018.
35. Duffy MJ, Harbeck N, Nap M, Molina R, Nicolini A, Senkus E, Cardoso F. Clinical use of biomarkers in breast cancer: Updated guidelines from the European Group on Tumor Markers (EGTM). Eur J Cancer. 2017;75:284–98.
36. Meng S, Tripathy D, Shete S, Ashfaq R, Haley B, Perkins S, Beitsch P, Khan A, Euhus D, Osborne C, Frenkel E. HER-2 gene amplification can be acquired as breast cancer progresses. Proc Natl Acad Sci U S A. 2004;101(25):9393–8.
37. Yardley DA, Kaufman PA, Huang W, Krekow L, Savin M, Lawler WE, Zrada S, Starr A, Einhorn H, Schwartzberg LS, Adams JW. Quantitative measurement of HER2 expression in breast cancers: comparison with 'real-world' routine HER2 testing in a multicenter Collaborative Biomarker Study and correlation with overall survival. Breast Cancer Res. 2015;17(1):41. https://doi.org/10.1186/s13058-015-0543-x.
38. Soliman NA, Yussif SM. Ki-67 as a prognostic marker according to breast cancer molecular subtype. Cancer Biol Med. 2016;13(4):496–504.
39. Yerushalmi R, Woods R, Ravdin PM, Hayes MM, Gelmon KA. Ki67 in breast cancer: prognostic and predictive potential. Lancet Oncol. 2010;11(2): 174–83.
40. Cronin M, Sangli C, Liu ML. Analytical validation of the Oncotype DX genomic diagnostic test for recurrence prognosis and therapeutic response prediction in node-negative, estrogen receptor-positive breast cancer. Clin Chem. 2007;53(6):1084–91.
41. Peethambaram PP, Hoskin TL, Day CN, Goetz MP, Habermann EB, Boughey JC. Use of 21-gene recurrence score assay to individualize adjuvant chemotherapy recommendations in ER+/HER2− node positive breast cancer—A National Cancer Database study. NPJ Breast Cancer. 2017;3(1):41. https://doi.org/10.1038/s41523-017-0044-4.
42. Ma XJ, Wang Z, Ryan PD, et al. A two-gene expression ratio predicts clinical outcome in breast cancer patients treated with tamoxifen. Cancer Cell. 2004;5(6):607–16.
43. Jansen MP, Sieuwerts AM, Look MP, et al. HOXB13-to-IL17BR expression ratio is related with tumor aggressiveness and response to tamoxifen of recurrent breast cancer: a retrospective study. J Clin Oncol. 2007;25(6):662–8.
44. Ma XJ, Salunga R, Dahiya S, et al. A five-gene molecular grade index and HOXB13:IL17BR are complementary prognostic factors in early stage breast cancer. Clin Cancer Res. 2008;14(9):2601–8.
45. Hequet D, Callens C, Gentien D, Albaud B, Mouret-Reynier MA, Dubot C, Cottu P, Huchon C, Zilberman S, Berseneff H, Foa C. Prospective, multicenter French study evaluating the clinical impact of the Breast Cancer Intrinsic Subtype-Prosigna® Test in the management of early-stage breast cancers. PLoS One. 2017;12(10):e0185753. https://doi.org/10.1371/journal.pone.0185753.
46. Lænkholm AV, Jensen MB, Eriksen JO, Rasmussen BB, Knoop AS, Buckingham W, Ferree S, Schaper C, Nielsen TO, Haffner T, Kibøl T. PAM50 risk of recurrence score predicts 10-year distant recurrence in a comprehensive Danish cohort of postmenopausal women allocated to 5 years of endocrine therapy for hormone receptor–positive early breast cancer. J Clin Oncol. 2018; https://doi.org/10.1200/JCO.2017.74.6586.
47. Buus R, Sestak I, Kronenwett R, Denkert C, Dubsky P, Krappmann K, Scheer M, Petry C, Cuzick J, Dowsett M. Comparison of EndoPredict and EPclin with oncotype DX recurrence score for prediction of risk

of distant recurrence after endocrine therapy. J Natl Cancer Inst. 2016;108(11) https://doi.org/10.1093/jnci/djw149.
48. Duffy MJ, McGowan PM, Harbeck N, Thomssen C, Schmitt M. uPA and PAI-1 as biomarkers in breast cancer: validated for clinical use in level-of-evidence-1 studies. Breast Cancer Res. 2014;16(4):428. https://doi.org/10.1186/s13058-014-0428-4.
49. Desmedt C, Voet T, Sotiriou C, Campbell PJ. Next generation sequencing in breast cancer: First take home messages. Curr Opin Oncol. 2012;24(6):597. https://doi.org/10.1097/CCO.0b013e328359554e.
50. Nassar FJ, Nasr R, Talhouk R. MicroRNAs as biomarkers for early breast cancer diagnosis, prognosis and therapy prediction. Pharmacol Ther. 2015;172:34–49.
51. Bertoli G, Cava C, Castiglioni I. MicroRNAs: new biomarkers for diagnosis, prognosis, therapy prediction and therapeutic tools for breast cancer. Theranostics. 2015;5(10):1122. https://doi.org/10.7150/thno.11543.
52. Saadeh Y, Leung T, Vyas A, Chaturvedi LS, Perumal O, Vyas D. Applications of nanomedicine in breast cancer detection, imaging, and therapy. J Nanosci Nanotechnol. 2014;14(1):913–23.
53. Sharma A, Jain N, Sareen R. Nanocarriers for diagnosis and targeting of breast cancer. Biomed Res Int. 2013;2013:960821. https://doi.org/10.1155/2013/960821.
54. Singh AK, Pandey A, Tewari M, Kumar R, Sharma A, Pandey HP, Shukla HS. Prospects of nano–material in breast cancer management. Pathol Oncol Res. 2013;19(2):155–65.
55. Baskin Y, Yigitbasi T. Clinical proteomics of breast cancer. Curr Genomics. 2012;11(7):528–36.
56. Bertucci F, Birnbaum D, Goncalves A. Proteomics of breast cancer principles and potential clinical applications. Mol Cell Proteomics. 2006;5(10):1772–86.
57. Gast MC, Schellens JH, Beijnen JH. Clinical proteomics in breast cancer: a review. Breast Cancer Res Treat. 2009;116(1):17–29.
58. Qin XJ, Ling BX. Proteomic studies in breast cancer. Oncol Lett. 2012;3(4):735–43.
59. Hudler P, Kocevar N, Komel R. Proteomic approaches in biomarker discovery: new perspectives in cancer diagnostics. Sci World J. 2014;2014 https://doi.org/10.1155/2014/260348.
60. Wang DL, Xiao C, Fu G, Wang X, Li L. Identification of potential serum biomarkers for breast cancer using a functional proteomics technology. Biomark Res. 2017;5(1):11. https://doi.org/10.1186/s40364-017-0092-9.
61. Lourenco AP, Benson KL, Henderson MC, Silver M, Letsios E, Tran Q, Gordon KJ, Borman S, Corn C, Mulpuri R, Smith W. A noninvasive blood-based combinatorial proteomic biomarker assay to detect breast cancer in women under the age of 50 years. Clin Breast Cancer. 2017;17(7):516–25.
62. Porto-Mascarenhas EC, Assad DX, Chardin H, Gozal D, Canto GD, Acevedo AC, Guerra EN. Salivary biomarkers in the diagnosis of breast cancer: a review. Crit Rev Oncol Hematol. 2017;110:62–73.
63. Shaheed SU, Tait C, Kyriacou K, Linforth R, Salhab M, Sutton C. Evaluation of nipple aspirate fluid as a diagnostic tool for early detection of breast cancer. Clin Proteomics. 2018;15(1):3. https://doi.org/10.1186/s12014-017-9179-4.
64. Beretov J, Wasinger VC, Millar EK, Schwartz P, Graham PH, Li Y. Proteomic analysis of urine to identify breast cancer biomarker candidates using a label-free LC-MS/MS approach. PLoS One. 2015;10(11):e0141876. https://doi.org/10.1371/journal.pone.0141876.
65. Lebrecht A, Boehm D, Schmidt M, Koelbl H, Schwirz RL, Grus FH. Diagnosis of breast cancer by tear proteomic pattern. Cancer Genomics Proteomics. 2009;6(3):177–82.

Molecular Diagnostics in Non-Hodgkin Lymphoma

7

Suraj Pratap and Teresa A. Scordino

7.1 Introduction

Non-Hodgkin lymphomas (NHLs) represent a heterogeneous group of malignancies that originate in B-lymphocytes, T-lymphocytes, or natural killer (NK) lymphocytes. In the developed world, B-cell lymphomas represent about 85% of all cases, T-cell lymphomas represent about 15% and NK lymphomas are very rare [1, 2]. Within the subset of B-cell lymphomas, diffuse large B-cell lymphoma (DLBCL) is the most prevalent subtype globally. According to the estimate by Surveillance, Epidemiology and End Results (SEER) program, a total of 72,240 new cases of NHL were diagnosed in USA in 2017. A recent study analyzed the data from the UK population-based Haematological Malignancy Research Network (HMRN) over a period of 8 years and found that the cumulative incidence of diffuse large B-cell lymphoma (DLBCL), follicular lymphoma (FL) and marginal zone lymphoma (MZL) was about three-fourths of all lymphomas [3] (Fig. 7.1). Cancer registries of developing nations, like India, show that their NHL patients tend to have relatively higher frequency of DLBCL, lower frequency of FL and T-cell lymphoma, and poorer performance statuses at diagnosis when compared to developed nations [4, 5]. Although there is geographical variation in the prevalence of individual subtypes of NHL it is indisputably a major cause of morbidity and mortality worldwide. Recent progress in molecular genetics has significantly deepened our understanding of the biology of this complex disease.

7.2 Clinical Presentation

NHLs present with widely varying signs and symptoms depending upon the subtype and areas of involvement. Some NHLs behave indolently with lymphadenopathy gradually enlarging over years, while others can be highly aggressive, causing life-threatening complications within weeks if left untreated. Indolent lymphomas typically evolve slowly, often presenting only with intermittent lymphadenopathy, hepatomegaly, splenomegaly, or cytopenias. Examples of indolent lymphomas include follicular lymphoma (FL), chronic lymphocytic leukemia (CLL)/ small lymphocytic lymphoma (SLL), and splenic marginal zone lymphoma (MZL). On the other

S. Pratap (✉)
Jimmy Everest Section of Pediatric Hematology-Oncology, University of Oklahoma Health Sciences Center, Oklahoma City, OK, USA
e-mail: Suraj-pratap@ouhsc.edu

T. A. Scordino
Department of Pathology, University of Oklahoma Health Sciences Center, Oklahoma City, OK, USA
e-mail: Teresa-Scordino@ouhsc.edu

K. K. Shukla et al. (eds.), *Molecular Diagnostics in Cancer Patients*,
https://doi.org/10.1007/978-981-13-5877-7_7

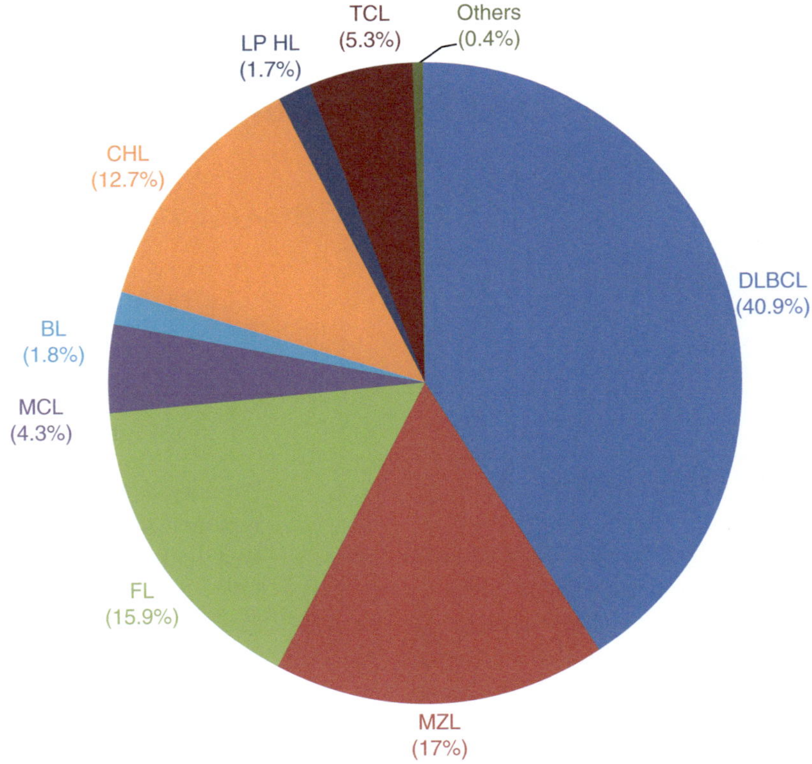

PREVALENCE OF LYMPHOMAS

Fig. 7.1 Incidence of lymphomas from 2004 to 2012 determined from the UK's population-based Haematological Malignancy Research Network (*DLBCL* diffuse large B cell lymphoma, *MZL* marginal zone lymphoma, *FL* follicular lymphoma, *MCL* Mantle cell lymphoma, *BL* Burkitt lymphoma, *CHL* classical Hodgkin lymphoma, *LP HL* lymphocyte predominant Hodgkin lymphoma, *TCL* T cell Lymphoma)

hand, aggressive lymphomas become symptomatic relatively quickly, often present with rapidly growing masses, with variable systemic B symptoms (fever, night sweats, weight loss), and may have elevation in serum lactate dehydrogenase (LDH) and uric acid. Lymphomas that generally have aggressive presentations include diffuse large B-cell lymphoma (DLBCL), Burkitt lymphoma (BL), adult T-cell leukemia/lymphoma, and B and T lymphoblastic leukemia/lymphoma. It is important to point out that the natural history of these tumors shows significant patient-to-patient variability.

About half of all the patients develop secondary extranodal disease and up to a third have primary extranodal lymphoma at diagnosis [6]. Presenting symptoms are generally nonspecific but can, at times, point to the location of primary tumor. Anorexia, malabsorption, vomiting, abdominal pain, bowel obstruction, or even acute perforations have been seen in patients with primary gastrointestinal lymphoma. Patients with primary lymphoma of the central nervous system (CNS) can present with headaches, lethargy, focal neurologic deficits, paralysis, seizures, aseptic meningitis or other symptoms of raised intracranial pressure. Uncommon presentations include skin rash, pruritus, hypersensitivity to insect bites, fever of unknown origin, and effusions.

Occasionally NHL can present with oncologic emergencies that may require immediate interventions. These can include tumor lysis syndrome, spinal cord compression, pericardial tamponade, superior vena cava syndrome, venous thromboembolism, hypercalcemia, hyperleukocytosis, acute airway obstruction, CNS mass lesions, intestinal obstruction and acute renal injury due to ureteral obstruction. Some patients with NHL can develop an acquired form of C1 inhibitor deficiency causing angioedema that may require treatment with infused C1 inhibitor concentrates. The potential for these emergent complications depend on the size, type and location of the primary tumor. The oncologist must keep these in consideration during the initial workup and evaluation as any delay in either their recognition or prompt implementation of corrective measures can have grave consequences.

7.3 Initial Evaluation

7.3.1 Laboratory Investigations

The laboratory investigations used to diagnose NHL include testings performed in hematology, chemistry, flow cytometry, cytogenetics, molecular diagnostics, and histology. Complete blood counts and basic electrolytes are generally within their age appropriate reference ranges early in the disease. As the disease progresses, it can infiltrate into the bone marrow leading to anemia, thrombocytopenia, leukopenia or pancytopenia in the patients. Occasionally lymphocytosis with circulating malignant cells and thrombocytosis can also be seen. Blood chemistries can show an elevated lactate dehydrogenase (LDH) and uric acid levels. If tumor burden is high or tumor lysis is ongoing, patients may develop hyperkalemia, hyperphosphatemia as well as hypercreatininemia due to renal involvement. Abnormal liver function tests that occur secondary to hepatic involvement can be also seen in advanced disease. Association of different types of NHL with monoclonal gammopathy, positive Coomb's test, or hypogammaglobulinemia was also found in some studies [7]. In patients where diagnosis is in question, appropriate tests to exclude other common ailments should be done. Such a workup depends on the type of lymphoma, site of the tumor and sometimes on geographical prevalence of other disease. It can consist of, but is not limited to, HIV serology, TB testing, serological tests for endemic mycoses, et cetera.

7.3.2 Histology

A well-processed hematoxylin and eosin (H&E) stained section of the excised mass is still the gold standard for confirming a diagnosis of NHL. The biopsy must be obtained urgently if an aggressive NHL is suspected and the evaluation should be performed by a hematopathologist or a pathologist with expertise in this field. The morphological features of NHL depend on the subtype and the site where the malignant lympho-proliferation begins. The abnormal lymphocytes in the tumor can be categorized as small, intermediate or large cells, cleaved or non-cleaved and can have a follicular or diffuse pattern. Figure 7.2a, b show typical histological appearances of some of the common non-Hodgkin lymphoma subtypes.

It is important to mention here that statistically, most patients presenting with enlarged lymph nodes have benign reactive lymphadenopathy. Many centers therefore routinely use fine needle aspiration as an initial screening test. FNA can be a useful tool for distinguishing reactive processes from clonal mature B-cell neoplasms when coupled with comprehensive immunophenotyping. However, apart from these selected situations where FNA can aid in confirming the presence of malignancy, the general consensus is that a precise histopathologic evaluation of lymphoma requires an intact tissue biopsy and not a needle aspiration [8–10].

Immunophenotyping of lymphoma cells has become a standard practice all over the world. This is done either by immunohistochemistry on sections of fixed tissues or by flow cytometry conducted on fresh unfixed single cell suspensions. Thanks to the advances in immunohistochemistry, a pathologist can now detect almost all diagnostically relevant lymphoid markers in formalin-fixed paraffin-embedded tissues. A notable exception is that stains for surface immunoglobulin light chains, which are helpful in determining the clonality of B-cell proliferations, are challenging and are best evaluated by flow cytometry. For genetic and molecular studies, fresh frozen tissues are probably the best source of high quality DNA and RNA although many of these tests can now be conducted on formalin-fixed paraffin-embedded tissues as well. A list of common stains used in immunohistochemical staining of NHL is given in Table 7.1.

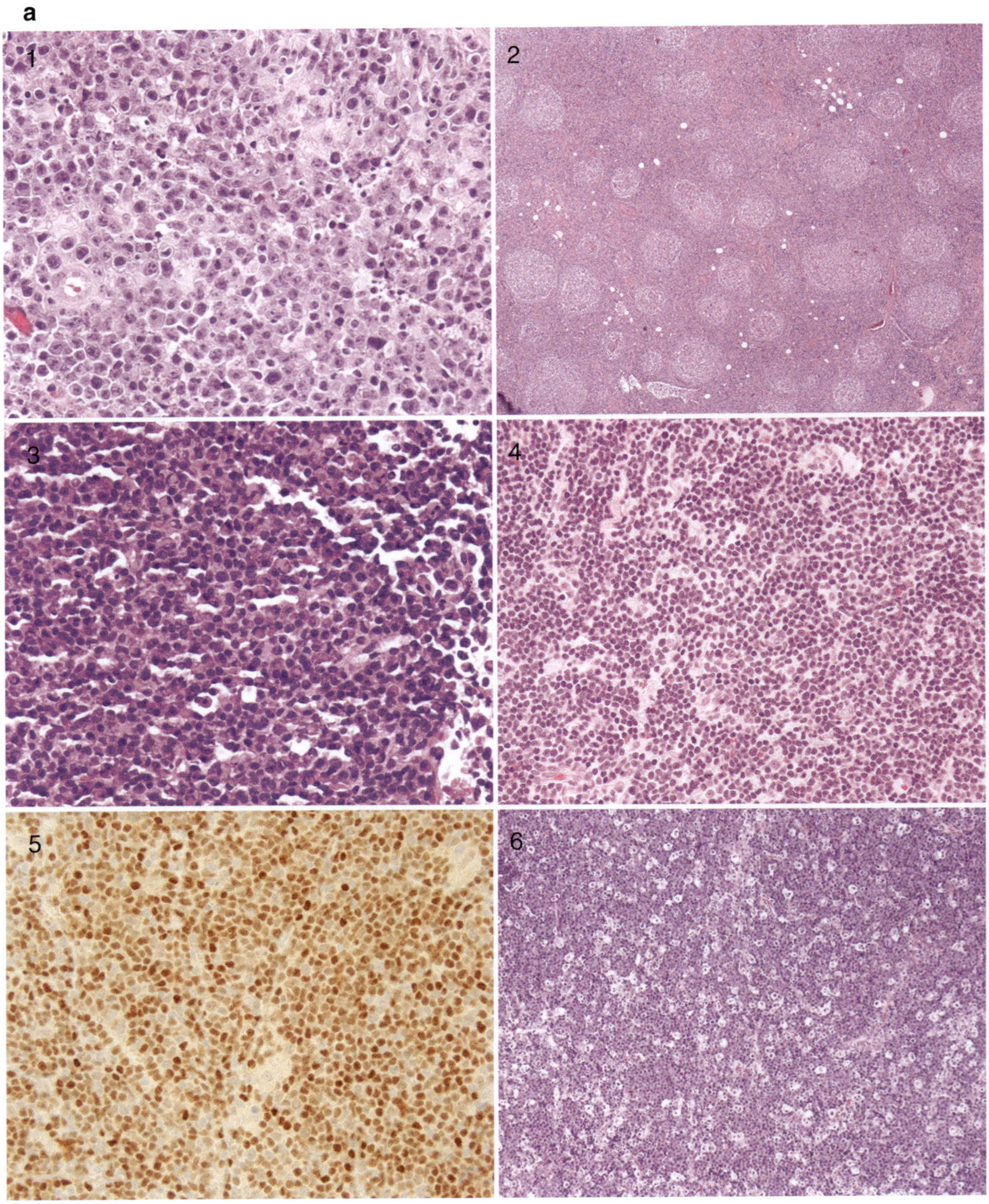

Fig. 7.2 (**a**) Histological images of some common Non-Hodgkin Lymphomas 1. Diffuse large B-cell lymphoma (H&E, 400×) 2. Follicular lymphoma (H&E, 100×) 3. Extranodal marginal zone lymphoma of breast with prominent plasmacytic differentiation (H&E, 400×) 4. Mantle cell lymphoma (H&E, 400×) 5. Mantle cell lymphoma (Cyclin D1 stain, 400×) 6. High grade B-cell lymphoma (H&E, 100×). (**b**) Histological images of some common Non-Hodgkin Lymphomas 7. Burkitt lymphoma (H&E, 400×) 8. Burkitt lymphoma (Wright-Giemsa, 1000×) 9. Chronic lymphocytic leukemia (Wright, 400×) 10. Anaplastic large cell lymphoma (H&E, 400×) 11. Anaplastic large cell lymphoma (ALK stain, 400×) 12. Hairy cell leukemia (Wright, 1000×)

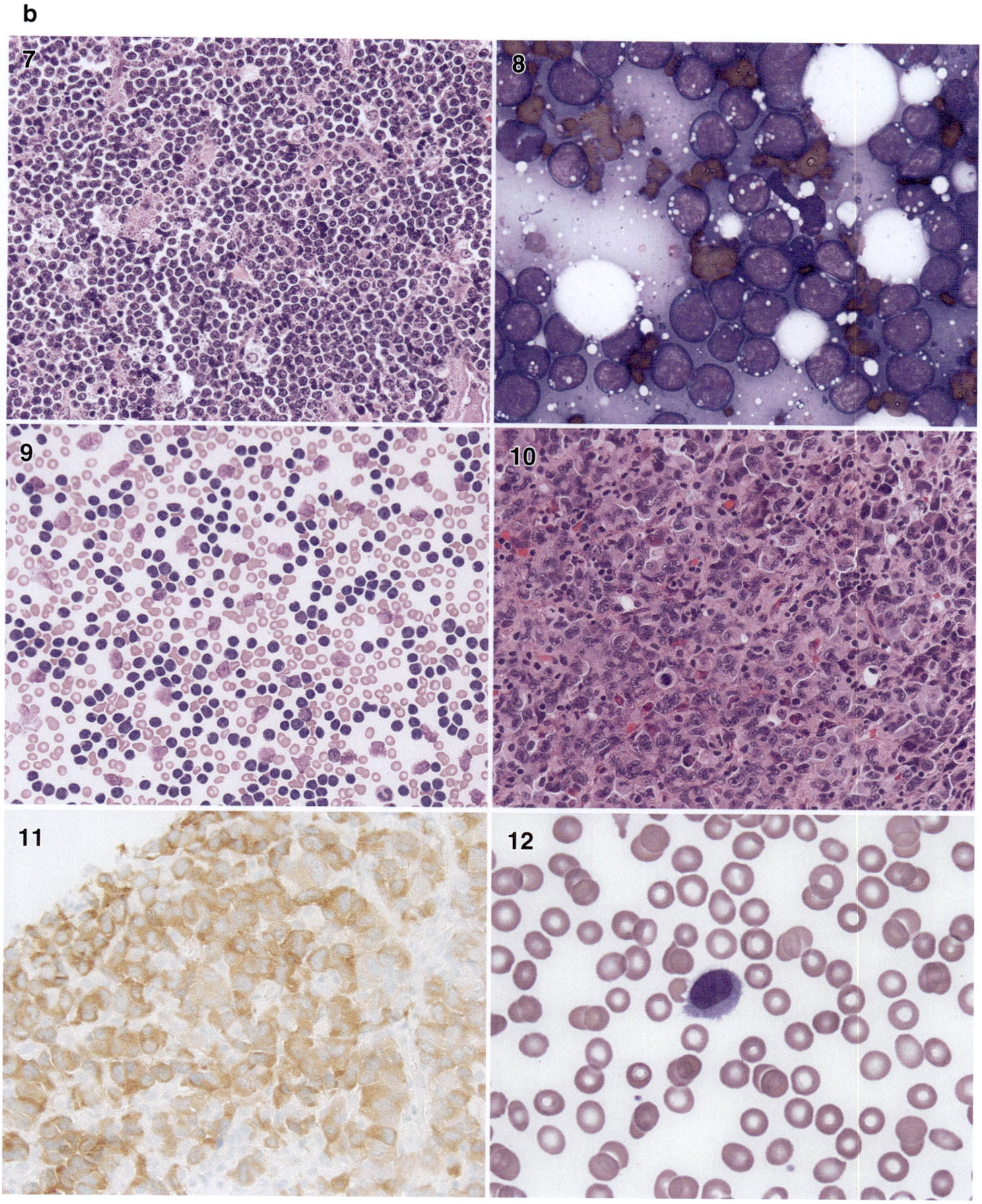

Fig. 7.2 (continued)

Table 7.1 Immunophenotype and cytogenetic features of common NHL types

Common types of lymphoma	Immunophenotype and cytogenetics
Diffuse large B-cell lymphoma (DLBCL), NOS	PanB+, surface or cytoplasmic IGM > IGG > IGA, CD45+/–, CD5–/+, CD10+/–, BCL6 +/–, 3q27 region abnormalities involving *BCL6* seen in 30% of cases, t(14;18) involving BCL2 seen in 20–30% of cases, *MYC* rearrangement seen in 10% of cases
Follicular lymphoma (FL)	sIG+ (usually IGM +/– IGD, IGG, IGA), PanB+, CD10+/–, CD5–/+, CD23–/+, CD43-, CD11c-, CD25-; overexpression of BCL2+ (useful to distinguish from reactive follicles), BCL6+; *IGH* and *IGL* gene rearrangements, t(14;18)(q32;q21) with rearranged *BCL2* gene (70–95% in adults)
Primary mediastinal (Thymic) large B-cell lymphoma	sIG–/+, PanB+, (especially CD20, CD79a), CD45+/–, CD15-, CD30–/+ (weak), IRF4/MUM1 +/–, BCL2+/–, BCL6+/–, CD23+, MAL+; *IGH* and *IGL* gene rearrangements, translocations of *CIITA* with *PDL1* and *PDL2*, gains of 9p24.1 (*JAK2/PDL1/PDL2*), gains of 2p16.1 (*REL* and *BCL11A);* gene expression profiling similarities with classical Hodgkin lymphoma
Extranodal marginal zone lymphoma of MALT	sIG+ (IGM or IGA or IGG), sIGD-, cIG–/+, PanB+, CD5-, CD10-, CD23-, CD43–/+; IGH and IGL gene rearrangements, trisomy 3 or t(11;18)(q21;q21) and other translocations may be present.
Mantle cell lymphoma (MCL)	sIGM+, sIGD+, lambda>kappa, PanB+, CD5+, CD10–/+, CD23-, CD43+, CD11c-, CD25-, cyclin D1+; IGH and IGL gene rearrangements, t(11;14)(q13;q32); *CCND1* gene rearrangements (cyclinD1) common
Burkitt lymphoma (BL)	sIGM+, PanB+, CD5-, CD10+, BCL6+, CD38+, CD77+, CD43+, CD23-; Ki-67 (95–100%), BCL2-; TdT-, IGH and IGL gene rearrangements, t(8;14)(q24;q32) and variants t(2;8)(p12;q24) and t(8;22)(q24;q11); rearranged *MYC* gene; EBV common (95%) in endemic cases and infrequent (15–20%) in sporadic cases, intermediate incidence (30–40%) in HIV-positive cases
Hairy cell leukemia (HCL)	sIG+ (IGM, IGD, IGG, or IGA), PanB+, CD79a+, CD79b-, DBA44+, CD123+, CD5-, CD10-, CD23-, CD11c+, CD25+, FMC7+, CD103+ (mucosal lymphocyte antigen as detected by B-ly7), TRAP+; *IGH* and *IGL* gene rearrangements, *BRAF* V600E mutation, no specific cytogenetic findings
Lymphoplasmacytic lymphoma (LPL)	sIGM+, sIGD–/+, cIG+, PanB+, CD19+, CD20+, CD138+ (in plasma cells), CD79a+, CD5-, CD10-, CD43+/–, CD25–/+; *IGH* and *IGL* gene rearrangements, no specific cytogenetic findings, *MYD88* L265P mutation
Chronic lymphocytic leukemia (CLL)/small lymphocytic lymphoma (SLL)	Faint sIGM+, sIGD+/–, cIG–/+, panB+ (CD19+, CD20+), CD5+, CD10-, CD23+, CD43+, CD11c–/+; *IGH* and *IGL* gene rearrangements; trisomy 12; del 13q, del(17p), or del(11q) can be seen
High-grade B-cell lymphoma	sIG +/–, PanB+, CD10+, BCL6+, BCL2–/+, IRF4/MUM1-, Ki-67 (50–100%), 8q24/*MYC* translocation with *BCL2* translocation and/or BCL6 translocation (so-called "double-hit" or "triple hit" lymphoma); complex karyotypes, *TP53* mutations
B-cell lymphoma, unclassifiable, with features intermediate between DLBCL and classical Hodgkin lymphoma	CD45+/–, CD20+/–, CD79a+/–, CD30+/–, CD15+/–, PAX-5+/–, OCT-2+/–, BOB.1+/–, CD10–, ALK–, gains/amplifications of *JAK2* and *PDL2* loci at 9p24.1, gains / amplifications of *REL* (2p16.1), breaks in *CIITA* locus (16p13.13), gains of *MYC*
Anaplastic large cell lymphoma, ALK positive	CD30+, ALK+, EMA+/–, CD3–/+, CD2+/–, CD4+/–, CD5+/–, CD8–/+, CD43+/–, CD25+, CD45+/–, CD45RO+/–, TIA1+/–, granzyme+/–, perforin+/–, EBV-, TCR gene rearrangements+/–, t(2;5)(p23;35) in 80% of cases, t(1;2)(q25;p23) in 10–15% of cases. Other variant *ALK* translocations can also be seen.

Table 7.1 (continued)

Common types of lymphoma	Immunophenotype and cytogenetics
Anaplastic large cell lymphoma, ALK negative	CD30+ (strong/intense staining), CD2+/−, CD3+/−, CD5−/+, CD4+/−, CD8−/+, CD43+, TIA1+/−, granzyme B+/−, perforin +/−, ALK−, TCR gene rearrangements +, *DUSP22* rearrangements (30%), *TP63* rearrangements (8%).
Peripheral T-cell lymphoma, NOS	PanT variable (CD2+/−, CD3+/−, CD5−/+, CD7−/+), most cases CD4+, some cases CD8+, a few cases are CD4−/CD8−, or CD4+/CD8+; TCR gene rearrangements+
Angioimmunoblastic T-cell lymphoma	PanT+, CD4+, TFH markers (CD10/ICOS/CXCL13/BCL6/PD1) in 60–100%, EBV+ B-cell proliferation may be present, TCR gene rearrangement +, IG gene rearrangements in ~30%; mutations in *IDH2, TET2, DNMT3A, CLTA4-CD28* fusions may be present

Use of flow cytometry has become a fundamental step in the diagnosis and classification of most forms of NHL. It offers some unique advantages such as rapid turnaround, higher sensitivity, ability to detect multiple markers simultaneously and the option to apply a standard panel and diagnostic algorithms to samples. Since lymphoid neoplasms are divided according to their derivation (B, T, or NK cell) the expression of lymphoid differentiation antigens on the cell surface is an efficient way to distinguish between B and T-cells at various developmental stages.

Bone marrow aspirations are primarily performed for assessing the extent of the disease but occasionally they can be important for primary immunophenotypic, cytogenetic and molecular investigations. The aspiration is often accompanied with a trephine biopsy which may aid in the diagnosis of NHL, particularly the marrow infiltrating low-grade lymphoma. Apart from being an important part of the staging procedure, marrow aspirations and biopsies are also useful for assessing the response to treatment. In rare cases it is possible that the lymph node biopsy is not available, either because the primary tumor could not be identified or it is not easily accessible, and assessment of bone marrow infiltration may be the only mode to establish a precise diagnosis.

7.3.3 Radiology

Imaging studies are an essential part of the workup of NHL patients. Apart from providing vital information about the extent of disease, they may sometimes help identify the optimum site for biopsy. A positron emission tomography (PET) with computed tomography (CT) is the preferred modality for majority of patients since most NHLs are Fluorodeoxyglucose (FDG)-avid. Less commonly, for FDG-non avid lymphomas (chronic lymphocytic leukemia, lymphoplasmacytic lymphoma, mycosis fungoides, and marginal zone lymphoma) CT alone is preferred.

PET scan works by differential uptake of FDG by the lymphoma cells (and other metabolically active tissues like sites of infection or inflammation) versus the normal tissue. By superimposing the FDG avidity on the images obtained by CT scan the quality of data is further augmented. Whether a particular site is considered positive or negative on PET scan is determined by the using a 5-point scale (Deauville score). Using a standardized scale to convert visual data to numeric scale allows the interpretation and comparison of scans done at different time points during therapy. It also minimizes the variability due to use of different scanning machines at different centers. PET scans are generally considered highly sensitive and specific for detecting NHL in nodal and extranodal sites, albeit less reliable for assessment of marrow disease. In certain situations where meticulous visualization of the tumor bed is important for surgeons, a dedicated contrast-enhanced CT scan or magnetic resonance imaging (MRI) may be required in addition to the PET/CT scan. PET scans performed at diagnosis serve as a crucial baseline image with which all future scans are compared. The importance of this imaging modality is evident by the fact that most new treatment protocols have incorporated PET scans at initial presentation, at interim time points, at the end of therapy and even for long term follow up. Indeed the increasing availability and relative convenience of this powerful imaging modality has greatly enhanced the ability of an oncologist to identify poorly responding patients much earlier than by conventional histological means. This in turn should translate into better outcomes since the ability to accurately monitor response to treatment is crucial to select patients who require intensification of therapy.

7.4 Diagnosis

The first step in the management of any patient with NHL is obtaining a detailed medical history, thorough clinical examination, analysis of the blood smear and results of laboratory and radiological investigations. Once these preliminary evaluations are complete the most important next step is to establish an accurate pathologic diagnosis. The basic initial pathologic assessment is similar to other solid tumors and involves an incisional or excisional lymph node biopsy to establish the diagnosis of NHL. As previously mentioned, core needle biopsies and fine needle aspiration (FNA) biopsies are discouraged unless warranted by the patient's clinical status, as they are ineffective in elucidating the microarchitecture of the tissue. The 2017 NCCN guidelines recommend that FNA results alone should not be used for making an initial diagnosis of NHL, although they may be sufficient to establish relapse [11]. However, in practice, often the selection of initial biopsy technique is governed by other parameters like the clinical status of the patient or accessibility of the tumor and a combination of core biopsy and FNA in conjunction with ancillary techniques (polymerase chain reaction for gene rearrangements and florescence in-situ hybridization for major translocations) is a plausible option to reach a diagnosis. This is truer for certain subtypes of NHL, like small lymphocytic lymphoma, than others like follicular lymphoma.

Immunophenotypic analysis has now become mandatory for diagnosis and classification of NHL and may also provide information about prognosis and potential therapeutic targets. It can be performed using flow cytometry and immunohistochemistry depending on the antigenic expression of the suspected lymphoma, availability of antibodies and the expertise of hematopathologist. Cytogenetic and molecular genetic analysis may be necessary under certain circumstances, to identify the recurrent chromosomal translocations that have been shown to be associated with certain subtypes of NHL.

The availability of next generation sequencing (NSG) and gene expression profiling (GEP) has led to the discovery of novel oncogenic pathways involved in the process of malignant transformation. Deeper analysis of these molecular mechanisms have helped identify many new lymphoma subtypes that were histologically considered indistinguishable. Understanding the nuances of molecular lymphomagenesis and distinguishing the subtypes of NHL has now begin to translate into clinical gains as we are now able to better predict the outcomes of distinct subtypes that were once considered same and tailor the therapy accordingly. It is anticipated that in time, NSG and GEP will become routine applications which will help further refine the classification and treatment of malignant lymphomas.

7.5 Classification

The classification of NHL has undergone significant changes over the years and it continues to be a topic of scientific and clinical discussion. Developed in 1960s, one of the earliest classifications, the Rappaport system used growth patterns (diffuse vs. nodular) and cytology (undifferentiated vs. differentiated) as the basic criteria for disease definitions [12]. A plethora of classification systems using either histology, anatomy or spread of the disease were popular in different parts of the world at different times. In fact one of the reasons why clinical trials from different regions could not be compared in that era was because of vastly different disease classifications. It was not until 1990s that the International Lymphoma Study Group undertook a major effort to overcome this conundrum and to create a uniform classification of NHL based on on biologic principles, called the Revised European-American Classification of Lymphoid Neoplasms (REAL) classification [13]. The REAL classification then paved way for the WHO classification of tumors of the hematopoietic and lymphoid tissues produced in 2002 (revised in 2008 and 2016) which is the most extensively used classification system at present [1, 14]. The WHO classification divides lymphomas according to the lineage (B, T, or NK cell) and then further stratifies the subtypes within each lineage based on a combination of morphology, immunophenotype, genetic features, and clinical features (Table 7.2). For practical purposes oncologists also group NHL subtypes based

Table 7.2 WHO classification of hematological malignancies

Mature B-cell neoplasms
Chronic lymphocytic leukemia/small lymphocytic lymphoma
Monoclonal B-cell lymphocytosis[a]
B-cell prolymphocytic leukemia
Splenic marginal zone lymphoma
Hairy cell leukemia
Splenic B-cell lymphoma/leukemia, unclassifiable
Splenic diffuse red pulp small B-cell lymphoma
Hairy cell leukemia-variant
Lymphoplasmacytic lymphoma
Waldenström macroglobulinemia
Monoclonal gammopathy of undetermined significance (MGUS), IgM[a]
μ heavy-chain disease
γ heavy-chain disease
α heavy-chain disease
Monoclonal gammopathy of undetermined significance (MGUS), IgG/A[a]
Plasma cell myeloma
Solitary plasmacytoma of bone
Extraosseous plasmacytoma
Monoclonal immunoglobulin deposition diseases[a]
Extranodal marginal zone lymphoma of mucosa-associated lymphoid tissue (MALT lymphoma)
Nodal marginal zone lymphoma
Pediatric nodal marginal zone lymphoma
Follicular lymphoma
In situ follicular neoplasia[a]
Duodenal-type follicular lymphoma[a]
Pediatric-type follicular lymphoma[a]
Large B-cell lymphoma with IRF4 rearrangement[a]
Primary cutaneous follicle center lymphoma
Mantle cell lymphoma
In situ mantle cell neoplasia[a]
Diffuse large B-cell lymphoma (DLBCL), NOS
Germinal center B-cell type[a]
Activated B-cell type[a]
T-cell/histiocyte-rich large B-cell lymphoma
Primary DLBCL of the central nervous system (CNS)

(continued)

Table 7.2 (continued)

Primary cutaneous DLBCL, leg type
EBV⁺ DLBCL, NOS[a]
EBV+ mucocutaneous ulcer[a]
DLBCL associated with chronic inflammation
Lymphomatoid granulomatosis
Primary mediastinal (thymic) large B-cell lymphoma
Intravascular large B-cell lymphoma
ALK⁺ large B-cell lymphoma
Plasmablastic lymphoma
Primary effusion lymphoma
HHV8+ DLBCL, NOS[a]
Burkitt lymphoma
Burkitt-like lymphoma with 11q aberration[a]
High-grade B-cell lymphoma, with *MYC* and *BCL2* and/or *BCL6* rearrangements[a]
High-grade B-cell lymphoma, NOS[a]
B-cell lymphoma, unclassifiable, with features intermediate between DLBCL and classical Hodgkin lymphoma
Mature T and NK neoplasms
T-cell prolymphocytic leukemia
T-cell large granular lymphocytic leukemia
Chronic lymphoproliferative disorder of NK cells
Aggressive NK-cell leukemia
Systemic EBV⁺ T-cell lymphoma of childhood[a]
Hydroa vacciniforme–like lymphoproliferative disorder[a]
Adult T-cell leukemia/lymphoma
Extranodal NK–/T-cell lymphoma, nasal type
Enteropathy-associated T-cell lymphoma
Monomorphic epitheliotropic intestinal T-cell lymphoma[a]
Indolent T-cell lymphoproliferative disorder of the GI tract[a]
Hepatosplenic T-cell lymphoma
Subcutaneous panniculitis-like T-cell lymphoma
Mycosis fungoides
Sézary syndrome
Primary cutaneous CD30⁺ T-cell lymphoproliferative disorders
Lymphomatoid papulosis
Primary cutaneous anaplastic large cell lymphoma
Primary cutaneous γδ T-cell lymphoma
Primary cutaneous CD8+ aggressive epidermotropic cytotoxic T-cell lymphoma
Primary cutaneous acral CD8+ T-cell lymphoma[a]
Primary cutaneous CD4+ small/medium T-cell lymphoproliferative disorder[a]
Peripheral T-cell lymphoma, NOS
Angioimmunoblastic T-cell lymphoma
Follicular T-cell lymphoma[a]
Nodal peripheral T-cell lymphoma with TFH phenotype[a]
Anaplastic large-cell lymphoma, ALK⁺
Anaplastic large-cell lymphoma, ALK⁻[a]
Breast implant–associated anaplastic large-cell lymphoma[a]
Hodgkin lymphoma
Nodular lymphocyte predominant Hodgkin lymphoma
Classical Hodgkin lymphoma
Nodular sclerosis classical Hodgkin lymphoma
Lymphocyte-rich classical Hodgkin lymphoma
Mixed cellularity classical Hodgkin lymphoma
Lymphocyte-depleted classical Hodgkin lymphoma

Table 7.2 (continued)

Posttransplant lymphoproliferative disorders (PTLD)
Plasmacytic hyperplasia PTLD
Infectious mononucleosis PTLD
Florid follicular hyperplasia PTLD[a]
Polymorphic PTLD
Monomorphic PTLD (B- and T-/NK-cell types)
Classical Hodgkin lymphoma PTLD
Histiocytic and dendritic cell neoplasms
Histiocytic sarcoma
Langerhans cell histiocytosis
Langerhans cell sarcoma
Indeterminate dendritic cell tumor
Interdigitating dendritic cell sarcoma
Follicular dendritic cell sarcoma
Fibroblastic reticular cell tumor
Disseminated juvenile xanthogranuloma
Erdheim-Chester disease[a]

Provisional entities are listed in italics
[a]Changes from the 2008 classification

on the speed of disease progression. Aggressive lymphomas constitute about 60% of all NHLs with diffuse large B-cell lymphoma (DLBCL) being the most common type. Indolent lymphomas have a tendency to grow slower, remain asymptomatic for a longer time and are often diagnosed late. They represent about 40 percent of all NHL cases with follicular lymphoma (FL) being the commonest type of indolent NHL.

7.6 Staging

One of the most widely used staging system for NHL is the Ann Arbor staging. While originally developed for staging of Hodgkin lymphoma almost half a century ago, it forms the basis of anatomic staging in non-Hodgkin Lymphomas as well. It has undergone many modifications over past four decades with the Cotswolds modification in 1988 being the most prominent one (Table 7.3). Despite remaining a popular staging system for Non-Hodgkin lymphoma, the Ann Arbor system has a number of shortcomings. Most of these are due to the inherent difference in the clinical features between NHL and HL. For example, the Ann-Arbor classification subdivides patients according to the absence (A) or presence (B) of disease-related symptoms. While such a stratification may have relevance for Hodgkin lymphoma most clinicians will agree that such a distinction is often absent in NHL. Another example is the primary extranodal disease which is rare in HL but frequently seen in certain types of NHLs. The increased use of systemic and multimodality approaches has also reduced the role of Ann Arbor stage as a determinant of therapy.

Due to these reasons the 11th International Conference on Malignant Lymphoma in Lugano recommended modifications to the Ann Arbor staging system [15]. The fundamental change was the use prognosis and risk factors as the primary determinant of the stage and removal of designations like A, B or X (bulky disease). Basically the Stages I and II are now considered as limited forms of disease while Stages III and IV are considered advanced disease. PET-CT scans are used to ascertain the extent of disease for FDG-avid lymphomas while CT alone suffices for non-avid histologies. Stage II bulky disease can be treated as either limited or advanced disease based on histology and associated prognostic factors.

Table 7.3 Ann Arbor Classification of lymphomas with Cotswolds Modifications

Stage	Features
I	Involvement of a single lymph node region or lymphoid structure
II	Involvement of two or more lymph node regions on the same side of the diaphragm
III	Involvement of lymph regions or structures on both sides of the diaphragm
IV	Involvement of extranodal site(s) beyond that designated as 'E'
For all stages	
A	No symptoms
B	Fever (≥38 °C), night sweats, weight loss (≥10% body weight over 6 months)
For stages I to III	
E	Involvement of a single, extranodal site contiguous or proximal to known nodal site
Cotswolds modifications	Massive mediastinal disease has been defined as maximum transverse mass diameter greater than or equal to one-third of the internal transverse thoracic diameter measured at the T5/T6 intervertebral disc level on chest radiography. The number of anatomic regions involved should be indicated by a subscript (e.g., II_3). Stage III may be subdivided into: III_1, with or without splenic, hilar, celiac, or portal nodes; III_2, with Para-aortic, iliac, mesenteric nodes. Staging should be identified as clinical stage (CS) or pathologic stage (PS). A new category of response to therapy, unconfirmed/uncertain complete remission (CR) can be introduced because of the persistent radiologic abnormalities of uncertain significance.

7.7 Pathological Features

Malignant cells share some biological, histological and immunophenotypic features with the normal cells belonging to their respective lineages. The same is true for lymphomas which are derived from B and T lymphocytes or NK cells at varying stages of maturation. This grouping, however, is far from being black-and-white, as some NHLs derived from different cells or at different stages of maturation are classified in the same category. Also, for some NHL subtypes there may be no identified cell of origin (like hairy cell leukemia). Another instance of such lack of distinction is seen in cases of some NK/T-cell lymphomas that share immunophenotypic and functional features with NK cells as well as T lymphocytes [16].

B-cell lymphomas can arise from any stage of B-lymphocyte development. B-cells originate in the bone marrow as progenitor cells and then migrate to secondary lymphoid organs (lymph nodes, spleen) where they are exposed to antigens. A subset of these mature B-cells migrate to the germinal centers of lymphoid organs while a smaller number of cells are released into the peripheral blood. Naive mature B-cells in the mantle zone are thought to give rise to mantle cell lymphomas while antigen-exposed B-cells in the germinal center give rise to germinal center B-cell (GCB) lymphomas and follicular lymphomas. As the name suggests marginal zone lymphoma arises from B-cells residing in the marginal zone (Fig. 7.3). Plasmablasts are thought to give rise to activated B-cell (ABC) like diffuse large B-cell lymphoma and plasma cells give rise to multiple myeloma. T-cell and NK-cell lymphomas can also arise from any stage of normal T or NK cell development. For cases in which this distinction is unclear, the term 'NK/T-cell' NHL is used. The prothymocytes originate in bone marrow and produce lymphoid progenitors that travel to the thymus and mature to become antigen-naïve T-cells. NK cells originate in the bone marrow and travel to the spleen, mucosa, and peripheral blood without transiting through the thymus. Thymic T-cells are thought to give rise to lymphoblastic T-cell NHLs while post-thymic T-cells and NK cells are thought to give rise to the other peripheral T-cell NHLs.

Molecular techniques like florescence microscopy, DNA amplification, next generation sequencing, gene expression profiling, and cytogenetic testing have become integral to lymphoma evaluation. While morphological assessment is still the basis of the lymphoma diagnosis, ancillary studies are now needed in most cases. Molecular genetic abnormalities are ubiquitous in hematological malignancies. However, unlike

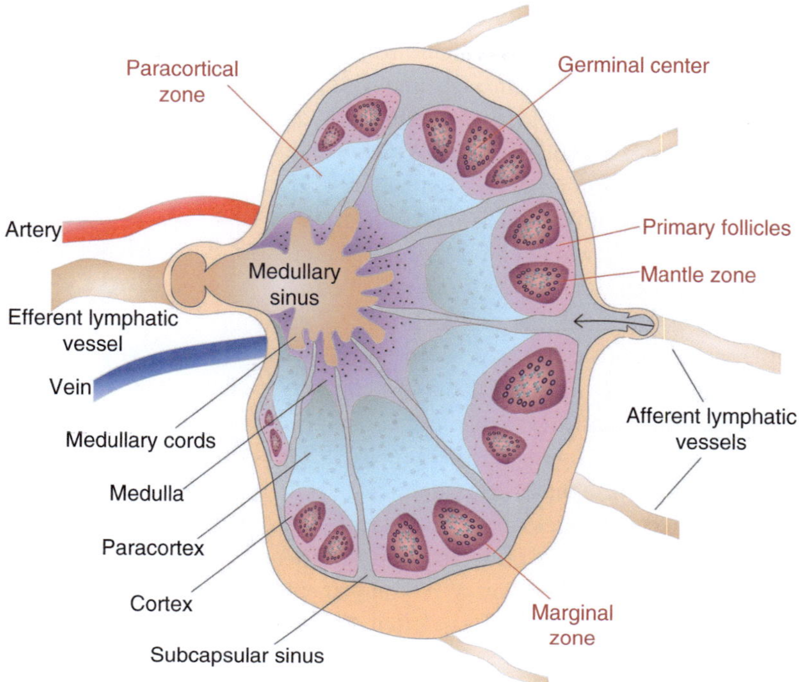

Fig. 7.3 Structure of a healthy lymph node

leukemia where many subtypes need to be genotyped for diagnosis, genetic changes in lymphoma are more commonly used for prognostication and therapy selection. Many recurrent molecular genetic abnormalities in NHL are associated with better or worse prognosis and therefore can guide the clinicians in choosing the appropriate therapy. As newer molecularly targeted therapies become available these genetic alterations can also become potential therapeutic targets.

The objective of using ancillary studies in lymphoma diagnosis is to evaluate for clonality and genetic mutations. Assessment of clonality is done by using tools like flow cytometry, polymerase chain reaction (PCR), and immunocytochemistry. The detection of chromosomal translocations can help support or refute a diagnosis and is generally done by karyotyping, FISH or PCR. Flow cytometry, a laser based technology, is the method of choice for analyzing the cell size, surface receptor expression and intracellular molecules. After staining with fluorochrome-labeled antibodies, the operator feeds the sample to the flow cytometer which generates a hydrodynamic stream of single cell suspension which is then analyzed. The flow cytometer characterizes different cell types in a heterogeneous cell population and assesses the purity of isolated subpopulations on the basis of cell size, complexity and fluorescence. The ability to simultaneously measure multiple different parameters of a cell greatly increases the utility of this technique.

PCR is based on the concept of nucleic acid amplification by utilizing the ability of DNA polymerase, obtained from a thermophilic bacterium *Thermus aquaticus*, to catalyze the reproduction of a specific DNA sequence. In order to do so the enzyme substrate mixture is exposed through a thermal cycling system where the denatured strands of target DNA bind to carefully designed primers at lower temperature followed by elongation of the complementary strand by DNA polymerase enzyme at a higher temperature. At the completion of a PCR, millions of identical copies of an original DNA target sequence are generated which have same electrical charge as well as molecular weight. When tested by gel electrophoresis these DNA copies migrate simultaneously, forming a single identifiable band, thereby making the target DNA easily identifiable. PCR can be used to identify monoclonal genetic rearrangements and translocations.

FISH is a molecular cytogenetic technique that uses fluorescent probes which bind to complimentary regions of the chromosome with high fidelity. The use of FISH in evaluation can identify complex karyotypic changes which often characterize certain types of lymphomas. By using single or differentially labeled probes, FISH can identify whole chromosomes or chromosomal loci on tissue spreads or even in paraffin wax- embedded tissue sections. Many different types of probes have been engineered for the purpose of 'fishing' such as whole chromosome, arm specific, centromere specific, gene specific, and low copy sequence probes. FISH performed in metaphase can identify genetic changes (like microdeletions) associated with particular diseases and require appropriate DNA probe selection. Enumeration or rearrangements involving specific DNA probes are often detected via interphase FISH studies. The technique of FISH has also been combined with other diagnostic tools to tailor it to specific needs. For instance Q-FISH, which combines FISH with synthetic nucleic acids and quantifies the fluorescence intensity, can be used to study telomeric length. Similarly Flow-FISH can quantify the copy number of specific repetitive elements in the cellular genome of test samples by integrating flow cytometry with FISH.

Next generation sequencing (NGS), which until recently was just a research tool, is now increasingly being used for clinical application. It allows assessment of the expression rate of up to hundreds of genes in a particular sample simultaneously using miniaturized and parallelized platforms. An emerging tool for Gene expression profiling (GEP), called Microarray, employs a "gene chip" consisting of a small glass plate encased in plastic. The surface of each chip contains hundreds of wells that are embedded with synthetic single-stranded DNA sequences which are complimentary to known DNA sequences or genes. Data from NGS and GEP studies has shed light on the pathobiology of non-Hodgkin lymphomas, allowed more precise classification of lymphoma subtypes, and identified potential therapeutic targets. Due to increasing availability and accuracy of whole genome sequencing novel mutations are increasingly being recognized as either the driver or the accomplice of lymphomagenesis. In the following section we have tried to summarize the important cytogenetic changes associated with some common types of NHLs.

7.8 Molecular Biology and Cytogenetics

The majority of B-cell and T-cell neoplasms show clonal rearrangement of their immunoglobulin (*IG*) and T-cell receptor (*TCR*) genes, respectively. Demonstration of a clonal immunoglobulin heavy chain (*IGH*), immunoglobulin kappa (*IGK*), immunoglobulin lambda (*IGL*) or T-cell receptor (*TCR*) gene rearrangement is generally not required to make a diagnosis of NHL, but can be useful to help confirm malignancy in cases where morphologic and immunophenotypic findings are inconclusive. It should be noted that clonal antigen receptor gene rearrangements are not detectable in all cases of NHL and that clonal rearrangements are sometimes detected in benign lymphoid proliferations [17].

7.8.1 B-Cell Lymphomas

7.8.1.1 Diffuse Large B-Cell Lymphoma (DLBCL)

Most DLBCL patients demonstrate rearrangement of the immunoglobulin heavy and light chain genes and somatic mutations of the variable regions of these genes [18, 19]. The pathogenesis of DLBCL is believed to be guided by at least 2 distinct mechanisms - a transformative pathway and the de novo pathway. The B-cell lymphoma 6 gene (*BCL6*), located on chromosome 3, can be mutated in up to 40% cases with mutations in 5′ noncoding region commonly present [20, 21]. The 5′ noncoding mutations hamper the negative auto-regulation by the transcriptional repressor protein BCL6. Numerous translocations have also been identified which replace the *BCL6* promoter with constitutively active promoters derived from other genes. The constellation of *BCL6* and similar genes represent the de novo pathway of

DLBCL origin. The *BCL2* rearrangement, which is considered a marker of follicular lymphomas is also found in about 20–30 percent cases of DLBCL. It is widely held that many of these DLBCL cases are a result of histologic transformations in a prior follicular lymphoma, though de novo cases of DLBCL may also have this rearrangement. Mutations of *TP53* and 9p21 are frequently detected in cases of histologic transformation [22–24]. On the basis of gene expression DLBCLs can be divided into two groups each corresponding to a different stage of B-cell differentiation. One group has high expression of genes that are commonly seen in germinal center B-cells (GCB-type), while the other group follows the gene expression pattern normally seen in activated peripheral B-cells (ABC type). Common genetic alterations seen in GCB type DLBCL are *BCL2* translocation, *REL* amplification, mutations of *EZH2*, and gains of 12q12 [25–28]. Mutations frequently seen in ABC type DLBCL are trisomy 3, gains of 3q and 18q21-q22, losses of 6q21-q22, and mutations of genes regulating the NF-κB pathway (*TRAF3*, *TRAF5*, *MAP 3 K7*, *TNFAIP3* and *MYD88*) [24, 26, 29–31]. There is also a significant prognostic difference between these two groups as GCB type DLBCL patients have a better 5 year overall survival (OS) as compared to the ABC type [32]. Truncating or DNA-binding domain mutations of *TP53*, mutations of *CDNK2A*, and alterations of the NOTCH pathway have been associated with worse outcomes [33].

Recent comprehensive genetic analyses have identified multiple genetic subtypes or clusters of DLBCL, defined by shared genetic changes. A study of over 500 DLBCL biopsy samples described four genetic subtypes: EZB, associated with EZH2 mutations, GCB-like gene expression profiles, and a relatively favorable prognosis; BN2, associated with BCL6 fusions, NOTCH2 mutations, unclassified gene expression profiles, and a favorable prognosis; N1, associated with NOTCH1 mutations, ABC-like gene expression profiles, and a less favorable prognosis; and MCD, associated with MYD88 L265P and CD79B mutations, ABC-like gene expression profiles, and less favorable outcomes [34]. BN2 tumors were noted to show changes associated with marginal zone lymphoma. The MCD-type tumors shared genetic changes previously described in primary extranodal large B cell lymphomas and tended to present with extranodal disease. Another study of 304 primary DLBCLs has found five genetic subsets (clusters C1-C5) [35]. Cluster 1 was associated with BCL6 structural variants, NOTCH2 mutations, mutations in NF-κB pathway members BCL10 and TNFAIP3, and frequent FAS mutations. These tumors were associated with favorable outcomes despite having predominantly ABC-like gene expression profiles and their genetic profiles were similar to marginal zone lymphoma. Cluster 2 tumors had frequent biallelic TP53 inactivation by mutation and/or copy loss, loss of 9p21.13/CDKN2A, and loss of 13q14.2/RB1; this cluster included both ABC and GCB-like tumors. Cluster 3 was characterized by frequent BCL2 mutations and structural variants, mutations in chromatin modifiers, including EZH2 and PTEN alterations, and were associated with a worse prognosis, though the majority were GCB-type. Cluster 4 tumors had a favorable prognosis, were predominantly GCB-type, and had mutations in multiple linker and core histone genes, BRAF, STAT3, genes encoding immune-evasion molecules such as CD58, CD70, and CD83, and NF-κB regulators including CARD11. Cluster 5 tumors had a worse prognosis, tended to be ABC-type, and were characterized by gains of 18q (possibly affecting BCL2 and MALT1). Similar to the MCD-type described by Schmitz et al., C5 tumors had frequent mutations in MYD88 (L265P), CD79B, and other genes associated with primary extranodal tumors.

MYC rearrangement is found in up to 10–15% cases of diffuse large B-cell lymphoma [36]. However, approximately 50% of *MYC*-rearranged large B-cell lymphomas have additional rearrangements involving the *BCL2* and/or *BCL6* genes, and are now classified separately as high-grade B-cell lymphoma with *MYC* and/or *BCL2* rearrangements [37]. These high-grade B-cell lymphomas often have complex karyotypes and *TP53* mutations, and a poor response to standard chemotherapy regimens including Rituximab [38, 39].

7.8.1.2 Follicular Lymphoma (FL)

FL is a B-cell neoplasm with germinal center differentiation. Most cases of FL show a translocation between the long arm of chromosome 18, which is the site of the *BCL2* oncogene, and an immunoglobulin (*IG*) gene locus [40, 41]. The translocation t(14;18)(q32;q21) involving the *IG* heavy chain gene is seen in up to 90% cases of FL. Mechanistically this translocation juxtaposes the *BCL2* gene on chromosome 18 with the *IGH* promoter sequence on chromosome 14 resulting in inappropriately high expression of the anti-apoptotic protein BCL2. Involvement of the kappa or lambda light chain genes, t(2;18)(q11;q21) and t(18;22)(q21;q21) respectively, is much less common [42, 43]. The majority of patients have additional mutations such as breaks in chromosomes 1, 2, 4, 5, 13, and 17 or trisomies affecting chromosomes X, 7, 12, and 18 [44, 45]. About 10 percent of FL patients have abnormalities or rearrangements affecting the 3q27 region, which contains *BCL6* and is essential for normal germinal center development [46]. These patients tend to have more aggressive disease and worse prognosis.

Deep RNA sequencing data from NHL patients has revealed that genes with role in histone modification are frequent targets of somatic mutations in DLBCL and FL. About 30% of DLBCL and 90% of FL cases were found to be carrying somatic mutations in *KTM2D* (previously *MLL2*), a gene that encodes a histone methyltransferase and over 10% of both DLBCL and FL cases have mutations in *MEF2B*, a calcium-regulated gene that contributes to histone acetylation [47]. Recently scientists also observed that FL patients carry mutations in genes encoding transcription factors and proteins that are involved in epigenomic regulation (*EZH2*, *ARID1A*, *EP300*) [47, 48]. One study showed that many FL patients also carry mutations affecting the *CREBBP* gene, which codes for a histone acetyl transferase protein that might play a role in regulating the expression of *BCL6* [49]. These findings suggest that alterations in chromatin structure plays an important pathogenic role in FL.

7.8.1.3 Mantle Cell Lymphoma (MCL)

MCL is a mature B-cell lymphoma that occurs in middle aged to elderly patients. The malignant cells are small to intermediate in size, with irregular nuclear contours and condensed chromatin, and express CD19, CD20, CD22, FMC-7, CD5, CD43, and BCL-2. Nuclear expression of cyclin D1 is detected in greater than 95% of cases and SOX11 is present in greater than 90% [50]. The immunoglobulin heavy chain variable region (*IGHV)* genes are unmutated or minimally/borderline mutated in the majority of cases [50]. Greater than 95% of cases of mantle cell lymphoma have a t(11;14)(q13;q32) translocation involving *CCND1* (which encodes cyclin D1) and the *IGH* gene. Rare variant translocations involving light chain genes have been reported [50]. These rearrangements result in increased expression of cyclin D1, leading to activation of cyclin-dependent kinases CDK4 and CDK6, which counteract retinoblastoma protein (RB) dependent cell cycle inhibition [51]. Secondary genetic changes are common which include losses of 1p, 6q (*TNFAIP3*), 8p, 9p (*CDKN2A*), 9q, 11q (*ATM*), 13q, and 17p (*TP53*) and gains of 3q, 7p21, 8q24 (*MYC*), and 12q [50, 52]. *TP53* mutations are present in approximately 20% of MCL, and are associated with higher proliferative rates and poor response to chemotherapy [53]. *CCND1*, *NOTCH1*, and *NOTCH2* mutations have also been associated with a poor prognosis [54].

Rare cases of cyclin D1-negative mantle cell lymphoma lack *IGH-CCND1* rearrangements. Approximately half of these cases have rearrangements involving *CCND2,* and cyclin D3 expression is seen in a subset of cases [50].

7.8.1.4 Marginal Zone Lymphoma (MZL)

According to the 2016 WHO classification of lymphoid neoplasms the MZL includes three distinct diseases (nodal, extra-nodal and splenic MZL) that seem to arise from post-germinal center marginal zone B-cells. MZLs show a typical immunophenotype that is positive for CD19, CD20, and CD22 and negative for CD5 and CD10 [1]. Extranodal marginal zone lymphoma of mucosa-associated lymphoid tissue (MALT lymphoma) is the most common type of marginal zone lymphoma and accounts for approximately 5–8% of B-cell lymphomas. Immunoglobulin genes are often rearranged in these patients with frequent somatic mutations in the variable region which is consistent with a post-germinal center stage of B-cell development [55]. MALT lymphoma often arises in the sites of chronic inflammation, generally in the setting of infectious or autoimmune disease. The stomach is the most commonly involved site. Gastric MALT lymphomas arise in the setting of *Helicobacter pylori* infection and often regress in response to H. pylori eradication [56, 57]. Translocation t(11;18)(q21;q21) (*BIRC3-MALT1*) is the commonest cytogenetic abnormality in gastric and lung MALT lymphomas and is associated with resistance to *H. pylori* eradication when it occurs in gastric lesions [58]. Translocation t(14;18)(q32;q21) (*IGH-MALT1*) is most frequent in MALT lymphomas of the lung, ocular adnexa, orbit, and salivary gland and t(1;14)(p22;q32) (*IGH-BCL10*) is seen in the lung, stomach, and intestine [56, 58]. Most cytogenetic mutations seen in MALT lymphomas seem to dysregulate the NF-κB pathway. Translocation t(3;14)(p14.1;q32) (*IGH-FOXP1*) occurs in less than 5% of MALT lymphomas and is most commonly seen in ocular adnexa, thyroid, and skin lesions [56, 58]. Deletion of the *TNFAIP3* gene on chromosome 6q23 (seen in 15–30% of cases) and *MYD88* mutations (seen in 6–10%) also lead to NF-κB activation. Trisomies of chromosomes 3 or 18 may also be present [56, 58].

Splenic marginal zone lymphoma and nodal marginal zone lymphoma are less common than extranodal marginal zone lymphoma. The most common genetic abnormalities observed in splenic marginal zone lymphoma include deletion of chromosome 7q, gain of 3q, *NOTCH2* and *KLF2* mutations [59]. Nodal marginal zone lymphoma may show gains of chromosomes 3 or 18 or deletion of 6q23. Increased expression of NF-κB-related genes has been shown by gene expression profiling. Rarely *MYD88* L265P mutation, which involves substitution of proline for leucine at amino acid position 265, can be present [60].

7.8.1.5 Burkitt Lymphoma (BL)

BL accounts for about 2% of all human lymphomas but it is a major lymphoid malignancy of childhood and young adulthood. Three distinct forms of BL are well recognized: the endemic form which affects children in equatorial Africa (peak age 4–7 years, male:female ratio 2:1), the sporadic form which is commonly seen in US and Europe (peak age 11 years) and the immunodeficiency associated BL which is generally seen in HIV infected patients or organ transplant recipients. BL is associated with a pathognomonic translocation between the *c-MYC* oncogene (8q24) and one of three locations on immunoglobulin (*IG*) genes. About 80% patients have involvement of the *IGH* gene on chromosome 14 or t(8;14)(q24;q32) [61]. Translocations affecting the kappa and lambda light chain genes are involved in all the other cases, namely t(2;8)(p12;q24) and t(8;22)(q24;q11). The *c-MYC* gene encodes for a transcription factor (MYC protein) which is a multifunctional phosphoprotein capable of altering the overall behavior of the cell by regulating cell cycle progression, apoptosis and cellular transformation. The location of *MYC* breakpoints is fairly variable depending on the type of *IG* partner. In patients with sporadic or immunodeficiency associated BL the breakpoints are generally within *MYC* or nearby while endemic BL patients can have their breakpoints dispersed farther making them difficult to identify in some break-apart FISH assays. BL patients also show high frequency of mutations in 5′ noncoding region of the *BCL-6* gene (like DLBCL) [62]. Epstein-Barr virus (EBV) genomes can be isolated in up to a third of all cases associated with acquired immune deficiency syndrome [63]. Recent studies using next-generation sequencing have demonstrated that mutations in the transcription factor TCF3 and ID3 (a negative regulator of TCF3) are also frequently seen in BL [64].

7.8.1.6 Chronic Lymphocytic Leukemia (CLL)/Small Lymphocytic Lymphoma (SLL)

CLL is the most common adult leukemia in Western countries [65, 66]. CLL is a neoplastic proliferation of small mature B lymphocytes with coarsely clumped chromatin and scant cytoplasm. The malignant cells express CD5, CD19, CD20, CD23, CD43, and CD200. CD20 and surface immunoglobulin expression are often relatively weak and FMC-7 expression is generally absent [65]. ZAP-70, CD49d, and CD38 expression is seen in a subset of cases and is associated with a poor prognosis [65]. The same neoplastic cell population is present in CLL and SLL. The disease is classified as CLL if there are greater than 5×10^9 circulating neoplastic cells in the peripheral blood, SLL if there is nodal/tissue involvement with fewer than 5×10^9/L circulating neoplastic cells, and monoclonal B-cell lymphocytosis (MBL) if there are fewer than 5×10^9/L circulating neoplastic cells in the absence of lymphadenopathy or other extramedullary involvement [67, 68]. Cases of MBL with $<0.5 \times 10^9$/L circulating clonal cells (low-count MBL) tend not to progress, whereas high-count MBL has a risk of progression to overt CLL (approximately 1–2% per year) [65, 69, 70].

Cytogenetic abnormalities are present in the majority of cases of CLL, but there is no disease defining mutation. Deletion of chromosome 13q14.3 is the most common abnormality, seen in approximately one half of cases. This deletion typically involves microRNAs 16–1 and 15a, which normally play a role in downregulating *BCL2* gene [71]. Del(13q) as the sole cytogenetic abnormality is generally associated with a good prognosis; however, some studies have shown a worse prognosis when the deletion is present in ≥80% of cells [65, 72]. Trisomy 12 is seen in approximately 16–20% of cases and is associated with atypical cytological features including irregular or cleaved nuclei, increased prolymphocytes, and lymphoplasmacytoid morphology [65, 71, 73]. Deletion of chromosome 11q22–23 is present in 18–20% of cases. This deletion involves the *ATM* gene, with variable involvement of other genes, including *BIRC3*. Patients with 11q22–23 deletions may present with prominent lymphadenopathy and have a poor outcome [66, 74]. Deletion of 17p13 is associated with loss of the *TP53* gene, lack of response to fludarabine-containing chemotherapy regimens, and a poor prognosis [65, 66]. The mutational status of the immunoglobulin heavy chain variable region (*IGHV*) genes has been shown to be prognostically important in CLL. Unmutated *IGHV* genes (at least 98% homology with germline) are associated with a worse prognosis than mutated *IGHV* genes (<98% homology with germline) [75]. Zap-70 and CD38 expression are associated with unmutated IGHV status [76, 77]. Expression of *IGHV3–21* is also associated with poor outcomes, regardless of *IGHV* mutational status [78, 79]. *NOTCH1* and *SF3B1* mutations are also associated with aggressive disease [66, 80].

7.8.1.7 Hairy Cell Leukemia (HCL)

Hairy cell leukemia is a rare B-cell neoplasm characterized by infiltrates of atypical, mature lymphocytes involving the peripheral blood, bone marrow, and spleen [81]. Hairy cell leukemia is generally a disease of middle aged to elderly adults and has a marked male preponderance [1]. Patients frequently present with cytopenias and splenomegaly [81]. The malignant cells have characteristic hair-like cytoplasmic projections and express the B-cell markers CD19, CD20, and CD22, as well as CD11c, CD25, CD103, CD123, CD200, TRAP, TBX21, and annexin A1 [81]. Immunohistochemical staining for cyclin D1 is positive, in the absence of *CCND1* gene rearrangement [81, 82]. The gene expression profile of hairy cell leukemia is more closely related to memory B-cells than naïve B-cells. Expression of chemokine receptors CCR7 and CXCR5, which are involved in homing to lymph nodes and entry into lymphoid follicles, is downregulated in hairy cell leukemia, which may help explain the distribution of disease [83]. Nearly all cases of hairy cell leukemia have a V600E mutation in the *BRAF* gene, causing constitutive activation of the MAP kinase signaling pathway [84, 85]. This mutation is highly sensitive and specific for hairy cell leukemia. The *BRAF* V600E mutation can be detected by a variety of molecular methods, including Sanger sequencing, allele specific PCR, and next-generation sequencing; both qualitative and quantitative assays are available [86]. Mutation-specific antibodies for immunohistochemistry have also been developed and show good correlation with molecular studies [86, 87].

7.8.1.8 Lymphoplasmacytic Lymphoma (LPL)

Lymphoplasmacytic lymphoma is a rare, low grade B-cell neoplasm. The neoplastic cells are a mixture of small lymphocytes, plasmacytoid lymphocytes, and plasma cells. The lymphoid component expresses the B-cell markers CD19, CD20, CD22, and CD79a, usually without co-expression of CD5 or CD10. The plasma cell component expresses CD19 and CD138, and is generally positive for CD45 [88, 89]. The bone marrow is usually involved, with occasional involvement of the lymph nodes and spleen [90]. In most cases, an IgM paraprotein is also present, fulfilling diagnostic criteria for Waldenstrom macroglobulinemia [88, 91]. A point mutation in the *MYD88* gene (L265P) is present in greater than 90% of cases of LPL [88, 92, 93]. This mutation causes activation of the NF-κB signaling pathway [93]. While the *MYD88* L265P mutation can also be seen in some types of large B-cell lymphoma, it is rare in other small B-cell lymphomas and therefore testing for this mutation can be useful to confirm a diagnosis of LPL [90]. Truncating mutations in *CXCR4* are seen in 27–30% of LPL, and have been associated with increased disease activity and resistance to ibrutinib [88, 94, 95]. Mutations in the gene encoding the chromatin remodeling protein ARID1A are seen in approximately 17% of cases of LPL [88, 96]. LPL is associated with a low risk of progression to large B-cell lymphoma; when this occurs, it is often associated with *TP53* deletion or mutation [90].

7.8.2 T-Cell Lymphomas

T-cell lymphomas are much less common than B-cell lymphomas, with the commonest subtypes being peripheral T-cell lymphoma, not otherwise specified (PTCL-NOS) and anaplastic large cell lymphoma (ALCL) [97]. Rearrangements of *TCR* gene with germline *IG* genes are frequently seen. Translocations affecting the *TCR* genes in PTCLs are much less frequent than the translocations affecting the *IG* (B-cell receptor) genes in BCL. The translocations most frequently associated with TCL are t(7;14), t(11;14), and t(14;14). Gene expression profiling is increasingly being used to further characterize PTCL by focusing on transcription factors (like *GATA*) which play vital role in the differentiation of helper T lymphocytes into TH1 and TH2 cells [98].

7.8.2.1 Anaplastic Large Cell Lymphoma, ALK-Positive (ALK^+ ALCL)

ALK^+ ALCL accounts for approximately 7% of T-cell lymphomas [99] and 10–20% of childhood lymphomas [100]. Though the morphologic features are somewhat variable, all cases contain at least some characteristic "hallmark" cells with abundant cytoplasm and horseshoe or kidney-bean-shaped nuclei [100]. The neoplastic cells express CD30. Though CD3 is frequently negative, expression of one or more other T-cell-associated markers such as CD2, CD4, and CD5 is often present. Cytotoxic T-cell markers may be expressed [100]. Rearrangement of the *TCR* genes is present in approximately 90% of anaplastic large cell lymphomas, even when T-cell markers are not expressed [101]. ALK^+ ALCLs have rearrangements involving the anaplastic lymphoma kinase (*ALK*) gene on chromosome 2p23, resulting in constitutive activation of the ALK tyrosine kinase [102]. *ALK* regulates multiple pathways, including RAS-MAPK, PI3K-AKT, mTOR, SHH, STAT3, STAT5b, and others, that have effects on cell growth, differentiation and anti-apoptotic signaling [103, 104]. The most common *ALK* translocation partner, involved in approximately 80% of cases, is *NPM1* on chromosome 5q35 [100, 102]. The second most frequent translocation is t(1;2)(q21.3;p23) (*TPM3-ALK*), occurring in approximately 13% of cases. Less common translocation partners include *ATIC* (2q35), *TFG* (3q12.2), *TRAF1* (9q33.2), *CLTC* (17q23.1), *ALO17/RNF213* (17q25.3), *TPM4* (19p13.12), *MYH9* (22q12.3), and *MSN* (Xq12) [102, 103]. Cytogenetic analysis is not required to diagnose ALK^+ ALCL, as

ALK expression can be detected by immunohistochemistry. The common *NPM1-ALK* rearrangement results in nuclear and cytoplasmic ALK staining, while the variant translocations result in cytoplasmic or membranous staining [100]. Gene expression profiling studies have revealed a common gene signature for ALK^+ and ALK^- ALCL that allows their distinction from peripheral T-cell lymphoma, not otherwise specified. The common ALCL signature includes *TNFRSF8* (CD30), *BATF*, *TMOD1*, and *p53* transcriptional targets, with downregulation of genes associated with T-cell receptor signaling [98]. Genes that are overexpressed in ALK^+ ALCL include genes involved in ALK signaling, *BCL6*, *CEBPB*, *PTPN1*, and *SERPINA* [105]. ALK^+ ALCL is usually BCL2 negative and has slightly better prognosis than ALK^- types although this could be confounded by the varying age distribution of the two types.

7.8.2.2 Anaplastic Large Cell Lymphoma, ALK-Negative (ALK^- ALCL)

ALK^- ALCL shares morphologic and immunophenotypic features with ALK^+ ALCL, but lacks ALK expression. ALK^- ALCL tends to affect an older patient population and is associated with a worse prognosis than ALK^+ ALCL [100]. A subset of ALK^- ALCLs have genetic alterations that lead to constitutive activation of the JAK-STAT3 pathway, including activating mutations of *JAK1* and/or *STAT3*, or fusions involving transcriptional regulators and tyrosine kinases (*NFKB1-ROS1*, *NCOR2-ROS1*, or *NFKB1-TYK2)* [106]. *CCR7*, *CNTFR*, *IL22*, and *IL21* are overexpressed in ALK^- ALCL [105]. Losses of *TP53* and *PRDM1/BLIMP1* are more common in ALK^- ALCL than ALK^+ ALCL and are associated with poor outcomes [100]. Translocations involving the *DUSP22* gene on chromosome 6p25.3 are present in approximately 30% of ALK^- ALCL [107]. The most common translocation involves the *FRA7H* fragile site on chromosome 7q32.3 [100]. The t(6;7)(p25.3;q32.3) translocation results in downregulation of *DUSP22* expression and increased expression of microRNAs in the *MIR29* cluster [108]. *DUSP22* rearrangements have been associated with a more favorable prognosis, with 5-year OS rates similar to ALK^+ ALCL [107]. Rearrangements involving the *TP63* gene on 3q28 are present in approximately 8% of ALK^- ALCL, often in the setting of inv. (3)(q26q28), resulting in a *TBL1XR1-TP63* fusion [100, 107, 108]. *TP63* rearrangements are associated with a particularly poor prognosis [107].

7.8.2.3 Peripheral T-Cell Lymphoma, Not Otherwise Specified (PTCL-NOS)

PTCL-NOS is a heterogeneous group of mature T-cell neoplasms that almost always affects adult patients. Advanced stage disease, aggressive course and complex abnormal karyotypes are common in PTCL-NOS [109]. There are no specific gene mutations or rearrangements for PTCL NOS, but patients often have chromosomal gains in 7q, 8q, 17q, and 22q, and chromosomal losses in 4q, 5q, 6q, 9p, 10q, and 12q [110]. Complex abnormal karyotypes are common in PTCL-NOS. A subset of PTCL-NOS show increased expression of *GATA3* and its target genes (*CCR4, IL18RA, CXCR7, IK*), while another subset is characterized by increased expression of *TBX21* (*T-bet*). High expression of *GATA3* has been associated with adverse prognosis [98]. *VAV1* rearrangements have been described in approximately 7% of cases, involving the VAV1 guanine nucleotide exchange factor, which has a role in T-cell receptor signaling [111].

7.9 Conclusion

Our understanding of the molecular pathogenesis of NHL has significantly broadened in recent years. Technological innovations in biochemistry and biophysics have revolutionized the diagnosis and classification of NHL. Novel genetic changes that dictate the nature and therapeutic response of lymphoma cells will continue to be discovered at a very fast pace in the coming decade. This enrichment in the knowledge of molecular mechanisms has, in turn, lead to an improvement in the overall survival of NHL patients. This is primarily because of early recognition of patients that have a tendency to respond poorly and therefore require intensification of therapy. Substantial gains have also been made in identifying molecularly targeted agents that are more specific in their cytotoxicity towards a particular cancer subtype when compared to conventional chemotherapy. The rituximab paradigm has convinced scientific and medical community that molecularly directed therapy can be meaningfully used to improve the outcomes in patients with certain NHL subtypes. It is expected that continued improvements in diagnosis and characterization of non-Hodgkin lymphoma will dramatically change the prognostication and treatment options for patients in near future.

Disclosure The authors certify that they have NO affiliations with or involvement in any organization or entity with any financial interest (such as honoraria; educational grants; participation in speakers' bureaus; membership, employment, consultancies, stock ownership, or other equity interest; and expert testimony or patent licensing arrangements), or non-financial interest (such as personal or professional relationships, affiliations, knowledge or beliefs) in the subject matter or materials discussed in this manuscript.

References

1. Steven H, Swerdlow EC, Harris NL, et al. WHO classification of tumours of haematopoietic and lymphoid tissues. Lyon: International Agency for Research on Cancer; 2008. p. 274–88.
2. Perry AM, Jacques D, Nathwani BN, et al. Classification of non-Hodgkin lymphoma in seven geographic regions around the world: review of 4539 cases from the international non-Hodgkin lymphoma classification Project. Blood. 2015;126:1484.
3. Smith A, Crouch S, Lax S, et al. Lymphoma incidence, survival and prevalence 2004–2014: subtype analyses from the UK's Haematological Malignancy Research Network. Br J Cancer. 2015;112(9):1575–84.
4. Naresh K, Srinivas V, Soman C. Distribution of various subtypes of non-Hodgkin's lymphoma in India: a study of 2773 lymphomas using REAL and WHO Classifications. Ann Oncol. 2000;11(suppl_1):S63–7.
5. Arora N, Manipadam MT, Nair S. Frequency and distribution of lymphoma types in a tertiary care hospital in South India: analysis of 5115 cases using the World Health Organization 2008 classification and comparison with world literature. Leuk Lymphoma. 2013;54(5):1004–11.
6. Anderson T, Chabner BA, Young RC, et al. Malignant lymphoma I. The histology and staging of 473 patients at the National Cancer Institute. Cancer. 1982;50(12):2699–707.
7. Economopoulos T, Papageorgiou S, Pappa V, et al. Monoclonal gammopathies in B-cell non-Hodgkin's lymphomas. Leuk Res. 2003;27(6):505–8.
8. Jeffers M, Milton J, Herriot R, McKean M. Fine needle aspiration cytology in the investigation on non-Hodgkin's lymphoma. J Clin Pathol. 1998;51(3):189–96.
9. Hehn ST, Grogan TM, Miller TP. Utility of fine-needle aspiration as a diagnostic technique in lymphoma. J Clin Oncol. 2004;22(15):3046–52.
10. Dong HY, Harris NL, Preffer FI, Pitman MB. Fine-needle aspiration biopsy in the diagnosis and classification of primary and recurrent lymphoma: a retrospective analysis of the utility of cytomorphology and flow cytometry. Mod Pathol. 2001;14(5):472–81.
11. Horwitz SM, Zelenetz AD, Gordon LI, et al. NCCN guidelines insights: non-Hodgkin's lymphomas, version 3.2016. J Natl Compr Cancer Netw. 2016;14(9):1067–79.
12. Byrne G Jr. Rappaport classification of non-Hodgkin's lymphoma: histologic features and clinical significance. Cancer Treat Rep. 1977;61(6):935–44.
13. Harris NL, Jaffe ES, Stein H, et al. A revised European-American classification of lymphoid neoplasms: a proposal from the International Lymphoma Study Group. Blood. 1994;84(5):1361–92.
14. Harris NL, Jaffe ES, Diebold J, et al. World Health Organization classification of neoplastic diseases of the hematopoietic and lymphoid tissues: report of the Clinical Advisory Committee meeting—Airlie House, Virginia, November 1997. J Clin Oncol. 1999;17(12):3835–49.
15. Cheson BD, Fisher RI, Barrington SF, et al. Recommendations for initial evaluation, staging, and response assessment of Hodgkin and non-Hodgkin lymphoma: the Lugano classification. J Clin Oncol. 2014;32(27):3059–67.
16. Jaffe E. Classification of natural killer (NK) cell and NK-like T-cell malignancies [editorial; comment]. Blood. 1996;87:1207–10.
17. Van Dongen J, Langerak A, Brüggemann M, et al. Design and standardization of PCR primers and protocols for detection of clonal immunoglobulin and T-cell receptor gene recombinations in suspect lymphoproliferations: report of the BIOMED-2 concerted action BMH4-CT98-3936. Leukemia. 2003;17(12):2257–317.
18. Klein U, Goossens T, Fischer M, et al. Somatic hypermutation in normal and transformed human B cells. Immunol Rev. 1998;162:261–80.
19. Kuppers R, Rajewsky K, Hansmann ML. Diffuse large cell lymphomas are derived from mature B cells carrying V region genes with a high load of somatic

mutation and evidence of selection for antibody expression. Eur J Immunol. 1997;27(6):1398–405.
20. Kuppers R, Zhao M, Hansmann ML, Rajewsky K. Tracing B cell development in human germinal centres by molecular analysis of single cells picked from histological sections. EMBO J. 1993;12(13):4955–67.
21. Shen HM, Peters A, Baron B, Zhu X, Storb U. Mutation of BCL-6 gene in normal B cells by the process of somatic hypermutation of Ig genes. Science. 1998;280(5370):1750–2.
22. Lo Coco F, Gaidano G, Louie DC, Offit K, Chaganti RS. Dalla-Favera R. p53 mutations are associated with histologic transformation of follicular lymphoma. Blood. 1993;82(8):2289–95.
23. Elenitoba-Johnson KS, Gascoyne RD, Lim MS, Chhanabai M, Jaffe ES, Raffeld M. Homozygous deletions at chromosome 9p21 involving p16 and p15 are associated with histologic progression in follicle center lymphoma. Blood. 1998;91(12):4677–85.
24. Tagawa H, Suguro M, Tsuzuki S, et al. Comparison of genome profiles for identification of distinct subgroups of diffuse large B-cell lymphoma. Blood. 2005;106(5):1770–7.
25. Huang JZ, Sanger WG, Greiner TC, et al. The t (14; 18) defines a unique subset of diffuse large B-cell lymphoma with a germinal center B-cell gene expression profile. Blood. 2002;99(7):2285–90.
26. Pasqualucci L, Dalla-Favera R. The genetic landscape of diffuse large B-cell lymphoma. Paper presented at Seminars in Hematology, 2015.
27. Rosenwald A, Wright G, Chan WC, et al. The use of molecular profiling to predict survival after chemotherapy for diffuse large-B-cell lymphoma. N Engl J Med. 2002;346(25):1937–47.
28. Houldsworth J, Olshen AB, Cattoretti G, et al. Relationship between REL amplification, REL function, and clinical and biologic features in diffuse large B-cell lymphomas. Blood. 2004;103(5):1862–8.
29. Bea S, Zettl A, Wright G, et al. Diffuse large B-cell lymphoma subgroups have distinct genetic profiles that influence tumor biology and improve gene-expression-based survival prediction. Blood. 2005;106(9):3183–90.
30. Compagno M, Lim WK, Grunn A, et al. Mutations of multiple genes cause deregulation of NF-κB in diffuse large B-cell lymphoma. Nature. 2009;459(7247):717–21.
31. Kato M, Sanada M, Kato I, et al. Frequent inactivation of A20 in B-cell lymphomas. Nature. 2009;459(7247):712–6.
32. Alizadeh AA, Eisen MB, Davis RE, et al. Distinct types of diffuse large B-cell lymphoma identified by gene expression profiling. Nature. 2000;403(6769):503–11.
33. Karube K, Enjuanes A, Dlouhy I, et al. Integrating genomic alterations in diffuse large B-cell lymphoma identifies new relevant pathways and potential therapeutic targets. Leukemia. 2018;32(3):675–84.
34. Schmitz, Roland, et al. "Genetics and pathogenesis of diffuse large B-cell lymphoma." New England Journal of Medicine 378.15 (2018): 1396–1407.
35. Chapuy, Bjoern, et al. "Molecular subtypes of diffuse large B cell lymphoma are associated with distinct pathogenic mechanisms and outcomes." Nature medicine 24.5 (2018):679.
36. Cigudosa JC, Parsa NZ, Louie DC, et al. Cytogenetic analysis of 363 consecutively ascertained diffuse large B-cell lymphomas. Genes Chromosomes Cancer. 1999;25(2):123–33.
37. Gascoyne RDCE, Jaffe ES, et al. Diffuse large B cell lymphoma NOS. In: Swerdlow S, Campo E, Harris N, et al., editors. WHO classification of tumours of haematopoietic and lymphoid tissues. Revised 4th ed. Lyon: IARC Press; 2017. p. 291–7.
38. Kluin PMHN, Stein H, et al. High-grade B cell lymphoma. In: Swerdlow S, Campo E, Harris N, et al., editors. WHO classification of tumours of haematopoietic and lymphoid tissues. Revised 4th ed. Lyon: IARC Press; 2017. p. 335–40.
39. Barrans S, Crouch S, Smith A, et al. Rearrangement of MYC is associated with poor prognosis in patients with diffuse large B-cell lymphoma treated in the era of rituximab. J Clin Oncol. 2010;28(20):3360–5.
40. Rowley JD. Chromosome studies in the non-Hodgkin's lymphomas: the role of the 14;18 translocation. J Clin Oncol. 1988;6(5):919–25.
41. Bloomfield CD, Arthur DC, Frizzera G, Levine EG, Peterson BA, Gajl-Peczalska KJ. Nonrandom chromosome abnormalities in lymphoma. Cancer Res. 1983;43(6):2975–84.
42. Leroux D, Monteil M, Sotto J, et al. Variant t (2; 18) translocation in a follicular lymphoma. Br J Haematol. 1990;75(2):290–2.
43. Lin P, Jetly R, Lennon PA, Abruzzo LV, Prajapati S, Medeiros LJ. Translocation (18; 22)(q21; q11) in B-cell lymphomas: a report of 4 cases and review of the literature. Hum Pathol. 2008;39(11): 1664–72.
44. Johnson NA, Al-Tourah A, Brown C, Connors JM, Gascoyne RD, Horsman DE. Prognostic significance of secondary cytogenetic alterations in follicular lymphomas. Genes Chromosom Cancer. 2008;47(12):1038–48.
45. Tilly H, Rossi A, Stamatoullas A, et al. Prognostic value of chromosomal abnormalities in follicular lymphoma. Blood. 1994;84(4):1043–9.
46. Bosga-Bouwer AG, van Imhoff GW, Boonstra R, et al. Follicular lymphoma grade 3B includes 3 cytogenetically defined subgroups with primary t (14; 18), 3q27, or other translocations: t (14; 18) and 3q27 are mutually exclusive. Blood. 2003;101(3):1149–54.
47. Morin RD, Mendez-Lago M, Mungall AJ, et al. Frequent mutation of histone-modifying genes in non-Hodgkin lymphoma. Nature. 2011;476(7360): 298–303.
48. Pastore A, Jurinovic V, Kridel R, et al. Integration of gene mutations in risk prognostication for patients

receiving first-line immunochemotherapy for follicular lymphoma: a retrospective analysis of a prospective clinical trial and validation in a population-based registry. Lancet Oncol. 2015;16(9): 1111–22.
49. Pasqualucci L, Dominguez-Sola D, Chiarenza A, et al. Inactivating mutations of acetyltransferase genes in B-cell lymphoma. Nature. 2011;471(7337): 189–95.
50. Swerdlow SHCE, Seto M, et al. Mantle cell lymphoma. In: Swerdlow S, Campo E, Harris N, et al., editors. WHO classification of tumours of haematopoietic and lymphoid tissues. revised 4th ed. Lyon: IARC Press; 2017. p. 285–90.
51. Musgrove EA, Caldon CE, Barraclough J, Stone A, Sutherland RL. Cyclin D as a therapeutic target in cancer. Nat Rev Cancer. 2011;11(8):558–72.
52. Espinet B, Salaverria I, Beà S, et al. Incidence and prognostic impact of secondary cytogenetic aberrations in a series of 145 patients with mantle cell lymphoma. Genes Chromosom Cancer. 2010;49(5):439–51.
53. Eskelund CW, Dahl C, Hansen JW, et al. TP53 mutations identify younger mantle cell lymphoma patients who do not benefit from intensive chemoimmunotherapy. Blood. 2017;130(17):1903–10.
54. Onaindia A, Medeiros LJ, Patel KP. Clinical utility of recently identified diagnostic, prognostic, and predictive molecular biomarkers in mature B-cell neoplasms. Mod Pathol. 2017;30(10):1338–66.
55. Du M, Diss TC, Xu C, Peng H, Isaacson PG, Pan L. Ongoing mutation in MALT lymphoma immunoglobulin gene suggests that antigen stimulation plays a role in the clonal expansion. Leukemia. 1996;10(7):1190–7.
56. Cook JRIP, Chott A, Nakamura S, Muller-Hermelink HK, Harris NL, Swerdlow SH. Extranodal marginal zone lymphoma of mucosa-assoiated lymphoid tissue (MALT lymphoma). In: Swerdlow S, Campo E, Harris N, et al., editors. WHO classification of tumours of haematopoietic and lymphoid tissues. Revised 4th ed. Lyon: IARC Press; 2017.
57. Zucca E, Bertoni F. The spectrum of MALT lymphoma at different sites: biological and therapeutic relevance. Blood. 2016;127(17):2082–92.
58. Thieblemont C, Bertoni F, Copie-Bergman C, Ferreri AJ, Ponzoni M. Chronic inflammation and extranodal marginal-zone lymphomas of MALT-type. Paper presented at Seminars in Cancer Biology, 2014.
59. Pyris MAIP, Swerdlow SH, Thieblemont C, Pittaluga S, Rossi D, Harris NL. Splenic marginal zone lymphoma. In: Swerdlow S, Campo E, Harris N, et al., editors. WHO classification of tumours of haematopoietic and lymphoid tissues. Revised 4th ed. Lyon: IARC Press; 2017. p. 223–5.
60. Campo EPS, Jaffe ES, Nathwani BN, Stein H, Muller-Hermelink HK. Nodal marginal zone lymphoma. In: Swerdlow S, Campo E, Harris N, et al., editors. WHO classification of tumours of haematopoietic and lymphoid tissues. Revised 4th ed. Lyon: IARC Press; 2017. p. 263–5.
61. Dalla-Favera R, Bregni M, Erikson J, Patterson D, Gallo RC, Croce CM. Human c-myc onc gene is located on the region of chromosome 8 that is translocated in Burkitt lymphoma cells. Proc Natl Acad Sci. 1982;79(24):7824–7.
62. Capello D, Carbone A, Pastore C, Gloghini A, Saglio G, Gaidano G. Point mutations of the BCL-6 gene in Burkitt's lymphoma. Br J Haematol. 1997;99(1):168–70.
63. Hamilton-Dutoit SJ, Pallesen G, Franzmann MB, et al. AIDS-related lymphoma. Histopathology, immunophenotype, and association with Epstein-Barr virus as demonstrated by in situ nucleic acid hybridization. Am J Pathol. 1991;138(1):149–63.
64. Schmitz R, Ceribelli M, Pittaluga S, Wright G, Staudt LM. Oncogenic mechanisms in Burkitt lymphoma. Cold Spring Harb Perspect Med. 2014;4(2).
65. Campo EGP, Montserrat E, Harris NL, Muller-Hermelink HK, Stein H, Swerdlow SH. Chronic lymphocytic leukaemia/small lymphocytic lymphoma. In: Swerdlow S, Campo E, Harris N, et al., editors. WHO classification of tumours of haematopoietic and lymphoid tissues. Revised 4th ed. Lyon: IARC Press; 2017. p. 216–21.
66. Rai KR, Jain P. Chronic lymphocytic leukemia (CLL)—then and now. Am J Hematol. 2016;91(3):330–40.
67. Hallek M, Cheson BD, Catovsky D, et al. Guidelines for the diagnosis and treatment of chronic lymphocytic leukemia: a report from the International Workshop on chronic lymphocytic leukemia updating the National Cancer Institute–working group 1996 guidelines. Blood. 2008;111(12):5446–56.
68. Marti GE, Rawstron AC, Ghia P, et al. Diagnostic criteria for monoclonal B-cell lymphocytosis. Br J Haematol. 2005;130(3):325–32.
69. Rawstron AC, Bennett FL, O'Connor SJ, et al. Monoclonal B-cell lymphocytosis and chronic lymphocytic leukemia. N Engl J Med. 2008;359(6):575–83.
70. Fazi C, Scarfò L, Pecciarini L, et al. General population low-count CLL-like MBL persists over time without clinical progression, although carrying the same cytogenetic abnormalities of CLL. Blood. 2011;118(25):6618–25.
71. Hsi ED. Pathologic and molecular genetic features of chronic lymphocytic leukemia. Paper presented at Seminars in Oncology, 2012.
72. Rodríguez AE, Hernández JÁ, Benito R, et al. Molecular characterization of chronic lymphocytic leukemia patients with a high number of losses in 13q14. PLoS One. 2012;7(11):e48485.
73. Matutes E, Oscier D, Garcia-Marco J, et al. Trisomy 12 defines a group of CLL with atypical morphology: correlation between cytogenetic, clinical and

laboratory features in 544 patients. Br J Haematol. 1996;92(2):382–8.
74. Puiggros A, Blanco G, Espinet B. Genetic abnormalities in chronic lymphocytic leukemia: where we are and where we go. Biomed Res Int. 2014;2014:1–13.
75. Hamblin TJ, Davis Z, Gardiner A, Oscier DG, Stevenson FK. Unmutated Ig V H genes are associated with a more aggressive form of chronic lymphocytic leukemia. Blood. 1999;94(6):1848–54.
76. Dürig J, Naschar M, Schmücker U, et al. CD38 expression is an important prognostic marker in chronic lymphocytic leukaemia. Leukemia. 2002;16(1):30–5.
77. Wiestner A, Rosenwald A, Barry TS, et al. ZAP-70 expression identifies a chronic lymphocytic leukemia subtype with unmutated immunoglobulin genes, inferior clinical outcome, and distinct gene expression profile. Blood. 2003;101(12):4944–51.
78. Amaya-Chanaga CI, Rassenti LZ. Biomarkers in chronic lymphocytic leukemia: clinical applications and prognostic markers. Best Pract Res Clin Haematol. 2016;29(1):79–89.
79. Ghia EM, Jain S, Widhopf GF, et al. Use of IGHV3–21 in chronic lymphocytic leukemia is associated with high-risk disease and reflects antigen-driven, post–germinal center leukemogenic selection. Blood. 2008;111(10):5101–8.
80. Rossi D, Rasi S, Spina V, et al. Integrated mutational and cytogenetic analysis identifies new prognostic subgroups in chronic lymphocytic leukemia. Blood. 2013;121(8):1403–12.
81. Foucar KFB, Stein H. Hairy cell leukaemia. In: Swerdlow S, Campo E, Harris N, et al., editors. WHO classification of tumours of haematopoietic and lymphoid tissues. Revised 4th ed. Lyon: IARC Press; 2017. p. 226–8.
82. Bosch F, Campo E, Jares P, et al. Increased expression of the PRAD-1/CCND1 gene in hairy cell leukaemia. Br J Haematol. 1995;91(4):1025–30.
83. Basso K, Liso A, Tiacci E, et al. Gene expression profiling of hairy cell leukemia reveals a phenotype related to memory B cells with altered expression of chemokine and adhesion receptors. J Exp Med. 2004;199(1):59–68.
84. Tiacci E, Trifonov V, Schiavoni G, et al. BRAF mutations in hairy-cell leukemia. N Engl J Med. 2011;364(24):2305–15.
85. Tiacci E, Schiavoni G, Forconi F, et al. Simple genetic diagnosis of hairy cell leukemia by sensitive detection of the BRAF-V600E mutation. Blood. 2012;119(1):192–5.
86. Turakhia S, Lanigan C, Hamadeh F, Swerdlow SH, Tubbs RR, Cook JR. Immunohistochemistry for BRAF V600E in the differential diagnosis of hairy cell leukemia vs other splenic B-cell lymphomas. Am J Clin Pathol. 2015;144(1):87–93.
87. Andrulis M, Penzel R, Weichert W, von Deimling A, Capper D. Application of a BRAF V600E mutation-specific antibody for the diagnosis of hairy cell leukemia. Am J Surg Pathol. 2012;36(12):1796–800.
88. Swerdlow SHCJ, Sohani AR, Pileri SA, Harris NL, Jaffe ES, Stein H. Lymphoplasmacytic lymphoma. In: Swerdlow S, Campo E, Harris N, et al., editors. WHO classification of tumours of haematopoietic and lymphoid tissues. Revised 4th ed. Lyon: IARC Press; 2017. p. 232–5.
89. Morice WG, Chen D, Kurtin PJ, Hanson CA, McPhail ED. Novel immunophenotypic features of marrow lymphoplasmacytic lymphoma and correlation with Waldenström's macroglobulinemia. Mod Pathol. 2009;22(6):807–16.
90. Swerdlow SH, Kuzu I, Dogan A, et al. The many faces of small B cell lymphomas with plasmacytic differentiation and the contribution of MYD88 testing. Virchows Arch. 2016;468(3):259–75.
91. Owen RG, Barrans SL, Richards SJ, et al. Waldenström macroglobulinemia: development of diagnostic criteria and identification of prognostic factors. Am J Clin Pathol. 2001;116(3):420–8.
92. Treon SP, Cao Y, Xu L, Yang G, Liu X, Hunter ZR. Somatic mutations in MYD88 and CXCR4 are determinants of clinical presentation and overall survival in Waldenström macroglobulinemia. Blood. 2014;123(18):2791–6.
93. Treon SP, Xu L, Yang G, et al. MYD88 L265P somatic mutation in Waldenström's macroglobulinemia. N Engl J Med. 2012;367(9):826–33.
94. Schmidt J, Federmann B, Schindler N, et al. MYD88 L265P and CXCR4 mutations in lymphoplasmacytic lymphoma identify cases with high disease activity. Br J Haematol. 2015;169(6):795–803.
95. Cao Y, Hunter ZR, Liu X, et al. CXCR4 WHIM-like frameshift and nonsense mutations promote ibrutinib resistance but do not supplant MYD88L265P-directed survival signalling in Waldenström macroglobulinaemia cells. Br J Haematol. 2015;168(5):701–7.
96. Hunter ZR, Xu L, Yang G, et al. The genomic landscape of Waldenström macroglobulinemia is characterized by highly recurring MYD88 and WHIM-like CXCR4 mutations, and small somatic deletions associated with B-cell lymphomagenesis. Blood. 2014;123(11):1637–46.
97. Swerdlow SH, Campo E, Pileri SA, et al. The 2016 revision of the World Health Organization classification of lymphoid neoplasms. Blood. 2016;127(20):2375–90.
98. Iqbal J, Wright G, Wang C, et al. Gene expression signatures delineate biological and prognostic subgroups in peripheral T-cell lymphoma. Blood. 2014;123(19):2915–23.
99. Harris ME. International peripheral T-cell and natural killer/T-cell lymphoma study: pathology findings and clinical outcomes. J Clin Oncol. 2008;26:4124–30.
100. Falini BL-RL, Campo E, Jaffe ES, Gascoyne RD, Stein H, Muller-Hermelink HL, Kinney MC. Anaplastic large cell lymphoma, ALK-positive.

In: Swerdlow S, Campo E, Harris N, et al., editors. WHO classification of tumours of haematopoietic and lymphoid tissues. Revised 4th ed. Lyon: IARC Press; 2017. p. 413–8.

101. Foss H-D, Anagnostopoulos I, Araujo I, et al. Anaplastic large-cell lymphomas of T-cell and null-cell phenotype express cytotoxic molecules. Blood. 1996;88(10):4005–11.
102. van der Krogt J-A, Bempt MV, Ferreiro JF, et al. Anaplastic lymphoma kinase-positive anaplastic large cell lymphoma with the variant RNF213-, ATIC-and TPM3-ALK fusions is characterized by copy number gain of the rearranged ALK gene. Haematologica. 2017;102(9):1605–16.
103. Hallberg B, Palmer RH. Mechanistic insight into ALK receptor tyrosine kinase in human cancer biology. Nat Rev Cancer. 2013;13(10):685–700.
104. Werner MT, Zhao C, Zhang Q, Wasik MA. Nucleophosmin-anaplastic lymphoma kinase: the ultimate oncogene and therapeutic target. Blood. 2017;129(7):823–31.
105. Lamant L, De Reynies A, Duplantier M-M, et al. Gene-expression profiling of systemic anaplastic large-cell lymphoma reveals differences based on ALK status and two distinct morphologic ALK+ subtypes. Blood. 2007;109(5):2156–64.
106. Crescenzo R, Abate F, Lasorsa E. T-cell project: prospective collection of data in patients with peripheral T-cell lymphoma and the AIRC 5xMille consortium "Genetics-Driven Targeted Management of Lymphoid Malignancies". *Convergent mutations and kinase fusions lead to oncogenic STAT3 activation in anaplastic large cell lymphoma*. Cancer Cell. 2015;27(5):744.
107. Castellar ERP, Jaffe ES, Said JW, et al. ALK-negative anaplastic large cell lymphoma is a genetically heterogeneous disease with widely disparate clinical outcomes. Blood. 2014;124(9):1473–80.
108. Zeng Y, Feldman AL. Genetics of anaplastic large cell lymphoma. Leuk Lymphoma. 2016;57(1):21–7.
109. Pileri SAWD, Sng I, et al. Peripheral T cell lymphoma, NOS. In: Swerdlow S, Campo E, Harris N, et al., editors. WHO classification of tumours of haematopoietic and lymphoid tissues. Revised 4th ed. Lyon: IARC Press; 2017. p. 403–7.
110. Nelson M, Horsman DE, Weisenburger DD, et al. Cytogenetic abnormalities and clinical correlations in peripheral T-cell lymphoma. Br J Haematol. 2008;141(4):461–9.
111. Boddicker RL, Razidlo GL, Dasari S, et al. Integrated mate-pair and RNA sequencing identifies novel, targetable gene fusions in peripheral T-cell lymphoma. Blood. 2016;128(9):1234–45.

Molecular Diagnosis of Cervical Cancer

8

Balraj Mittal and Saurabh Yadav

8.1 Introduction

Cervical carcinoma is a type of preventable cancer, still it is fourth-most common cancer amongst women. About 528,000 women are diagnosed with cervical cancer contributing to around 266,000 deaths across the globe every year. Out of these, 85% deaths occur in the developing countries [1];. Every year in India, 122,844 women are diagnosed with cervical cancer and 67,477 die from the disease (ICO Information Centre on HPV and cancer, Human Papillomavirus (HPV) and Related Diseases in India. Summary Report 2014-08-22). India has a population of 432.2 million women aged 15 years and older are at risk of developing cancer. Cervical cancer is the second most common in women aged 15–44 years. India also has the highest age standardized incidence of cervical cancer in South Asia at 22, compared to 19.2 in Bangladesh, 13 in Sri Lanka, and 2.8 in Iran. The recently reported NCRP data shows that incidence and prevalence of cervical cancer show great variability within India [2]. In 2009–2011, Aizawl district in the north eastern region of India had the highest levels of cervical cancer at an age-adjusted rate of 24.3, followed by Barshi Expanded at 19.5 and Bangalore at 18.9 (Fig. 8.1). A decline in cervical cancer incidences has been observed across various registries. In the Bangalore registry, the age-adjusted rate fell from 32.4 in 1982 to 18.7 in 2009, in Barshi from 22.1 in 1988 to 14.1 in 2010, in Chennai from 41 to 16.7 in 2009, and in Thiruvananthapuram from 9.2 in 2005 to 7.7 in 2011.

The cervical cancer development is a slow process which takes place over several years. The detection of this cancer mostly takes place in later stages when it has already progressed because the symptoms do not appear in early stages. Vaginal bleeding and pain during sexual intercourse or pelvic pain are some of the most common later symptoms of the cervical cancer [1, 3].

8.2 Screening for Cervical Cancers

Cervical cancer was leading cause of the deaths in women but in recent years, there is decrease in cervical cancer-related deaths [4]. This reduction in cancer mortality is the results of early detection of cervical cancer lesions due to intense screening programs [5]. The screening of

B. Mittal (✉)
Department of Biotechnology, Babasaheb Bhimrao Ambedkar University, Lucknow, Uttar Pradesh, India

S. Yadav
Department of Surgical Gastroenterology, Sanjay Gandhi Postgraduate Institute of Medical Sciences, Lucknow, Uttar Pradesh, India

K. K. Shukla et al. (eds.), *Molecular Diagnostics in Cancer Patients*,
https://doi.org/10.1007/978-981-13-5877-7_8

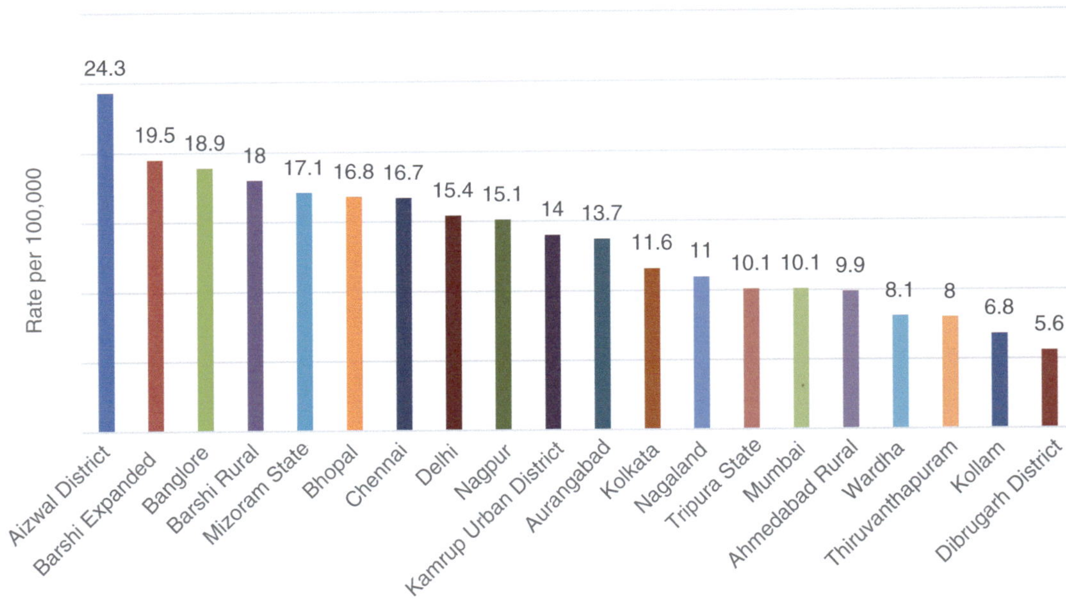

Fig. 8.1 Prevalence of cervical cancer reported across various cancer registries in India (NCRP report)

cervical cancer involves detection of the early precancerous changes which may progress to cancer if left untreated. There are two major screening modalities, cytology and HPV test. In cytology, cells are scraped from the squamo-columnar junction of the cervix and fixed on a glass slide for reading by a trained cytologist. HPV testing involves detection of HPV DNA/RNA by molecular methods.

8.2.1 Pap Test

The Papanicolaou test is commonly referred as Pap test. The test is also called cervical smear and is one of the most common methods for screening of cervical cancer. The Pap test is based on cytological investigation to detect abnormal cells which are precancerous or cancerous cells present in the cervix. During a Pap test, cervix is scraped and brushed to take the cells and the smear is prepared. The smear is analyzed microscopically according to a uniform standardized system known as the Bethesda System. An abnormal Pap smear may show precancerous changes before cancer develops. Any abnormal findings in Pap testing are usually followed up by more sensitive diagnostic procedures. If the abnormality requires closer scrutiny, the patient may be referred for detailed inspection of the cervix by colposcopy.

Pap smear test is typically done every three to five years for those who have not had previous abnormal smears. The test, when combined with a regular program of screening and appropriate follow-up, can reduce cervical cancer deaths up to 80%. However, Pap tests may not always detect cell changes. This may be because the area from where sample has been taken does not contain abnormal cells which may be present on other part of the cervix. Also, some samples are hard to interpret. For example, blood or mucus in the smear may make it hard to visualize cells. Moreover, abnormal cells are sometime missed under the microscope. Adenocarcinoma of the cervix which accounts for about 15% of all cervical cancers is not discernible by Pap tests [6].

As the first cancer screening test of the modern era, the Pap smear was never initially scrutinized through a standard evidence based approach as many of our modern screening tests are today. However, the epidemiologic data are convincing. In nations that have adopted cytologic screening programs, the incidence and mortality from cervical cancer has declined dramatically [7]. Because of its success in cervical cancer prevention, the Pap smear has come to be known as the archetype of screening tests [8]. The Pap test had a profound effect on cervical cancer morbidity and mortality in an era of highly prevalent cervical disease, however cytologic screening has inherent limitations, particularly as the patterns of incidence have changed and the morbidity from overtreatment is now fully appreciated.

8.2.1.1 The Limitation of Pap Smears

Despite recognition of Pap smear as primary screening method for cervical cancer, the test has shown a high false negative rate because it misses considerable number of cases of cervical intraepithelial neoplasia (CIN2+). Studies have shown that 20% to 40% of new cervical cancer cases are diagnosed in women who had been consistently Pap negative [9, 10]. As data from population based trials have emerged, the Pap smear has shown variable sensitivity depending on woman's age, highest in the 50 and older age group. In a meta-analysis by Spence et al., average false negative rate of cytologic testing was as high as 35.5% [11]. The test has lower specificity for high-grade CIN than low-grade lesions, which can lead to overtreatment [12, 13]. Since the sensitivity of cervical smears for adenocarcinoma is lower than for squamous cell carcinoma [14], significant number of cervical cancer cases can be missed [14–16].

Pap smear limitations also include failure to acquire adequate specimens, inter-observer bias, and misinterpretations. Inflammation, scant cellularity, and blood contaminating samples have all been cited as reasons for inadequate or unsatisfactory samples. Approximately 1–8% of Pap smears have been reported as unsatisfactory [17, 18]. Even with satisfactory samples, cytologic interpretation is subject to inter-observer variability despite international standards. Even with experienced cytologists and adequate samples, varied interpretations continue to reduce cytologic testing's diagnostic accuracy.

The most effective screening tests must achieve a balance between high sensitivity and acceptable specificity. Equally important is identifying a screening interval that is frequent enough to detect lesions before they become invasive while still minimizing cost and morbidity associated with overtreatment. Because of its low sensitivity, cytologic testing alone requires regular exams with diligent follow-up. Therefore, a screening test with a high negative predictive value, which safely allows for extension of screening intervals, is of greatest benefit.

8.2.2 HPV DNA Test

In 1976, Harald zur Hausen proposed that Human papillomavirus (HPV) plays an important role in causation of cervical cancer. In 1983–1984, two subtypes of HPV, HPV16 and HPV18 were identified in cervical cancer [19]. HPV is now accepted as a necessary factor in the development of pre-invasive and invasive cancer of the cervix [20]. HPVs are DNA viruses from the papillomavirus family, of which over 170 types with different variations in their genetic and oncogenic potential are known [21]. These viruses largely spread through sexual contact and mainly infect the anus and genitals.

HPV is part of an ancient family of pathogens which are known to infect epithelial tissues of various organisms. HPVs are a small double-stranded circular DNA virus with a genome of approximately 8000 base pairs with three distinct regions: the early region (E), late region (L), and upstream regulatory region (URR) (Fig. 8.2). The URR is found between the E and L regions and contains promoter and enhancer DNA sequences that are critical for regulating viral replication and transcription of both viral and cellular genes The HPV virion infects epithelial tissues, where it associates with putative receptors such as alpha integrins and laminins on cell surface, entering through clathrin-mediated endocytosis and/or caveolin-mediated endocytosis depending on the type of HPV. The viral genome transports into the host nucleus and establishes itself at a copy number of 10–200 viral genomes per cell.

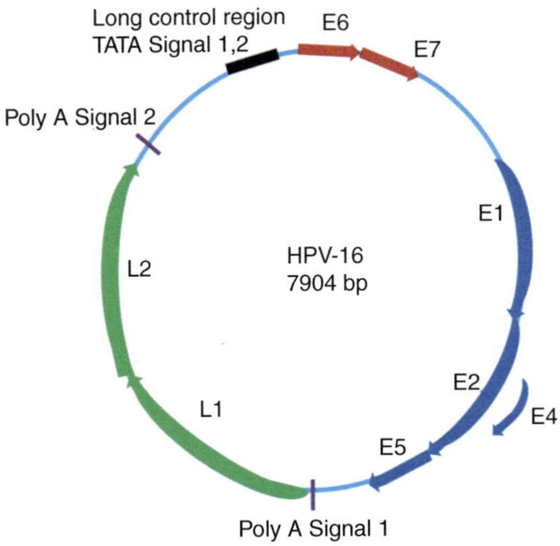

Fig. 8.2 Genomic organisation of HPVs. Cartoon depiction of the genomic organization of a high-risk HPV. HPV genome consists of early and late regions. The name early and late is used due to their timing of expression during the viral life cycle and the positions of the genes within the genome. The early region genes such as E2, E1, E6, and E7 play key role in transcription and viral replication. The E6 and E7 genes encode proteins E6 and E7 that are critical for HPV life cycle and these also play crucial role as a major transforming proteins. The late region contains L1 and L2 that encode for viral structural proteins, with L1 encodes major capsid protein and L2 encodes the minor capsid protein. The upstream regulatory region (URR) controls of transcription and replication of early genes, it contains promoter, viral origin of replication and enhancer elements. Assembly of transcriptional apparatus takes place at URR, resulting in transcription of polycistronic transcripts utilizing the early polyadenylation signal

8.2.2.1 Life Cycle of HPV

HPV can integrate into DNA or stays as non-integrated episomes in the host. Some of the "early genes" carried by the HPV virus, such as genes E6 and E7, act as oncogenes that promote tumor growth and malignant transformation [22]. The viral oncogenes E6/E7 proteins inactivate host's tumor suppressor proteins, p53 is inactivated by E6 and pRb is inactivated by E7. E6 and E7 are believed to modify host cellular machinery in a state that is favorable to the amplification of viral genome replication [23]. Normally, p53 acts to prevent cell growth, and promotes cell death in the presence of DNA damage. However, inactivation of p53 by E6 promotes unregulated cell division, cell growth, and cell survival, which are typical characteristics of cancer. E7 in oncogenic HPVs acts as the primary transforming protein. E7 binds to retinoblastoma protein (pRb) releasing transcription factor E2F to transactivate its targets, therefore leading the cell cycle forward.

8.2.2.2 Sexually Transmitted HPV Types: Two Categories

Low risk HPVs: These low-risk HPVs do not cause cancer but can cause skin warts on or around the genitals and anus. HPV types 6 and 11 cause 90% of all genital warts but are considered low risk for cervical cancer [24].

High risk HPVs: This category comprises HPVs which can potentially cause cancer. Majority of cervical cancer cases are caused by high risk HPVs. HPV types, namely 16, 18, 31, 33, 35, 39, 45, 51, 52, 56, 58, 59, 68, 73, and 82 have been implicated in carcinogenesis [24]. Only HPV 16 and 18 account for approximately 70% of cervical cancer incidences. HPV type 16 has been found to be most carcinogenic strain. It may, however, be noted that majority of high-risk HPV infections may not cause any symptoms and the infection generally goes away automatically within 1–2 years, However, some HPV infections can persist for many years and, can progress to cancer, if left untreated. Environment factors such as tobacco can enhance the risk of HPV-related cancers [25]. During last two decades, epidemiologic information and better molecular understanding of malignant transformation has led to the development of many strategies for detection and early intervention. Specific tests for oncogenic HPVs have made it possible to predict the risk of future development of cervical cancer.

8.3 HPV Testing

The HPV is DNA virus, and most of the tests are based on detecting viral DNA. There are many sub-types of HPV, and sequence-specific discrimination is required for specific type of testing. Since HPV 16 and 18 are responsible for most of cervical-cancer cases, specific tests are available to detect these two subtypes. Other tests can detect DNA from several high-risk HPV types and can indicate whether HPV-16 or HPV-18 is present. A different test detects RNA from the most common high-risk HPV types and can detect HPV infections before cell abnormalities are evident [26].

Initially, molecular tests were based on DNA hybridization, using dot blot or Southern hybridization (Table 8.1). Although Southern blot was considered gold standard for HPV DNA detection but the test proved to be cumbersome and time-consuming for routine diagnosis [27]. Subsequently, signal amplification by polymerase chain reaction (PCR) combined with restriction fragment length polymorphism came into usage. The HPV-PCR protocols use consensus primers which target conserved regions of the HPV genome, such as the L1 capsid gene [28]. Researchers have used a type-specific PCR, with primers that amplify the long control region L1 and E6/E7 [29]. After amplification, the HPV genotypes are done by restriction-fragment length polymorphism (RFLP). In this technique, the amplified DNA is digested by restriction enzymes, resulting in DNA fragments of various lengths which can be resolved by electrophoresis. Common restriction enzymes such as BamHI, Dd6eI, HaeIII, HinfI, PstI and RsaI are usually required [30, 31]. The test can identify single or multiple infections. The methodology is simple, and well suited for limited resource settings.

For identifying various subtypes of HPV present, DNA sequencing of PCR product can be carried out for high resolution HPV typing. HPV genome sequencing can be performed by classical DNA sequencing methods. The Sanger dideoxy chain-termination technique is carried

Table 8.1 Laboratory based tests for human papilloma virus (HPV)

Method	Benefits	Weaknesses	Comments
Southern blot hybridization	It is gold standard for HPV	Low sensitivity, time consuming, require relatively large amounts of purified intact DNA	Not suitable for routine diagnosis
Dot blot	Easy to perform on multiple samples	Low sensitivity, HPV typing still cumbersome	No longer popular in diagnostics
PCR PCR/RFLP Type-specific PCR	The HPV-PCR protocols use consensus primers After amplification, genotypes are done by restriction-fragment length polymorphism (RFLP) Type-specific PCR also used	May show false negative results for multiple type infections that are contained in samples at lower copy numbers Sometimes, additional, labor-intensive procedures, such as type-specific PCR are required Contamination with previously amplified material can lead to false positives	Particularly suited for limited resource settings
Real-time PCR	Quantitative Reliable, sensitive, and specific diagnostic tool Ability to detect viral load	Equipment is moderately expensive	Reproducible, rapid, and applicable to clinical samples
PCR-sequencing	Sanger Dideoxy sequencing Pyro-sequencing	Expensive	Used mainly in research setting
Microarray	This assay detects and genotypes multiple HPV types in a single reaction. Detection of multiple infections, and may be considered a reliable screening test	Cost is still relatively high, and it requires specific apparatus	Cost factor deters its usage in routine diagnostics
Next generation sequencing (NGS)	High-throughput technology for detection of viral DNA in circulation	Still under development for clinical settings	High cost

out using fluorescently labeled nucleotides on automated instrument; however, it is mainly used in research setting and has not been validated for clinical applications. Another sequencing method, pyrosequencing is applicable to any source of DNA or RNA that can be amplified by PCR. The sequencing reaction detects pyrophosphate released during DNA synthesis. The major advantage of pyrosequencing method is its simplicity in read out and it is faster and less expensive [32].

The amplification based tests along with hybridization have also been developed. These tests with several variations are commercially available. The primers or probes labeled with biotin can detect HPV subtypes with great sensitivity. These tests are either qualitative or semi-quantitative and do not provide accurate information on viral loads. Therefore, real-time PCR is replacing simple PCR for screening. Using different fluorochromes that emit fluorescence at different wave lengths, the reactions can be performed in multiples and can amplify different nucleic-acid targets. Here, the viral nucleic acids can be detected even when present in very small concentrations. The method is extremely reproducible, rapid, and well-suited for clinical samples [33, 34]. However, viral load tests do not always appear to be advantageous over cytology, and testing for high viral load levels may not be clinically useful, except in the case of HPV-16 [35, 36].

After infection, HPV-DNA is usually present in extrachromosomal or episomal form in beginning. Subsequently, viral DNA integrates into the host genome and leads to morphological changes. HPV integration can be detected by PCR, fluorescence *in situ* hybridization, and Real-Time PCR [37].

Due to large scale screening programmes, a standardized assay is required to provide consistency across various centers. Therefore, various commercial kits have been developed, and many of them have been approved by FDA (USA).

8.4 Commercial Kits for HPV (Table 8.2)

8.4.1 Hybrid Capture 2 (HC2)

First commercial test for HPV, Hybrid Capture 2 (HC2) developed by Qiagen/Digene, was introduced in 2003. It is an Food and Drug Administration (FDA, USA) approved test to be used as an adjunct to Pap testing. It detects the DNA of 13 "high-risk" HPV types that most commonly affect the cervix, but it does not tell the specific HPV types. Hybrid Capture 2 has been the most widely investigated commercially available HPV assay and the many of the population-based screening have utilized this particular test [38, 39].

8.4.2 Cobas HPV Test

In 2011, FDA approved Cobas HPV test, developed by Roche. It specifically identifies types HPV 16 and HPV 18 while simultaneously detecting the rest of the high-risk HPV types [40]. The test was evaluated in the ATHENA trial, involving routine cervical cancer screening among more than 47,000 U.S. women 21 years old and older. The trial demonstrated that 1 in 10 women, age 30 and older, who tested positive for HPV 16 and/or 18, actually had cervical pre-cancer lesions even though they tested negative by Pap smear [41].

8.4.3 CLART Human Papillomavirus 2

The CLART Human Papillomavirus 2 by Genomica, Madrid, Spain utilizes biotinylated primers to amplify a 450 bp fragment within the HPV L1 region. Amplified DNA is detected by hybridization using low-density microarray. This method demonstrated excellent sensitivity, specificity, and reproducibility [42].

Table 8.2 List of commercially available detection tests for human papilloma virus (HPV)

Name of the test	Principle	Specificity	Comments
Hybrid Capture 2 Qiagen/ Digene Germany	Also called the *digene* HPV Test Allows rapid, testing of HPV in virtually any laboratory setting It employs specific RNA probes, hybridization, antibody capture, and signal amplification that utilizes qualitative chemiluminescent detection	Detects the DNA of 13 "high-risk" HPV types that most commonly affect the cervix Does not tell the specific HPV types	Approved by FDA for follow-up testing of women with abnormal Pap test results or cervical cancer screening in combination with a Pap test Most widely studied commercially available HPV assay and for population-based screening
Cobas® HPV test Roche Molecular Systems, Inc	The tests utilize amplification of target DNA PCR followed by nucleic acid hybridization	Detect 14 high-risk HPV Tests simultaneously provide pooled results on high-risk genotypes and individual results on the highest-risk genotypes, HPV 16 and HPV 18, at clinically relevant infection levels	Semi-quantitative results can be obtained in an automatic reader with highly comparable outcomes, showing excellent sensitivity, specificity, and reproducibility
CLART® human papillomavirus 2 Genomica, Madrid, Spain	Uses biotinylated primers that amplify a 450 bp fragment within the HPV L1 region. Co-amplification of an 892 bp region of the FTR gene and a 1.202 bp fragment of a transformed plasmid as control for DNA adequacy and PCR efficiency Amplicons are detected by hybridization in a low-density microarray	35 HPV types (-6, -11, -16, -18, -26, -31, -33, -35, -39, -40, -42, -43, -44, -45, -51, -52, -53, -54, -56, -58, -59, -61, -62, -66, -68, -70, -71, -72, -73, -81, -82, -83, -84, -85 and -89). are detected	
PapilloCheck® assay (Greiner Bio-One GmbH, Frickenhausen, Germany)	The assay utilizes a multiplex PCR with fluorescent primers to amplify a 350 bp fragment of the E1 gene of HPV, comprising 28 probes, on a DNA chip. Co-amplification of the human *ADAT1* gene is used as internal control	Detects and genotypes 24 HPV types in a single reaction (HPV -6, -11, -16, -18, -31, -33, -35, -39, -40, -42, -43, -44, -45, -51, -52, -53, -55, -56, -58, -59, -66, -68, -70, -73, and -82)	The main advantages is HR/LR-HPV identification, and detection of multiple infections. Reliable screening test but this assay does not amplify HPV -35 and -53. It requires specific apparatus which is expensive
INNO-LiPA (FujirebioDiagnostics Sweden)	It is based on the co-amplification of the 65 bp region of the HPV L1 gene and the 270 bp of the human HLA-DP1 gene using SPF10 biotinylated primers, followed by genotyping	This assay genotypes all 14 HPV that are covered by Real-Time PCR Can reliably detect HPV in cervical-swab, brushes, tampons, and lavage specimens, including archival clinical specimens	Some carcinogenic genotypes such as HPV-35, -39, -52, -56 and -66 are not covered by this method Not effective for HPV-42 and -59 genotyping

(continued)

Table 8.2 (continued)

Name of the test	Principle	Specificity	Comments
The Linear array® HPV Genotyping (Roche Molecular Diagnostics, Pleasanton, CA, USA)	The Linear Array® is a PCR-based assay coupled with a reverse line blot hybridization	Allows the discrimination of 36 HPV types	
Clinicalarrays® HPV kit (Genomica SAU, Madrid, Spain)	Employs biotinylated primers to amplify 451 nucleotides within the polymorphic L1 region of the HPV genome. A human CFTR gene and control plasmids are used as internal controls	Allows detection of 35 genotypes that are individually associated with both high-risk- (-16, -18, -26,-31, -33, -35, -39, -45, -51, -52, -53, -56, -58, -59, -66, -68, -70, -73, -82 and -85) as well as low risk- (-6, -11, -40, -42, -43, -44, -54, -61, -62, -71, -72, -81, -83, -84 and -89) HPVs	It is possible to identify simple or co-infections
Microplate colorimetric hybridization assay (MCHA) (Boehringer Mannheim, Germany)	The MCHA is based on the amplification of the 150 bp fragment within the L1 region by consensus primers GP5+/6+, followed by colorimetric hybridization to six type-specific probes on microwell plates	For identifying six HR-HPV (-16, -18, -31, -33, -39 and -45) High sensitivity in identifying HPV -16/18 Including extra probes, HPV-35, -52, -56 and 58 can also be detected	
The Pretect® HPV-Proofer assay (NorChip AS, Klokkarstua, Norway)	Detect mRNA for E6/E7 oncogenes	Detects E6/E7 mRNA from five HR-HPV (-16, -18, -31,-33, and -45)	Clinical studies have shown high sensitivity
The APTIMA® HPV assay (Gen-Probe, San Diego, CA, USA)	Detect mRNA for E6/E7 oncogenes	Detects E6/E7 mRNA of the 14 HR (-16, -18, -31, -33, -35, -39, -45, -51, -52, -56, -58, -59, -66, and -68)	Better sensitivity than the Proofer test, which detects only 5 HR-HPV

8.4.4 PapilloCheck Assay (Greiner Bio-One GmbH, Frickenhausen, Germany)

It detects and genotypes 24 HPV types in a single PCR reaction. The assay utilizes a multiplex PCR with fluorescent primers to amplify a 350 bp fragment of the E1 gene of HPV, comprising 28 probes, on a DNA chip. The hybridized microarray chip, is automatically scanned and analyzed.

8.4.5 INNO-LiPA

INNO-LiPA by LiPA HBV GT; Innogenetics, genotypes 14 HPVs by Real-Time PCR [43, 44]. It amplifies 65 bp region of the HPV L1 gene and the 270 bp of the human HLA-DP1 gene (internal control) using biotinylated primers. The method can detect HPV in samples taken with swabs, brushes, tampons, and lavage.

8.4.6 The Linear Array

Roche Linear Array HPV Genotyping is a PCR-based assay combined with reverse line blot hybridization. This assay types 36 HPV, including 15 HR Colored signals on strips can be read by naked eye and interpreted according to the Linear Array reference guide [45].

8.4.7 Clinical Arrays HPV

This kit from Genomica SAU allows the detection and genotyping of 35 high and low risk HPV. The biotinylated primers amplify 451 nucleotides within the polymorphic L1 region of the HPV genome and Human CFTR co-amplification is used as internal control [46].

8.4.8 Microplate Colorimetric Hybridization Assay (MCHA)

The MCHA from Boehringer Mannheim identifies six high risk -HPV (-16, -18, -31, -33, -39 and -45). The test is based on the amplification by PCR of the 150 bp fragment within the L1 region and consensus primers GP5+/6+, The colorimetric hybridization with type-specific probes is carried out on microwell plates [47].

8.4.9 PreTect HPV Proofer the Test by PreTect

AS, KLOKKARSTUA, Norway is based on transcription-mediated amplification of full-length E6/E7 transcripts preempted by target capture. This assay uses Real-Time multiplex PCR and is more specific for high-gradesquamous intraepithelial lesions. It detects E6/E7 mRNA from five high risk -HPV (-16, -18, -31, -33, and -45). Clinical studies have shown high sensitivity [48, 49].

8.4.10 The APTIMA HPV

The assay from Gen-Probe, San Diego detects HPV E6/E7 mRNA of the 14 high risk HPVs, to provide better sensitivity than the Proofer test, which detects only 5 HR-HPV [49]. This assay has numerous advantages over the other HPV tests such as higher sensitivity and non-cross reactivity with low risk -HPV types. The test is compatible with a fully automated processing system. The test was approved by FDA in 2011.

8.5 Screening and Prevention of Cervical Cancer

In the current scenario, invasive cervical cancer is largely a preventable disease. In the light of Pap smear limitations and better understanding of the role of HPV in cervical carcinogenesis, prevention has primarily shifted its focus on high-risk HPV (HR-HPV) testing and HPV vaccination. Several studies have shown a benefit of HPV testing for the primary detection of cervical dysplasia [50]. HPV DNA testing has increased sensitivity with acceptable specificity and high negative predictive values for detecting CIN 2/3 relative to cervical cytology [51]. Several international trials have provided strong evidence that primary HPV testing alone has better sensitivity than cytology [52]. HPV testing is also more objective and reproducible than the other cervical cancer screening tests [53]. It can be automated, centralized, and be quality-checked for large specimen input while avoiding the subjective interpretation in cytology based tests [54]. In low resource settings, HPV testing in women over 30 may be an effective large-scale method of cervical cancer screening [51].

Despite these facts, American Society for Colposcopy and Cervical Pathology (ASCCP) has not yet adopted primary screening with HPV testing because of concerns for an evidence based approach to subsequent follow-up. ASCCP, however, recommended HR-HPV testing in a variety of situations. These include “Co-testing” with cytology in women over thirty years old. In women over thirty, HPV DNA testing combined with cytology, known as “co-testing”, was approved for screening in the US in 2006. The combined test improved detection of pre-invasive and invasive lesions. The natural history of HPV infection has shown decreased incidence in women over the age of 30. Testing specifically for HPV 16 and 18 is also emerging as an important test for further triage of women greater than 30 years of age who are high risk-HPV positive but cytology negative. Therefore, combining cytology with HR-HPV testing in this age group also allows for extended screening intervals if both tests are negative, given its high negative predictive value [55–57].

HPV- Cytology Triage approach is currently utilized in many European nations and is being evaluated in the USA. It involves primary HR-HPV testing followed with cytology triage. In this screening, a woman with positive high risk-HPV test is subjected to Pap test. Patients with abnormal cytology then proceed with colposcopic evaluation. With this method, the test with the higher sensitivity (HPV testing) is followed by the test with the higher specificity (cytology), thus improving detection rates while eliminating false positive results.

A prospective Finnish trial demonstrated that primary HPV DNA screening with cytology triage improved sensitivity and equivalent specificity for detection of CIN 2/3. Moreover, in women 35 years or older, HPV testing with cytology triage was more specific than cytology alone and decreased colposcopy referrals and follow-up tests [58]. "Reflex" testing (HPV testing when cytology is abnormal) in postmenopausal women with Low grade squamous intraepithelial lesion (LSIL) cytology was first studied and found to be a viable option for screening in the ASC-US/LSIL Triage Study (ALTS) trial. The ALTS trial found that testing for HPV after an ASC-US Pap smear was a sensitive and cost effective strategy. HPV testing detected CIN 3 with a sensitivity of 96% and it decreased the number of colposcopies by 50% [52].

In India, population-based cervical cancer screening is largely nonexistent in most regions due to competing healthcare priorities, insufficient financial resources and a limited number of trained providers [59]. In recent years, many recommendations have emerged for screening of various cancers including cervical cancer in India [60]. However, pilot HPV DNA testing has been carried out at several locations in India. The reported test sensitivity varies from 45.7 to 80.9% for detection of cervical intraepithelial neoplasia grade 2. HPV testing is expensive and requires relatively sophisticated laboratory infrastructure, although it is the most reproducible of all cervical screening tests [61].

Other than the availability of screening tests, there are numerous other factors that influence uptake. Age, education, marital status, income, number of children, use of contraception, lack of knowledge about screening of cervical cancer and its prevention, personal and lifestyle factors, attitudes, limited family support, ease of access, and lack of patient-friendly health services are factors affecting screening [62]. There is long interval between initial infection and cancer. It is believed that other factors such as sexual habits, reproductive factors, other sexually transmitted diseases, coinfection with HIV, smoking, nutritional deficiency, genetic susceptibility, use of hormonal contraceptives, and high parity. A meta-analysis of social inequality and the risk of cervical cancer showed increased risk in the low-social-class categories for the development of invasive cervical cancer. Although this difference was observed in all countries, it was stronger in low- and middle-income countries [63]. In India, even after diagnosis of advanced cervical cancer, completed treatment consisting of radiation and brachytherapy is low due to various factors such as advanced age, high cost of treatment and non-availability of treatment facilities in remote areas [2].

8.6 Future Prospectus

Improved screening algorithms, which may in the future include primary HPV testing, followed by cytology triage will likely continue to change as data from large prospective trials emerge. This method has shown promise by maintaining high sensitivity, prolonged screening intervals, and may ultimately prove to be more efficacious. Other areas of current research include identification of other novel molecular markers associated with protein expression and cell cycle regulators that are present in high-grade lesions. E6 and E7 viral oncogenes are necessary for HPV carcinogenesis and tests for E6/E7 mRNA, already commercially available, could help identify women at higher risk for developing cancer [64], Staining for p16 overexpression has already shown promise in the triage of abnormal cytology, specifically in those with ASC-US, ASC-H, and LSIL cytology [65]. Additionally, high-grade lesions have genetic expression profiles that resemble invasive disease. Therefore, DNA micro-array analysis may be able to better stratify a woman's risk in the setting of a positive high risk-HPV test.

The utilization of the Pap smear in preventive care and cervical cancer screening has been a cornerstone in women's health for over 70 years. Decline of cervical cancer rates after implementation of cytology programs is considered one of the greatest successes in cancer prevention of all time. Through a better understanding of the role of HPV in cervical cancer carcinogenesis and the development of HR-HPV tests, cervical cancer screening strategies have already shown a drastic shift from conventional annual cytology to a more complex interplay of HPV triage, extended screening intervals, and varying methods of follow-up. These changes likely represent just the beginning of a paradigm shift in cervical cancer prevention. As we move forward with cervical cancer screening programs, HPV testing will likely emerge as a primary screening method followed by triage with either cytology, HPV genotyping, or other genetic profiling, which will more efficiently guide clinicians in the prevention of invasive disease [66].

Biopsies are critical to the diagnosis and treatment of cancer. Conventional approaches involve collection of the tissue for the examination using several methods. Because cancer cells can release genetic material into the bloodstream, blood can help us learn earlier if there's cancer in the body, before it causes symptoms or grows enough to be seen through imaging. This is currently most helpful to monitor if cancer has returned after treatment. Blood also can reveal genetic information about the cancer that's present. Liquid biopsies scan for particular genetic alterations, can aid in the prognosis and suggest appropriate treatment, including targeted therapies in advanced cervical cancer patients [67, 68].

Acknowledgements B.M. is Emeritus Medical Scientist of Indian Council of Medical Research (ICMR), New Delhi, and S.Y. is a senior research fellow, Council of Scientific and Industrial Research (CSIR).

References

1. de Sanjosé S, et al. Human papillomavirus (HPV) and related cancers in the global alliance for vaccines and immunization (GAVI) countries. Vaccine. 2012;30:D1–D83. http://www.ncbi.nlm.nih.gov/pubmed/23510764.
2. Sreedevi A, Javed R, Dinesh A. Epidemiology of cervical cancer with special focus on India. Int J Women's Health. 2015;7:405–14. http://www.ncbi.nlm.nih.gov/pubmed/25931830.
3. Dutta S, Biswas N, Muhkherjee G. Evaluation of socio-demographic factors for non-compliance to treatment in locally advanced cases of cancer cervix in a Rural Medical College Hospital in India. Indian J Palliat Care. 2013;19(3):158–65. http://www.jpalliativecare.com/text.asp?2013/19/3/158/121530.
4. Siegel R, Naishadham D, Jemal A. Cancer statistics, 2012. CA Cancer J Clin. 2012;62(1):10–29. http://www.ncbi.nlm.nih.gov/pubmed/22237781.
5. Wright TC, et al. 2001 Consensus Guidelines for the management of women with cervical cytological abnormalities. JAMA. 2002;287(16):2120–9. http://www.ncbi.nlm.nih.gov/pubmed/11966387.
6. DeMay RM. Practical principles of cytopathology. American Society for Clinical Pathology Press; 2007. ISBN 978-0-89189-549-7.
7. Tota JE, et al. The road ahead for cervical cancer prevention and control. Curr Oncol. 2014;21(2):255. http://www.ncbi.nlm.nih.gov/pubmed/24764711.
8. Sawaya GF, et al. Current approaches to cervical-cancer screening. N Engl J Med. 2001;344(21):1603–7. http://www.ncbi.nlm.nih.gov/pubmed/11372013.
9. Leyden WA, et al. Cervical cancer in women with comprehensive health care access: attributable factors in the screening process. J Natl Cancer Inst. 2005;97(9):675–83. http://academic.oup.com/jnci/article/97/9/675/2544234/Cervical-Cancer-in-Women-With-Comprehensive-Health.
10. Subramaniam A, et al. Invasive cervical cancer and screening: what are the rates of unscreened and underscreened women in the modern era? J Low Genit Tract Dis. 2011;15(2):110–3. https://insights.ovid.com/crossref?an=00128360-201104000-00007.
11. Spence AR, Goggin P, Franco EL. Process of care failures in invasive cervical cancer: systematic review and meta-analysis. Prev Med. 2007;45(2–3):93–106. http://linkinghub.elsevier.com/retrieve/pii/S0091743507002514.
12. Elfgren K, et al. Colposcopic and histopathologic evaluation of women participating in population-based screening for human papillomavirus deoxyribonucleic acid persistence. Am J Obstet Gynecol. 2005;193(3 Pt 1):650–7. http://linkinghub.elsevier.com/retrieve/pii/S0002937805001778.
13. Nanda K, et al. Accuracy of the Papanicolaou test in screening for and follow-up of cervical cytologic abnormalities: a systematic review. Ann Intern Med. 2000;132(10):810–9. http://www.ncbi.nlm.nih.gov/pubmed/10819705.

14. Scheiden R, et al. Atypical glandular cells in conventional cervical smears: incidence and follow-up. BMC Cancer. 2004;4(1):37. http://www.ncbi.nlm.nih.gov/pubmed/15257755.
15. Howlader N, et al. SEER Cancer Statistics Review, 1975-2009 (Vintage 2009 Populations), National Cancer Institute. Bethesda, MD. http://seer.cancer.gov/csr/1975_2009_pops09/, based on November 2011 SEER data submission, posted to the SEER web site, April 2012, 2011.
16. Silverberg SG, Ioffe OB. Pathology of cervical cancer. Cancer J. 2003;9(5):335–47. http://www.ncbi.nlm.nih.gov/pubmed/14690308.
17. Bentz JS, et al. The unsatisfactory ThinPrep Pap test: missed opportunity for disease detection? Am J Clin Pathol. 2002;117(3):457–63. https://academic.oup.com/ajcp/article-lookup/doi/10.1309/XMQP-9AJD-104W-07C8.
18. Islam S, et al. Reprocessing unsatisfactory ThinPrep Papanicolaou test specimens increases sample adequacy and detection of significant cervicovaginal lesions. Cancer. 2004;102(2):67–73. https://doi.org/10.1002/cncr.11932.
19. zur Hausen H. Papillomaviruses and cancer: from basic studies to clinical application. Nat Rev Cancer. 2002;2(5):342–50. http://www.ncbi.nlm.nih.gov/pubmed/12044010.
20. Walboomers JMM, et al. Human papillomavirus is a necessary cause of invasive cervical cancer worldwide. J Pathol. 1999;189(1):12–9. http://www.ncbi.nlm.nih.gov/pubmed/10451482.
21. Faridi R, et al. Oncogenic potential of Human Papillomavirus (HPV) and its relation with cervical cancer. Virol J. 2011;8(1):269. http://www.ncbi.nlm.nih.gov/pubmed/21635792.
22. Lu B, et al. Epidemiologic factors associated with seropositivity to human papillomavirus type 16 and 18 virus-like particles and risk of subsequent infection in men. Cancer Epidemiol Biomarkers Prev. 2010;19(2):511–6. http://cebp.aacrjournals.org/cgi/doi/10.1158/1055-9965.EPI-09-0790.
23. Ganguly N, Parihar SP. Human papillomavirus E6 and E7 oncoproteins as risk factors for tumorigenesis. J Biosci. 2009;34(1):113–23. http://www.ncbi.nlm.nih.gov/pubmed/19430123.
24. Burd EM. Human papillomavirus and cervical cancer. Clin Microbiol Rev. 2003;16(1):1–17. http://www.ncbi.nlm.nih.gov/pubmed/12525422.
25. Kumar R, et al. Alcohol and tobacco increases risk of high risk HPV infection in head and neck cancer patients: Study from North-East Region of India. PLoS One. 2015;10(10):e0140700. http://dx.plos.org/10.1371/journal.pone.0140700.
26. Cuschieri K, Wentzensen N. Human papillomavirus mRNA and p16 detection as biomarkers for the improved diagnosis of cervical neoplasia. Cancer Epidemiol Biomarkers Prev. 2008;17(10):2536–45. http://www.ncbi.nlm.nih.gov/pubmed/18842994.
27. Villa LL, Denny L. CHAPTER 7 Methods for detection of HPV infection and its clinical utility. Int J Gynecol Obstet. 2006;94:S71–80. https://www.sciencedirect.com/science/article/pii/S0020729207600137.
28. Lungu O, Wright TC, Silverstein S. Typing of human papillomaviruses by polymerase chain reaction amplification with L1 consensus primers and RFLP analysis. Mol Cell Probes. 1992;6(2):145–52. http://www.ncbi.nlm.nih.gov/pubmed/1355266.
29. Carvalho Nde O, et al. Comparison of HPV genotyping by type-specific PCR and sequencing. Mem Inst Oswaldo Cruz. 2010;105(1):73–8. http://www.ncbi.nlm.nih.gov/pubmed/20209333.
30. Naqvi SH, Wajid S, Mitra AB. Restriction fragment length polymorphism of L1 amplicon using Rsa 1 detects five different human papillomavirus types and their co-infections among women attending a gynaecological outpatient department. J Virol Methods. 2004;117(1):91–5. http://linkinghub.elsevier.com/retrieve/pii/S0166093403004002.
31. Santiago E, et al. Full HPV typing by a single restriction enzyme. J Clin Virol. 2006;37(1):38–46. http://linkinghub.elsevier.com/retrieve/pii/S1386653206001910.
32. Novais RC, Thorstenson YR. The evolution of Pyrosequencing® for microbiology: from genes to genomes. J Microbiol Methods. 2011;86(1):1–7. http://www.ncbi.nlm.nih.gov/pubmed/21514329.
33. Roberts I, et al. Critical evaluation of HPV16 gene copy number quantification by SYBR green PCR. BMC Biotechnol. 2008;8(1):57. http://bmcbiotechnol.biomedcentral.com/articles/10.1186/1472-6750-8-57.
34. Yoshida T, et al. Quantitative real-time polymerase chain reaction analysis of the type distribution, viral load, and physical status of human papillomavirus in liquid-based cytology samples from cervical lesions. Int J Gynecol Cancer. 2008;18(1):121–7. https://doi.org/10.1111/j.1525-1438.2007.00979.x.
35. Gravitt PE, et al. High load for most high risk human papillomavirus genotypes is associated with prevalent cervical cancer precursors but only HPV16 load predicts the development of incident disease. Int J Cancer. 2007;121(12):2787–93. https://doi.org/10.1002/ijc.23012.
36. Lowe B, et al. Distribution of Human papillomavirus load in clinical specimens. J Virol Methods. 2011;173(1):150–2. http://www.ncbi.nlm.nih.gov/pubmed/21295613.
37. Kulmala S-MA, et al. Early integration of high copy HPV16 detectable in women with normal and low grade cervical cytology and histology. J Clin Pathol. 2006;59(5):513–7. https://doi.org/10.1136/jcp.2004.024570.
38. Bozzetti M, et al. Comparison between hybrid capture II and polymerase chain reaction results among women at low risk for cervical cancer. Ann Epidemiol. 2000;10(7):466. http://www.ncbi.nlm.nih.gov/pubmed/11018389.

39. Hwang SJ, Shroyer KR. Biomarkers of cervical dysplasia and carcinoma. J Oncol. 2012;2012:1–9. http://www.ncbi.nlm.nih.gov/pubmed/22131995.
40. Heideman DAM, et al. Clinical validation of the cobas 4800 HPV test for cervical screening purposes. J Clin Microbiol. 2011;49(11):3983–5. http://jcm.asm.org/lookup/doi/10.1128/JCM.05552-11.
41. Katki HA, et al. Cervical cancer risk for women undergoing concurrent testing for human papillomavirus and cervical cytology: a population-based study in routine clinical practice. Lancet Oncol. 2011;12(7):663–72. http://www.ncbi.nlm.nih.gov/pubmed/21684207.
42. Pista A, Verdasca N, Oliveira A. Clinical performance of the CLART human papillomavirus 2 assay compared with the hybrid capture 2 test. J Med Virol. 2011;83(2):272–6. https://doi.org/10.1002/jmv.21952.
43. Kocjan BJ, Seme K, Poljak M. Comparison of the Abbott RealTime High Risk HPV test and INNO-LiPA HPV Genotyping Extra test for the detection of human papillomaviruses in formalin-fixed, paraffin-embedded cervical cancer specimens. J Virol Methods. 2011;175(1):117–9. http://linkinghub.elsevier.com/retrieve/pii/S0166093411001443.
44. van Hamont D, et al. Evaluation of the SPF10-INNO LiPA human papillomavirus (HPV) genotyping test and the roche linear array HPV genotyping test. J Clin Microbiol. 2006;44(9):3122–9. https://doi.org/10.1128/JCM.00517-06.
45. Martínez SB, et al. Comparison of the Cobas 4800 Human Papillomavirus test against a combination of the Amplicor Human Papillomavirus and the Linear Array tests for detection of HPV types 16 and 18 in cervical samples. J Virol Methods. 2012;180(1–2):7–10. http://linkinghub.elsevier.com/retrieve/pii/S0166093411004794.
46. Kotsopoulos IC, et al. Implication of human papillomavirus-66 in vulvar carcinoma: a case report. J Med Case Reports. 2011;5(1):232. http://jmedicalcasereports.biomedcentral.com/articles/10.1186/1752-1947-5-232.
47. Barcellos RB, et al. Evaluation of a novel microplate colorimetric hybridization genotyping assay for human papillomavirus. J Virol Methods. 2011;177(1):38–43. http://linkinghub.elsevier.com/retrieve/pii/S0166093411002746.
48. Alaghehbandan R, et al. Performance of proex c and pretect hpv-proofer e6/e7 mrna tests in comparison with the hybrid capture 2 hpv dna test for triaging ascus and lsil cytology. Diagn Cytopathol. 2013;41(9):767–75. http://www.ncbi.nlm.nih.gov/pubmed/23341349.
49. Dockter J, et al. Analytical characterization of the APTIMA HPV Assay. J Clin Virol. 2009;45(Suppl 1):S39–47. http://linkinghub.elsevier.com/retrieve/pii/S1386653209700071.
50. Sahasrabuddhe VV, Luhn P, Wentzensen N. Human papillomavirus and cervical cancer: biomarkers for improved prevention efforts. Future Microbiol. 2011;6(9):1083–98. http://www.ncbi.nlm.nih.gov/pubmed/21958146.
51. Boone JD, Erickson BK, Huh WK. New insights into cervical cancer screening. J Gynecol Oncol. 2012;23(4):282–7. http://www.ncbi.nlm.nih.gov/pubmed/23094132.
52. Solomon D, et al. Comparison of three management strategies for patients with atypical squamous cells of undetermined significance: baseline results from a randomized trial. J Natl Cancer Inst. 2001;93(4):293–9. http://www.ncbi.nlm.nih.gov/pubmed/11181776.
53. Sankaranarayanan R, et al. HPV screening for cervical cancer in rural India. N Engl J Med. 2009;360(14):1385–94. http://www.ncbi.nlm.nih.gov/pubmed/19339719.
54. Franco EL, et al. Chapter 20: Issues in planning cervical cancer screening in the era of HPV vaccination. Vaccine. 2006;24:S171–7. http://www.ncbi.nlm.nih.gov/pubmed/16844268.
55. Bulkmans NWJ, et al. Human papillomavirus DNA testing for the detection of cervical intraepithelial neoplasia grade 3 and cancer: 5-year follow-up of a randomised controlled implementation trial. Lancet. 2007;370(9601):1764–72. http://linkinghub.elsevier.com/retrieve/pii/S0140673607614500.
56. Naucler P, et al. Human Papillomavirus and Papanicolaou tests to screen for cervical cancer. N Engl J Med. 2007;357(16):1589–97. http://www.ncbi.nlm.nih.gov/pubmed/17942872.
57. Ronco G, et al. Efficacy of human papillomavirus testing for the detection of invasive cervical cancers and cervical intraepithelial neoplasia: a randomised controlled trial. Lancet Oncol. 2010;11(3):249–57. http://www.ncbi.nlm.nih.gov/pubmed/20089449.
58. Leinonen M, et al. Age-specific evaluation of primary human papillomavirus screening vs conventional cytology in a randomized setting. J Natl Cancer Inst. 2009;101(23):1612–23. https://academic.oup.com/jnci/article-lookup/doi/10.1093/jnci/djp367.
59. Mishra GA, Pimple SA, Shastri SS. Prevention of cervix cancer in India. Oncology. 2016;91(1):1–7. http://www.ncbi.nlm.nih.gov/pubmed/27463969.
60. Rajaraman P, et al. Recommendations for screening and early detection of common cancers in India. Lancet Oncol. 2015;16(7):e352–61. http://linkinghub.elsevier.com/retrieve/pii/S1470204515000789.
61. Denny L, Sankaranarayanan R. CHAPTER 6 Secondary prevention of cervical cancer. Int J Gynecol Obstet. 2006;94(S1):S65–70. https://doi.org/10.1016/S0020-7292%2807%2960012-5.
62. Aswathy S, et al. Cervical cancer screening: Current knowledge and practice among women in a rural population of Kerala, India. Indian J Med Res. 2012;136(2):205–10. http://www.ncbi.nlm.nih.gov/pubmed/22960886.

63. Parikh S, Brennan P, Boffetta P. Meta-analysis of social inequality and the risk of cervical cancer. Int J Cancer. 2003;105(5):687–91. http://www.ncbi.nlm.nih.gov/pubmed/12740919.
64. Cuzick J, et al. Chapter 10: new dimensions in cervical cancer screening. Vaccine. 2006;24(Suppl 3):S3/90–7. http://linkinghub.elsevier.com/retrieve/pii/S0264410X06007316.
65. Reuschenbach M, et al. Performance of p16INK4a-cytology, HPV mRNA, and HPV DNA testing to identify high grade cervical dysplasia in women with abnormal screening results. Gynecol Oncol. 2010;119(1):98–105. http://linkinghub.elsevier.com/retrieve/pii/S0090825810004622.
66. Marlow L, Waller J. The changing landscape of cervical screening—what does the future hold for primary care? Eur J Cancer Care. 2017;26(3):e12693. https://doi.org/10.1111/ecc.12693.
67. Chung TKH, et al. Liquid biopsy of PIK3CA mutations in cervical cancer in Hong Kong Chinese women. Gynecol Oncol. 2017;146(2):334–9. http://linkinghub.elsevier.com/retrieve/pii/S0090825817308946.
68. Gradíssimo A, Burk RD. Molecular tests potentially improving HPV screening and genotyping for cervical cancer prevention. Expert Rev Mol Diagn. 2017;17(4):379–91. https://www.tandfonline.com/doi/full/10.1080/14737159.2017.1293525.

Molecular Diagnostics in Colorectal Cancer

9

Sandeep Agrawal, Aditi Bhattacharya, Janvie Manhas, and Sudip Sen

9.1 Introduction

Colorectal cancer (CRC) is a leading cause of cancer related mortality worldwide. Despite being one of the best characterized models of carcinogenesis with distinct molecular events in the adenoma to carcinoma sequence, mortality rate of CRC is high. Globally it is the third most common cancer in men and second in women. Mortality rate is around 8.5% with poor survival in the developing countries and high incidence rates in the developed countries [1]. The risk of getting CRC increases with increasing age and most of the new cases occur in patients older than 50 years. Almost 5–6% CRC occur in patients before the age of 30, mostly due to hereditary CRC syndromes. The mean 5-year survival rate in CRC patients is approximately 65%. Most of the cases of CRC are diagnosed at an advanced stage; responsible for low 5-year survival rates. Patients with localized CRC have 5-year survival approaching 90% which worsens significantly with regional and distant metastasis [2].

CRC presents in one of the three major patterns: sporadic, inherited and familial. Sporadic disease accounts for almost 70% of all CRCs, have no family history, presents commonly after the age of 50 years and generally associated with dietary and environmental factors. Inherited form of CRC accounts for less than 10% of all CRCs and is subdivided on the basis of colonic polyps as a major disease manifestation. All these conditions are associated with high risk of developing CRC. The cases having polyposis as major manifestation are familial adenomatous polyposis (FAP), MUTYH associated polyposis (MAP) and certain hamartomatous polyposis syndromes. The hereditary cases without polyposis are referred to as hereditary nonpolyposis CRC (HNPCC; Lynch syndrome). The most unclear pattern of CRC is seen with familial CRC, which accounts for up to 25% of total cases. These patients have a family history of CRC but the pattern is not consistent with the above discussed inherited syndromes. Nevertheless, the risk of developing CRC is high in these cases [3] (Fig. 9.1).

The risk factors for development of CRC can be divided into modifiable and non-modifiable categories. The former includes: diet rich in unsaturated fats and low in fibers, obesity, physical inactivity, alcohol consumption and smoking. Non-modifiable risk factors are age above 50 years, family history of CRC or hereditary syndromes associated with CRC, ulcerative colitis and Crohn's disease [4]. CRC patients are generally asymptomatic until advanced stages of the disease. The most common symptoms include changes in bowel habits with either diarrhea or constipation, feeling of incomplete evacuation

S. Agrawal (✉) · A. Bhattacharya · J. Manhas
S. Sen
Department of Biochemistry, All India Institute of Medical Sciences, New Delhi, India

K. K. Shukla et al. (eds.), *Molecular Diagnostics in Cancer Patients*,
https://doi.org/10.1007/978-981-13-5877-7_9

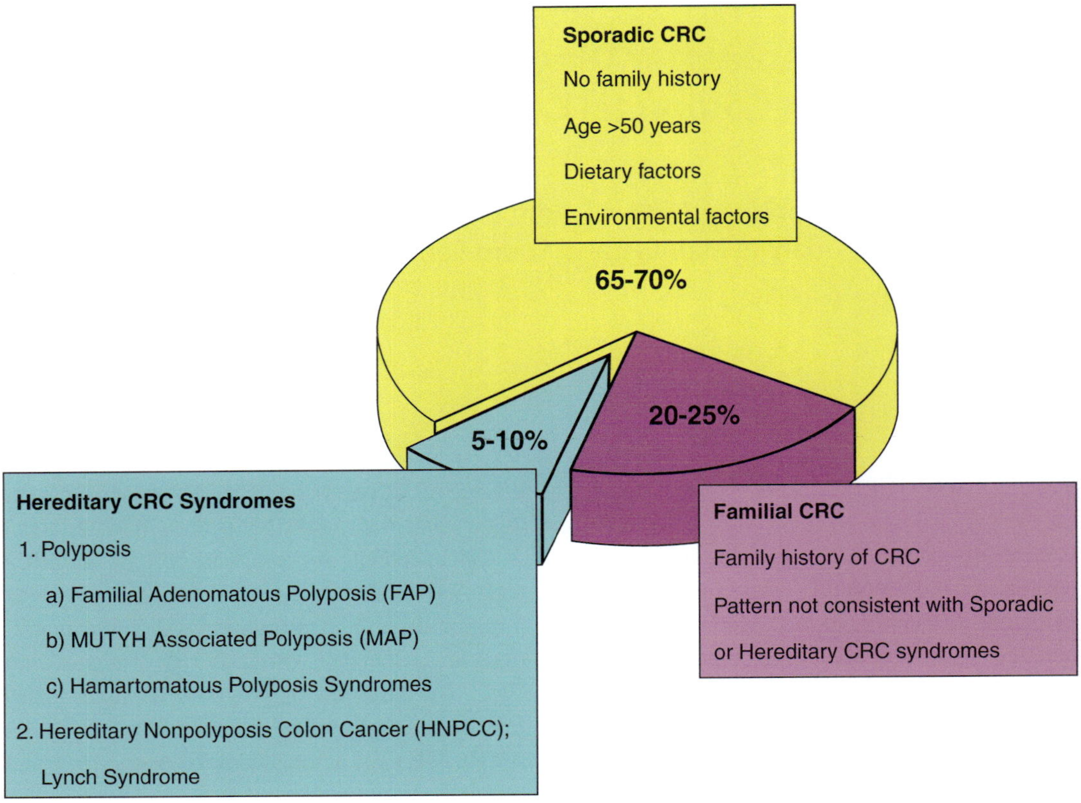

Fig. 9.1 Types of colorectal cancer

and bloating. Blood in stool, abdominal pain, unexplained weight loss, weakness, constant tiredness and unexplained iron deficiency anemia are other important clinical features. Sign and symptoms also vary with location of the tumor in colon [5].

The importance of screening and early diagnosis of CRC lies in the fact that it is generally asymptomatic until advanced stages and it is potentially a preventable and curable disease if high risk adenomas and early stage tumors are detected and removed at an appropriate time. Therefore, improved screening practices aimed at early diagnosis is vital to reduce the incidence and mortality rates. In the past few decades many efforts have been made to understand the molecular characteristics of CRC. It is a heterogeneous disease resulting from complex multifactorial processes leading to alteration of normal colon epithelial rejuvenation cycle. The three major molecular mechanisms involved in colorectal carcinogenesis are; chromosomal instability (CIN), microsatellite instability (MSI) and CpG island methylator phenotype (CIMP). In this chapter we will discuss molecular pathways and mutations involved in development of CRC and methods available to detect them. These molecular methods not only have role in screening and early detection of disease but are also important for prognosis and to predict response to therapy in CRC.

9.2 Molecular Pathways of Colorectal Carcinogenesis

9.2.1 Chromosomal Instability

Chromosomal instability is characterized by change in chromosomal copy number or their structure. It is the commonest type of genomic instability which is found in approximately

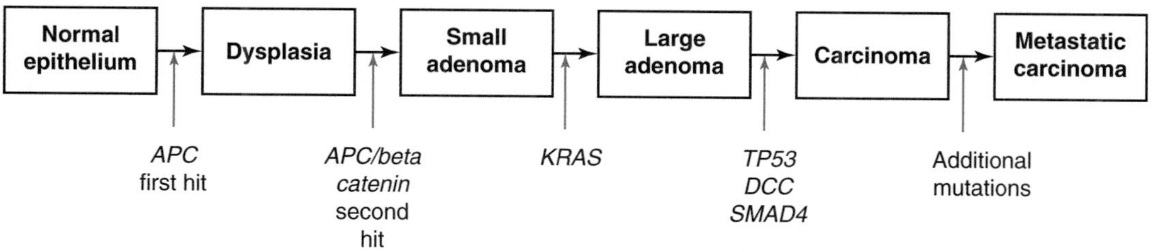

Fig. 9.2 Simplified adenoma-carcinoma sequence for CRC. (Modified from: Fearon ER, Vogelstein B. A genetic model for colorectal tumorigenesis. Cell. 1990;61(5):759–67)

80–85% of all CRC and adenoma cases. According to adenoma-carcinoma sequence model, germline or somatic mutations are needed for malignant transformation and it is the accumulation of multiple mutations which determines the biological characteristics of the tumor [6]. CIN induced changes leads to either loss of tumor suppressor genes like *APC, TP53* or activation of certain oncogenes like *KRAS*, resulting in improved survival and proliferation of cells and inhibition of apoptosis. CIN is generally associated with poor prognosis of CRC (Fig. 9.2).

9.2.1.1 RAS

The *RAS* oncogenes encode for a family of small G proteins which bind downstream of the EGFR in the PI3K/PTEN/AKT and RAF/MEK/ERK signaling pathways, transmitting extracellular growth signals to the nucleus. *RAS* exists as three cellular variants, *HRAS, KRAS* and *NRAS* but *KRAS* is most commonly mutated in CRC. These proteins normally cycle between a GDP-bound inactive state and a GTP-bound active state. Mutations in *RAS* lead to constitutively activated GTP-bound protein with a continuous growth stimulus to the cells. *RAS* mutations are found in approximately 50% of sporadic CRC cases. Activating mutations of *KRAS* are mostly seen in codon 12 and 13 and less commonly in codon 61 [7–9]. These mutations are associated with lack of response to anti-EGFR (cetuximab, panitumumab) therapy and poor prognosis in patients of metastatic CRC.

9.2.1.2 BRAF

BRAF gene encodes for a serine/threonine protein kinase, which is an immediate downstream effector of KRAS in the MAP kinase signaling pathway. Oncogenic activating BRAF mutation (V600E) is found in approximately 5–22% of CRC cases. This mutation is seen almost exclusively in MSI-H, CIMP+ CRCs with wild type *KRAS. BRAF* mutation is frequently detected in smokers with sporadic CRCs. Additional *BRAF* mutation in MSI-H CRCs may be associated with adverse prognosis. This mutation is also thought to be responsible for a proportion of CRC patients with wild type *KRAS*, who fail to respond to anti-EGFR therapy [10–15].

9.2.1.3 APC and Wnt Pathway

The most critical event in the early development of CRC is allelic loss or loss of heterozygosity (LOH) of *APC* (located at 5q21), a tumor suppressor gene. Somatic mutation in both the alleles of APC is found in almost 80% of sporadic CRCs. Germline mutations occur in familial adenomatous polyposis (FAP), an autosomal dominant syndrome characterized by development of hundreds of colorectal polyps early in the adult life [16, 17]. Normally APC plays a crucial role in Wnt/Wingless pathway and, is critically important for controlling the proliferation of colonic epithelial cells. Normal APC is thought to prevent the accumulation of cytosolic and nuclear beta-catenin by mediating its phosphorylation and degradation. Somatic or germline mutation in *APC* gene leads to accumulation of beta-catenin in nucleus and resultant activation of transcription factor Tcf-4, which results in proliferation of colonic epithelial cells by inhibiting terminal differentiation and providing resistance to apoptosis [18–21]. Mutation of *APC* gene is associated with chromosomal instability which

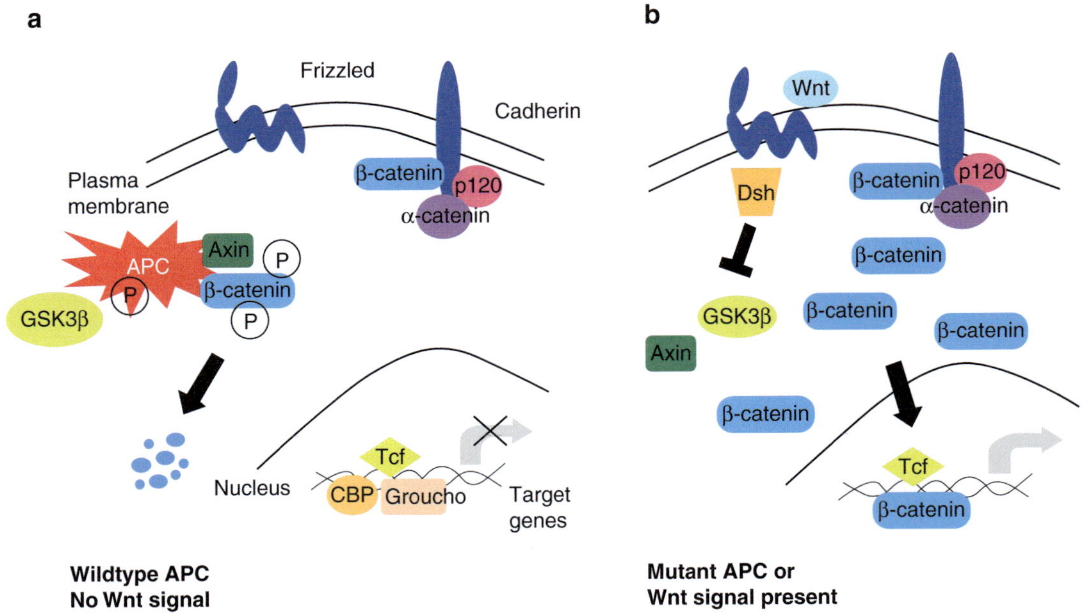

Fig. 9.3 Wnt pathway: (**a**) with wild type APC and absence of Wnt signal, (**b**) mutant APC and presence of Wnt signal. (Reproduced from: Goss KH, Groden J. Biology of the adenomatous polyposis coli tumor supressor. J Clin Oncol 2000; 18:1967. Copyright © 2000 American Society of Clinical Oncology. Permission Requested)

predisposes the cell to malignant transformation by mutation in other genes [22].

Wnt pathway is an evolutionarily conserved pathway, which plays a vital role during embryonic development. It is also important for intestinal epithelial cell renewal by maintaining stem cell population in the intestinal crypts [23]. Wnt signaling regulates signal transduction by controlling the levels of beta-catenin through phosphorylation and proteasomal degradation. In the absence of Wnt ligand, beta-catenin is phosphorylated by GSK3β in a cytoplasmic complex containing axin, APC and beta-catenin. Subsequently, beta-catenin is ubiquitinated and degraded in proteasomes (Fig. 9.3).

Binding of Wnt ligand to frizzled receptor leads to inactivation of GSK3β kinase through Dishevelled, creating a cytosolic pool of free beta-catenin. Beta-catenin is translocated to the nucleus, where it binds to Tcf family of transcription factors to regulate Wnt target gene transcription [20].

Mutations resulting in upregulation of Wnt signaling pathway leads to carcinogenesis including CRC. Multiple mutations including APC, β-catenin and axin have been observed in cases of CRC [24].

Additionally, epigenetic silencing of Wnt inhibitors and β-catenin destruction complex proteins by hypermethylation is also suggested to be the common mechanism of activation of Wnt pathway in CRC [25]. Wnt pathway represents a final common pathway for colorectal carcinogenesis because many other abnormalities in several other signaling pathways converge to it.

9.2.1.4 TP53

p53 acts as "guardian of genome" and guards the cell from genetic changes [26]. Approximately 50–70% of CRCs are associated with mutated *TP53* gene (located on chromosome 17p) coding for p53 protein which normally acts as a transcriptional activator of growth inhibitory genes, particularly when cells are under stress [27–29]. Due to mutation in *TP53,* G1 checkpoint does not function properly, defective DNA can replicate, perpetuating mutations and DNA rearrangements that are passed on to daughter cells. This can result in transformation into cancerous and metastatic cells. p53 loss of function mutations can also result in inhibition of apoptosis, contributing to survival of transformed cells. More than 70% of human cancers have a defect in *TP53* gene [30–32].

9.2.1.5 DCC, SMAD4 and SMAD2

DCC (deleted in colon carcinoma), *SMAD4* and *SMAD2* genes are located on chromosome 18q and, are mutated in certain proportion of CRC patients. *DCC* is thought to have a role in cell-cell or cell-matrix adhesion, although its exact function is not known [27, 33–36]. TGF-beta signaling normally has growth inhibitory effects by binding to TGFBR1 and TGFBR2 transmembrane receptors. *SMAD4* and *SMAD2* encode for protein which is thought to have important role in TGF-beta signaling cascade and mutation in these genes lead to increased cell proliferation [37–41].

9.2.2 Microsatellite Instability (MSI)

Mutations in the DNA mismatch repair genes (MMR), *MLH1, MSH2, MSH6* and *PMS2* lead to accumulation of abnormalities in highly repeated DNA sequences called microsatellites. MSI is seen in almost all cases of an autosomal dominant inherited cancer syndrome called Lynch syndrome or hereditary non-polyposis colorectal cancer (HNPCC) which is associated with a germline mutation in MMR gene followed by a somatic mutation leading to loss of both the alleles of the affected gene. MSI is also observed in 10–15% cases of sporadic CRC but rather than gene mutation in MMR system, epigenetic methylation induced silencing of *MLH1* gene is responsible [42–45]. MSI is exemplified by frameshift mutations in some critical growth regulatory genes like *TGFBR2* and *BAX* which contain microsatellites in their promoter region [46–48]. MSI is identified by studying PCR of a panel of five nucleotide markers and tumor is considered MSI-high (MSI-H) if two or more of these markers are found mutated and MSI-low (MSI-L) if only one is mutated. Tumors showing no microsatellite mutations are classified as microsatellite stable or MSS [42].

9.2.3 CpG Island Methylator Phenotype (CIMP)

DNA methylation is usually responsible for epigenetic gene silencing. On the basis of extent of aberrant hypermethylation in a large number of gene promoters, CRCs can be classified into two groups, CpG island methylator phenotype (CIMP) positive and CIMP negative. Approximately 35–40% of sporadic CRC cases are CIMP+ [49, 50]. DNA methylation in humans occurs at the fifth carbon of the cytosine residues of the CpG dinucleotides. The CpG dinucleotides are not spread uniformly across the chromosome but tend to cluster in certain regions called as CpG island (CGI). CpG rich regions are found near the promoter of more than 50% of the genes. Aberrant hypermethylation of CpG island results in colorectal carcinogenesis by silencing certain critical tumor suppressor genes like *p16, p14, MGMT* and *MLH1* [51]. Epigenetic silencing of *MLH1* gene can lead to MSI in some cases of sporadic CRCs as mentioned before. Studying CIMP in CRC patients may prove to be an important diagnostic and prognostic tool.

9.2.4 POLE Mutation

POLE encodes for catalytic subunit of DNA polymerase ε, which is involved in the synthesis of leading strand during DNA replication [52]. Proofreading activity of *POLE* is necessary to ensure the fidelity of DNA replication. *POLE* mutations are rare in CRC and seen in less than 2% of cases [24, 53]. *POLE* mutations lead to a high burden of single nucleotide variants (SNVs) in human cancers, notably cancers of endometrium and CRC. Patients with stage II/III CRC with *POLE* mutation have good prognosis, which can be explained by potent cytotoxic T cell response because of enriched antigenic neoepitopes resulting from mutations of *POLE* [54]. These mutations are significantly associated with male sex, occurrence at a young age and location in the right colon. Patients with this mutation have shown better prognosis with reduced recurrence risk and high disease-free survival in both endometrial and colorectal cancers [55].

9.3 Molecular Diagnostic Tests in Colorectal Cancer

The survival and prognosis in patients of CRC is highly dependent on the stage at which it is diagnosed but the fact is most of CRC cases are diagnosed at advanced stages. Historically, a number of diagnostic procedures have been in use for CRC. These procedures include colonoscopy, flexible sigmoidoscopy, barium enema, MRI and CT colonography. Colonoscopy is an invasive procedure, which is regarded as the reference method with high sensitivity and specificity for detection of CRC and premalignant adenomas. It is also possible to take a biopsy specimen from suspected lesion during colonoscopy. However, it is not always possible to do colonoscopy in a suspected CRC case because of poor tolerance to the procedure and need for appropriate bowel preparation. Other diagnostic methods have their own limitations in terms of sensitivity and specificity [56]. Molecular diagnostic methods are thought to be more sensitive and specific than these methods and can also detect genetic defects involved in the carcinogenesis. The molecular markers can predict the response to particular therapy in addition to having diagnostic and prognostic significance. Extensive efforts have been made in the past and are currently underway for development of molecular markers in CRC. An ideal molecular marker should be unique, noninvasive, safe and affordable with high sensitivity and specificity; aimed at early detection of CRC to facilitate better clinical decision making.

9.3.1 Tests for Tumor Based Molecular Markers

These markers can be used to classify CRC cases based on the underlying molecular defects in order to help clinicians to make the best treatment decision for the patients. These markers can also assess prognosis and predict response to chemotherapeutic drugs.

9.3.1.1 Identification of Chromosomal Instability

A number of point mutations are involved in chromosomal instability leading to carcinogenesis as mentioned above. Mutation in the *APC* gene is an early event in FAP associated CRCs, as such it can be an important screening tool for identifying individuals with risk of CRC in patient's family so as to guide the CRC surveillance intervals and indications for prophylactic surgery. *KRAS* and *BRAF* mutations are mutually exclusive of each other. Mutational analysis for *KRAS, NRAS* and *BRAF* is an important tool to predict the response to anti-EGFR monoclonal antibodies (cetuximab, panitumumab). Growing evidence suggests that patients of sporadic CRC with these mutations fail to respond to anti-EGFR therapy (Fig. 9.4) [13, 57, 58]. Current guidelines from American Society for Clinical Oncology (ASCO) suggest that, tumors of stage IV sporadic CRC patients must undergo mutation testing for *KRAS* before administering any anti-EGFR therapy [11, 59–61].

These mutations can be detected by DNA sequencing and PCR based methods. Allele-specific PCR detects specific known mutations in a gene. In cases where the specific point mutations are not known, Sanger sequencing can be applied. Both the methods can be used for the detection of mutations in genes such as *APC* and *KRAS, NRAS* and *BRAF*.

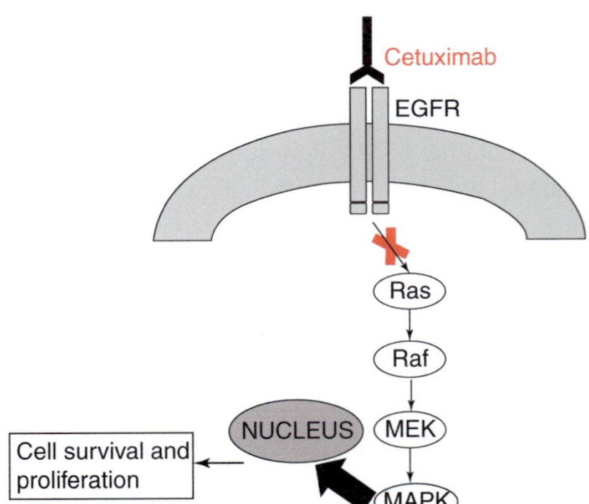

Fig. 9.4 EGFR pathway inhibited by cetuximab

With Sanger sequencing, it is also possible to detect both known and novel changes including insertions, deletions, nucleotide substitution. However, the long turnover time and high cost of processing each sample make it inappropriate for routine clinical applications. The development of fluorophore based quantitative real time PCR system and pyrosequencing are improved methods with greater sensitivity and specificity with shorter turnover time.

9.3.1.2 Identification of Microsatellite Instability (MSI)

Sporadic CRC tumors with MSI-H are mainly located in proximal colon and are poorly differentiated. MSI is also associated with mucinous nature of tumor and abundant tumor infiltrating lymphocytes [62, 63]. MSI status of CRC may prove to be an important prognostic factor in sporadic CRC as accumulating evidence suggests that patients with MSI-H phenotype have better survival, less recurrence and less propensity for metastatic disease [64–67]. Several studies have concluded that, these patients do not benefit from 5-fluorouracil (5-FU) while respond better to irinotecan-containing regimens, highlighting the predictive significance of MSI testing in CRC patients in addition to its diagnostic importance in patients of HNPCC [68–73]. *BRAF* somatic mutation (V600E) testing may be indicated in MSI-H cases as this mutation is specifically seen with sporadic MSI-H but absent in HNPCC cases. *BRAF* mutation seems to nullify the good prognosis characteristically seen with MSI-H CRCs [74, 75].

In MSI CRC cases, comparison between amplification of microsatellite regions in tumor and nearby normal cells can be taken as an indicator. Based on Bethesda guidelines for diagnosis of HNPCC, a panel of five markers are used for PCR based detection of MSI. It includes two mononucleotide (BAT25 and BAT26) and three dinucleotide (D2S123, D5S346, and D17S250) markers [42]. The mononucleotide markers are more sensitive than dinucleotide microsatellites and later a pentaplex of mononucleotide repeats (BAT-25, BAT-26, NR-21, NR-24 and MONO-27) was proposed with sensitivity and specificity more than 95% for detection of defective MMR genes in CRC [76]. The DNA samples from a tumor and normal tissue specimen from the patient are amplified for microsatellite markers in a fluorescent multiplex PCR based system and products are analyzed by capillary electrophoresis [77]. Genotype pattern of normal and tumor specimen are compared with each other and scored as MSI-H, MSI-L or MSS.

9.3.1.3 Identification of CpG Island Methylator Phenotype (CIMP)

Hypermethylation induced silencing of tumor suppressor genes can lead to carcinogenesis. In cases of Lynch syndrome after germline mutation in one of the alleles of MMR gene, the second normal allele can be inactivated by an epigenetic silencing by hypermethylation. Approximately 35–40% of sporadic CRC are CIMP+. Hypermethylation induced CRC are noted to be more common in women and are associated with *BRAF* mutations. They are generally located in proximal colon with mucinous nature and, are poorly differentiated [78–82].

DNA hypermethylation induced silencing of genes in CRC can be detected by bisulfite conversion of DNA followed by methylation specific PCR. Pyrosequencing technique can also be employed to detect hypermethylated DNA [83]. The panel of methylation specific markers for detection of CIMP in CRC has not yet been standardized but in future it can prove to be an important diagnostic and prognostic tool.

9.3.2 Immunohistochemistry (IHC) for CRC Biomarkers

Molecular testing of CRC tissue has important implications in diagnosis, prognosis and ascertaining the response to chemotherapy. Tumor tissues are obtained by colonoscopic biopsy or surgery and fixated usually by 10% formaldehyde buffering solution. The latter is made into paraffin blocks or formalin-fixed paraffin-embedded tissues (FFPET). These can be used for histological examination for characterization of tumor and immunohistochemistry to analyze the expression of proteins related to mismatch repair, microsatellite and chromosomal instability. IHC is particularly important for diagnosis of Lynch syndrome involving testing for MLH1, MSH2, MSH6 and PMS2. Colonic adenomas and adenocarcinomas show similar immunohistochemical staining characteristics. Almost all of them show positive staining with CK20 while some are focally positive for CK7 [84]. Other IHC biomarkers for CRC include CDX-2, beta-catenin, cadherin-17 [85], villin and SATB2 [86]. EGFR expression is associated with increased likelihood of metastatic disease but it also predicts response to anti-EGFR (therapy). Loss of expression of SMAD4 is associated with poor prognosis in cases of CRC [87]. Data from our own lab suggests that immunohistochemical staining for CD44 and CD166 are robust markers of cancer stem cells (CSC), which are thought to be involved in invasion, metastasis, therapeutic responsiveness and recurrence of CRC [88].

9.3.3 Tests for Stool Based CRC Biomarkers

Stool contains exfoliated and secreted colon cells which are shed in the colorectal lumen [89]. Fecal occult blood tests (FOBT) are based on detection of pseudoperoxidase activity of heme coming from bleeding in CRCs. Bleeding from CRCs can be intermittent therefore, in order to be sensitive this test has to be performed at frequent intervals [90–92]. Fecal immunochemical test (FIT) is based on enzyme linked immunosorbent assay (ELISA) which detects the globin of hemoglobin molecule in fecal blood [93, 94]. Fecal blood based tests have low sensitivity and specificity because other non-neoplastic gastrointestinal conditions also bleed and not all CRCs and adenoma will bleed in colorectal lumen. Extensive work has been done to detect CRC specific DNA markers in stool which are thought to be very specific as they are derived directly from the tumor cells but available tests show low sensitivity and specificity to detect CRC.

9.3.4 Tests for Serum CRC Biomarkers

The idea of a serum biomarker which can detect CRC at an early stage has attracted a lot of researchers to work on but so far, little success has been achieved in this area. Most of the currently available candidate serum based tumor markers for CRC are mostly detected in advanced stages of disease. Carcinoembryonic antigen (CEA) is a high molecular weight glycoprotein, found in embryonic tissues and colorectal malignancies. It is the only acceptable tumor marker and, is only useful to monitor tumor recurrence after treatment. High CEA levels are associated with poor prognosis of resectable CRC and correlate with advanced stage of disease. CEA is not specific for CRC and can be elevated in pancreaticobiliary diseases, inflammatory bowel disease (IBD) and other malignancies [95, 96]. Extensive efforts have been made to identify circulating nucleic acids, proteins and tumor cells as candidate biomarkers specific for CRC but search for a noninvasive serum tumor marker with high sensitivity and specificity is still incomplete.

MicroRNAs (miRNAs) are small (19–23 nucleotides) noncoding RNA which are relatively stable in blood and formalin fixed tissue specimens attributing to their small size [97]. miRNAs are involved in post-transcriptional regulation of gene expression. Certain specific miRNAs have been shown to be associated with CRCs and circulate in bloodstream in stable and free form [98]. Detection of CRC associated miRNA in bloodstream can prove to be an important noninvasive tumor marker in future [99]. The candidate miRNA associated with CRC are miR-135a, miR-135b, miR-92a, miR-17-3p and miR-211 [100–102]. MicroRNA profiling can be done by PCR based methods and microarrays [103–105]. A lateral flow nucleic acid based assay has been described for detection of miRNA, which can be used as a point of care testing (POCT) tool [106–108].

Secretion of certain tumor related proteins in the tumor microenvironment and bloodstream can serve as potential tumor marker for early

Table 9.1 Key features of three major CRC pathways

	Chromosomal instability (CIN)	Microsatellite instability (MSI)	CpG island methylator phenotype (CIMP)
Prevalence	80–85% of all CRCs	Almost all cases of HNPCC	35–40% of sporadic CRCs
Molecular defect	Loss of TSG: *APC, TP53*; Activation of proto-oncogenes: *KRAS, BRAF, DCC, SMAD4*	Defects in DNA mismatch repair system: *MLH1, MSH2, MSH6, PMS2*	DNA hypermethylation induced gene silencing of critical TSG: *p16, p14, MGMT* and *MLH1*
Testing method	DNA sequencing, Allele specific PCR	Mononucleotide repeats (BAT-25, BAT-26, NR-21, NR-24 and MONO-27) are amplified by PCR and then sized by capillary electrophoresis Immunohistochemistry	Bisulfite conversion of DNA followed by methylation specific PCR
Significance	Screening of at risk individuals in FAP by detecting APC gene mutation Identification of candidate for anti-EGFR therapy in metastatic CRC (Tumors with *KRAS* mutation do not respond)	Diagnosis of HNPCC MSI-H is associated with favorable prognosis but reduced response to 5-FU based regimens and improved response to irinotecan based regimens	More common in women Associated with BRAF mutation

CRC detection. Mass spectrometry based approach for proteomic profiling of serum from CRC patient can be used to define a distinct CRC serum proteomic signature. This method may help to diagnose CRC at an early stage [109].

9.4 Conclusion

CRC can occur in both inherited and sporadic form resulting from different carcinogenic molecular pathways including CIN, MSI and CIMP. Molecular techniques are applied for diagnosing CRC cases, so as to classify the disease based on the molecular defects involved which can predict the characteristic, prognosis and response to particular chemotherapeutic drugs. The main techniques involved in molecular testing for CRC are PCR based methods, DNA sequencing and immunohistochemistry analysis of tissue sections. These methods are currently used for diagnosis of Lynch syndrome by detection of MSI phenotype and discriminating them from sporadic CRC by looking for *BRAF* mutation. To identify the candidates for anti-EGFR therapy in metastatic disease, checking for *KRAS* mutation is now included in clinical guidelines (Table 9.1). Currently available blood and stool based tumor markers for early detection of CRC are not satisfactory in terms of sensitivity and specificity. CEA is used in clinical settings to monitor the risk of recurrence after surgical resection of CRC tumor but it has its own limitations. The search for a noninvasive, sensitive, specific serum biomarker which is highly acceptable to patients is still continuing. The advances in genomics, transcriptomics and proteomics techniques like quantitative PCR, microarrays, next generation sequencing (NGS) and mass spectrometry are being employed in development of novel markers and better understanding of the pathways involved in carcinogenesis using high throughput analysis.

References

1. Globocan Database. International Agency for Research on Cancer. 2012. http://globocan.iarc.fr/Pages/fact_sheets_cancer.aspx?cancer=colorectal. Accessed 18 Feb 2018.
2. Colorectal cancer facts & figures 2014-2016. 2014. American Cancer Society. Atlanta.
3. Lindor NM. Familial colorectal cancer type X: the other half of hereditary nonpolyposis

colon cancer syndrome. Surg Oncol Clin N Am. 2009;18(4):637–45.
4. Wei EK, Giovannucci E, Wu K, Rosner B, Fuchs CS, Willett WC, et al. Comparison of risk factors for colon and rectal cancer. Int J Cancer. 2004;108(3):433–42.
5. Jass JR. Classification of colorectal cancer based on correlation of clinical, morphological and molecular features. Histopathology. 2007;50(1):113–30.
6. Fearon ER, Vogelstein B. A genetic model for colorectal tumorigenesis. Cell. 1990;61(5):759–67.
7. Shibata D, Schaeffer J, Li ZH, Capella G, Perucho M. Genetic heterogeneity of the c-K-ras locus in colorectal adenomas but not in adenocarcinomas. J Natl Cancer Inst. 1993;85(13):1058–63.
8. Tortola S, Marcuello E, Gonzalez I, Reyes G, Arribas R, Aiza G, et al. p53 and K-ras gene mutations correlate with tumor aggressiveness but are not of routine prognostic value in colorectal cancer. J Clin Oncol. 1999;17(5):1375–81.
9. Takayama T, Ohi M, Hayashi T, Miyanishi K, Nobuoka A, Nakajima T, et al. Analysis of K-ras, APC, and beta-catenin in aberrant crypt foci in sporadic adenoma, cancer, and familial adenomatous polyposis. Gastroenterology. 2001;121(3):599–611.
10. Roth AD, Tejpar S, Delorenzi M, Yan P, Fiocca R, Klingbiel D, et al. Prognostic role of KRAS and BRAF in stage II and III resected colon cancer: results of the translational study on the PETACC-3, EORTC 40993, SAKK 60-00 trial. J Clin Oncol. 2010;28(3):466–74.
11. Di Nicolantonio F, Martini M, Molinari F, Sartore-Bianchi A, Arena S, Saletti P, et al. Wild-type BRAF is required for response to panitumumab or cetuximab in metastatic colorectal cancer. J Clin Oncol. 2008;26(35):5705–12.
12. Richman SD, Seymour MT, Chambers P, Elliott F, Daly CL, Meade AM, et al. KRAS and BRAF mutations in advanced colorectal cancer are associated with poor prognosis but do not preclude benefit from oxaliplatin or irinotecan: results from the MRC FOCUS trial. J Clin Oncol. 2009;27(35):5931–7.
13. De Roock W, Claes B, Bernasconi D, De Schutter J, Biesmans B, Fountzilas G, et al. Effects of KRAS, BRAF, NRAS, and PIK3CA mutations on the efficacy of cetuximab plus chemotherapy in chemotherapy-refractory metastatic colorectal cancer: a retrospective consortium analysis. Lancet Oncol. 2010;11(8):753–62.
14. Samowitz WS, Sweeney C, Herrick J, Albertsen H, Levin TR, Murtaugh MA, et al. Poor survival associated with the BRAF V600E mutation in microsatellite-stable colon cancers. Cancer Res. 2005;65(14):6063–9.
15. Deng G, Bell I, Crawley S, Gum J, Terdiman JP, Allen BA, et al. BRAF mutation is frequently present in sporadic colorectal cancer with methylated hMLH1, but not in hereditary nonpolyposis colorectal cancer. Clin Cancer Res. 2004;10(1 Pt 1):191–5.
16. Spirio LN, Samowitz W, Robertson J, Robertson M, Burt RW, Leppert M, et al. Alleles of APC modulate the frequency and classes of mutations that lead to colon polyps. Nat Genet. 1998;20(4):385–8.
17. Lamlum H, Ilyas M, Rowan A, Clark S, Johnson V, Bell J, et al. The type of somatic mutation at APC in familial adenomatous polyposis is determined by the site of the germline mutation: a new facet to Knudson's 'two-hit' hypothesis. Nat Med. 1999;5(9):1071–5.
18. Korinek V, Barker N, Morin PJ, van Wichen D, de Weger R, Kinzler KW, et al. Constitutive transcriptional activation by a beta-catenin-Tcf complex in APC-/- colon carcinoma. Science. 1997;275(5307):1784–7.
19. Morin PJ, Sparks AB, Korinek V, Barker N, Clevers H, Vogelstein B, et al. Activation of beta-catenin-Tcf signaling in colon cancer by mutations in beta-catenin or APC. Science. 1997;275(5307):1787–90.
20. Goss KH, Groden J. Biology of the adenomatous polyposis coli tumor suppressor. J Clin Oncol. 2000;18(9):1967–79.
21. Kim PJ, Plescia J, Clevers H, Fearon ER, Altieri DC. Survivin and molecular pathogenesis of colorectal cancer. Lancet. 2003;362(9379):205–9.
22. Fodde R, Kuipers J, Rosenberg C, Smits R, Kielman M, Gaspar C, et al. Mutations in the APC tumour suppressor gene cause chromosomal instability. Nat Cell Biol. 2001;3(4):433–8.
23. Schepers A, Clevers H. Wnt signaling, stem cells, and cancer of the gastrointestinal tract. Cold Spring Harb Perspect Biol. 2012;4(4):a007989.
24. Cancer Genome Atlas Network. Comprehensive molecular characterization of human colon and rectal cancer. Nature. 2012;487(7407):330–7.
25. Rawson JB, Manno M, Mrkonjic M, Daftary D, Dicks E, Buchanan DD, et al. Promoter methylation of Wnt antagonists DKK1 and SFRP1 is associated with opposing tumor subtypes in two large populations of colorectal cancer patients. Carcinogenesis. 2011;32(5):741–7.
26. Lane DP. Cancer. p53, guardian of the genome. Nature. 1992;358(6381):15–6.
27. Vogelstein B, Fearon ER, Hamilton SR, Kern SE, Preisinger AC, Leppert M, et al. Genetic alterations during colorectal-tumor development. N Engl J Med. 1988;319(9):525–32.
28. Soussi T. The p53 tumor suppressor gene: from molecular biology to clinical investigation. Ann N Y Acad Sci. 2000;910:121–37; discussion 37–9.
29. Baker SJ, Preisinger AC, Jessup JM, Paraskeva C, Markowitz S, Willson JK, et al. p53 gene mutations occur in combination with 17p allelic deletions as late events in colorectal tumorigenesis. Cancer Res. 1990;50(23):7717–22.
30. Kastan MB, Onyekwere O, Sidransky D, Vogelstein B, Craig RW. Participation of p53 protein in the cellular response to DNA damage. Cancer Res. 1991;51(23 Pt 1):6304–11.

31. Kuerbitz SJ, Plunkett BS, Walsh WV, Kastan MB. Wild-type p53 is a cell cycle checkpoint determinant following irradiation. Proc Natl Acad Sci U S A. 1992;89(16):7491–5.
32. Woods DB, Vousden KH. Regulation of p53 function. Exp Cell Res. 2001;264(1):56–66.
33. Hedrick L, Cho KR, Fearon ER, Wu TC, Kinzler KW, Vogelstein B. The DCC gene product in cellular differentiation and colorectal tumorigenesis. Genes Dev. 1994;8(10):1174–83.
34. Chan SS, Zheng H, Su MW, Wilk R, Killeen MT, Hedgecock EM, et al. UNC-40, a C. elegans homolog of DCC (Deleted in Colorectal Cancer), is required in motile cells responding to UNC-6 netrin cues. Cell. 1996;87(2):187–95.
35. Thiagalingam S, Lengauer C, Leach FS, Schutte M, Hahn SA, Overhauser J, et al. Evaluation of candidate tumour suppressor genes on chromosome 18 in colorectal cancers. Nat Genet. 1996;13(3):343–6.
36. Cho KR, Oliner JD, Simons JW, Hedrick L, Fearon ER, Preisinger AC, et al. The DCC gene: structural analysis and mutations in colorectal carcinomas. Genomics. 1994;19(3):525–31.
37. Goyette MC, Cho K, Fasching CL, Levy DB, Kinzler KW, Paraskeva C, et al. Progression of colorectal cancer is associated with multiple tumor suppressor gene defects but inhibition of tumorigenicity is accomplished by correction of any single defect via chromosome transfer. Mol Cell Biol. 1992;12(3):1387–95.
38. Reiss M, Santoro V, de Jonge RR, Vellucci VF. Transfer of chromosome 18 into human head and neck squamous carcinoma cells: evidence for tumor suppression by Smad4/DPC4. Cell Growth Differ. 1997;8(4):407–15.
39. Riggins GJ, Thiagalingam S, Rozenblum E, Weinstein CL, Kern SE, Hamilton SR, et al. Mad-related genes in the human. Nat Genet. 1996;13(3):347–9.
40. Xie W, Rimm DL, Lin Y, Shih WJ, Reiss M. Loss of Smad signaling in human colorectal cancer is associated with advanced disease and poor prognosis. Cancer J. 2003;9(4):302–12.
41. Zhou XP, Woodford-Richens K, Lehtonen R, Kurose K, Aldred M, Hampel H, et al. Germline mutations in BMPR1A/ALK3 cause a subset of cases of juvenile polyposis syndrome and of Cowden and Bannayan-Riley-Ruvalcaba syndromes. Am J Hum Genet. 2001;69(4):704–11.
42. Boland CR, Thibodeau SN, Hamilton SR, Sidransky D, Eshleman JR, Burt RW, et al. A National Cancer Institute Workshop on Microsatellite Instability for cancer detection and familial predisposition: development of international criteria for the determination of microsatellite instability in colorectal cancer. Cancer Res. 1998;58(22):5248–57.
43. Syngal S, Weeks JC, Schrag D, Garber JE, Kuntz KM. Benefits of colonoscopic surveillance and prophylactic colectomy in patients with hereditary nonpolyposis colorectal cancer mutations. Ann Intern Med. 1998;129(10):787–96.
44. Shibata D, Peinado MA, Ionov Y, Malkhosyan S, Perucho M. Genomic instability in repeated sequences is an early somatic event in colorectal tumorigenesis that persists after transformation. Nat Genet. 1994;6(3):273–81.
45. Kane MF, Loda M, Gaida GM, Lipman J, Mishra R, Goldman H, et al. Methylation of the hMLH1 promoter correlates with lack of expression of hMLH1 in sporadic colon tumors and mismatch repair-defective human tumor cell lines. Cancer Res. 1997;57(5):808–11.
46. Markowitz S, Wang J, Myeroff L, Parsons R, Sun L, Lutterbaugh J, et al. Inactivation of the type II TGF-beta receptor in colon cancer cells with microsatellite instability. Science. 1995;268(5215):1336–8.
47. Ionov Y, Peinado MA, Malkhosyan S, Shibata D, Perucho M. Ubiquitous somatic mutations in simple repeated sequences reveal a new mechanism for colonic carcinogenesis. Nature. 1993;363(6429):558–61.
48. Fujiwara T, Stolker JM, Watanabe T, Rashid A, Longo P, Eshleman JR, et al. Accumulated clonal genetic alterations in familial and sporadic colorectal carcinomas with widespread instability in microsatellite sequences. Am J Pathol. 1998;153(4):1063–78.
49. Legolvan MP, Taliano RJ, Resnick MB. Application of molecular techniques in the diagnosis, prognosis and management of patients with colorectal cancer: a practical approach. Hum Pathol. 2012;43(8):1157–68.
50. Kanwal R, Gupta S. Epigenetic modifications in cancer. Clin Genet. 2012;81(4):303–11.
51. Kanthan R, Senger JL, Kanthan SC. Molecular events in primary and metastatic colorectal carcinoma: a review. Patholog Res Int. 2012;2012:597497.
52. Pursell ZF, Isoz I, Lundstrom EB, Johansson E, Kunkel TA. Yeast DNA polymerase epsilon participates in leading-strand DNA replication. Science. 2007;317(5834):127–30.
53. Rayner E, van Gool IC, Palles C, Kearsey SE, Bosse T, Tomlinson I, et al. A panoply of errors: polymerase proofreading domain mutations in cancer. Nat Rev Cancer. 2016;16(2):71–81.
54. van Gool IC, Eggink FA, Freeman-Mills L, Stelloo E, Marchi E, de Bruyn M, et al. POLE proofreading mutations elicit an antitumor immune response in endometrial cancer. Clin Cancer Res. 2015;21(14):3347–55.
55. Domingo E, Freeman-Mills L, Rayner E, Glaire M, Briggs S, Vermeulen L, et al. Somatic POLE proofreading domain mutation, immune response, and prognosis in colorectal cancer: a retrospective, pooled biomarker study. Lancet Gastroenterol Hepatol. 2016;1(3):207–16.
56. De Rosa M, Pace U, Rega D, Costabile V, Duraturo F, Izzo P, et al. Genetics, diagnosis and management of colorectal cancer (Review). Oncol Rep. 2015;34(3):1087–96.

57. Cunningham D, Humblet Y, Siena S, Khayat D, Bleiberg H, Santoro A, et al. Cetuximab monotherapy and cetuximab plus irinotecan in irinotecan-refractory metastatic colorectal cancer. N Engl J Med. 2004;351(4):337–45.
58. Douillard JY, Oliner KS, Siena S, Tabernero J, Burkes R, Barugel M, et al. Panitumumab-FOLFOX4 treatment and RAS mutations in colorectal cancer. N Engl J Med. 2013;369(11):1023–34.
59. Kislitsin D, Lerner A, Rennert G, Lev Z. K-ras mutations in sporadic colorectal tumors in Israel: unusual high frequency of codon 13 mutations and evidence for nonhomogeneous representation of mutation subtypes. Dig Dis Sci. 2002;47(5):1073–9.
60. De Roock W, De Vriendt V, Normanno N, Ciardiello F, Tejpar S. KRAS, BRAF, PIK3CA, and PTEN mutations: implications for targeted therapies in metastatic colorectal cancer. Lancet Oncol. 2011;12(6):594–603.
61. Fornaro L, Lonardi S, Masi G, Loupakis F, Bergamo F, Salvatore L, et al. FOLFOXIRI in combination with panitumumab as first-line treatment in quadruple wild-type (KRAS, NRAS, HRAS, BRAF) metastatic colorectal cancer patients: a phase II trial by the Gruppo Oncologico Nord Ovest (GONO). Ann Oncol. 2013;24(8):2062–7.
62. Jass JR, Walsh MD, Barker M, Simms LA, Young J, Leggett BA. Distinction between familial and sporadic forms of colorectal cancer showing DNA microsatellite instability. Eur J Cancer. 2002;38(7):858–66.
63. Iacopetta B, Grieu F, Amanuel B. Microsatellite instability in colorectal cancer. Asia Pac J Clin Oncol. 2010;6(4):260–9.
64. Gryfe R, Kim H, Hsieh ET, Aronson MD, Holowaty EJ, Bull SB, et al. Tumor microsatellite instability and clinical outcome in young patients with colorectal cancer. N Engl J Med. 2000;342(2):69–77.
65. Popat S, Hubner R, Houlston RS. Systematic review of microsatellite instability and colorectal cancer prognosis. J Clin Oncol. 2005;23(3):609–18.
66. Sinicrope FA, Rego RL, Halling KC, Foster N, Sargent DJ, La Plant B, et al. Prognostic impact of microsatellite instability and DNA ploidy in human colon carcinoma patients. Gastroenterology. 2006;131(3):729–37.
67. Benatti P, Gafa R, Barana D, Marino M, Scarselli A, Pedroni M, et al. Microsatellite instability and colorectal cancer prognosis. Clin Cancer Res. 2005;11(23):8332–40.
68. Jo WS, Carethers JM. Chemotherapeutic implications in microsatellite unstable colorectal cancer. Cancer Biomark. 2006;2(1–2):51–60.
69. Jover R, Castells A, Llor X, Andreu M. Predictive value of microsatellite instability for benefit from adjuvant fluorouracil chemotherapy in colorectal cancer. Gut. 2006;55(12):1819–20.
70. Guastadisegni C, Colafranceschi M, Ottini L, Dogliotti E. Microsatellite instability as a marker of prognosis and response to therapy: a meta-analysis of colorectal cancer survival data. Eur J Cancer. 2010;46(15):2788–98.
71. Ribic CM, Sargent DJ, Moore MJ, Thibodeau SN, French AJ, Goldberg RM, et al. Tumor microsatellite-instability status as a predictor of benefit from fluorouracil-based adjuvant chemotherapy for colon cancer. N Engl J Med. 2003;349(3):247–57.
72. Bertagnolli MM, Niedzwiecki D, Compton CC, Hahn HP, Hall M, Damas B, et al. Microsatellite instability predicts improved response to adjuvant therapy with irinotecan, fluorouracil, and leucovorin in stage III colon cancer: Cancer and Leukemia Group B Protocol 89803. J Clin Oncol. 2009;27(11):1814–21.
73. Fallik D, Borrini F, Boige V, Viguier J, Jacob S, Miquel C, et al. Microsatellite instability is a predictive factor of the tumor response to irinotecan in patients with advanced colorectal cancer. Cancer Res. 2003;63(18):5738–44.
74. French AJ, Sargent DJ, Burgart LJ, Foster NR, Kabat BF, Goldberg R, et al. Prognostic significance of defective mismatch repair and BRAF V600E in patients with colon cancer. Clin Cancer Res. 2008;14(11):3408–15.
75. Ogino S, Nosho K, Kirkner GJ, Kawasaki T, Meyerhardt JA, Loda M, et al. CpG island methylator phenotype, microsatellite instability, BRAF mutation and clinical outcome in colon cancer. Gut. 2009;58(1):90–6.
76. Xicola RM, Llor X, Pons E, Castells A, Alenda C, Pinol V, et al. Performance of different microsatellite marker panels for detection of mismatch repair-deficient colorectal tumors. J Natl Cancer Inst. 2007;99(3):244–52.
77. Shi C, Washington K. Molecular testing in colorectal cancer: diagnosis of Lynch syndrome and personalized cancer medicine. Am J Clin Pathol. 2012;137(6):847–59.
78. Aaltonen LA, Peltomaki P, Mecklin JP, Jarvinen H, Jass JR, Green JS, et al. Replication errors in benign and malignant tumors from hereditary nonpolyposis colorectal cancer patients. Cancer Res. 1994;54(7):1645–8.
79. Lipkin SM, Wang V, Stoler DL, Anderson GR, Kirsch I, Hadley D, et al. Germline and somatic mutation analyses in the DNA mismatch repair gene MLH3: evidence for somatic mutation in colorectal cancers. Hum Mutat. 2001;17(5):389–96.
80. Lynch HT, de la Chapelle A. Hereditary colorectal cancer. N Engl J Med. 2003;348(10):919–32.
81. Wheeler JM, Loukola A, Aaltonen LA, Mortensen NJ, Bodmer WF. The role of hypermethylation of the hMLH1 promoter region in HNPCC versus MSI+ sporadic colorectal cancers. J Med Genet. 2000;37(8):588–92.
82. Issa JP. Colon cancer: it's CIN or CIMP. Clin Cancer Res. 2008;14(19):5939–40.
83. Herbst A, Kolligs FT. Detection of DNA hypermethylation in remote media of patients with colorectal

cancer: new biomarkers for colorectal carcinoma. Tumour Biol. 2012;33(2):297–305.
84. Bayrak R, Yenidunya S, Haltas H. Cytokeratin 7 and cytokeratin 20 expression in colorectal adenocarcinomas. Pathol Res Pract. 2011;207(3):156–60.
85. Ordonez NG. Cadherin 17 is a novel diagnostic marker for adenocarcinomas of the digestive system. Adv Anat Pathol. 2014;21(2):131–7.
86. Magnusson K, de Wit M, Brennan DJ, Johnson LB, McGee SF, Lundberg E, et al. SATB2 in combination with cytokeratin 20 identifies over 95% of all colorectal carcinomas. Am J Surg Pathol. 2011;35(7):937–48.
87. Isaksson-Mettavainio M, Palmqvist R, Forssell J, Stenling R, Oberg A. SMAD4/DPC4 expression and prognosis in human colorectal cancer. Anticancer Res. 2006;26(1B):507–10.
88. Manhas J, Bhattacharya A, Agrawal SK, Gupta B, Das P, Deo SV, et al. Characterization of cancer stem cells from different grades of human colorectal cancer. Tumour Biol. 2016;37(10):14069–81.
89. Osborn NK, Ahlquist DA. Stool screening for colorectal cancer: molecular approaches. Gastroenterology. 2005;128(1):192–206.
90. Mandel JS, Bond JH, Church TR, Snover DC, Bradley GM, Schuman LM, et al. Reducing mortality from colorectal cancer by screening for fecal occult blood. Minnesota Colon Cancer Control Study. N Engl J Med. 1993;328(19):1365–71.
91. Hardcastle JD, Chamberlain JO, Robinson MH, Moss SM, Amar SS, Balfour TW, et al. Randomised controlled trial of faecal-occult-blood screening for colorectal cancer. Lancet. 1996;348(9040):1472–7.
92. Kronborg O, Fenger C, Olsen J, Jorgensen OD, Sondergaard O. Randomised study of screening for colorectal cancer with faecal-occult-blood test. Lancet. 1996;348(9040):1467–71.
93. Oort FA, Terhaar Sive Droste JS, Van Der Hulst RW, Van Heukelem HA, Loffeld RJ, Wesdorp IC, et al. Colonoscopy-controlled intra-individual comparisons to screen relevant neoplasia: faecal immunochemical test vs. guaiac-based faecal occult blood test. Aliment Pharmacol Ther. 2010;31(3):432–9.
94. van Rossum LG, van Rijn AF, van Munster IP, Jansen JB, Fockens P, Laheij RJ, et al. Earlier stages of colorectal cancer detected with immunochemical faecal occult blood tests. Neth J Med. 2009;67(5):182–6.
95. Locker GY, Hamilton S, Harris J, Jessup JM, Kemeny N, Macdonald JS, et al. ASCO 2006 update of recommendations for the use of tumor markers in gastrointestinal cancer. J Clin Oncol. 2006;24(33):5313–27.
96. Hundt S, Haug U, Brenner H. Blood markers for early detection of colorectal cancer: a systematic review. Cancer Epidemiol Biomark Prev. 2007;16(10):1935–53.
97. Rossi S, Di Narzo AF, Mestdagh P, Jacobs B, Bosman FT, Gustavsson B, et al. microRNAs in colon cancer: a roadmap for discovery. FEBS Lett. 2012;586(19):3000–7.
98. Ng EK, Chong WW, Jin H, Lam EK, Shin VY, Yu J, et al. Differential expression of microRNAs in plasma of patients with colorectal cancer: a potential marker for colorectal cancer screening. Gut. 2009;58(10):1375–81.
99. Timoneda O, Balcells I, Cordoba S, Castello A, Sanchez A. Determination of reference microRNAs for relative quantification in porcine tissues. PLoS One. 2012;7(9):e44413.
100. Nagel R, le Sage C, Diosdado B, van der Waal M, Oude Vrielink JA, Bolijn A, et al. Regulation of the adenomatous polyposis coli gene by the miR-135 family in colorectal cancer. Cancer Res. 2008;68(14):5795–802.
101. Dong Y, Wu WK, Wu CW, Sung JJ, Yu J, Ng SS. MicroRNA dysregulation in colorectal cancer: a clinical perspective. Br J Cancer. 2011;104(6):893–8.
102. Pu XX, Huang GL, Guo HQ, Guo CC, Li H, Ye S, et al. Circulating miR-221 directly amplified from plasma is a potential diagnostic and prognostic marker of colorectal cancer and is correlated with p53 expression. J Gastroenterol Hepatol. 2010;25(10):1674–80.
103. Kroh EM, Parkin RK, Mitchell PS, Tewari M. Analysis of circulating microRNA biomarkers in plasma and serum using quantitative reverse transcription-PCR (qRT-PCR). Methods. 2010;50(4):298–301.
104. Chen C, Ridzon DA, Broomer AJ, Zhou Z, Lee DH, Nguyen JT, et al. Real-time quantification of microRNAs by stem-loop RT-PCR. Nucleic Acids Res. 2005;33(20):e179.
105. Li W, Ruan K. MicroRNA detection by microarray. Anal Bioanal Chem. 2009;394(4):1117–24.
106. Hou SY, Hsiao YL, Lin MS, Yen CC, Chang CS. MicroRNA detection using lateral flow nucleic acid strips with gold nanoparticles. Talanta. 2012;99:375–9.
107. Mao X, Xu H, Zeng Q, Zeng L, Liu G. Molecular beacon-functionalized gold nanoparticles as probes in dry-reagent strip biosensor for DNA analysis. Chem Commun (Camb). 2009;21(21):3065–7.
108. He Y, Zhang S, Zhang X, Baloda M, Gurung AS, Xu H, et al. Ultrasensitive nucleic acid biosensor based on enzyme-gold nanoparticle dual label and lateral flow strip biosensor. Biosens Bioelectron. 2011;26(5):2018–24.
109. de Noo ME, Mertens BJ, Ozalp A, Bladergroen MR, van der Werff MP, van de Velde CJ, et al. Detection of colorectal cancer using MALDI-TOF serum protein profiling. Eur J Cancer. 2006;42(8):1068–76.

Molecular Diagnostics in Pancreatic Cancer

10

Shruti Mishra, Vipin Rai, Abhai Kumar, Sushil Kumar Aggarwal, and Subash Chandra Gupta

10.1 Introduction

Pancreatic cancer (PaCa) originates with the formation of malignant (cancerous) cells in the lining of the ductal cells or the islets cells of the pancreas [1]. The most common form of pancreatic cancer is the ductal adenocarcinoma that originate from the epithelial tissue of the exocrine pancreas [2]. Although PaCa is less common in India compared to western countries, an increase in the incidence of the disease has been reported during the recent years. The disease normally remains silent and is diagnosed at a very advanced stage. Despite significant advances in the diagnosis, prevention and treatment during the recent years, the overall 5-year survival rate is less than 5% [3].

S. Mishra · V. Rai · S. C. Gupta (✉)
Laboratory for Translational Cancer Research, Department of Biochemistry, Institute of Science, Varanasi, India
e-mail: sgupta@bhu.ac.in; http://www.bhu.ac.in/science/biochemistry/sg.php

A. Kumar
Interdisciplinary School of Life Sciences, Institute of Science, Varanasi, India

S. K. Aggarwal
Department of Otorhinolaryngology, Institute of Medical Sciences, Banaras Hindu University, Varanasi, India

Pancreatic ductal adenocarcinoma, a high stage tumor, is associated with genetic alterations of several oncogenes and tumor suppressors such as K-ras, p53, p16, deleted in pancreatic cancer, locus 4 (DPC4), BRCA2, microsatellite instability and telomerase [4]. The activation of telomerase and inactivation of the p53 and DPC4 occur at the late stage of the PaCa. Accumulating evidence suggests that functional activity of K-ras and telomerase can be used as molecular markers for the diagnosis of pancreatic cancer. Similarly, alterations in p53 and p16 activities can be used as a potent prognostic marker for PaCa [4]. In this chapter, we discuss the advantages and limitations of molecular diagnostics in PaCa patients. The specificity and sensitivity associated with these molecular markers are also discussed.

10.2 Genetic Alterations Encompassing Pancreatic Cancer

It is now well known that pancreatic cancer like other cancers is caused by dysregulation of multiple genes. The microenvironment plays a crucial role in the development of PaCa. It is also well established that microenvironment of pancreatic cancer is inflammatory. The pro-inflammatory transcription factors, nuclear factor (NF)-κB and signal transducer and activa-

K. K. Shukla et al. (eds.), *Molecular Diagnostics in Cancer Patients*, https://doi.org/10.1007/978-981-13-5877-7_10

tor of transcription 3 (STAT3) are two transcription factors that control the expression of gene products involved in inflammation [5]. Numerous lines of evidence suggest that NF-κB plays a major role in the growth and chemoresistance of PaCa. Studies have indicated that NF-κB is constitutively active in PaCa cells but not in immortalized, nontumorigenic pancreatic ductal epithelial cells [6]. NF-κB and STAT3 activation promote PaCa growth via the induction of mitogenic gene products, such as c-myc and cyclin D1 [7]. The latter is overexpressed in human PaCa tissue and inversely correlated with patient survival [8]. Additionally, NF-κB and STAT3 enhance the angiogenic potential of PaCa cells via increased expression of proangiogenic factors, including vascular endothelial growth factor (VEGF), whereas other NF-κB-regulated gene products promote the migration and invasion of PaCa cells [9]. Furthermore, strong activation of NF-κB and of NF-κB–regulated gene products such as cyclooxygenase 2 (COX2), VEGF, and 5-lipoxygenase (5-LOX) was found in patients with PaCa [7]. Finally, NF-κB plays a pivotal role in promoting gemcitabine resistance in PaCa. Implication of these evidences suggest that NF-κB and STAT3 contribute to PaCa growth. The other common genes dysregulated in PaCa are discussed below:

10.3 Pancreatic Cancer Related Genes

10.3.1 KRAS2

KRAS2 belongs to the member of the GTPase superfamily that is frequently mutated in PaCa. KRAS2 gene is located on chromosome 12p12.1. In adenocarcinoma, the activated KRAS2 undergoes point mutation by substitution of an amino acid at codon 12 or 13 [10, 11]. This genetic alteration is sufficient to lock the KRAS2 in a GTP-bound active conformation. Subsequently, this leads to the aberrant signaling downstream to phosphoinositide-3-kinase (PI3K) and RAF-mitogen activated Protein kinase (MAPK) pathways [12].

10.3.2 p16/CDKN2A

The p16/CDKN2A act as an inhibitor of cyclin-dependent-kinase (CDK) at the G1/S checkpoint of cell cycle. This result in the suppression of Rb phosphorylation by CDKs and cyclin-CDK complexes [13, 14]. The functional loss of p16/CDKN2A gene (INK4A) is the most commonly observed tumor suppressor deficiency found in almost all PaCa [15].

10.3.3 p53

p53 also known as TP53 is a tumor suppressor protein. The inactivation in TP53 is reported in almost 70% of pancreatic cancer [16]. TP53 plays a role during cell cycle and the DNA damage response. Interestingly, mutation in p53 is known to suppress the transcriptional activity of 14-3-3σ and p21 [17, 18].

10.3.4 DPC4/SMAD4

SMAD4 also termed DPC4, a tumor suppressor, is known to regulate transforming growth factor beta (TGF-β) signal transduction pathway by phosphorylation. SMAD4 is also involved in the nuclear trafficking of SMAD transcription factors and produces growth inhibitory effects [19, 20]. The SMAD4 is inactivated in approximately 55% of pancreatic cancers, either by homozygous deletion (30%) or by intragenic mutations and loss of second allele (25%) [21].

10.4 Pancreatic Tumor Markers

Several markers have been evaluated for their potential in the diagnosis and prognosis of PaCa. However, only few of them have been recommended for clinical use. The serum carbohydrate antigen 19-9 (CA 19-9) and microsatellite RNA are the only marker recommended for clinical use. In the following section, we discuss the advantages and limitations associated with serum markers, protein markers and pancreatic juice markers.

10.4.1 Serum Markers

10.4.1.1 Carbohydrate Antigen 19-9 (CA-19-9)

Carbohydrate antigen 19-9 (CA 19-9) is a modified Lewis (a) blood group antigen. Serum CA 19-9 is known to be elevated in patients with cholangiocarcinoma, colon cancer and pancreatic cancer [22]. To our knowledge, serum CA19-9 is the only FDA-approved biomarker for pancreatic ductal adenocarcinoma. However, its utility as a prognostic marker remains to be explored [23–25]. Later in 2006, it was proved by the American Society of Clinical Oncology (ASCO) that CA-19-9 in combination with other markers can be of greater diagnostic value [26].

Although CA-19-9 has been used as a diagnostic tool for PaCa, its use as a single molecule is associated with several limitations. For example, elevation in CA-19-9 has been reported during several other conditions such as chronic pancreatitis, cholangitis, and hepatic cirrhosis [27, 28]. Nevertheless, CA-19-9 remains the standard in combination with other markers.

10.4.1.2 Carbohydrate Antigen 242 (CA-242)

CA-242 is a protein that was first isolated from immunization of mice with COLO205, a human colon adenocarcinoma cell line [29]. The proposed antigenic determinant of CA-242 reveals its sialylated carbohydrate structure related to type I chain [30]. In comparison to CA-19-9, the efficacy, diagnostic utility, and clinical usefulness of CA-242 suggest that its expression is independent of Lewis-a secretor status [27].

10.4.1.3 CAM17.1

CAM17.1 is a monoclonal antibody and a mucin-based marker that detects a mucous glycoprotein epitope of a sialylated blood group antigen [31]. It was first reported in pancreatic cancer with the help of an enzyme-linked antibody sandwich assay in combination with CA-19-9 assay [32]. CAM 17.1 is found to be overexpressed in pancreatic cancer as compared to those in normal ductal cells and chronic pancreatitis.

10.4.1.4 Tissue Inhibitor of Matrix Metalloproteinase 1 (TIMP-1)

The matrix metalloproteinase (MMP) family of enzymes are known to degrade the extracellular matrix thus promoting the progression and invasion of the cancer [33]. TIMP-1 gene counteract the effect of MMP by encoding the inhibitor protein [34]. An overexpression of TIMP-1 in the tumor and serum of pancreatic cancer patients has been associated with a decrease in the invasive potential of both cancer cells [35]. In one study, TIMP-1 was significantly higher in the serum from pancreatic cancer patients as compared to normal controls [36–38]. This suggest that elevated serum TIMP-1 could be used as a diagnostic marker for pancreatic cancer.

10.4.1.5 Macrophage Inhibitory Cytokine 1 (MIC-1)

MIC-1 belongs to the family of transforming growth factor beta (TGF-β) superfamily. It is located on chromosome 19p13.11 [39]. MIC-1 has been reported to be significantly overexpressed in the cytoplasm of pancreatic tumor cells. As a single marker, MIC-1 has been reported to be more effective as compared to CA-19-9 [40]. In combination with other markers, the diagnostic accuracy of MIC-1 is further increased [40]. MIC-1 is reported to have better sensitivity and specificity. However, MIC-1 cannot discriminate between chronic pancreatitis and pancreatic adenocarcinoma.

10.4.1.6 Osteopontin (OPN)

The genes for OPN are located on chromosome 4q22.1. OPN is frequently overexpressed in pancreatic adenocarcinoma tumors and other cancer types [41]. It encodes for an adhesive glycoprotein identified as a sialoprotein in bone. OPN is known to play a role in tumor progression and promotes metastases by facilitating anchorage independent growth in transformed cells [42, 43]. OPN is reported to have diagnostic potential due to its elevated level in the serum and tissues produced by the pancreatic cancer cells. The elevated level of OPN was first identified in pancreatic cancer in 2002 by the global gene expression profiling technology [44].

10.4.2 Pancreatic Juice Markers

10.4.2.1 DNA Methylation Alterations

DNA methylation is an epigenetic mark related with transcriptional regulation and genome structure. DNA methylation of pancreatic developmental genes has shown strong correlation with patient survival. These markers have been tested in a variety of settings for their utility in normal and tumor tissues. Genome-wide studies of CpG islands have revealed thousands of loci where demethylation and hypermethylation can segregate pancreatic tumor tissue from normal tissue [45, 46]. These sites have been involved in cell-fate determination in the pancreas. In one study, pancreatic juice from 155 suspected patients was collected and analyzed using conventional methylation specific PCR (MSP) analysis [47]. The use of six most promising markers within this panel [cyclin D2, forkhead box E1 (FOXE1), neuronal pentraxin 2 (NPTX2), ppENK, p16, and tissue factor pathway inhibitor 12 (TFP12)] detected pancreatic cancer with 82% sensitivity and 100% specificity through quantitative MSP [47]. In another study, three candidate genes [NPTX2, secreted apoptosis-related protein (SARP2), and claudin 5 (CLDN5)] were selected and evaluated for methylation status in pancreatic cancer and pancreatic juice in comparison to normal epithelia. Of three genes, aberrant methylation of at least one gene was detected in 100% of primary pancreatic carcinoma and in 75% of pancreatic juice in known cases of cancer [48]. Implication of all these observations suggest that DNA methylation can help in determining the molecular diagnosis of pancreatic cancer.

10.4.2.2 KRAS Mutations in DNA

Point mutation in the proto-oncogene Kirsten rat sarcoma viral oncogene homolog (KRAS) at an early stage of pancreatic adenocarcinoma, could represent a biomarker to diagnose the disease. The mutations affect the hotspot codons 12 or 13. The substitution of specific amino acid, decides the mRNA expression patterns, biochemical activity and transforming capacity [49, 50]. About 90% of tumors harbor mutations of KRAS, its detection in circulating free tumor DNA (cftDNA) could represent a biomarker to monitor chemotherapy response. A study comprising of three groups (no pancreatic disease, benign pancreatic disease, and pancreatic cancer) was designed to assess the presence of KRAS mutations in the pancreatic juice. The analysis was done using PCR mediated restriction length polymorphism (PCR/RFLP). Observations suggest the presence of 0% KRAS mutations in the groups with no pancreatic disease and benign pancreatic conditions. Interestingly, KRAS mutations were detected in 77% of patients known to possess malignant pancreatic cancer [51]. A number of studies has compared the diagnostic potential of mutant KRAS and mutant p53 in the pancreatic juice. In such studies, mutant KRAS has been found to outperform the mutation in the p53 gene [52].

10.4.3 Other Protein Markers

10.4.3.1 hENT1

Human equilibrative transporter 1 (hENT1) is a member of nucleoside-transporter proteins, which mediates cellular entry of cytotoxic chemotherapies such as gemcitabine [53]. Being one of the most abundant proteins, hENT1 is also a major route for gemcitabine transport. Therefore, hENT1 may potentially be a predictive marker for gemcitabine effectiveness [54]. The role of hENT1 as a predictive marker for gemcitabine effectiveness in pancreatic cancer with increased overall survival in patients with high epithelial hENT1 expression has also been reported [55, 56].

10.4.3.2 SPARC

Secreted protein, acidic, and rich in cysteine (SPARC) is a protein that is involved in cell-matrix interaction, cell migration, proliferation and angiogenesis [57].The overexpression of SPARC has been reported in pancreatic cancer and its peritumoral stroma. Conversely, some study suggest that SPARC expression cannot be used as a prognostic biomarker in advanced pancreatic cancer patients [57, 58].

10.4.3.3 Mucins

Mucins belong to a group of glycosylated proteins of the epithelia and are often overexpressed in pancreatic cancer. Mucins function as a protective barrier in the mucosal system by forming a gel like structure. Mucins are able to form a protective coat around cancer cells, critically associated with resistance to cytotoxic drugs, invasiveness, metastases and cell proliferation. A number of studies has demonstrated that mucins are dysregulated in pancreatic cancer and thus could serve as a prognostic biomarker [59]. Employing in situ hybridization and immunohistochemistry, mucin-1 (MUC1) was found to be predominantly expressed in the normal pancreas [60, 61]. In another study, MUC1 was expressed in more than 60% of PaCa that correlated with tumor size and dysplasia [59, 62–65]. In cancer cells, MUC1 attaches to epidermal growth factor receptor (EGFR), β-catenin and NF-κB to intensify cell proliferation through the MAPK, Akt or Wnt/β-catenin pathways [62, 65, 66]. MUC4 is another member of mucin family. MUC4 is known to activate a number of proliferative pathways such as MAPK, PKC and RAS-REK, all of which are known to induce cell growth and differentiation. MUC4 is known to be expressed in more than 70% of pancreatic tumor tissue, while it was undetectable in normal pancreas and chronic pancreatitis [67].

10.5 Conclusions

Despite significant advances in the diagnosis, prognosis and therapy, the overall 5-year survival rate due to pancreatic cancer is less than 5%. As discussed in this chapter, several markers have been examined by pre-clinical and clinical studies. However, only few of them have been recommended for human use. Furthermore, most of these biomarkers are based on invasive assays. It is our hope that the ongoing studies across the world will help to identify novel markers for the early diagnosis and prognosis of pancreatic cancer. Subsequently, this will help to improve the life of pancreatic cancer patients.

Acknowledgement The authors would like to acknowledge the financial support from Science and Engineering Research Board (ECR/2016/000034), and University Grants Commission [No. F.30-112/2015 (BSR)]. SM is an ICMR-JRF (3/1/3/JRF-2016/LS/HRD-65-80388).

References

1. Coppola D. Molecular prognostic markers in pancreatic cancer. Cancer Control. 2000;7(5):421–7.
2. Furukawa T, Duguid WP, Rosenberg L, Viallet J, Galloway DA, Tsao M-S. Long-term culture and immortalization of epithelial cells from normal adult human pancreatic ducts transfected by the E6E7 gene of human papilloma virus 16. Am J Pathol. 1996;148(6):1763.
3. Siegel R, Naishadham D, Jemal A. Cancer statistics, 2012. CA Cancer J Clin. 2012;62(1):10–29.
4. Inoue S, Tezel E, Nakao A. Molecular diagnosis of pancreatic cancer. Hepatogastroenterology. 2001;48(40):933–8.
5. Aggarwal BB. Nuclear factor-κB: the enemy within. Cancer Cell. 2004;6(3):203–8.
6. Liptay S, Weber CK, Ludwig L, Wagner M, Adler G, Schmid RM. Mitogenic and antiapoptotic role of constitutive NF-κB/Rel activity in pancreatic cancer. Int J Cancer. 2003;105(6):735–46.
7. Aggarwal BB, Vijayalekshmi R, Sung B. Targeting inflammatory pathways for prevention and therapy of cancer: short-term friend, long-term foe. Clin Cancer Res. 2009;15(2):425–30.
8. Kornmann M, Ishiwata T, Itakura J, Tangvoranuntakul P, Beger HG, Korc M. Increased cyclin D1 in human pancreatic cancer is associated with decreased postoperative survival. Oncology. 1998;55(4):363–9.
9. Yebra M, Filardo E, Bayna E, Kawahara E, Becker J, Cheresh D. Induction of carcinoma cell migration on vitronectin by NF-kappa B-dependent gene expression. Mol Biol Cell. 1995;6(7):841–50.
10. Almoguera C, Shibata D, Forrester K, Martin J, Arnheim N, Perucho M. Most human carcinomas of the exocrine pancreas contain mutant cK-ras genes. Cell. 1988;53(4):549–54.
11. Hruban RH, Van Mansfeld A, Offerhaus G, Van Weering D, Allison DC, Goodman SN, et al. K-ras oncogene activation in adenocarcinoma of the human pancreas. A study of 82 carcinomas using a combination of mutant-enriched polymerase chain reaction analysis and allele-specific oligonucleotide hybridization. Am J Pathol. 1993;143(2):545.
12. Hingorani SR, Tuveson DA. Ras redux: rethinking how and where Ras acts. Curr Opin Genet Dev. 2003;13(1):6–13.
13. Russo AA, Tong L, Lee J-O, Jeffrey PD, Pavletich NP. Structural basis for inhibition of the cyclin-dependent kinase Cdk6 by the tumour suppressor p16 INK4a. Nature. 1998;395(6699):237.

14. Liggett WH Jr, Sidransky D. Role of the p16 tumor suppressor gene in cancer. J Clin Oncol. 1998;16(3):1197–206.
15. Schutte M, Hruban RH, Geradts J, Maynard R, Hilgers W, Rabindran SK, et al. Abrogation of the Rb/p16 tumor-suppressive pathway in virtually all pancreatic carcinomas. Cancer Res. 1997;57(15):3126–30.
16. Redston MS, Caldas C, Seymour AB, Hruban RH, Da Costa L, Yeo CJ, et al. p53 mutations in pancreatic carcinoma and evidence of common involvement of homocopolymer tracts in DNA microdeletions. Cancer Res. 1994;54(11):3025–33.
17. Hermeking H, Lengauer C, Polyak K, He T-C, Zhang L, Thiagalingam S, et al. 14-3-3σ is a p53-regulated inhibitor of G2/M progression. Mol Cell. 1997;1(1):3–11.
18. Chan TA, Hermeking H, Lengauer C, Kinzler KW, Vogelstein B. 14-3-3σ is required to prevent mitotic catastrophe after DNA damage. Nature. 1999;401(6753):616.
19. Massagué J, Blain SW, Lo RS. TGFβ signaling in growth control, cancer, and heritable disorders. Cell. 2000;103(2):295–309.
20. Siegel PM, Massagué J. Cytostatic and apoptotic actions of TGF-β in homeostasis and cancer. Nat Rev Cancer. 2003;3(11):807.
21. Hahn SA, Schutte M, Hoque AS, Moskaluk CA, Da Costa LT, Rozenblum E, et al. DPC4, a candidate tumor suppressor gene at human chromosome 18q21.1. Science. 1996;271(5247):350–3.
22. Koprowski H, Steplewski Z, Mitchell K, Herlyn M, Herlyn D, Fuhrer P. Colorectal carcinoma antigens detected by hybridoma antibodies. Somatic Cell Genet. 1979;5(6):957–71.
23. Berger AC, Garcia M Jr, Hoffman JP, Regine WF, Abrams RA, Safran H, et al. Postresection CA 19-9 predicts overall survival in patients with pancreatic cancer treated with adjuvant chemoradiation: a prospective validation by RTOG 9704. J Clin Oncol. 2008;26(36):5918.
24. Pelzer U, Hilbig A, Stieler J, Sinn M, Bahra M, Dörken B, et al. Value of carbohydrate antigen 19-9 in predicting response and therapy control in patients with metastatic pancreatic cancer undergoing first-line therapy. Front Oncol. 2013;3:155.
25. Shah UA, Saif MW. Tumor markers in pancreatic cancer: 2013. JOP. 2013;14(4):318–21.
26. Locker GY, Hamilton S, Harris J, Jessup JM, Kemeny N, Macdonald JS, et al. ASCO 2006 update of recommendations for the use of tumor markers in gastrointestinal cancer. J Clin Oncol. 2006;24(33):5313–27.
27. Lamerz R. Role of tumour markers, cytogenetics. Ann Oncol. 1999;10(Suppl 4):S145–S9.
28. Goonetilleke K, Siriwardena A. Systematic review of carbohydrate antigen (CA 19-9) as a biochemical marker in the diagnosis of pancreatic cancer. Eur J Surg Oncol. 2007;33(3):266–70.
29. Lindholm L, Johansson C, Jansson E, Hallberg C, Nilsson O. An immunoradiometric assay (IRMA) for the CA 50 antigen. Tumor Marker Antigens Lund: Studentlitteratur; 1985. p. 122–33.
30. Nilsson O, Johansson C, Glimelius B, Persson B, Nørgaard-Pedersen B, Andrén-Sandberg Å, et al. Sensitivity and specificity of CA242 in gastro-intestinal cancer. A comparison with CEA, CA50 and CA 19-9. Br J Cancer. 1992;65(2):215.
31. Eccleston D, Milton J, Hoffman J, Bara J, Rhodes J. Pancreatic tumour marker anti-mucin antibody CAM 17.1 reacts with a sialyl blood group antigen, probably I, which is expressed throughout the human gastrointestinal tract. Digestion. 1998;59(6):665–70.
32. Parker N, Makin C, Ching C, Eccleston D, Taylor O, Milton D, et al. A new enzyme-linked lectin/mucin antibody sandwich assay (CAM 17.1/WGA) assessed in combination with CA 19-9 and peanut lectin binding assay for the diagnosis of pancreatic cancer. Cancer. 1992;70(5):1062–8.
33. Kessenbrock K, Plaks V, Werb Z. Matrix metalloproteinases: regulators of the tumor microenvironment. Cell. 2010;141(1):52–67.
34. Olson MW, Gervasi DC, Mobashery S, Fridman R. Kinetic analysis of the binding of human matrix metalloproteinase-2 and-9 to tissue inhibitor of metalloproteinase (TIMP)-1 and TIMP-2. J Biol Chem. 1997;272(47):29975–83.
35. Zhou W, Sokoll LJ, Bruzek DJ, Zhang L, Velculescu VE, Goldin SB, et al. Identifying markers for pancreatic cancer by gene expression analysis. Cancer Epidemiol Biomarkers Prev. 1998;7(2):109–12.
36. Mroczko B, Lukaszewicz-Zajac M, Wereszczynska-Siemiatkowska U, Groblewska M, Gryko M, Kedra B, et al. Clinical significance of the measurements of serum matrix metalloproteinase-9 and its inhibitor (tissue inhibitor of metalloproteinase-1) in patients with pancreatic cancer: metalloproteinase-9 as an independent prognostic factor. Pancreas. 2009;38(6):613–8.
37. Poruk KE, Firpo MA, Scaife CL, Adler DG, Emerson LL, Boucher KM, et al. Serum osteopontin and TIMP-1 as diagnostic and prognostic biomarkers for pancreatic adenocarcinoma. Pancreas. 2013;42(2):193.
38. Gress T, Müller-Pillasch F, Lerch M, Friess H, Büchler M, Adler G. Expression and in-situ localization of genes coding for extracellular matrix proteins and extracellular matrix degrading proteases in pancreatic cancer. Int J Cancer. 1995;62(4):407–13.
39. Bootcov MR, Bauskin AR, Valenzuela SM, Moore AG, Bansal M, He XY, et al. MIC-1, a novel macrophage inhibitory cytokine, is a divergent member of the TGF-β superfamily. Proc Natl Acad Sci. 1997;94(21):11514–9.
40. Koopmann J, Buckhaults P, Brown DA, Zahurak ML, Sato N, Fukushima N, et al. Serum macrophage inhibitory cytokine 1 as a marker of pancreatic and other periampullary cancers. Clin Cancer Res. 2004;10(7):2386–92.
41. Harsha H, Kandasamy K, Ranganathan P, Rani S, Ramabadran S, Gollapudi S, et al. A compendium of

potential biomarkers of pancreatic cancer. PLoS Med. 2009;6(4):e1000046.
42. Rittling S, Chambers A. Role of osteopontin in tumour progression. Br J Cancer. 2004;90(10):1877.
43. Wu Y, Denhardt D, Rittling S. Osteopontin is required for full expression of the transformed phenotype by the ras oncogene. Br J Cancer. 2000;83(2):156.
44. Iacobuzio-Donahue CA, Maitra A, Shen-Ong GL, Van Heek T, Ashfaq R, Meyer R, et al. Discovery of novel tumor markers of pancreatic cancer using global gene expression technology. Am J Pathol. 2002;160(4):1239–49.
45. Vincent A, Omura N, Hong S-M, Jaffe A, Eshleman JR, Goggins M. Genome-wide analysis of promoter methylation associated with gene expression profiles of pancreatic adenocarcinomas. Clin Cancer Res. 2011;17(13):4341–54.
46. Nones K, Waddell N, Song S, Patch AM, Miller D, Johns A, et al. Genome-wide DNA methylation patterns in pancreatic ductal adenocarcinoma reveal epigenetic deregulation of SLIT-ROBO, ITGA2 and MET signaling. Int J Cancer. 2014;135(5):1110–8.
47. Matsubayashi H, Canto M, Sato N, Klein A, Abe T, Yamashita K, et al. DNA methylation alterations in the pancreatic juice of patients with suspected pancreatic disease. Cancer Res. 2006;66(2):1208–17.
48. Sato N, Fukushima N, Maitra A, Matsubayashi H, Yeo CJ, Cameron JL, et al. Discovery of novel targets for aberrant methylation in pancreatic carcinoma using high-throughput microarrays. Cancer Res. 2003;63(13):3735–42.
49. Cully M, Downward J. SnapShot: Ras signaling. Cell. 2008;133(7):1292.
50. Stolze B, Reinhart S, Bulllinger L, Fröhling S, Scholl C. Comparative analysis of KRAS codon 12, 13, 18, 61, and 117 mutations using human MCF10A isogenic cell lines. Sci Rep. 2015;5:8535.
51. Berthelemy P, Bouisson M, Escourrou J, Vaysse N, Rumeau JL, Pradayrol L. Identification of K-ras mutations in pancreatic juice in the early diagnosis of pancreatic cancer. Ann Intern Med. 1995;123(3):188–91.
52. Lu X, Xu T, Qian J, Wen X, Wu D. Detecting K-ras and p53 gene mutation from stool and pancreatic juice for diagnosis of early pancreatic cancer. Chin Med J. 2002;115(11):1632–6.
53. Farrell JJ, Elsaleh H, Garcia M, Lai R, Ammar A, Regine WF, et al. Human equilibrative nucleoside transporter 1 levels predict response to gemcitabine in patients with pancreatic cancer. Gastroenterology. 2009;136(1):187–95.
54. Kim R, Tan A, Lai KK, Jiang J, Wang Y, Rybicki LA, et al. Prognostic roles of human equilibrative transporter 1 (hENT-1) and ribonucleoside reductase subunit M1 (RRM1) in resected pancreatic cancer. Cancer. 2011;117(14):3126–34.
55. Calegari M, Orlandi A, Cocomazzi A, Martini M, Bagala C, Indellicati G, et al. P-164 Gemcitabine versus FOLFIRINOX in patients with advanced pancreatic adenocarcinoma HENT1 positive: back to the future. Ann Oncol. 2015;26(Suppl 4):iv47–iv8.
56. Renouf DJ, Karasinska J, Kalloger S, Peixoto RDA, O'Connor K, Schaeffer D. The association of epithelial expression of hENT1 and survival from adjuvant gemcitabine in pancreatic ductal adenocarcinoma (PDAC). J Clin Oncol. 2015;33(3 Suppl):296.
57. Von Hoff DD, Ramanathan RK, Borad MJ, Laheru DA, Smith LS, Wood TE, et al. Gemcitabine plus nab-paclitaxel is an active regimen in patients with advanced pancreatic cancer: a phase I/II trial. J Clin Oncol. 2011;29(34):4548.
58. Ormanns S, Haas M, Baechmann S, Remold A, Quietzsch D, Clemens MR, et al. Impact of SPARC expression level on outcome in patients with advanced pancreatic cancer not receiving nab-paclitaxel: a pooled analysis from prospective clinical and translational trials. Br J Cancer. 2016;115(12):1520–9.
59. Jonckheere N, Skrypek N, Van Seuningen I. Mucins and pancreatic cancer. Cancers. 2010;2(4):1794–812.
60. Balagué C, Gambús G, Carrato C, Porchet N, Aubert J-P, Kim YS, et al. Altered expression of MUC2, MUC4, and MUC5 mucin genes in pancreas tissues and cancer cell lines. Gastroenterology. 1994;106(4):1054–61.
61. Terada T, Ohta T, Sasaki M, Nakanuma Y, Kim YS. Expression of MUC apomucins in normal pancreas and pancreatic tumours. J Pathol. 1996;180(2):160–5.
62. Tréhoux S, Duchêne B, Jonckheere N, Van Seuningen I. The MUC1 oncomucin regulates pancreatic cancer cell biological properties and chemoresistance. Implication of p42–44 MAPK, Akt, Bcl-2 and MMP13 pathways. Biochem Biophys Res Commun. 2015;456(3):757–62.
63. Tréhoux S, Lahdaoui F, Delpu Y, Renaud F, Leteurtre E, Torrisani J, et al. Micro-RNAs miR-29a and miR-330-5p function as tumor suppressors by targeting the MUC1 mucin in pancreatic cancer cells. Biochim Biophys Acta. 2015;1853(10):2392–403.
64. Yonezawa S, Higashi M, Yamada N, Yokoyama S, Goto M. Significance of mucin expression in pancreatobiliary neoplasms. J Hepatobiliary Pancreat Sci. 2010;17(2):108–24.
65. Besmer DM, Curry JM, Roy LD, Tinder TL, Sahraei M, Schettini J, et al. Pancreatic ductal adenocarcinoma mice lacking mucin 1 have a profound defect in tumor growth and metastasis. Cancer Res. 2011;71(13):4432–42.
66. Nath S, Roy LD, Grover P, Rao S, Mukherjee P. Mucin 1 regulates Cox-2 gene in pancreatic cancer. Pancreas. 2015;44(6):909.
67. Andrianifahanana M, Moniaux N, Schmied BM, Ringel J, Friess H, Hollingsworth MA, et al. Mucin (MUC) gene expression in human pancreatic adenocarcinoma and chronic pancreatitis: a potential role of MUC4 as a tumor marker of diagnostic significance. Clin Cancer Res. 2001;7(12):4033–40.

Molecular Diagnostics in Head and Neck Squamous Cell Carcinoma

11

Nuzhat Husain and Azfar Neyaz

11.1 Introduction

HNSCC is the sixth most common cancer diagnosed in the world [1] and is one of the most common malignancies throughout the Asia Pacific region (South Asia, South East Asia, East Asia and Oceania) accounting for 40–50% of all cancers [2]. Oral squamous cell carcinoma [OSCC] is the most prevalent malignancy in India accounting for about 30% of all cancer [3]. It ranks number one in terms of incidence among men and third among women [4]. Recent studies have shown a rising incidence of Squamous Cell Carcinoma (SCC) of the oropharynx, despite the reduction of tobacco use in several of these countries. This suggests increasing the prevalence of another risk factor, now clearly identified as persistent infection with so-called "high risk" types of human papillomavirus (HPV) [5].

Head and neck squamous cell carcinoma (HNSCC) has complex poorly understood genetic and epigenetic alterations. Diverse etiological factors produce genetic diversity and multiple oncogenic pathways are involved. Our understanding of the mutational spectrum of Oral squamous cell carcinoma (OSCC) and Oropharyngeal Squamous cell Carcinoma (OPSCC) is evolving with the discovery of several oncogene mutations evident in squamous cell carcinoma. UV light, tobacco (both smoked and unsmoked), areca nut, alcohol and poor nutritional status have been implicated in the etiology of Head and Neck Squamous Cell Carcinoma HNSCC. Hundreds of genes are involved however diagnostic molecular markers used in practice are related to HPV. HNSCC has many other promising molecular markers including p53, cyclin D1, p16, cyclooxygenase-2 (COX-2), epidermal growth factor (EGF), and vascular endothelial growth factor (VEGF). Few companion diagnostic assays are used in the routine clinical setting. In terms of current day, application HPV is now a mandatory marker for categorizing OPSCC. Its role at other sites in HNSCC is controversial however there is growing evidence that it may be related to other neoplasia.

Several genes which form targets for therapy have been found to be overexpressed in HNSCC and prominent among these are EGFR and VEGF. Some of these oncogenes like PIK3 though evident in a small percentage of cases (5–10%) form targets for therapy. Clinical trials of targeted therapy have been initiated and some have some promising results.

N. Husain (✉) · A. Neyaz
Department of Pathology, Dr. Ram Manohar Lohia Institute of Medical Sciences, Lucknow, Uttar Pradesh, India

K. K. Shukla et al. (eds.), *Molecular Diagnostics in Cancer Patients*,
https://doi.org/10.1007/978-981-13-5877-7_11

11.2 Genetic Risk factors

Inherited germline mutations have also been implicated in HNSCC. These rare syndromes with inherited germline gene mutations include

(a) Familial Atypical Multiple melanoma Syndrome (FAMMMS) an autosomal dominant disorder caused by a mutation in the *CDKN2A* gene mutation. These patients also share a melanoma and pancreatic carcinoma risk.
(b) ATR gene mutations: these cases are also at a risk of developing cervical, skin, and breast carcinomas.
(c) Fanconi anemia: associated with mutations in the Fanconi anemia genes resulting in chromosomal instability.

Familial genetic risk factors may be associated with combinations of specific single nucleotide polymorphisms resulting in high mutagen sensitivity phenotype.

11.3 Molecular Markers and Tobacco-Related OSCC and OPSCC (Non-HPV Associated HNSCC)

Diverse and mutation intensive complex genetic cancers with the involvement of more than hundred mutated genes. Most of these genes function as tumour suppressors. Several pathways may be involved including the biotransformation pathways, detoxification, DNA repair, Apoptosis, Bilirubin-related pathway, Transcription factor TEAD2 pathway. Certain mitochondrial DNA polymorphisms and miRNA variation increase susceptibility. The most commonly mutated genes include *TP53, CDKN2A, PIK3CA, FAT1, KMT2D/KMT2B, NOTCH2, NOTCH3, CASP8, HLA-A, HRAS, TP63* [6].

p53 is a tumor suppressor gene, located on chromosome 17p13.1, plays a role in cell cycle progression, DNA repair, cellular differentiation, and apoptosis. The frequency of p53 mutation in oral cancers is 25–72% [7, 8]. Most TP53 alterations are missense mutations that occur in a hot spot region located in the DNA-binding domain, from codon 238 to codon 248 and abolish the transcriptional activity of p53. Such gain of function activities of the mutant p53 protein includes the ability to transform cells, increase tumorigenicity, increased half-life of p53 protein during immunohistochemical examination and modulate the sensitivity of cancer cells to drugs [9, 10]. P53 mutation commonly arises as a result of alcohol or tobacco exposure, and their presence is associated with the early recurrence and development of second primary tumors [11]. The mutation of the p53 is common in OSCC and its overexpression has been correlated with poor prognosis [12].

The Cancer Genome Atlas (TCGA) project has revealed four molecular subtypes including Classical, Basal, mesenchymal and atypical based on multi-gene profiling of 300 cases. The altered gene expression profiles overlap that in Lung squamous cell carcinoma. The TCGA profiling identified at least 18 targetable mutations including EGFR, FGFR1, FGFR2, MET, ERBB2. The project identified the oxidative pathway in addition to other altered pathways in HNSCC (Table 11.1).

11.3.1 Molecular Margins and Field Carcinogenesis

Widespread exposure to carcinogens results in mucosa adjacent to cancer also showing molecular alterations known as **field cancerization** effect. This phenomenon has been used for molecular testing of the margins. The presence of molecular alterations at the margins confers an increased risk of recurrence [38].

Molecular margins: Traditionally surgeons utilize intraoperative frozen section and subsequent paraffin sections to detect the involvement of surgical margins and lymph node by tumour. If margins are positive, patients may be subjected to further resection. Post-operative H& E stained FFPE sections define margins as clear, close or involved for further therapeutic management. Quick, reliable, and sensitive molecular detection

Table 11.1 Comparison of demographic, pathology, genetic and prognostic factors in HPV-OPSCC vs. tobacco associated OPSCC[a]

Features	HPV+ OPSCCs	HPV− OSCCs	References
Age (mean)	Younger age (40–60)	Older age at presentation (>60)	Fakhry et al. [13]
Race	White ≫ Non white	Non white > White	Fakhry et al. [13]
Geographical distribution	Northern Europe and North America	Asia-Pasific	Forte et al. [14]
Gender	Men > Females (8:1)	Men > Females (3:1)	Gillison ML et al. [15]
Socioeconomic status	Higher	Low-middle	Gillison ML et al. [15]
Prevalence estimates and trend	Variable in regions 13–56%, Increasing	Stable	Hwang et al. [16], Gillison ML [15]
Etiologic factors	Nine subtypes of HPV 90–95%-HPV-16	Known risk factors induce molecular changes and precancer No known etiologic factors	Gillison ML et al. [17]
Risk factors	Sexual behavior (high number of sexual partners, history of oral-genital sex, and history of oral-anal sex)	Smoking, alcohol, areca nut, smokeless tobacco, betel quid chewing	Gillison ML et al. [18] Heck et al. [19]
Cofactors	Marijuana (Cannabinoids) smoking immunosuppression	Diet, oral hygiene, stress	Marks et al. [20]
Site of origin	Reticulated epithelium lining the tonsillar crypts	Squamous epithelium at all sites in oral and oropharyngeal cavity	El-Mofty and Patil [21]
Preneoplastic condition	Lack precancerous HPV+ve mucosal changes	Keratinizing squamous dysplasia, field cancerization	Wenig [22]
Anatomical sites	Lingual and palatine tonsils, base of tongue	All sites	Heck et al. [19]
Pathological findings	Unassociated with dysplasia of the surface epithelium Exhibit non keratinizing morphology, or varinat morphology basaloid, papillary, lympheoithelial, adenoqumous, spindle cell cystic cervical nodes, ciliated cells, prominent infiltrating lymphocytes	Associated with dysplasia of surface epithelium, Keratinizing SCC which may be well, moderaely or poorly differentiated	Westra [23] Wenig et al. [22] Lewis JJ. Modern Pathology (2017), S44–S53; https://doi.org/10.1038/modpathol.2016.152
Regional lymph node involvement	Frequent, cystic	Frequent but less than HPV+ OPSCCs Necrotising or Solid	Yasui et al. [24]
Prognosis	Favourable	Unfavourable	Ang et al. [25] Kraft et al. [26]
T stage	Early T stage (T3&T4~42%)	More advanced T stage (T3&T4~67%)	Fakhry et al. [13]
Nodal stage	Advance N stage (N2-N3 = 66%)	Early N stage (N2-N3 = 50%)	Fakhry et al. [13]
Oncoprotein expression: Viral oncoproteins E6&E7 p53 gene mutation Rb gene tumor repression function p-16 gene product	Expressed Usually Wild type Impaired less frequently Overexpressed	Not present Frequently mutated Impaired more frequently Usually not evident	Gondim et al. [27], El-Mofty and Patil [21]

(continued)

Table 11.1 (continued)

Features	HPV+ OPSCCs	HPV− OSCCs	References
Molecular Phenotype **Cell cycle and survival:** TP53 mutation PI3K3CA EGFR FGFR1 PTEN HPV E6/E7 MET CCND1 CDKN2A Let-7c E2F1 MYC **Cell death** TRAF3 CASP8 FADD **Differentiation** NOTCH1 TP63 FAT1 AJUBA **Oxidative stress** NFE2L2	% 03 56 06 00 06 100 00 03 00 17 19 03 22 03 06 17 19 03 00 00	% 84 34 15 10 12 09 02 31 58 40 02 14 01 01 32 26 28 32 07 14	Agrawal et al. [28] Cancer Genome Atlas Network [29] Lechner et al. [30]
IHC signature molecule	p16^{INK4a}	p53overexpression, Cyclin D1 overexpression, Rb gene deletion	Ndiaye et al. [31]
mRNA signature	E6/E7 mRNA		Ndiaye et al. [31]
Epigenetic changes: MiRNA signature	**Up-regulated:** miR-320a miR-222-3p miR-93-5p **Downregulated:** miR-199a-3p//miR-199b-3p, miR-143, miR-145, and miR-126a	**Age:** hsa-miR-99a-5p hsa-miR-301b hsa-miR-182-5p hsa-miR-455-3p hsa-let-7c hsa-miR-32-5p hsa-miR-18a-5p hsa-miR-100-5p hsa-miR-130b-3p hsa-miR-331-3p **Smoking:** hsa-miR-1228-5p* hsa-miR-1207-5p hsa-miR-1224-5p hsa-miR-92b-5p hsa-miR-339-5p hsa-miR-1471 hsa-miR-324-5p hsa-miR-93-5p	Miller et al. [32]
Epigenetic changes : DNA methylation of genes	CDKN2A, DAP kinase (DAPK), MGMT and MLH1	CDKN2A, RARb, RASSF1, MGMT, and GATA4	Anayannis et al. [33]
Chromosomal alterations	Chromosome 11q deletion Prominence of amplification of 3q Amplification at 20q11	Focal amplification on chromosome 7	Hayes et al. [34]

Table 11.1 (continued)

Features	HPV+ OPSCCs	HPV− OSCCs	References
Mutation signature	TpC mutations (C > T), Increased APOBEC cytosine deaminase activity, PIK3CA mutations in two hotspots (E542K, E545K)	Mutation at CpG sites more frequent, *PIK3CA*mutations are seen throughout the gene and are seen much less commonly in the hot spots	Hayes et al. [34]
Tumor surveillance	PCR, ISH techniques, IHC detection of HPV and surrogate markers	Evidence of keratinizing dysplasia, molecular alterations in p53, Cyclin D1	Smeets et al. [35]
3 year overall survival (months)	82.4% (95% CI, 77.2–87.6)	57.1% (95% CI, 48.1–66.1)	Ang et al. [25]
3-year progression-free survival (months)	73.7% (95% CI, 67.7–79.8)	43.4% (95% CI, 34.4–52.4)	Ang et al. [25]
Overall response to treatment 2-Year OS (%) 2-Year PFS (%)	94 (95% CI, 87–100) 85 (95% CI, 74–99)	58 (95% CI, 49–74) 53 (95% CI, 36–67)	Marur et al. [36]

[a]Modified from Husain and Neyaz [37] (Husain N, Neyaz A. Human papillomavirus associated head and neck squamous cell carcinoma: Controversies and new concepts. J Oral Biol Craniofac Res. 2017 Sep-Dec;7(3):198–205)

techniques would augment management. Published studies have used p53 mutation detection, immunohistochemical expression of p53 protein, and methylation markers specifically p16 promoter gene hypermethylation and other mutations listed in an epigenetic changes to assess the presence of positive molecular margins. The clinical implications of detecting a positive molecular margin have, however, not been defined [39, 40].

11.3.2 Molecular Gene Alterations in Early Detection of HNSCC (Precancer and Molecular Changes)

Tumorigenesis is a multistep process involving serial increase and accumulation of multiple genetic and epigenetic alterations. Genetic susceptibility to HNSCC determines occurrence in a small percentage of cases as discussed earlier. The progression of disease from hyperplasia to the precancer stages like dysplasia or squamous intraepithelial neoplasia is a feature of HPV associated cancers, EGFR amplification is an early even evident in hyperplastic epithelium also. Chromosomal alterations 1p, 9p and 17p with p16 inactivation and epigenetic changes accompany Squamous Intraepithelial Neoplasia which progresses from grade 1 to grade 3 or carcinoma in situ accompanied by alterations in chromosome 11p, 13p, 14p with p53 mutation and cyclin D1 amplification. Frank HNSCC also shows chromosomal 6p and 4 p losses [41, 42].

11.3.3 Molecular Markers of Lymph Node Metastasis in HNSCC

Cervical lymph node metastasis is the single adverse independent prognostic indicator for local recurrence and/or distant metastasis in HNSCC [43]. Presence of several conventional factors like depth of invasion, lymphovascular invasion, perineural invasion, the pattern of invasion among others have been used in predicting metastasis to regional lymph nodes in OSCC [44]. The neoplastic squamous cell gets a selective growth advantage, which drives the development of the primary tumor and metastasis. Several groups have attempted genetic prediction of lymph node metastases trying to identify a metastatic signature in primary tumor tissues versus matched lymph node metastasis [45]. These include genes that have also been correlated with metastatic behavior and organ-specific metastasis in other cancers of epithelial origin. Several of these genes (ENPP2, CXCR4, LTF, S100A2, and IL24) have been identified as mechanistically important in the cascade of events that drives metastasis in HNSCC [46, 47]. The *p53* tumor suppressor gene is mutated in more than 72% of OSCC tumors [7], but the large variety of mutations limits its applicability as a quick and reliable method of detection [12]. Molecular metastasis detection in nodal micrometastasis, as well as defining molecular alterations at the resection margins first, targeted TP53 mutations [48, 49]. The number of metastasis positive nodes may double using molecular techniques however the clinical implications of detecting molecular involvement without the demonstration of cytological metastasis is not defined.

mRNA expression of squamous cell carcinoma antigen (SCAA) has also been detected in nested PCR. The mRNA for this antigen has also been detected in 18.7% of negative nodes of which on additional sectioning a micrometastatic focus 4.6% [50]. Other studies have investigated *MUC1* gene, *E48*, cytokeratin 14 (CK14), CK20 primarily using RT-PCR. Ferris and associates published promising reports of four qRT-PCR markers for intraoperative nodal diagnosis. They found four markers, that is pemphigus vulgaris antigen, SCCA1/2, parathyroid hormone-related protein (PTHrP), and tumor-associated calcium signal transducer 1 (TACSTD1), discriminated between positive and benign nodes with accuracy greater than 97% [51]. Each study has been shown to successfully uncover subclinically node-positive patients. However, although the clinical management of head and neck cancer dictates that patients with even a slight risk of nodal metastasis based on tumor site and staging receive therapy that treats the nodal basins of the neck with either radiation therapy or surgical node dissection, this increased fidelity in finding regional lymph node disease has not translated to improved regional control or survival [6].

11.4 Viruses and HNSCC

11.4.1 HPV and HNSCC

Recent studies have shown a rising incidence of Squamous Cell Carcinoma (SCC) of the oropharynx, despite the reduction of tobacco use in several of these countries. This suggests increasing prevalence of another risk factor, now clearly identified as persistent infection with so-called "high risk" types of human papillomavirus (HPV) [15–17, 52]. HPV is a small, non-enveloped, double-stranded closed circular DNA virus that presents tropism for epithelial cells. Historically, HPV is one of the most common causes of sexually transmitted diseases in both men and women around the world and associated with 90–100% of cervical cancer cases [53]. The first evidence of HPV in the oral and oropharyngeal carcinogenesis was proposed in 1983 by Syrjanen et al., since then numerous studies have been conducted to identify the evidence of HPV in the etiology of HNSCC and reported its strongest association with cancer of the tonsillar region and other parts of the oropharynx [54]. Today, more than 150 different HPV types have been cataloged and about 40 can infect the epithelial lining of the anogenital tract and other mucosal areas of the human body. HPVs are divided into **high-risk [HR-HPV]** and **low-risk [LR-HPV]** types based on their oncogenic potential. **HR-HPV types**, highlighting HPV 16 and 18, is associated with the occurrence of pre-malignant and malignant cervical lesions, penile, vulvar, anal and HNSCC and contribute to over 40% of oral cancers [53, 55, 56]. The HPV genome, in benign warts, is interestingly maintained in a nonintegrated episomal form, while in cancers the HPV viral genome is integrated into the host genome, suggesting that integration of viral genome is a significant event in malignant transformation. The integration site is random and there is no consistent association with any specific host proto-oncogene. The mechanism of carcinogenesis is attributed to the interruption of the viral DNA within the E1/E2 open reading frame, leading to loss of the E2 viral repressor and overexpression of the oncoproteins E6 and E7. In fact the

oncogenic potential of HPV can be predominantly explained by the activities of the two viral genes encoding E6 and E7. Two viral oncoproteins E6 and E7 have the ability to deregulate the tumor suppressor function of p53 and pRb proteins. E6 binds to a cellular ubiquitin ligase-E6AP and simultaneously to the tumor suppressor protein p53, resulting in ubiquitination and proteasomal degradation of p53 that ultimately cause abrogation of p53 function [57]. E7 attaches with retinoblastoma protein (pRb) preventing its binding to E2F transcription factor, thereby leaving E2F available to promote the cell to S-phase and cause cell-cycle progression and malignant transformation. Moreover functional inactivation of pRb results in a reciprocal over-expression of p16 protein [58].

11.4.2 HPV vs Non-HPV OPSCC

Clinical morphological and molecular differences apart from having a different epidemiology and aetiology, the HPV-positive HNSCC showed distinct clinico-pathological characteristics with discrete histopathology. They are generally never married; tend to be younger at time of diagnosis [<40 years] with less and/or no exposure to tobacco and alcohol, but have had more marijuana exposure and/or higher numbers of sexual partners [18, 59]. Tobacco-associated OSCC are more frequent in men, while equal risk of HPV associated OSCC in both men and women. Clinically HPV-positive tumors present in loco-regionally advanced disease [stage III or IV] with early T stage and advanced nodal stage. The nodal metastases are usually cystic and multilevel regional involvement is common [60]. These are usually poorly differentiated, non-keratinizing and have prominent basaloid morphology in contrast to the HPV negative cases that is more moderately differentiated and keratinizing [23, 61]. Moreover, HPV-related cancers presenting p16 overexpression are very sensitive to radiotherapy, and have a better prognosis than those unrelated to HPV. In this context, p16 overexpression has been suggested to have a major impact on treatment response and survival in patients with HNSCC treated with conventional radiotherapy [62, 63], leading to the hypothesis that malignant tumors over-expressing p16 have higher radio-sensitivity. In other words, positive HPV/p16 status has been consistently found to be a favorable prognostic factor in terms of loco-regional control and overall survival irrespective of treatment modality. Until now, it remains unclear why HPV-related oropharyngeal squamous cell carcinomas show better outcome than their HPV-negative counterparts. HPV positive oral cancer represents a distinct molecular phenotype with a unique mechanism of tumorigenesis independent of the mutagenic effect of tobacco and alcohol. The typical genetic alterations that results from long exposure of tobacco and alcohol may not be found in HPV-positive tumors. HPV-positive cancers are characterized by loss of expression of pRb, cyclin D1 and over-expression of p16. In contrast, HPV-negative tumors consistently show over-expression of pRb and cyclin D1 and loss of p16. Mutation in the p53 gene is common in HPV-negative cancers whereas the inactivation of p53 gene that is more commonly seen in HPV-positive cancers. HPV-positive HNSCCs also differ from HPV-negative HNSCCs in their patterns of allelic and chromosomal loss and in their global gene expression profiles [64, 65].

11.4.3 HPV and OSCC

Oral cancer has been defined as a neoplasm involving the oral cavity which begins at the lip and ends at the anterior pillar of the fauces. The etiological role of Hr-HPV in OPSCC is well defined. The frequency of HPV in OSCC is low in Asia and worldwide and the majority of OSCC are associated with a tobacco habit. We have observed in our studies on OSCC and risk factors that HPV positive cases show a confounding effect with tobacco. Use of p16 protein as a surrogate marker to assess the potential etiological role of HPV in OSCC in our population is not reliable [66]. In our attempt to elicit the differences in the expression pattern of p16 and p53 in HPV-positive and HPV-negative OSCC, we observed that risk factors including oral tobacco

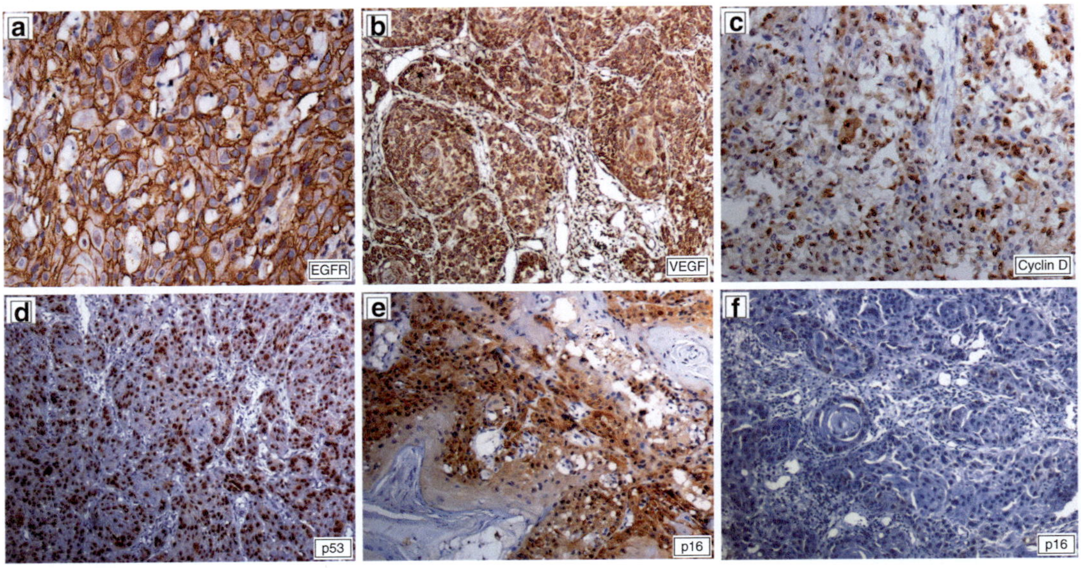

Fig. 11.1 Immunohistochemical detection of molecular markers in HNSCC: (**a**) Strong membranous EGFR expression (**b**) strong cytoplasmic and membraneous VEGF expression. (**c**) nuclear cyclin D1 in a fair number of cells (**d**) mutant type p53 expression and (**e**) block positivity for p16 in >75% cells, and (**f**) a negative p16 in a keratinizing SCC

consumption and alcohol were present in all of the ten p16-positive cases. Presence of mutant-type p53 and exposure to tobacco-related risk factors in both HPV-positive and negative cases suggest the existence of p53-related carcinogenesis in HPV-positive cases in Indian population. Further, we observed basaloid morphology in only one case of 31 positive cases while all other cases were keratinizing SCC (Fig. 11.1). The survival of our patients was not affected by HPV, p16 and p53 status. Hence unlike OPSCC, HPV positive OSCC do not form a separate prognostic and treatment group [12].

11.4.4 Detection of HPV Related OPSCC and Surrogate Markers

p16 is an important tumor suppressor gene which regulates gene expression at different levels by modifying functional equilibrium of transcription factors [67]. It is located on chromosome 9p21 of the human genome at INK4A locus. It is the negative regulator of cell cycle and inhibits the transition of the cell cycle from G1 to S phase as a component of a multi-protein regulatory complex. In normal oral epithelium, p16 is detected merely in the basal and suprabasal cell layers where the cells are actively proliferative. In tobacco-associated HNSCC, it has been observed that there is a lack of p16, hence, favoring cell cycle progression in cancer cells [68, 69]. p16 is a gene with the second most frequently altered expression after p53. In the current scientific literature, it has been postulated that HPV presence can be connected to an altered expression of p16. The overexpression of p16 has been demonstrated to be strongly related to the presence of HPV16, 18 and many investigators have suggested that the expression of p16 be a surrogate marker for HPV-related HNSCC [68–72].

(a) **Overexpression of p16 protein** is defined as a diffuse strong expression of p16 in tumor cells, which shows, in turn, a high correlation with HPV infection. Rare cases may be p16 negative. Oropharyngeal SCC is diffusely p16 positive but may be negative for HPV by FISH due its low sensitivity but high specificity. p16 diffusely positive Some cases of cutaneous squamous cell carcinoma or HNMSCC-non-HPV are p16 diffusely positive including when presenting in lymph nodes.

(b) **HPV (+) FISH/ISH**: Rare cases are p16 negative (~5%) but still behaves as well as cases. In Situ Hybridization for HPV may be required to confirm or exclude HPV infection. HPV 16 correlates with p16 immunohistochemistry. **Positive** cases showing nuclear dots, which may range from strongly and diffusely positive to only a rare positive cell. A single punctate nuclear dot or multiple nuclear dots may be seen in the tumor cell in HPV ISH. It is not detected in the normal tonsillar epithelium. May need to be hybridization signals in dysplastic epithelium to highlight tour.

(c) **HPV ISH mRNA E6/E7**: has also been used and comes positive when the viral genome is integrated and neoplastic conversion of the squamous cell has occurred. The findings are usually concordant with p16. IHC HPV ISH can be used on FNA cell block from metastatic lymph node.

(d) **Other HPV types have been detected**, including HPV 6, 18, 33, 35, 45, and 52/58.

11.4.5 EBV Associated Lymphoepithelial Carcinoma

It is a rare sinonasal tract carcinoma that is morphologically similar to its better known histological counterpart in the nasopharynx. A strong association with EBV is present ion these lesions frequently located in the nasal cavity than paranasal sinuses but may rarely originate in other upper aerodigestive mucosal sites. The tumour has a favorable prognosis owing to a good response to radiotherapy Neoplastic cells are present in trabeculae, cords, islands, lobules, and sheets include large round to oval nuclei, vesicular appearing chromatin, 1 or more prominent nucleoli, and abundant amphophilic to eosinophilic cytoplasm with absent keratinization. A prominent non-neoplastic dense lymphoplasmacytic cell infiltrate is present. Cytokeratin (AE1/AE3, CAM5.2), p63 (+) CD117 is expressed by tumour cells and In situ hybridization for EBV-encoded RNA (EBER) is positive. Serologic Testing for IgA against viral capsid antigen (VCA) and IgG against early EBV antigens have 70–90% sensitivity [73].

11.5 Genetic Diagnosis of New Tumour Entities

The 4th edition of the Classification of Head and Neck Tumors published by the World Health Organization included several new entities and emerging entities. Squamous cell related new entity (NUT carcinoma) and emerging entities (SMARCB1-deficient carcinoma and HPV-related carcinoma with adenoid cystic-like features) are briefly outlined below with emphasis on molecular diagnosis [74, 75].

11.5.1 HPV-Related Carcinoma with Adenoid Cystic-Like Features

Sino-nasal carcinoma with morphologic features suggestive of adenoid cystic carcinoma including the presence of myoepithelial differentiation but the presence of surface intraepithelial dysplasia, the absence of *MYB* gene rearrangement, and association with human papillomavirus (HPV) evidenced in presence of strong diffuse p16 reactivity and positive HPV DNA hybridization [16, 52, 76, 77].

11.5.2 NUT Carcinoma

It is a poorly differentiated SCC with sheets of monotonous small to medium-sized cells with round to oval nuclei with no pleomorphism and abrupt squamous differentiation. Necrosis, brisk mitosis and invasion are features of this lesion. The neoplastic cells both the small round and keratinized clusters express CK5/6, p40, p63. Diagnosis is based on strong diffuse speckled nuclear positivity for NUT protein. IHC carries 100% specificity and 87% sensitivity. BRD4-NUTM1 fusion (the majority of cases), BRD3-NUT or NUT variant fusions can be detected using FISH or RT-PCR. Interestingly NUT carcinomas have a simple karyotype lacking the complex cytogenetic rearrangements in other SCC [74, 78].

11.5.3 SMARC-D1 Deficient HNSCC

It is a highly aggressive poorly or undifferentiated sino-nasal carcinoma which contains varying proportions of plasmacytoid/rhabdoid cells with loss of SMARCB1/INI1 located on Chromosome 22q11 2. It constitutes 3.0% of sino-nasal tract carcinoma occurring mostly in the naso-ethmoid region locally advanced destructive. The cells are undifferentiated basaloid cells arranged in compact cohesive nests, sheets, lobules, cords with intermixed rhabdoid to plasmacytoid cells. Frank keratinization is absent but cells express cytokeratins including CK 5/6, p40, p16. P63. Loss of INI1 characteristic of a tumour leads to increased cellular proliferation via overexpression of cyclin-D1, resulting in phosphorylation and inactivation of Rb and cell cycle progression. Overexpression of cyclin-D1 is sufficient to induce rhabdoid morphology. IHC is preferred for detection of INI loss. FISH may also be used. Genetic testing shows Homozygous (biallelic) deletion *SMARCB1* gene deletion is most common. Co-loss of *SMARCA2* may be seen, but *ARID1A* generally not detected. Methylation of *SMARCB1/INI1* gene is not seen. *RASSF1* gene methylation is seen in *SMARCB1/INI1*-deficient tumors to much higher extent than *SMARCB1/INI1*-intact tumors [79, 80].

11.6 Chromosomal Alterations

A variety of chromosomal alterations are found in oral cancer. Table 11.1 shows common alterations in HNSCC. The impact of these alterations varies significantly and their cellular and clinical significance is uncertain. Alterations in TP53 in 17p13, RB1 in 13q14 or the CDKN2A gene in 9p21 occur in pre-malignant lesions or early stage oral cancer and show their considerable prognostic significance. High prevalence of LOH or homozygous deletions in 3p, 9p, 13q and 17p also reported in early oral lesions [81]. Chromosome 9 is believed to be one of the earliest target and allelic loss in 9p21 region, possibly associated with genes encoding the p16 and p14 cyclin-dependent-kinase inhibitors, are present in pre-malignant lesions [82] and in oral cancer [81]. Chromosome 3 frequently hosts allelic imbalance in several regions, especially 3p25, 3p21, and 3p13–14,103 although the underlying responsible genes are not yet entirely clear. Allelic losses in 5q21–22 [83], 22q13 [84], 4q, 11q, 18q and 21q [85] and Gains in 3q66 are usually associated with advanced tumor stage or poor differentiation.

11.7 Epigenetic Changes

Hypermethylation of CpG islands in the promoter region is the most associated with HNSCC formation and progression. Silenced expression of tumor suppressor genes such as *p16* and E-cadherin by hypermethylation has been observed in HNSCC. Further, acquisition of telomerase activity is associated with early tumorigenesis. Global methylation is associated with tobacco-associated OSCC [86]. Hypomethylation of Long interspersed nuclear elements family (LINES) is detected in early OSCC [87, 88]. Epigenetic changes observed in head and neck cancer are subsite dependent [89]. It has also been shown that subsets of epigenetic events associated with individual genes have prognostic value in HNSCC tumors [89]. The WISP1 gene (WNT-inducible-signaling pathway protein 1), has been identified to be associated with lymph node metastasis, [90] and promoter hypomethylation of BIRC5 (the gene that encodes survivin) is frequently found in OSCC, and leads to a more aggressive and invasive tumor phenotype [87]. Methylation of the promoter region of MGMT is associated with increased tumor recurrence and decreased patient survival, independent of other factors [91].

11.7.1 Tobacco Induced Epigenetic Changes

Tobacco smoke has been associated with DNA hypermethylation of CpG sites within promoter regions and exons of tumor suppressor genes, and with global hypomethylation of DNA in HNSCC (Baba S et al). A number of candidate genes with CpG-rich regions have been found to be hypermethylated. The strongest evidence for DNA hypermethylation (25–60%) exists for the promoter region of CDKN2A gene. Other tumor suppressor genes frequently hypermethylated in smoking-related cancers include RARb, RASSF1, MGMT, GATA4, TIMP3, FHIT, RUNX3, MLH1, and CHFR [86].

11.7.2 HPV Induced Epigenetic Changes

Wilson et al. have identified 43 hypermethylated promoter regions associated with HPV in HNSCC, including 3 cadherins of the polycomb group target genes [92]. Sartor and colleagues reported that promoter regions of polycomb repressive complex 2 (PRC2) target tend to be much more highly methylated in HPV-positive cancers [93]. The PRC2 complex protein EZH2 is a direct downstream target of viral oncoproteins, activating EZH2 at the transcriptional level via the E7-mediated release of E2F from pocket proteins [94]. PRC2 has also been shown to mediate H3K27me3 trimethylation and recruit the DNMTs, furthering the link between chromatin changes and DNA methylation [95]. Numerous studies have identified promoter DNA methylation of such genes as CDKN2A (p16), DAP kinase (DAPK), and DNA repair genes MGMT and MLH1 [96].

MicroRNAs are a class of non-coding RNAs that are well investigated in HNSCC, Genetic and epigenetic alterations in several miRNAs were correlated with cancer. Distinct molecular profiles of miRNA in HPV related vs tobacco-related cancers are shown in Table 11.1.

11.8 Screening

Conventionally several techniques have been used for early detection and screening of HNSCC. Vital staining techniques using acetic acid, toluidine blue methylene blue lugols iodine tolonium chloride have been used to highlight the cancerous foci. Light-based detection systems employing fluorescence-based imaging, and cyto-diagnosis using oral brush cytology and liquid-based cytology have been tested with varying sensitivity and specificity against histological biopsy [97]. ***Molecular screening*** involves screening for epigenetic and genetic alterations as described here especially those related to early molecular changes which accompany precancer in the oral cavity. The use of multigene panels for detection of genes involved in precancer in cells/biopsy obtained from the oral cavity can be a sensitive diagnostic modality for detection of Squamous intraepithelial neoplasia. Epigenetic changes related to early cancer developments and late progressive disease have also been defined.

Among potential biomarkers for oral carcinogenesis, HOXA9 (Homeobox A9) and NID2 (Nidogen 2) hold high promise due to their apparent sensitivity and specificity. The identification of epigenetic biomarkers is paving the road to more attractive and reliable screenings to identify the development of HNSCC [87]. Viral genome studies for detection of HR-HPV would require a modality similar to cervical cancer screening for HPV associated OPSCC. Immunohistochemical identification of p16 overexpression, p53, Cyclin D1, EGFR and other oncogenes can also be tested in biopsies [98].

11.9 Predictive Markers

Surgical excision and/or Systemic therapy has been the mainstay of treatment in HNSCC in stages II, III and IV and comprises of Platinum-based doublet including cisplatin or carboplatin and 5-fluorouracil [99]. Targeted therapy utilizing cellular pathways in clinical trials in HNSCC have applied strategies that might have the potential to change clinical routine within the near future (Table 11.2). The TCGA profiling identified at least 18 targetable mutations including EGFR, FGFR1, FGFR2, MET, ERBB2 [138].

Table 11.2 Molecular markers for targeted therapy in HNSCC: review of clinical trails

Broad category	Target	Mechanism of action	Drugs	Indication	FDA approval and trial phase	References
ErbB family	EGFR	**TKIs:** Reversible Irreversible (Pan-Her2 kinase inhibitors)	Erlotinib, Lapatininb, (Both EGFR & HER-2) Gefitinib Afatinib, Dacomitinib	LA HNSCC, R/M HNSCC LA HNSCC, R/M HNSCC R/M HNSCC LA HNSCC, R/M HNSCC R/M HNSCC	Randomized and Non-randomized, Phase II & III Randomized and Non-randomized, Phase III Phase III trial, limited activity Randomized, Phase II & III (eg. LUX-Head and Neck 1 trial) Non-randomized, Phase I & II (NCT01116843)	Siu et al. [100] Kim et al. [101] Del Campo et al. [102] de Souza et al. [103] Patel et al. [104] Argiris et al. [105] Machiels et al. [106] Cohen et al. [107] Machiels et al. [108] Abdul Razak et al. [109]
		Monoclonal antibody	Cetuximab, Panitumumab Zalutumumab Nimotuzumab	LA HNSCC, R/M HNSCC R/M HNSCC R/M HNSCC LA HNSCC	Randomized, phase III (eg, EXTREME trial) Only FDA approved drug Randomized, Phase II & III (eg, SPECTRUM trial) Randomized, Phase III (eg. DAHANCA 19) Randomized, Phase II & III (NCT01425736)	Bonner et al. [110] Bonner et al. [111] Burtness et al. [112] Yang et al. [113] Wirth et al. [114] Machiels et al. [115] Eriksen et al. [116] Rodriguez et al. [117] Basavaraj et al. [118]
	Her2/Neu	Monoclonal antiboby	Trastuzumab, Pertuzumab	R/M HNSCC	Phase II & III	Uno et al. [119] Pollock and Grandis [120]
Neo-angiogenesis markers	VEGF	Monoclonal antibody	Bevacizumab	R/M HNSCC	Phase II & III (eg. NCT00588770)	Cohen et al. [121, 122]
	VEGFR	Small molecule Kinase inhibitors	Sorafenib, Sunitinib, Vandetanib	R/M HNSCC R/M HNSCC R/M HNSCC	Phase II, Lack significant response Phase II, Lack significant response Randomized, Phase II (eg. NCT01414426)	Williamson et al. [123] Choong et al. [124] Machiels et al. [125] Limaye et al. [126]
STAT	Member of a family of transcription factors	STAT3 Decoy (soluble nucleic acid decoy)			Phase 0, proof of concept trial (NCT00696176) is underway to evaluate the effect.	Fung and Grandis [127]
Src family kinases (SFKs)	Mediate and enhance the downstream signaling of TKRs	Kinase inhibitors	Dasatininb, Saracatinib (AZD0530)	HNSCC	Phase II	Brooks et al. [128] Johnson et al. [129]

Mammalian target of rapamycin (mTOR)	Downstream effectors of Akt pathway	Rapamycin analogs (mTOR kinase inhibitor)	Everolimus Temsirolimus	HNSCC	Phase II, Evaluated in a panel of three HNSCC cell lines	Aissat et al. [130]
Immunotherapy	PD-1	Monoclonal antibody	Pembrolizumab, Nivolumab	R/M HNSCC R/M HNSCC	FDA Approved, (eg. KEYNOTE-012/048) FDA Approved, Randomized, Phase III (CheckMate 651/714)	Uppaluri et al. [131] Mehra et al. [132] Ferris et al. [133]
	PD-L1	Monoclonal antibody	Durvalumab	R/M HNSCC	Randomized, Phase II & III, (eg. KESTREL study)	Seiwert et al. [134]
	CTLA-4	Monoclonal antibody	Ipilimumab, Tremelimumab	Presurgical LA HNSCC R/M HNSCC R/M HNSCC Platinum-refractory HNSCC	Phase I. open label Phase III (eg. CheckMate 651 trial) Phase III, KESTREL study (NCT02551159) Randomised CONDOR trial	Ferris et al. [133] Seiwert et al. [134] Economopoulou et al. [135]
	TCR-8 agonist	Receptor agonist	Motolimod (VTX-2337)	HNSCC	Phase Ib, II (eg.NCT01836029)	Chow et al. [136] Chow et al. [137]

11.9.1 EGFR-Targeting Therapies

These therapies included two large categories of molecules one using monoclonal antibodies, which recognize the ligand-binding domain and interfere with receptor activation including Cetuximab, Panitumumab, Zalutumumab and two Tyrosine kinase inhibitors which bind to the cytoplasmic region and influence with downstream signaling events include Gefitinib, Erlotinib and Lapatinib. Vermorken et al. have demonstrated the superiority of adding cetuximab targeting epidermal growth factor receptor (EGFR), in combination with cisplatin/carboplatin and fluorouracil in patients with HNSCC [139] (Fig. 11.2).

11.9.2 Neo-angiogenesis Markers

In HNSCC, VEGF and VEGF receptor expression has been demonstrated in tumor tissue and is associated with a worse prognosis. Currently, the two dominant approaches to targeting angiogenesis are inhibition of VEGF ligand itself and small molecule inhibition of VEGF receptor tyrosine kinases. Bevacizumab is a humanized mAb that binds and sequesters all five isoforms of VEGF [140]. Small molecule inhibition of VEGFR is complicated by the fact that the agents closest to commercialization for HNSCC are generally thought to be less specific multikinase inhibitors. At this time, the three most promising VEGFR targeted TKIs are vandetanib, sunitinib and sorafenib. Vandetanib is a dual EGFR and VEGFR inhibitor that is awaiting marketing approval for NSCLC. Phase II studies in HNSCC are underway evaluating the combination of vandetanib with docetaxel (NCT00459043) and cisplatin (NCT00720083). Sorafenib and sunitinib are multikinase inhibitors with specificity for a broad array of tyrosine kinases including VEGFR [141].

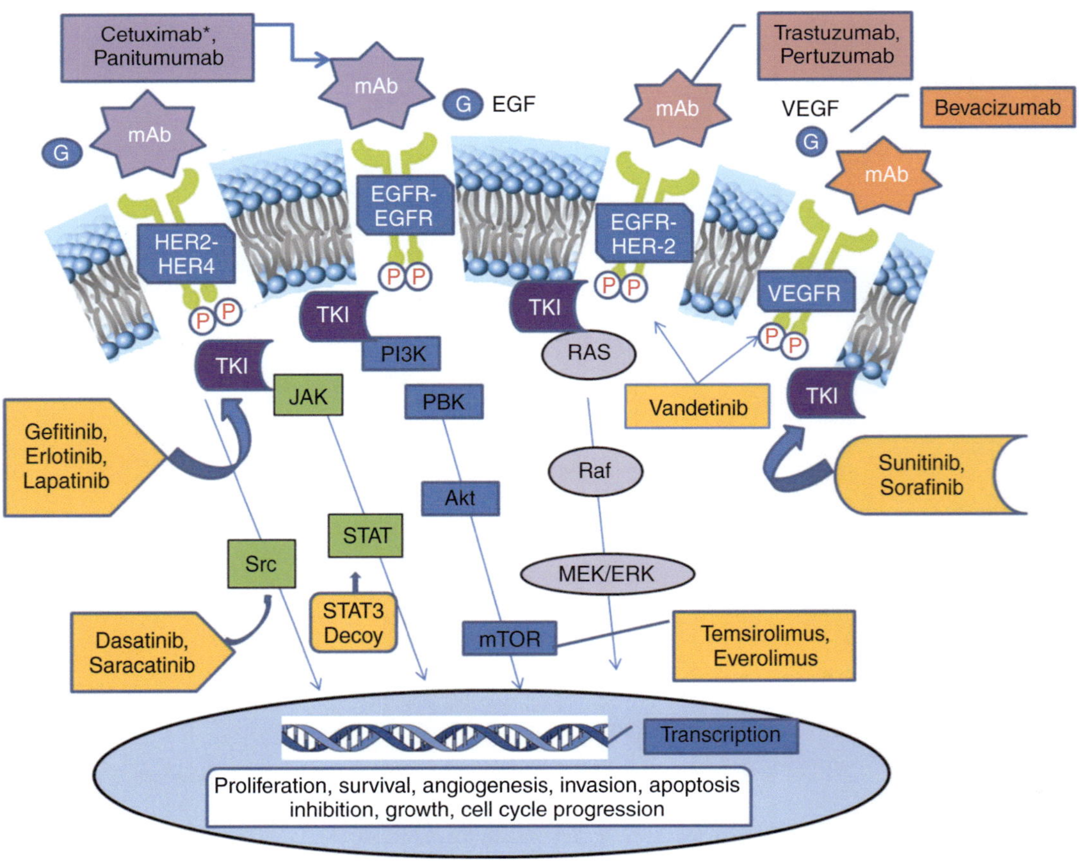

Fig. 11.2 Pathways of oncogenesis in HNSCC and targets for targeted therapy

11.9.3 Immunotherapies in HNSCC

Therapies Targeting PD-1, PD-L1, CTLA-4, TCR-8 Agonist have been utilized in separate trials. Efficacy of pembrolizumab, a mAb targeting programmed cell death 1 (PD-1), in KEYNOTE-012 trial has been demonstrated in heavily pre-treated patients with HNSCC [132, 142, 143].

11.9.4 Cell-Cycle Control Abnormalities

Up to 90% of squamous cell cancers of the head and neck may have abnormalities in the cyclin-D1/Rb/p16 pathway. Abnormalities in cyclin D1 and p16 have correlated with survival in two large studies; smaller studies have reported various results [7]. Various drugs that have an impact on cell-cycle control abnormalities in head and neck cancer clinical trials, including Ad5CMV-p53 (virally mediated transduction of the p53 gene), flavopiridol (a cyclin-dependent kinase inhibitor), and the proteasome inhibitor PS-341 (inhibits degradation of signaling or modulatory molecules, such as p53, p27, and I kappaB) are being targeted in HNSCC.

11.10 Liquid Biopsy

There is a strong need in the HNSCC for diagnostic tools which could be used to (1) identify patients at risk of developing metastasis early in order to escalate systemic treatment (2) assess the tumour heterogeneity to tailor treatment options and, (3) monitor for residual disease. Circulating Tumour Cells (CTC), circulating tumor DNA (ctDNA) and exosomes form a convenient and non invasive option in HNSCC patients. ctDNA is the more frequently studied parameter and enables specific complementary information for diagnosis, prognosis and management of treatment. Potential prognostic applications of cfDNA include in monitoring of response to therapy, emergence of treatment resistance, observation of residual disease and analysis of tumour dynamics and burden in metastatic patients [144, 145]. We believe that blood is an attractive medium for two reasons (1) reduced clonal heterogeneity as cfDNA and CTCs represent a large portion of tumour derivatives and (2) can be non-invasively sampled compared to a tissue biopsy. The liquid biopsy presents an option where HNSCC patients can be tracked in a non-invasive manner, allowing for serial sampling, informing of the tumour heterogeneity, response to treatment and residual disease ([146], abstract). Implementation of a liquid biopsy in HNSCC through serial blood samples has the potential to detect metastatic events earlier, thereby allowing better selection of appropriate treatment choices, predict prognosis in patients with potentially curable disease, monitor systemic therapies and residual disease post-treatment.

In a study by Agnieszka M. Mazurek et al. the comparison of the cfDNA levels in cancer patients and age-matched controls showed a noticeably higher level in HNSCC patients. In our analysis of a relationship between cfDNA concentration and clinical parameters showed a significantly higher level of cfDNA in patients with stage IV of the tumor or with N2-3 nodal disease ($p = 0.015$) [147]. We have also observed cfDNA was significantly increased in HNSCC compared to normal controls ($p < 0.001$). In a β-globin assay, the mean level of cfDNA in HNSCC was 14-fold higher than the healthy control group. In a follow-up of cases on chemoradiation therapy, the percentage decrease in cfDNA levels after chemo-therapy was 9.57 and 29.66% at 3 months of post-therapy follow up in the responders. In non responders, the percentage increase in the cfDNA levels after chemotherapy was 13.28% and 24.52% at 3 months of follow up [146].

11.11 Conclusion

The challenge for the pathologist is not just knowing the relevant mutation profiles for different tumors, but also in truly understanding the practical value for patient care and being able to assess the benefit of using a given mutation panel in a particular case. Perhaps the most important question that a pathologist can ask before ordering a molecular test is: how will this test result change the management of this patient? In the context of HNSCC molecular testing for HPV or detection of its surrogate markers like p16 in IHC is of definite clinical value for prognosticating and treatment planning. Specific mutations related to the diagnosis of variants like NUT carcinoma or SMARCD1-deficient carcinomas are required for diagnosis. Further predictive markers in cases undergoing targeted therapy are the need of the day. The future holds potential for implementation of molecular testing for screening, early diagnosis of precancer, molecular margins for predicting recurrence and molecular margins and metastasis detection. The scenarios where molecular testing is cost-effective and high-value addition to the diagnostic workup need to be worked out and implemented in a standardized manner in HNSCC as has been done is other several other solid tumours.

Acknowledgments Sources of support, including pharmaceutical and industry support that require acknowledgment: None.

Disclosure of funding: None.

Conflict of interest: None.

References

1. Parkin DM, et al. Global cancer statistics, 2002. CA Cancer J Clin. 2005;55(2):74–108.
2. D'Costa J, et al. Detection of HPV-16 genome in human oral cancers and potentially malignant lesions from India. Oral Oncol. 1998;34(5):413–20.
3. Sankaranarayanan R, et al. Trivandrum Oral Cancer Screening Study Group. Effect of screening on oral cancer mortality in Kerala, India: a cluster-randomised controlled trial. Lancet. 2005;365(9475):1927–33.
4. Byakodi R, et al. Oral cancer in India: an epidemiologic and clinical review. J Community Health. 2012;37(2):316–9.
5. Amin MB, et al. AJCC cancer staging manual. 8th ed. New York: Springer; 2017.
6. Koch WM. Early diagnosis and treatment of cancer series: head and neck cancers. 1st ed. New York: Elsevier; 2010. Chapter 1—Molecular gene alterations as early-detection markers; page 1–18.
7. Gupta S, et al. Understanding molecular markers in recurrent oral squamous cell carcinoma treated with chemoradiation. Heliyon. 2016;2(12):e00206. eCollection 2016 Dec.
8. Levine AJ, et al. The p53 tumour suppressor gene. Nature. 1991;351(6326):453–6.
9. Sigal A, Rotter V. Oncogenic mutations of the p53 tumor suppressor: the demons of the guardian of the genome. Cancer Res. 2000;60(24):6788–93.
10. Soussi T, Wiman KG. Shaping genetic alterations in human cancer: the p53 mutation paradigm. Cancer Cell. 2007;12(4):303–12.
11. Shin DM, et al. p53 expressions: predicting recurrence and second primary tumors in head and neck squamous cell carcinoma. J Natl Cancer Inst. 1996;88(8):519–29.
12. Singh V, et al. p16 and p53 in HPV-positive versus HPV-negative oral squamous cell carcinoma: do pathways differ? J Oral Pathol Med. 2017;46(9):744–51.
13. Fakhry C, et al. Improved survival of patients with human papillomavirus-positive head and neck squamous cell carcinoma in a prospective clinical trial. J Natl Cancer Inst. 2008;100(4):261–9.
14. Forte T, et al. Incidence trends in head and neck cancers and human papillomavirus (HPV)-associated oropharyngeal cancer in Canada, 1992-2009. Cancer Causes Control. 2012;23:1343–8.
15. Gillison ML, et al. Prevalence of oral HPV infection in the United States, 2009-2010. JAMA. 2012;307(7):693–703.
16. Hwang TZ, et al. Incidence trends of human papillomavirus-related head and neck cancer in Taiwan, 1995-2009. Int J Cancer. 2015;137:395–408.
17. Gillison ML, Alemany L, Snijders PJ, Chaturvedi A, Steinberg BM, Schwartz S, et al. Human papillomavirus and diseases of the upper airway: head and neck cancer and respiratory papillomatosis. Vaccine. 2012;30(Suppl 5):F34–54.
18. Gillison ML, D'Souza G, Westra W, Sugar E, Xiao W, Begum S, et al. Distinct risk factor profiles for human papillomavirus type 16-positive and human papillomavirus type 16-negative head and neck cancers. J Natl Cancer Inst. 2008;100(6):407–20.
19. Heck JE, et al. Sexual behaviours and the risk of head and neck cancers: a pooled analysis in the International Head and Neck Cancer Epidemiology (INHANCE) consortium. Int J Epidemiol. 2010;39(1):166–81.
20. Marks MA, et al. Association of marijuana smoking with oropharyngeal and oral tongue cancers: pooled analysis from the INHANCE consortium. Cancer Epidemiol Biomarkers Prev. 2014;23(1):160–71.
21. El-Mofty SK, Patil S. Human papillomavirus (HPV)-related oropharyngeal nonkeratinizing squamous cell carcinoma: characterization of a distinct phenotype. Oral Surg Oral Med Oral Pathol Oral Radiol Endod. 2006;101(3):339–45.
22. Wenig BM. Squamous cell carcinoma of the upper aerodigestive tract: dysplasia and select variants. Mod Pathol. 2017;30(s1):S112–8.
23. Westra WH. The morphologic profile of HPV-related head and neck squamous carcinoma: implications

for diagnosis, prognosis, and clinical management. Head Neck Pathol. 2012;6(Suppl 1):S48–54.
24. Yasui T, et al. Human papillomavirus and cystic node metastasis in oropharyngeal cancer and cancer of unknown primary origin. PLoS One. 2014;9(4):e95364.
25. Ang KK, et al. Human papillomavirus and survival of patients with oropharyngeal cancer. N Engl J Med. 2010;363(1):24–35.
26. Kraft S, et al. HPV-associated neuroendocrine carcinoma of the oropharynx: a rare new entity with potentially aggressive clinical behavior. Am J Surg Pathol. 2012;36(3):321–30.
27. Gondim DD, Haynes W, Wang X, Chernock RD, El-Mofty SK, Lewis JS Jr. Histologic typing in oropharyngeal squamous cell carcinoma: a 4-year prospective practice study with p16 and high-risk HPV mRNA testing correlation. Am J Surg Pathol. 2016;40(8):1117–24.
28. Agrawal N, et al. Exome sequencing of head and neck squamous cell carcinoma reveals inactivating mutations in NOTCH1. Science. 2011;333(6046):1154–7.
29. Cancer Genome Atlas Network. Comprehensive genomic characterization of head and neck squamous cell carcinomas. Nature. 2015;517(7536):576–82.
30. Lechner M, et al. Targeted next-generation sequencing of head and neck squamous cell carcinoma identifies novel genetic alterations in HPV+ and HPV- tumors. Genome Med. 2013;5(5):49.
31. Ndiaye C, et al. HPV DNA, E6/E7 mRNA, and p16INK4a detection in head and neck cancers: a systematic review and meta-analysis. Lancet Oncol. 2014;15(12):1319–31.
32. Miller DL, et al. Identification of a human papillomavirus-associated oncogenic miRNA panel in human oropharyngeal squamous cell carcinoma validated by bioinformatics analysis of the Cancer Genome Atlas. Am J Pathol. 2015;185(3):679–92.
33. Anayannis NV, et al. Epigenetic mechanisms of human papillomavirus-associated head and neck cancer. Arch Pathol Lab Med. 2015;139(11):1373–8.
34. Hayes DN, et al. Genetic landscape of human papillomavirus-associated head and neck cancer and comparison to tobacco-related tumors. J Clin Oncol. 2015;33(29):3227–34.
35. Smeets SJ, et al. A novel algorithm for reliable detection of human papillomavirus in paraffin embedded head and neck cancer specimen. Int J Cancer. 2007;121(11):2465–72.
36. Marur S, et al. HPV-associated head and neck cancer: a virus-related cancer epidemic. Lancet Oncol. 2010;11(8):781–9.
37. Husain N, Neyaz A. Human papillomavirus associated head and neck squamous cell carcinoma: controversies and new concepts. J Oral Biol Craniofac Res. 2017;7(3):198–205.
38. Mohan M, Jagannathan N. Oral field cancerization: an update on current concepts. Oncol Rev. 2014;8(1):244.
39. Nathan CO, et al. Molecular analysis of surgical margins in head and neck squamous cell carcinoma patients. Laryngoscope. 2002;112(12):2129–40.
40. Shaw RJ, et al. Molecular staging of surgical margins in oral squamous cell carcinoma using promoter methylation of p16(INK4A), cytoglobin, E-cadherin, and TMEFF2. Ann Surg Oncol. 2013;20(8):2796–802.
41. Dasgupta S, et al. Emerging strategies for the early detection and prevention of head and neck squamous cell cancer. J Cell Physiol. 2012;227(2):467–73.
42. Shakib K, et al. Stem cells in head and neck squamous cell carcinoma. Br J Oral Maxillofac Surg. 2011;49(7):503–6.
43. Ferlito A, et al. Prognostic significance of microscopic and macroscopic extracapsular spread from metastatic tumor in the cervical lymph nodes. Oral Oncol. 2002;38:747–51.
44. Arora A, et al. Development of a new outcome prediction model in early-stage squamous cell carcinoma of the oral cavity based on histopathologic parameters with multivariate analysis: the Aditi-Nuzhat Lymph-node Prediction Score (ANLPS) System. Am J Surg Pathol. 2017;41(7):950–60.
45. Colella S, et al. Molecular signatures of metastasis in head and neck cancer. Head Neck. 2008;30(10):1273–83.
46. Nam SW, et al. Autotaxin (ATX), a potent tumor motogen, augments invasive and metastatic potential of ras-transformed cells. Oncogene. 2000;19(2):241–7.
47. Yang L, Lin PC. Mechanisms that drive inflammatory tumor microenvironment, tumor heterogeneity, and metastatic progression. Semin Cancer Biol. 2017;47:185–95.
48. Goldenberg D, et al. Intraoperative molecular margin analysis in head and neck cancer. Arch Otolaryngol Head Neck Surg. 2004;130(1):39–44.
49. Partridge M, et al. Detection of minimal residual cancer to investigate why oral tumors recur despite seemingly adequate treatment. Clin Cancer Res. 2000;6(7):2718–25.
50. Hamakawa H, et al. Genetic diagnosis of micrometastasis based on SCC antigen mRNA in cervical lymph nodes of head and neck cancer. Clin Exp Metastasis. 1999;17(7):593–9.
51. Ferris RL, et al. Molecular staging of cervical lymph nodes in squamous cell carcinoma of the head and neck. Cancer Res. 2005;65(6):2147–56.
52. Hwang SJ, et al. Human papillomavirus-related carcinoma with adenoid cystic-like features of the inferior turbinate: a case report. Auris Nasus Larynx. 2015;42(1):53–5.
53. Muñoz N, et al. International Agency for Research on Cancer Multicenter Cervical Cancer Study Group. Epidemiologic classification of human papillomavirus types associated with cervical cancer. N Engl J Med. 2003;348(6):518–27.
54. Syrjänen KJ, Pyrhönen S. Demonstration of human papilloma virus (HPV) antigens in a case

of urethral condyloma. Scand J Urol Nephrol. 1983;17(3):267–70.
55. Bosch FX, et al. Epidemiology and natural history of human papillomavirus infections and type-specific implications in cervical neoplasia. Vaccine. 2008;26(Suppl 10):K1–16.
56. Stanley M. Pathology and epidemiology of HPV infection in females. Gynecol Oncol. 2010;117(2 Suppl):S5–10.
57. Münger K, et al. Mechanisms of human papillomavirus-induced oncogenesis. J Virol. 2004;78(21):11451–60.
58. Zaravinos A. An updated overview of HPV-associated head and neck carcinomas. Oncotarget. 2014;5(12):3956–69.
59. Smith EM, et al. Age, sexual behavior and human papillomavirus infection in oral cavity and oropharyngeal cancers. Int J Cancer. 2004;108(5):766–72.
60. Goldenberg D, et al. Cystic lymph node metastasis in patients with head and neck cancer: an HPV-associated phenomenon. Head Neck. 2008;30(7):898–903.
61. Begum S, Westra WH. Basaloid squamous cell carcinoma of the head and neck is a mixed variant that can be further resolved by HPV status. Am J Surg Pathol. 2008;32(7):1044–50.
62. Gupta T, et al. Radical radiotherapy with concurrent weekly cisplatin in loco-regionally advanced squamous cell carcinoma of the head and neck: a single-institution experience. Head Neck Oncol. 2009;1:17.
63. Lassen P, et al. Effect of HPV-associated p16INK4A expression on response to radiotherapy and survival in squamous cell carcinoma of the head and neck. J Clin Oncol. 2009;27(12):1992–8.
64. Braakhuis BJ, et al. Genetic patterns in head and neck cancers that contain or lack transcriptionally active human papillomavirus. J Natl Cancer Inst. 2004;96(13):998–1006.
65. Smeets SJ, et al. Genome-wide DNA copy number alterations in head and neck squamous cell carcinomas with or without oncogene-expressing human papillomavirus. Oncogene. 2006;25(17):2558–64.
66. Singh VS, et al. Do human papilloma viruses play any role in oral squamous cell carcinoma in north Indians? Asian Pac J Cancer Prev. 2015;16(16):7077–84.
67. Souza-Rodrígues E, et al. Proteomic analysis of p16ink4a-binding proteins. Proteomics. 2007;7(22):4102–11.
68. Pannone G, et al. Evaluation of a combined triple method to detect causative HPV in oral and oropharyngeal squamous cell carcinomas: p16 Immunohistochemistry, Consensus PCR HPV-DNA, and In Situ Hybridization. Infect Agent Cancer. 2012;7:4.
69. Singhi AD, Westra WH. Comparison of human papillomavirus in situ hybridization and p16 immunohistochemistry in the detection of human papillomavirus-associated head and neck cancer based on a prospective clinical experience. Cancer. 2010;116(9):2166–73.
70. Fregonesi PA, et al. p16(INK4A) immunohistochemical overexpression in premalignant and malignant oral lesions infected with human papillomavirus. J Histochem Cytochem. 2003;51(10):1291–7. PubMed PMID: 14500697.
71. Marklund L, Hammarstedt L. Impact of HPV in oropharyngeal cancer. J Oncol. 2011;2011:509036.
72. Weinberger PM, et al. Prognostic significance of p16 protein levels in oropharyngeal squamous cell cancer. Clin Cancer Res. 2004;10(17):5684–91.
73. Wenig BM. Lymphoepithelial-like carcinomas of the head and neck. Semin Diagn Pathol. 2015;32(1):74–86.
74. Stelow EB, et al. Update from the 4th Edition of the World Health Organization Classification of Head and Neck Tumours: Tumors of the nasal cavity, paranasal sinuses and skull base. Head Neck Pathol. 2017;11(1):3–15.
75. Thompson LDR, Franchi A. New tumor entities in the 4th edition of the World Health Organization classification of head and neck tumors: nasal cavity, paranasal sinuses and skull base. Virchows Arch. 2018;472(3):315–30.
76. Bishop JA, et al. Human papillomavirus-related carcinoma with adenoid cystic-like features: a peculiar variant of head and neck cancer restricted to the sinonasal tract. Am J Surg Pathol. 2013;37(6):836–44.
77. Wenig BM. Recently described sinonasal tract lesions/neoplasms: considerations for the new world health organization book. Head Neck Pathol. 2014;8(1):33–41.
78. Bishop JA. Recently described neoplasms of the sinonasal tract. Semin Diagn Pathol. 2016;33(2):62–70.
79. Agaimy A, et al. SMARCB1 (INI-1)-deficient sinonasal carcinoma: a series of 39 cases expanding the morphologic and clinicopathologic spectrum of a recently described entity. Am J Surg Pathol. 2017;41(4):458–71.
80. Agaimy A, et al. SMARCA4-deficient sinonasal carcinoma. Head Neck Pathol. 2017;11(4):541–5.
81. Rosin MP, et al. Use of allelic loss to predict malignant risk for low-grade oral epithelial dysplasia. Clin Cancer Res. 2000;6(2):357–62.
82. Jiang WW, et al. Accumulative increase of loss of heterozygosity from leukoplakia to foci of early cancerization in leukoplakia of the oral cavity. Cancer. 2001;92(9):2349–56.
83. Mao EJ, et al. Loss of heterozygosity at 5q21-22 (adenomatous polyposis coli gene region) in oral squamous cell carcinoma is common and correlated with advanced disease. J Oral Pathol Med. 1998;27(7):297–302.
84. Reis PP, et al. Quantitative real-time PCR identifies a critical region of deletion on 22q13 related to prognosis in oral cancer. Oncogene. 2002;21(42):6480–7.
85. Bockmühl U, et al. Distinct patterns of chromosomal alterations in high- and low-grade head

and neck squamous cell carcinomas. Cancer Res. 1996;56(23):5325–9.
86. Baba S, et al. Global DNA hypomethylation suppresses squamous carcinogenesis in the tongue and esophagus. Cancer Sci. 2009;100(7):1186–91.
87. Gasche JA, Goel A. Epigenetic mechanisms in oral carcinogenesis. Future Oncol. 2012;8(11):1407–25.
88. Subbalekha K, et al. Detection of LINE-1s hypomethylation in oral rinses of oral squamous cell carcinoma patients. Oral Oncol. 2009;45(2):184–91.
89. Noorlag R, et al. Promoter hypermethylation using 24-gene array in early head and neck cancer: better outcome in oral than in oropharyngeal cancer. Epigenetics. 2014;9(9):1220–7.
90. Clausen MJ, et al. Identification and validation of WISP1 as an epigenetic regulator of metastasis in oral squamous cell carcinoma. Genes Chromosomes Cancer. 2016;55(1):45–59.
91. Zuo C, et al. O6-methylguanine-DNA methyltransferase gene: epigenetic silencing and prognostic value in head and neck squamous cell carcinoma. Cancer Epidemiol. 2004;13(6):967–75.
92. Wilson GA, et al. Integrated virus-host methylome analysis in head and neck squamous cell carcinoma. Epigenetics. 2013;8(9):953–61.
93. Sartor MA, et al. Genome-wide methylation and expression differences in HPV(+) and HPV(-) squamous cell carcinoma cell lines are consistent with divergent mechanisms of carcinogenesis. Epigenetics. 2011;6(6):777–87.
94. Holland D, et al. Activation of the enhancer of zeste homologue 2 gene by the human papillomavirus E7 oncoprotein. Cancer Res. 2008;68(23):9964–72.
95. McCabe MT, et al. Cancer DNA methylation: molecular mechanisms and clinical implications. Clin Cancer Res. 2009;15(12):3927–37.
96. Maruya S, et al. Differential methylation status of tumor-associated genes in head and neck squamous carcinoma: incidence and potential implications. Clin Cancer Res. 2004;10(11):3825–30.
97. Carreras-Torras C, Gay-Escoda C. Techniques for early diagnosis of oral squamous cell carcinoma: systematic review. Med Oral Patol Oral Cir Bucal. 2015;20(3):e305–15.
98. Khan H, et al. Correlation between expressions of Cyclin-D1, EGFR and p53 with chemoradiation response in patients of locally advanced oral squamous cell carcinoma. BBA Clin. 2014;3:11–7.
99. Schantz SPHL, Forastiere A. Cancer: principles and practice of oncology. 6th ed. Philadelphia: Lippincott Williams & Wilkins; 2001. p. 797–860.
100. Siu LL, et al. Princess Margaret Hospital Phase II Consortium; National Cancer Institute of Canada Clinical Trials Group Study. Phase I/II trial of erlotinib and cisplatin in patients with recurrent or metastatic squamous cell carcinoma of the head and neck: a Princess Margaret Hospital phase II consortium and National Cancer Institute of Canada Clinical Trials Group Study. J Clin Oncol. 2007;25(16):2178–83.
101. Kim ES, et al. Final results of a phase II study of erlotinib, docetaxel and cisplatin in patients with recurrent/metastatic head and neck cancer. Presented at the American Society of Clinical Oncology Annual Meeting, June 1–5, 2007, Chicago.
102. Del Campo JM, et al. Effects of lapatinib monotherapy: results of a randomised phase II study in therapy-naive patients with locally advanced squamous cell carcinoma of the head and neck. Br J Cancer. 2011;105(5):618–27.
103. de Souza JA, et al. A phase II study of lapatinib in recurrent/metastatic squamous cell carcinoma of the head and neck. Clin Cancer Res. 2012;18(8):2336–43.
104. Patel PN, et al. Efficacy and toxicity of gefitinib in palliative treatment in recurrent squamous cell carcinoma of head and neck in poor performance elderly patients. Presented at the European Society of Medical Oncology Congress, September 29, 2014, Madrid.
105. Argiris A, et al. Phase III randomized, placebo-controlled trial of docetaxel with or without gefitinib in recurrent or metastatic head and neck cancer: an eastern cooperative oncology group trial. J Clin Oncol. 2013;31:1405–14.
106. Machiels JP, et al. LUX-H&N 1 investigators. Afatinib versus methotrexate as second-line treatment in patients with recurrent or metastatic squamous-cell carcinoma of the head and neck progressing on or after platinum-based therapy (LUX-Head & Neck 1): an open-label, randomised phase 3 trial. Lancet Oncol. 2015;16(5):583–94.
107. Cohen EEW, et al. Biomarker analysis in recurrent and/or metastatic head and neck squamous cell carcinoma (R/M HNSCC) patients (pts) treated with second-line afatinib versus methotrexate (MTX): LUX-Head and Neck 1 (LUX-H&N1). Presented at the American Society of Clinical Oncology Annual Meeting, May 29–June 2, 2015, Chicago.
108. Machiels JP, et al. Activity of afatinib administered in a window pre-operative study in squamous cell carcinoma of the head and neck (SCCHN): EORTC-90111. Presented at the American Society of Clinical Oncology Annual Meeting, June 3–7, 2016, Chicago.
109. Abdul Razak AR, et al. A phase II trial of dacomitinib, an oral pan-human EGF receptor (HER) inhibitor, as first-line treatment in recurrent and/or metastatic squamous-cell carcinoma of the head and neck. Ann Oncol. 2013;24:761–9.
110. Bonner JA, et al. Radiotherapy plus cetuximab for squamous-cell carcinoma of the head and neck. N Engl J Med. 2006;354(6):567–78.
111. Bonner JA, et al. Radiotherapy plus cetuximab for locoregionally advanced head and neck cancer: 5-year survival data from a phase 3 randomised trial, and relation between cetuximab-induced rash and survival. Lancet Oncol. 2010;11(1):21–8.
112. Burtness B, et al. Eastern Cooperative Oncology Group. Phase III randomized trial of cisplatin plus

placebo compared with cisplatin plus cetuximab in metastatic/recurrent head and neck cancer: an Eastern Cooperative Oncology Group study. J Clin Oncol. 2005;23(34):8646–54. Erratum in: J Clin Oncol. 2006;24(4):724.
113. Yang XD, et al. Development of ABX-EGF, a fully human anti-EGF receptor monoclonal antibody, for cancer therapy. Crit Rev Oncol Hematol. 2001;38(1):17–23.
114. Wirth LJ, et al. PARTNER: an open-label, randomized, phase 2 study of docetaxel/cisplatin chemotherapy with or without panitumumab as first-line treatment for recurrent or metastatic squamous cell carcinoma of the head and neck. Oral Oncol. 2016;61:31–40.
115. Machiels JP, et al. Zalutumumab plus best supportive care versus best supportive care alone in patients with recurrent or metastatic squamous-cell carcinoma of the head and neck after failure of platinum-based chemotherapy: an open-label, randomised phase 3 trial. Lancet Oncol. 2011;12(4):333–43.
116. Eriksen JG, et al. DAHANCA 19: first results of a randomized phase III study of the importance of the EGFR-inhibitor zalutumumab for the outcome of primary curative radiotherapy for squamous cell carcinoma of the head and neck. Late breaking abstract presented at: the European Cancer Congress, September 27–October 1, 2013, Amsterdam, Netherlands. Abstract 12.
117. Rodriguez MO, et al. Nimotuzumab plus radiotherapy for unresectable squamous-cell carcinoma of the head and neck. Cancer Biol Ther. 2010;9(5):343–9.
118. Basavaraj C, et al. Nimotuzumab with chemoradiation confers a survival advantage in treatment-naive head and neck tumors over expressing EGFR. Cancer Biol Ther. 2010;10(7):673–81.
119. Uno M, et al. Anti-HER2-antibody enhances irradiation-induced growth inhibition in head and neck carcinoma. Int J Cancer. 2001;94(4):474–9.
120. Pollock NI, Grandis JR. HER2 as a therapeutic target in head and neck squamous cell carcinoma. Clin Cancer Res. 2015;21(3):526–33.
121. Cohen EE, et al. Erlotinib and bevacizumab in patients with recurrent or metastatic squamous-cell carcinoma of the head and neck: a phase I/II study. Lancet Oncol. 2009;10(3):247–57.
122. Cohen R, et al. Bevacizumab and surgery: what is the real risk? Future Oncol. 2009;5(7):915–7.
123. Williamson SK, et al. A phase II trial of sorafenib in patients with recurrent and/or metastatic head and neck squamous cell carcinoma (HNSCC): a Southwest Oncology Group (SWOG) trial. 2007 ASCO Annual Meeting Proceedings Part I. J Clin Oncol. 2007;25(18S):6044.
124. Choong NW, et al. Phase II study of sunitinib malate in head and neck squamous cell carcinoma. Invest New Drugs. 2010;28(5):677–83.
125. Machiels JP, et al. Phase II study of sunitinib in recurrent or metastatic squamous cell carcinoma of the head and neck: GORTEC 2006-01. J Clin Oncol. 2010;28(1):21–8.
126. Limaye S, et al. A randomized phase II study of docetaxel with or without vandetanib in recurrent or metastatic squamous cell carcinoma of head and neck (SCCHN). Oral Oncol. 2013;49:835–41.
127. Fung C, Grandis JR. Emerging drugs to treat squamous cell carcinomas of the head and neck. Expert Opin Emerg Drugs. 2010;15(3):355–73.
128. Brooks HD, et al. Phase II study of dasatinib in the treatment of head and neck squamous cell carcinoma (HNSCC). J Clin Oncol. 2009;27(Suppl):15s. Abstract 6022.
129. Johnson FM, et al. Phase 1 pharmacokinetic and drug-interaction study of dasatinib in patients with advanced solid tumors. Cancer. 2010;116(6):1582–91.
130. Aissat N, et al. Antiproliferative effects of rapamycin as a single agent and in combination with carboplatin and paclitaxel in head and neck cancer cell lines. Cancer Chemother Pharmacol. 2008;62(2):305–13.
131. Uppaluri R, et al. Immunotherapy with pembrolizumab in surgically resectable. Presented at the American Society of Clinical Oncology Annual Meeting, June 3–7, 2016, Chicago.
132. Mehra R, et al. Efficacy and safety of pembrolizumab in recurrent/metastatic head and neck squamous cell carcinoma (R/M HNSCC): pooled analyses after long-term follow-up in KEYNOTE-012. Presented at the American Society of Clinical Oncology Annual Meeting, June 3–7, 2016, Chicago.
133. Ferris RL, et al. Nivolumab for recurrent squamous-cell carcinoma of the head and neck. N Engl J Med. 2016;375(19):1856–67.
134. Seiwert T, et al. A phase 3, randomized, open-label study of first-line durvalumab (MEDI4736) ± tremelimumab versus standard of care (SoC; EXTREME regimen) in recurrent/metastatic (R/M) SCCHN: KESTREL. Presented at the 2016 American Society of Clinical Oncology Annual Meeting, June 3–7, 2016, Chicago.
135. Economopoulou P, et al. The promise of immunotherapy in head and neck squamous cell carcinoma: combinatorial immunotherapy approaches. ESMO Open. 2017;1(6):e000122.
136. Chow LQM, et al. Phase Ib trial of TLR8 agonist VTX-2237 in combination with cetuximab in patients with recurrent or metastatic squamous cell carcinomas of the head and neck (SCCHN). Presented at the Multidisciplinary Head and Neck Cancer Symposium, 20–22 Feb 2014, Scottsdale.
137. Chow LQM, et al. Phase Ib trial of the toll-like receptor 8 agonist, motolimod (VTX-2337), combined with cetuximab in patients with recurrent or metastatic SCCHN. Clin Cancer Res. 2017;23(10):2442–50.
138. Chung CH, et al. Molecular classification of head and neck squamous cell carcinomas using patterns of gene expression. Cancer Cell. 2004;5(5):489–500.
139. Vermorken JB, et al. Platinum-based chemotherapy plus cetuximab in head and neck cancer. N Engl J Med. 2008;359:1116–27.

140. Ferrara N, et al. Discovery and development of bevacizumab, an anti-VEGF antibody for treating cancer. Nat Rev Drug Discov. 2004;3(5):391–400.
141. Stein MN, Flaherty KT. CCR drug updates: sorafenib and sunitinib in renal cell carcinoma. Clin Cancer Res. 2007;13(13):3765–70.
142. Chow LQM, et al. Antitumor activity of pembrolizumab in biomarker-unselected patients with recurrent and/or metastatic head and neck squamous cell carcinoma: results from the phase Ib KEYNOTE-012 expansion cohort. J Clin Oncol. 2016;34(32):3838–45.
143. Seiwert TY, et al. Safety and clinical activity of pembrolizumab for treatment of recurrent or metastatic squamous cell carcinoma of the head and neck (KEYNOTE-012): an open-label, multicentre, phase 1b trial. Lancet Oncol. 2016;17(7):956–65.
144. Gold B, et al. Do circulating tumor cells, exosomes, and circulating tumor nucleic acids have clinical utility? A report of the association for molecular pathology. J Mol Diagn. 2015;17:209–24.
145. Ignatiadis M, Dawson SJ. Circulating tumor cells and circulating tumor DNA for precision medicine: dream or reality? Ann Oncol. 2014;25:2304–13.
146. Husain, et al. Comparison of circulating cell-free DNA in serum as a biomarker for diagnosis and therapy monitoring in spectrum of tumors. Abstracts and Case Studies From the College of American Pathologists 2017 Annual Meeting (CAP17). Arch Pathol Lab Med. 2017;141(9):e2–191.
147. Mazurek AM, et al. Optimization of circulating cell-free DNA recovery for KRAS mutation and HPV detection in plasma. Cancer Biomark. 2013;13(5):385–94.

Molecular Diagnostic in Prostate Cancer

12

Mohammad Kaleem Ahmad, Soumya Srivastava, and Abbas Ali Mahdi

12.1 Introduction

In many developed countries, prostate cancer is the second leading cause of cancer-related deaths among men. The incidence of prostate cancer increases more with age than any other type of cancer [1].In India population of prostate cancer is second leading cancer among males in cities like Kolkata, Pune, Delhi [1]. Each year 232,090 men in the USA and 237,800 men in Europe are newly diagnosed with prostate cancer. Several emanating commercial molecular diagnostic assays have been proposed to provide more accurate risk stratification for early stage diagnosed prostate cancer. Unfamiliarity with molecular diagnostics may make it challenging for some clinicians to navigate and interpret the medical literature to ascertain whether particular assays are appropriately developed and validated for clinical use. Since there are no effective therapeutic options for advanced prostate cancer, early detection of this tumour is pivotal and can increase the curative success rate [1, 2]. Although the regular use of serum PSA testing has indubitably increased detection of prostate cancer, but the lack of specificity is the main downside that results in a high negative biopsy rate. Since prostate cancer is a heterogeneous disease, it has become clear that a defined set of markers will provide significantly more diagnostic information than any one biomarker. The list of potential prostate cancer biomarkers will continue to grow. Only when research groups use the proposed guidelines for biomarker development, then systematic evaluation and clinical investigation of these biomarkers will gain more insight into their true diagnostic potential. Prostate biopsy is currently the reference method for diagnosing prostate cancer. This method has high specificity, which means that the test seldom indicates a tumour in healthy men. Analysis of the tissue sample from a prostate tumour also provides some information about the possible severity level of the disease and guidance for treatment [2, 3]. However, clinicians are often uncertain whether the identified tumour requires intensive surgical treatment or radiation (accompanied by certain risks and discomfort), or if the tumour is actually harmless. The sensitivity of prostate biopsy is limited. Hence, there are chances of misdiagnosis and for many patients, prostate biopsies are uneasy and painful. The procedure also involves the risk for complications such as bleeding and infection. Molecular diagnosis reveals various changes that occur during the transformation of a normal cell to a tumour cell and capture this information as expression patterns. Molecular diagnostics are tests that detect genetic material, proteins, or related molecules

M. K. Ahmad (✉) · S. Srivastava · A. A. Mahdi
Department of Biochemistry, King George's Medical University, Lucknow, Uttar Pradesh, India
e-mail: mohdkaleemahmad@kgmcindia.edu

K. K. Shukla et al. (eds.), *Molecular Diagnostics in Cancer Patients*,
https://doi.org/10.1007/978-981-13-5877-7_12

that provide information about health or disease. These tests are most commonly run on samples of blood, saliva, or tumor tissue. Depending on the type of test, a molecular diagnostic may also be referred to as a gene panel, a gene signature panel, a gene signature test, or a gene expression panel, but molecular diagnostics is the broader term encompassing many different types of tests that examine DNA, RNA, and proteins.

For men with higher probability of prostate cancer, as reflected by PSA testing or rectal examination, diagnostic accuracy increases somewhat by adding the uPCA3 test. The higher the uPCA3 value, the higher the probability of cancer. A uPCA3 result above the threshold value implies a strong suspicion of prostate cancer. In some otherwise difficult-to-assess patients the test would contribute towards earlier biopsy and earlier diagnosis. The uPCA3 test cannot, however, rule out prostate cancer in men having a higher probability of the disease. Accuracy of the uPCA3 test is the same regardless of whether the individual had a previous biopsy with negative results, or never had a biopsy. The addition of the uPCA3 test to determine which patients should be biopsied involves a higher total cost than direct prostate biopsy of all men with an increased probability of prostate cancer as identified by PSA testing or rectal examination. The importance of the uPCA3 test in further investigation and its effects on disease course and mortality should be assessed in clinical studies [3]. To appraise the patient benefits of routine clinical use of uPCA3, better evidence is needed regarding the value of the extra information obtained from the test results in relation to other risk factors, *e.g.* PSA concentration, age, rectal examination, and the results of previous biopsies. The scientific evidence is insufficient to appraise the diagnostic accuracy of TMPRSS2: ERG and me-GSTP1 urine tests. Further studies are needed. Over-diagnosis of clinically insignificant prostate cancers will cause over-treatment, including incontinence and impotence that are side-effects of radical surgery and radiotherapy, and will negatively affect the patients' quality of life. Furthermore, PSA screening fails to detect a small proportion of highly aggressive prostate cancers, that are likely to be life threatening. Therefore, tests that can accurately identify men who have early stage, organ-confined prostate cancer and who would gain prolonged survival and improved quality of life from early radical intervention, are urgently needed [4, 5].

Some medical organizations recommend men consider prostate cancer screening in their 50s, or sooner for men who have risk factors for prostate cancer.

Prostate screening tests might include:

- **Digital rectal exam (DRE)**—In this procedure the doctor puts a gloved, lubricated finger inside the rectum to examine prostate, which is close to the rectum. If there is any abnormality in the, shape or size of the gland, textureit may require further tests.
- **Prostate-specific antigen (PSA) test**—In this test the blood sample is taken from a vein and evaluated for PSA, a substance which is naturally produced by prostate gland. It's normal for a small amount of PSA to be in bloodstream. But, if a higher level is found than the normal, it could be considered as the indicator of prostate infection, inflammation, enlargement or cancer.

The first PSA test from Hybritech (now Beckman Coulter) was released in 1985. It took an additional 9 years to obtain the FDA approval to use it in clinical practice for the detection of prostate cancer. Other markers are likely to follow PCA3DD3 and may add additional value in the diagnosis of prostate cancer. It was shown that the combination of PCA3DD3, Hepsin and PSMA was the best multivariate predictive model that distinguished 100% of the prostate cancer tissue specimens from the BPH tissue specimens. Additionally, such a set of genes combined with a set of markers for disease aggressiveness could aid the urologist in his decision which patient would benefit from curative treatment and which patient would benefit from other therapeutic approaches. The close collaboration and communication between clinicians and researchers is essential in clinical testing of these markers to assess their real diagnostic potential and to evaluate the impact of these tests on the reduction of unnecessary biopsies and disease mortality [5–8].

12.2 Recent Modifications in PSA Test

Scientists are continuously discovering methods to improve the PSA test to provide doctors a better way distinguish between cancerous and benign conditions. Till now, none has been proven to decrease the risk of death from prostate cancer. Some of the methods studied include:

- **Free versus total PSA**. The level of PSA in the blood that is "free" (not bound to other proteins) divided by the total amount of PSA (free plus bound) is denoted as the proportion of free PSA. Several reports suggested that a lower proportion of free PSA may be linked with more aggressive cancer.
- **PSA density of the transition zone**. The blood amount of PSA is divided by the volume of the transition zone that is, the interior part of the prostate that surrounds the urethra. Some data suggests that this may be more accurate at detecting prostate cancer.
- **Age-specific PSA reference ranges**. It has been suggested that the use of age-specific PSA reference ranges may increase the accuracy of PSA tests because a man's PSA level tends to increase with age. Although, age-specific reference ranges have not been generally considered because it could delay the detection of prostate cancer in many men.
- **PSA velocity and PSA doubling time**. This is the rate of change in a man's PSA level over time, expressed as ng/mL per year. PSA doubling time is the period of time over which a man's PSA level doubles. Several studies have suggested that increase in a man's PSA level may be helpful in predicting whether he has prostate cancer or not.
- **Pro-PSA**. It refers to several different inactive precursors of PSA. Some evidence shows that pro-PSA is more strongly associated with prostate cancer than with BPH.
- **Iso-PSA**. It is a structural forms (called isoforms) of PSA in the blood. The iso-PSA test, which measures the entire spectrum of PSA isoforms rather than the concentration of PSA in the blood, may improve the selection of men with prostate cancer for biopsy.
- **PSA in combination with other protein biomarkers**. Tests that combine measurements of PSA in blood with measurements of other biomarkers linked to prostate cancer in blood or urine are being studied for their ability to distinguish high-risk disease. These other biomarkers include kallikrein-related peptidase 2, prostate cancer antigen 3 (PCA3), and the TMPRSS2-ERG gene fusion [7–10].

Although in the recent era there have been so many modifications done in the prostate cancer diagnosis but unfortunately those tests are not able to make the diagnosis absolutely reliable. However, researchers evolved a new way for diagnosing prostate cancer as well others too and i.e., Molecular diagnosis. The molecular diagnosis is based on several parameters which we are going to discuss in this chapter.

12.3 Pathways Those Are Involved in the Progression of CaP

12.3.1 JAK/STAT Pathway

The JAK/STAT pathway plays an important role in mediating cell fates, such as apoptosis, differentiation and proliferation in response to growth promoting factors and cytokines. Upon binding their receptors, receptor-associated Janus Kinases (JAKS) phosphorylate tyrosine residues of the receptors, as well as the Signal Transducers and Activators of Transcription (STATs). The phosphorylated STAT forms homodimers by binding to other phosphorylated STAT. This dimer translocate to the nucleus and participate in transcription [6]. Deregulation of JAK/STAT pathway can lead to tumorogenesis directly and indirectly Fig. 12.1 [11, 12].

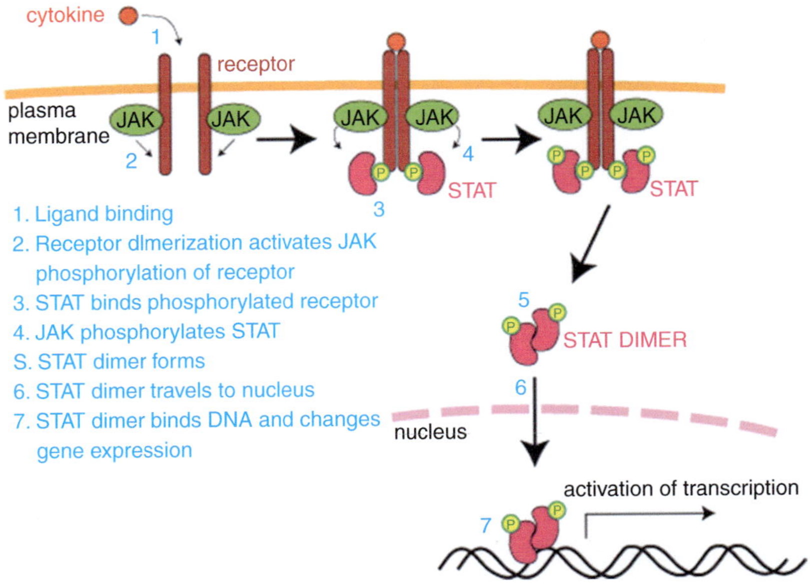

Fig. 12.1 Jak/stat pathway [11]

12.3.2 MAP KINASE/ERK Pathway

The RAS-Mitogen Activated Protein Kinase (MAPK) pathway promotes cell adhesion, proliferation, migration and survival. This pathway plays an important role in signaling from cytokines and growth factors through Receptor Tyrosine Kinases (RTK). RAS, a small membrane-bound GTPase switch proteins is central to this signaling cascade that shuttles between two conformational states: active GTP-bound and inactive GDP-bound [8]. It is activated by SOS which is a guanine exchange factor usually found in the cytoplasm of the cell. Activated GTP-bound RAS carries the activation of serine/threonine kinase RAF that activates mitogen-activated protein kinases (MAPK). It is also called extracellular signal regulated kinase (ERK). ERK1/2 gets translocated to the nucleus and there it activates Jun/Fos transcription factors leading to cell signaling [8]. Due to its vital role in cell proliferation, deregulation of the SOS-Ras-Raf-MAPK signaling cascade leads to a broad spectrum of human tumors (Fig. 12.2). Most of these mutations occur in RAS and RAF and result in constitutive pathway activation resulting in hyper proliferative state. RAS mutations are found in 45% of prostate cancers. RAF mutations, are found in two thirds of all melanoma approximately. This pathway is a target for therapeutic intervention and has got tremendous attention [11, 12].

12.3.3 NF-κB Pathway

The nuclear factor-kappa-B (NF-κB) pathway regulates genes involved in various cellular processes like, stress response, proliferation, innate immunity and inflammation (Fig. 12.3). In vertebrates, the NF-κB transcription factor family has p50/p105, p52/p100, c-Rel, RelA and RelB which regulate transcriptional expression of target genes. P105 and p100 are proteolytically processed to give rise to p50 and p52, respectively. c-Rel, RelA, RelB, p50 and p52 can form homo- and heterodimers, shuttle to the nucleus where they bind DNA regulatory κB sites [10]. In the absence of signaling, NF-κB dimers are located in the cytoplasm and inactivated by their interaction with I-κB inhibitory proteins. This pathway is activated by a variety of extracellular factors such as tumor necrosis factor-α (TNF-α), bacterial or viral infections, interleukin-1, oxidative stress, growth factors, and pharmaceutical compounds. In response to such stimuli, IκB is rapidly phosphorylated on serine 32 and 36 by the I-κB kinase (IKK). Phosphorylated I-κB is

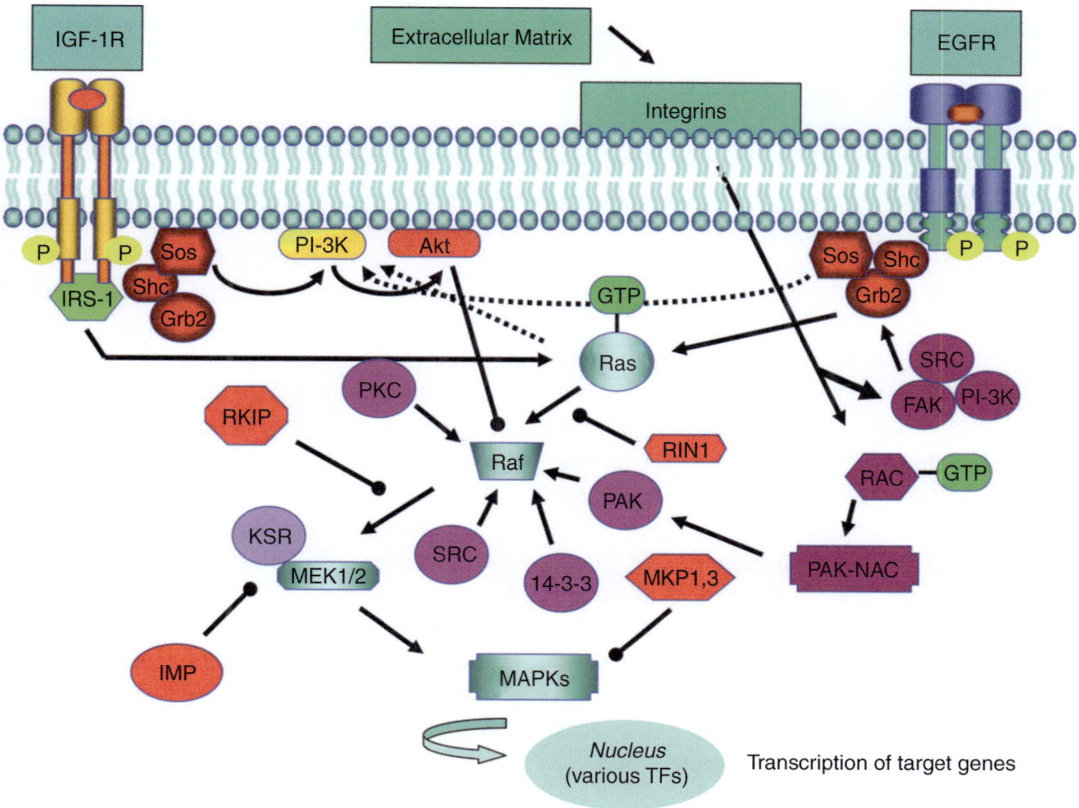

Fig. 12.2 MAP kinase/ERK pathway [7, 12]

Fig. 12.3 NF-κB pathway [13]

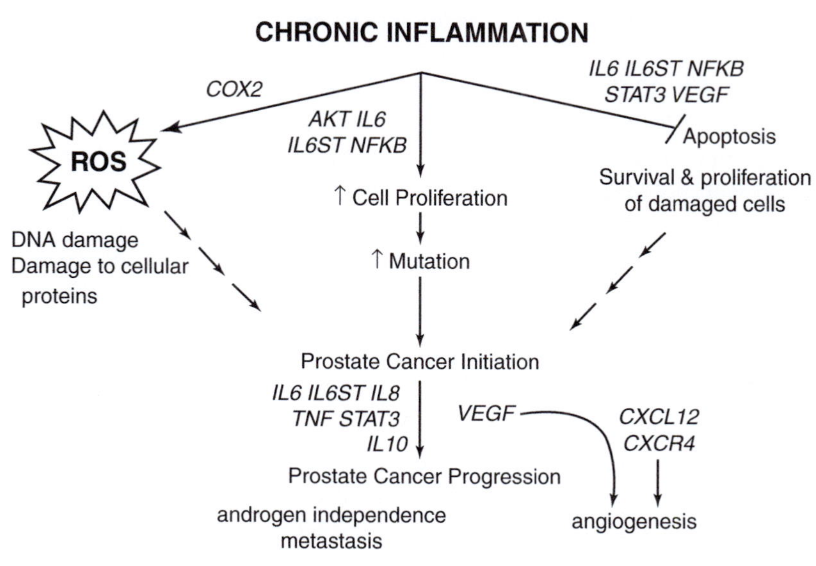

ubiquitinated by the E3 ubiquitin ligase complex and targeted for degradation by the 26S proteasome. The NF-κB dimers then move to the nucleus and activate target gene transcription [8]. Mutation in this pathway has been involved in a variety of cancers [11–13].

12.3.4 RAS

The *RAS* oncogenes encode for a family of small G proteins which bind downstream of the EGFR in the PI3K/PTEN/AKT and RAF/MEK/ERK signaling pathways, transmitting extracellular growth signals to the nucleus. *RAS* exists as three cellular variants, *HRAS, KRAS* and *NRAS* but *KRAS* is most commonly mutated in CaP. These proteins normally cycle between a GDP-bound inactive state and a GTP-bound active state (Fig. 12.2). Mutations in *RAS* lead to constitutively activated GTP-bound protein with a continuous growth stimulus to the cells. *RAS* mutations are found in approximately 50% of sporadic CaPcases [12, 13].

12.3.5 BRAF

BRAF gene encodes for a serine/threonine protein kinase, which is an immediate downstream effector of KRAS in the MAP kinase signaling pathway (Fig. 12.2). Oncogenic activating BRAF mutation (V600E) is found in approximately 5–22% of Cap cases. This mutation is seen almost exclusively in MSI-H, CIMP+ CaPs with wild type *KRAS. BRAF* mutation is frequently detected in smokers with sporadic Caps [13, 14].

12.4 Molecular Markers for CaP

There are various research is going on day by day to diagnose the cancer in the early stage and different markers are now being studied. In this era the molecular markers are being used to test the diagnosis of cancer i.e. molecular diagnostics. Molecular diagnostic test used for risk assessment is the blood test for the BRCA1 and BRCA2 genes. Alterations in either of these genes can increase the risk of breast, ovarian, and several other cancers. Many of us have heard the story of Angelina Jolie, the actress, filmmaker, and special envoy of the United Nations High Commissioner for Refugees. Angelina Jolie wrote several editorials for the New York Times explaining that she has a mutation in the BRCA1 gene. Her mother, grandmother, and aunt all died of cancer, and Ms. Jolie, chose to have her breasts and ovaries removed to prevent cancer of these organs. She stresses that the actions she took may not be right for everyone but that they were right for her [14–16].

Ms. Jolie's public acknowledgment of her BRCA1 mutation and her choice of preventive surgery helped raise awareness of the BRCA mutations and their potential to cause cancer. However, it is important to note that not everyone with a mutation in the BRCA1 or BRCA2 gene will get cancer. Moreover, many people diagnosed with breast cancer do not have either of these mutations and preventive surgery may not be the best choice for these individuals. Alternatives to preventive surgery are available, and each individual should discuss the options with her family and physician prior to making [15, 16] (Table 12.1).

Molecular gene based tests for Prostate Cancer—There are several genes which have their contribution in the molecular diagnosis of prostate cancer and they are as follow.

Tumor suppressor genes: The normal gene inhibits the growth of tumor cells. Initially, the loss of function of the gene was attributed to mutation or deletion of the two alleles, however, this has been revised to include epigenetic changes such as inactivation of one or both alleles by DNA methylation of CpG sites in gene promoters, heritably downregulated function, function compromised in a clonal fashion. Thus, the alteration of normal function can be by mutation, methylation of the promoter or by modification of the protein product. Various tumor suppressor genes have been identified, playing a role in prostate cancer development, progression and the emergence of androgen-independent phenotypes: a. p53 gene: This is the most commonly mutated

Table 12.1 Available techniques for biomarker determination

Type of assay	Technique	Target	Disadvantage	Advantage
Protein based assay	ELISA SELDI TOF-MS Western blot	Based on a single protein Based on a pattern of a protein Based on the size of the protein	Lack of standardization	Relatively easy to establish Recently validated by EDRN Good for further analysis
DNA based assay	Gene expression profile LOH MSP Sequence analysis	Based on expression of several gene Microsatellite alteration Epigenetic modification Evaluation of cancer specific mutation	Due to heterogeneity of prostate cancer only applicable in tissue specimens Not FDA approved Ineffective in detection of primary prostate cancers in general male population	
RNA based assay	Rt-PCR TMA	Specific mRNA	RNA degradation due to less stability	FDA approved Roche molecular system FDA approved Gen-probe

gene in human cancers. Because of its normal function, which is the prohibition of entrance into the synthetic phase of the cell cycle (phase S) and the promotion of apoptosis in cells that are disorganized or have damaged DNA, this gene is recognized as the 'guardian of the genome'. In primary prostate cancer a relatively low incidence (10–20%) of p53 gene mutations has been described, however, in advanced stages of the disease the p53 is mutated in 42% of the cases and it is associated with bone metastases and androgen-independent disease. Abnormal p53 expression correlates with high histological grade, high stage and clinical progression of the disease while, it is also correlated with reduced survival after radical prostatectomy and disease onset modulation [17].

Retinoblastoma (Rb) gene: The Rb gene plays an important role in the G1 phase of the cell cycle. Mutations and loss of Rb protein expression have been reported innomas. Studies have demonstrated at least 50% mutations of Rb gene in advanced prostate tumor. This gene has also been implicated in regulating apoptosis of prostate cells, especially in response to androgens Bcl-2: This gene is not expressed in the normal prostate, but is commonly expressed in prostate and other primary cancers. It promotes cell survival through the inhibition of the apoptotic pathway. Bcl-2 plays central role in the development of androgen independent prostate cancer because of its increased expression in the advanced stages of disease. It is suggested that androgen-mediated mechanisms may act through Bcl-2-mediated apoptotic pathways. The overexpression of Bcl-2 in prostate cancer safeguards the tumor cells from apoptosis [18].

PTEN: About 5–27% of localized and 30–60% of metastatic prostate tumors display PTEN mutations. The PTEN gene encodes a phospholipid phosphatase active against both protein and lipid substrates acting as a tumor suppressor gene by inhibiting the phosphatidylinositol 3-kinase-protein kinase B (PKB-Akt) signaling pathway which is essential for cell cycle progression and cell survival. PTEN is present in normal prostatic epithelial cells and in cells with prostatic intraepithelial neoplasia (PIN). In prostatic cancers, PTEN concentrations are reduced particularly in high grade or stage cancer. However, it has been shown that common genetic variants in PTEN do not substantially increase the risk of prostate cancer. A recent study suggested that germ-line variants in PTEN do not have a significant role in prostate cancer susceptibility. PTEN influences the levels of CDKN1B (p27) another tumor suppressor gene.

hPC1 or RNASEl: Located on chromosome 1q24-25 locus it was the first prostate cancer susceptibility gene to be identified. RNASEl is a ribonuclease that degrades viral and cellular RNA and can produce apoptosis in viral infection. Until now the RNASEl gene has been identified in many studies as the most important hereditary prostate cancer gene although other studies have not supported these findings [17, 18].

PCAP: This was the second prostate cancer gene to be identified located on chromosome 1q42.2-43 locus.

hPCX: This is an X-linked gene located on Xq27-28 and CAPB: This gene located on chromosome 1p36 and seems to be important in high-risk prostate cancer families with close relatives suffering from brain tumors.

hPC20: This is located on chromosome 20q13 and although it was identified as a prostate cancer susceptibility gene, others failed to support it, however it was suggested that the aforementioned locus may represent a low-penetrance prostate cancer predisposition gene [18].

PC2/ElAC2: This is located on chromosome 17p. Its function has been proposed as a metal dependent hydrolase. It was suggested as a prostate cancer susceptibility gene but this was not confirmed by subsequent studies. More recently, it has shown a minor effect, together with RNASEl, in prostate cancer risk in African American familial and sporadic cases. The association of one of hPC2/ElAC2 polymorphic variants (Thr541) with prostate cancer seems to be weak [19].

MSR1: This gene encodes a macrophage scavenger receptor responsible for cellular uptake of molecules, including bacterial cell wall products. Its role in hereditary prostate cancer is controversial since there are those who support it, while others have not provided evidence of such a role.

NBS1: This gene is involved in the rare human genetic disorder, the Nijmegen breakage syndrome, which is characterized by radiosensitivity, immunodeficiency, chromosomal instability and increased risk of lymphatic cancer. It encodes the protein nibrin, which is involved in the processing/repair of DNA double strand breaks and in cell cycle checkpoints.

ChEK2: This gene is an upstream regulator of p53 in the DNA damage signaling pathway. Mutations of this gene have been identified in hereditary prostate cancer and they are associated with a small increased risk for the disease. Despite the large number of studies seeking to determine a major prostate cancer susceptibility gene, this has not been achieved yet. Many mutations of the above genes have been identified in sporadic prostate cancer as well. Because of the high frequency of prostate cancer it is probably difficult to distinguish within families cases of sporadic tumors from true hereditary ones. Furthermore, the low penetrance of genes in hereditary prostate cancer may result from the fact that multiple genes are involved in hereditary prostate carcinogenesis exerting a small to moderate effect, which is increased by the proper genetic, dietary and environmental background [20].

Sporadic prostate cancer: Most of the prostate cancers are sporadic including various molecular pathways involved in the development, initiation, and spread of the disease:

CDKN1B (p27): It is an important tumor suppressor gene in prostate cancer. p27 is a cyclin dependent kinase inhibitor and its reduced levels are common in prostate cancer, especially in more aggressive tumors with a poor prognosis. This gene is located on chromosome 12p12-3 and the somatic loss of its sequences has been described in 23% of localized prostate cancers, in 30% of regional lymph node metastases and in 47% of distant metastases. Low p27 concentrations may be the result of both CDKN1B alterations and as mentioned before because of loss of PTEN function [19, 20].

NKX3.1: Its product binds to DNA and represses the expression of the PSA gene. The loss of function or deletion of this gene appears to be an early event in prostate cancer. It is present in androgen-sensitive cells but absent in androgen-independent prostate tumor. The loss of this gene may be involved in the increasing concentrations of PSA seen with prostate cancer progression. A study found that NKX3.1 was absent in 20% of PIN lesions, 6% of low stage prostate tumors, 22% of high stage prostate tumors, 34% of androgen-independent tumors and 78% of prostate cancer metastases.

12.4.1 Prostate Cancer Diagnosis Through micro RNAs (Abbr. miRNA)

A small non-coding RNA molecule encoded by eukaryotic nuclear DNA, found in plants and animals, functions in transcriptional and post-transcriptional regulation of gene expression. miRNAs function via base-pairing with complementary sequences within mRNA molecules, usually resulting in gene silencing via translational repression or target degradation. The human genome may encode over 1000 miRNAs, which may target about 60% of mammalian genes and are abundant in many human cell types. These days miRNAs are the emerging markers for the detection for various cancers such as prostate cancer. In 2006 Harris et al. conducted a research on the use of unique microRNA molecular profiles in lung cancer diagnosis and prognosis. They examined MicroRNA (miRNA) expression profiles for lung cancers to investigate miRNAs involvement in lung carcinogenesis. miRNA microarray analysis identified statistical unique profiles, which could discriminate lung cancers from noncancerous lung tissues as well as molecular signatures that differ in tumor histology. In 2007, William CS Cho presented a review on the importance of OncomiRs: the discovery and progress of microRNAs in cancers stating the function of miRNAs as tumor suppressors and oncogenes, and designating it as oncogenic miRNAs (oncomiRs). It has been reported that miRNAs play a crucial role in the initiation and progression of human cancer. Chen et al. reported on characterization of microRNAs in serum as a novel class of biomarkers for diagnosis of cancer and other diseases and the dysregulated expression of microRNAs (miRNAs) in various tissues is associated with a variety of diseases, including cancers. He and his colleagues demonstrated that the miRNAs are present in the serum and plasma of humans and other animals such as mice, rats, bovine foetuses, calves, and horses. The levels of miRNAs in serum are stable, reproducible, and consistent among individuals of the same species. In Prostate cancer, after failure of androgen deprivation therapy (ADT) and with the emergence of castration resistance, the survival period is limited but extremely variable between patients [21–24]. Knowledge of prognosis for individual patients in this stage has become critical because several therapeutic choices are available to control progression. Such prognostic factors are lacking in advanced PCa therapeutics, barring the presence of CTC counts, which are technically challenging and have not been widely adopted. Clinical prognostic factors used in several nomograms at the CRPC stage have yet to be validated in prospective studies [25, 26]. To overcome this short coming, the microRNAs are also helpful to predict prognosis because their up and down expression may be help in the predict in the transformation of lower grade prostate cancer to castration resistance prostate cancer (high grade prostate cancer). One of the good example, some report suggested that miR-21 up regulation involved in cancer progression and also helpful in prediction in castration résistance prostate cancer [27–29]. Following miRNAs have potential to be used as a marker for progression of prostate cancer:

12.4.2 miR-130b-3P

Some previous report suggested that the over expressed miR-130b caused tumorigenesis by targeting the tumor suppressor RUNX3 or TP53INP1 in hepato-carcinoma and PTEN in BCa. Zakaria et al. reported that mir-130b over expression in prostate cancer in comparison to control. Other study showed that expression of miR130b was down regulated in prostate cancer cell lines as well as clinical prostate cancer tissues [30, 31].

12.4.3 miR-183-5P

Most of previous studies also reported that the level of miR-183 expression in prostate cancer was described to be higher than adjacent normal tissues. Furthermore, miR-183 functions as an oncogene by targeting the transcription factor EGR1 and known prostate cancer tumor suppressor PTEN and promoting tumor cell migration in prostate cancer [32, 33]. Mihelich et al. reported that miR-183 was over expressed in prostate tissue and its expression regulates zinc homeostasis in prostate cells. The oncogenic miR-183 activates the Wnt/b-catenin pathway by directly inhibiting tumour suppressors Dkk-3 and SMAD4 in PC-3 cells [34, 35].

12.4.4 miR-329-3P

miR-329-3P (Chr14) is part of an extensive microRNA cluster which involved in prostate cancer pathogenesis. Yang et al. [35] found that miR-329-3p was down regulated in metastatic, neuroblastoma tumor tissue compared to the primary tumor [35–39]. MicroRNA-329-3p targets MAPK1 to suppress cell proliferation, migration and invasion in cervical cancer [36]. One promising target for miR-329-3P is KDM1A, which has been shown to be significantly up regulated in the androgen-dependent LnCaP prostate cell line [17, 37]. Upon depletion of KDMA1 using siRNA, VEGF-A expression was also decreased, which in turn blocked androgen-induced VEGF-A, PSA and Tmprss2 expression, suggesting a role for miR-329-3P as a tumor suppressor in prostate cancer.

12.4.5 miR-1827

Some earlier study showed that the deregulated expression of miR-1827 were responsible to different kind of melanoma as example colorectal cancer, lung cancer, chronic myeloid leukemia by the targeting MDM2, C-MYC gene [38–41]. Therefore, we were point out that mir-1827 provide a new area of research in prostate cancer grading as well as for biomarkers evaluation.

Clinical use of molecular diagnostics—Molecular diagnostics has become a novel and more relible technique for various diseases diagnosis and clinical trails. The various aspects of this are as follows (Fig. 12.4).

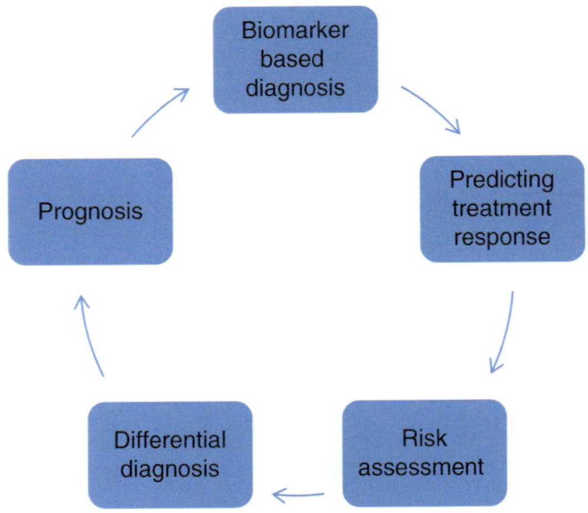

Fig. 12.4 Clinical use of molecular diagnostics

12.4.6 Prostate Cancer Diagnosis and Nanotechnology: Future Perspective

Prostate cancer nanotechnology is an integrative field of research which involves a vast and multiple array of devices like nano-vectors for the anticancer drugs targeted delivery and imaging contrast agents. Nanotechnology has emerged with broad applications for molecular diagnosis, molecular imaging and targeted drug therapy of cancer. It has central role in evolving the goals to recognize the populations of transforming cell early by in vivo imaging or ex vivo analysis. The basic rationale involved in cancer nanotechnology is that nanometer-sized particles, like iron oxide nanocrystals and semiconductor quantum dots, have magnetic, optical or structural properties that are not available from molecules or bulk solids. In the case of ligands which target the tumors such as peptides, monoclonal antibodies or small molecules, these nanoparticles can be used to target tumor antigens (biomarkers) as well as tumor vasculatures with high accuracy, specificity and affinity. Nanoparticles also have large surface areas and functional groups in the size range of 5–100 nm diameter, for conjugating to multiple diagnostic (e.g., optical, radioisotopic, or magnetic) and therapeutic (e.g., anticancer) agents. With very low amount of cancer cell sample preparation, substrate binding to even a small number of antibodies produces a measurable change in the device's conductivity, leading to a 100-fold increase in sensitivity over current diagnostic techniques. Nanoscale cantilevers, flexible, microscopic, beams that resemble a row of diving boards, are made up of semiconductor lithographic techniques. Nanocantilever and Nanowires arrays are the emerging approaches being developed for the early detection of precancerous and malignant lesions from biological fluids [41, 42].

12.5 Conclusion

Prostate cancer (PCa) is the most frequently diagnosed malignant tumor and the leading cause of cancer related deaths in men. As we discussed earlier in this chapter that, although PSA plays an important role in diagnosing PCa but due to low specificity and misdiagnosis it is now being considered as less significant for PCa detection. However, researches are trying to develop new approach to diagnose the PCa by studying molecular diagnostics. Moreover, they targeted on the molecular markers (genes/miRNA) that evolved in the progression of PCa for example—genes like Tumor suppressor genes, Sporadic prostate cancer, Pten and various miRNAs like miR-130b-3P, miR-183-5P, miR-329-3P, miR-1827 etc. In future, these molecular markers may be used in early diagnosis and helpful to check patient motility by prostate cancer. If we will be able to achieve our goals by using these molecular markers, it may be also helpful in the treatment of PCa patient. These molecular markers can be used as a diagnostic, prognostic biomarker and also helpful in therapy outcome. So we can say that use of molecular markers may enhance our potential to study tumor biology.

References

1. Ma S, Tang KH, Chan YP, et al. miR-130b Promotes CD133(+) liver tumor-initiating cell growth and self-renewal via tumor protein 53-induced nuclear protein 1. Cell Stem Cell. 2010;7:694–707. [PubMed: 21112564].
2. Goodman OB, Fink LM, Symanowski JT, Wong B, Grobaski B, Pomerantz D, Ma Y, Ward DC, Vogelzang NJ. Circulating tumor cells in patients with castration-resistant prostate cancer baseline values and correlation with prognostic factors. Cancer Epidemiol Biomarkers Prev. 2009;18:1904–13.
3. Feng DQ, Huang B, Li J, Liu J, Chen XM, Xu YM, Chen X, Zhang HB, Hu LH, Wang XZ. Selective miRNA expression profile in chronic myeloid leukemia K562 cell-derived exosomes. Asian Pac J Cancer Prev. 2013;14:7501–8.
4. Hessels D, Rittenhouse HG, Schalken JA. Molecular diagnosis in prostate cancer. 2009;6:255–61.
5. Bray F, Ren JS, Masuyer E, Ferlay J. Global estimates of cancer prevalence for 27 sites in the adult population in 2008. Int J Cancer. 2013;132:1133–45.
6. Wu K, Hu M, Chen Z, Xiang F, Chen G, Yan W, Peng Q, Chen X. Asiatic acid enhances survival of human AC16 cardiomyocytes under hypoxia by upregulating miR-1290. IUBMB Life. 2017;69(9):660–7.
7. Hessvik NP, Phuyal S, Brech A, Sandvig K, Llorente A. Profiling of microRNAs in exosomes released from PC-3 prostate cancer cells. Biochim Biophys Acta. 2012;1819:1154–63.
8. Zhao N, Yu H, Yu H, Sun M, Zhang Y, Xu M, Gao W. MiRNA-711-SP1-collagen-I pathway is involved in the anti-fibrotic effect of pioglitazone in myocardial infarction. Sci China Life Sci. 2013;56:431–9.
9. Huang X, Yuan T, Liang M, Du M, Xia S, Dittmar R, Wang D, See W, Costello BA, Quevedo F, Tan W. Exosomal miR-1290 and miR-375 as prognostic markers in castration-resistant prostate cancer. Eur Urol. 2015;67:33–41.
10. Shen J, Hruby GW, McKiernan JM, Gurvich I, Lipsky MJ, Benson MC, Santella RM. Dysregulation of circulating microRNAs and prediction of aggressive prostate cancer. Prostate. 2012;72:1469–77.
11. Liao A, Gao Tan LC, Zhou W, Hu H. RASSF1A inhibits gastric cancer cell proliferation by miR-711-mediated downregulation of CDK4 miR-1290 accurately distinguishes patients with low-stage pancreatic cancer from healthy and disease controls. expression. Oncotarget. 2016;7:5842.
12. Jackson RJ, Standart N. How do microRNAs regulate gene expression. Sci STKE. 2007;(367):re1. Kumar A. Epidemiology of prostate cancer in India. Meta Gene. 2014;29:596–605.
13. Karantanos T, Corn PG, Thompson TC. Prostate cancer progression after androgen deprivation therapy: mechanisms of castrate-resistance and novel therapeutic approaches. Oncogene. 2013;32:5501.

14. Li A, Yu J, Kim H, Wolfgang CL, Canto MI, Hruban RH, Goggins M. MicroRNA array analysis finds elevated serum. Clin Cancer Res. 2013;19(13):3600–10.
15. Ueno K, Hirata H, Shahryari V, Deng G, Tanaka Y, Tabatabai ZL, et al. microRNA-183 is an oncogene targeting Dkk-3 and SMAD4 in prostate cancer. Br J Cancer. 2013;108:1659–67.
16. Lin M, Shi C, Lin X, Pan J, Shen S, Xu Z, Chen Q. sMicroRNA-1290 inhibits cells proliferation and migration by targeting FOXA1 in gastric cancer cells. Gene. 2016;582:137–42.
17. Yang H, Li Q, Zhao W, Yuan D, Zhao H, Zhou Y. miR-329 suppresses the growth and motility of neuroblastoma by targeting KDM1A. FEBS Lett. 2014;588:192–7.
18. Abd Elmageed ZY, Yang Y, Thomas R, Ranjan M, Mondal D. Neoplastic reprogramming of patient-derived adipose stem cells by prostate cancer cell-associated exosomes. Stem Cells. 2014;32:983–97.
19. Lu J, Getz G, Miska EA, Alvarez-Saavedra E, Lamb J, Peck D, et al. MicroRNA expression profiles classify human cancers. Nature. 2005;435:834–8.
20. Ambs S, Prueitt RL, Yi M, Hudson RS, Howe TM, Petrocca F, et al. Genomic profiling of microRNA and messenger RNA reveals deregulated microRNA expression in prostate cancer. Cancer Res. 2008;68:6162–70.
21. Miao Y, Zheng W, Li N, Su Z, Zhao L, Zhou H, Jia L. MicroRNA-130b targets PTEN to mediate drug resistance and proliferation of breast cancer cells via the PI3K/Akt signaling pathway. Sci Rep. 2017;7:41942. https://doi.org/10.1038/srep41942.
22. Schaefer A, Jung M, Mollenkopf HJ, Wagner I, Stephan C, Jentzmik F, et al. Diagnostic and prognostic implications of microRNA profiling in prostate carcinoma. Int J Cancer. 2010;126:1166–76.
23. Ralfkiaer U, Hagedorn PH, Bangsgaard N, Løvendorf MB, Ahler CB, Svensson L, Kopp KL, Vennegaard MT, Lauenborg B, Zibert JR, Krejsgaard T. Diagnostic microRNA profiling in cutaneous T-cell lymphoma (CTCL). Blood. 2011;118:5891–900.
24. Ramalho-Carvalho J, Graça I, Gomez A, Oliveira J, Henrique R, Esteller M, et al. Downregulation of miR-130b~301b cluster is mediated by aberrant promoter methylation and impairs cellular senescence in prostate cancer. J Hematol Oncol. 2017;10:43.
25. Stuopelytė K, Daniūnaitė K, Jankevičius F, Jarmalaitė S. Detection of miRNAs in urine of prostate cancer patients. Medicina. 2016;52:116–24.
26. Rizos E, Siafakas N, Katsantoni E, Skourti E, Salpeas V, Rizos I, et al. Let-7, Mir-98 and Mir-181 as biomarkers for cancer and schizophrenia. PLoS One. 2015;10:e0123522.
27. Sabirzhanov B, Stoica BA, Zhao Z, Loane DJ, Wu J, Dorsey SG, Faden AI. miR-711 upregulation induces neuronal cell death after traumatic brain injury. Cell Death Differ. 2016;23:654–68.
28. Sarver AL, Li L, Subramanian S. MicroRNA miR-183 functions as an oncogene by targeting the transcription factor EGR1 and promoting tumor cell migration. Cancer Res. 2010;70:9570–80.
29. Mihelich BL, Khramtsova EA, Arva N, Vaishnav A, Johnson DN, Giangreco AA, et al. MiR-183-96-182 cluster is overexpressed in prostate tissue and regulates zinc homeostasis in prostate cells. J Biol Chem. 2011;286:44503–11.
30. Schröder FH, Hugosson J, Roobol MJ, Tammela TL, Ciatto S, Nelen V, et al. Screening and prostate-cancer mortality in a randomized European study. N Engl J Med. 2009;360:1320–8.
31. Hugosson J, Carlsson S, Aus G, Bergdahl S, Khatami A, Lodding P, et al. Mortality results from the Göteborg randomised population-based prostate-cancer screening trial. Lancet Oncol. 2010;11:725–32.
32. Siegel RL, Miller KD, Jemal A. Cancer statistics, 2016. CA Cancer J Clin. 2016;66:7–30.
33. Ribas J, Ni X, Haffner M, Wentzel EA, Salmasi AH, Chowdhury WH, Kudrolli TA, Yegnasubramanian S, Luo J, Rodriguez R, Mendell JT. miR-21: an androgen receptor–regulated microRNA that promotes hormone-dependent and hormone-independent prostate cancer growth. Cancer Res. 2009;69:7165–9.
34. Trang P, Weidhaas JB, Slack FJ. MicroRNAs as potential cancer therapeutics. Oncogene. 2008;27:S52–7.
35. Li W, Liang J, Zhang Z, Lou H, Zhao L, Xu Y, Ou R. MicroRNA-329-3p targets MAPK1 to suppress cell proliferation, migration and invasion in cervical cancer. Oncol Rep. 2017;37:2743–50.
36. Daniel R, Wu Q, Williams V, Clark G, Guruli G, Zehner Z. A panel of microRNAs as diagnostic biomarkers for the identification of prostate cancer. Int J Mol Sci. 2017;18:1281.
37. Xiong F, Wu C, Chang J, Yu D, Xu B, Yuan P, Zhai K, Xu J, Tan W, Lin D. Genetic variation in an miRNA-1827 binding site in MYCL1 alters susceptibility to small-cell lung cancer. Cancer Res. 2011;71:5175–81.
38. Xu L, Qi X, Duan S, Xie Y, Ren X, Chen G, et al. MicroRNAs: potential biomarkers for disease diagnosis. Biomed Mater Eng. 2014;24:3917–25.
39. Zhang C, Liu J, Tan C, Yue X, Zhao Y, Peng J, Wang X, Laddha SV, Chan CS, Zheng S, Hu W. microRNA-1827 represses MDM2 to positively regulate tumor suppressor p53 and suppress tumorigenesis. Oncotarget. 2016;7:8783.
40. Ye L, Jiang T, Shao H, Zhong L, Wang Z, Liu Y, Tang H, Qin B, Zhang X, Fan J. miR-1290 is a biomarker in DNA-mismatch-repair-deficient colon cancer and promotes resistance to 5-fluorouracil by directly targeting hMSH2. Mol Ther Nucleic Acids. 2017;7:453–64.
41. Liu R, Zhou Z, Huang J, Chen C. PMEPA1 promotes androgen receptor-negative prostate cell proliferation through suppressing the Smad3/4-c-Myc-p21 Cip1 signaling pathway. J Pathol. 2004;223:683–94.
42. Hu JY, Yi W, Zhang MY, Xu R, Zeng LS, Long XR, Zhou XM, Zheng XF, Kang Y, Wang HY. MicroRNA-711 is a prognostic factor for poor overall survival and has an oncogenic role in breast cancer. Oncol Lett. 2016;11:2155–63.

Molecular Diagnostics in Renal Cancer

13

Barkha Singhal Sanganeria, Radhieka Misra, and Kamla Kant Shukla

13.1 Introduction to Renal Cancer

Kidney (renal) cancer is an aggressive and incurable disease with a worldwide prevalence that ranks it to be twelfth most common type of cancer. According to world cancer, around 338,000 new kidney cancer incidences are diagnosed annually [1, 2] (Table 13.1). Kidney cancer is not a single disease instead is made up of a number of different types of cancer that occur in the kidney. Each is caused by mutation of a different gene, follows a different clinical course, has a different histology, and responds differently to therapy [3]. Most common type of kidney cancer in adults is renal cell carcinoma (RCC) (Fig. 13.1) and in children is Wilms (also called nephroblastoma) tumor, which majorly are unilateral in origin and only in 5% of the cases they may be bilateral [4]. RCC originates in the lining of renal tubules, located in the kidney and contributes to about 90% of all kidney cancers. The remaining 10% of kidney cancers start in the renal pelvis located in the center of the kidney, which is where urine collects. Globally RCC is the seventh and ninth most common malignancy in men and women, respectively and contributes to 6% of all cancers with an incidence peak between 60–70 years of age [4]. Kidney cancer has a high incidence and mortality rate but has attracted little public health attention because of its low ranking among other cancers as a cause of death. Since RCCs are highly recurrent and metastatic in tendency, recent treatments have just been able to increase the survival-rate by 5 years post-diagnosis or treatment but not cure the disease [5].

Kidney tumors can be (a) benign (noncancerous, can grow but will not spread), (b) indolent (cancerous but rarely spreads to other parts) or (c) malignant (cancerous and can spread to other parts of the body). Malignant tumor can grow uncontrollably and these tumor cells may metastasize to distant organs. Most of the kidney cancers are detected before they metastasize to near by venous flow or the lymph nodes and thus spread to different tissues and organs of the body, e.g. lungs; however, in many cases RCC can lead to bone or lung cancer.

Risk Factor RCC is a complicated and aggressive disease caused by both sporadic and familial factors. The common risk factors identified in RCC include several environmental,

B. S. Sanganeria (✉)
Centre for Transplant and Renal Research, Westmead Institute for Medical Research, Westmead, NSW, Australia

R. Misra
Era's Lucknow Medical College and Hospital, Lucknow, India

K. K. Shukla
Department of Biochemistry, All India Institute of Medical Sciences, Jodhpur, Rajasthan, India
e-mail: shuklakk@aiimsjodhpur.edu.in

K. K. Shukla et al. (eds.), *Molecular Diagnostics in Cancer Patients*,
https://doi.org/10.1007/978-981-13-5877-7_13

Table 13.1 GLOBOCON 2012: worlds estimated cancer incidence, mortality and 5-year prevalence of cancer in both sexes [1, 2]

	Incidence			Mortality			5-year prevalence		
Cancer	Number	(%)	ASR (W)	Number	(%)	ASR (W)	Number	(%)	Prop.
Lip, oral cavity	300,373	2.1	4.0	145,353	1.8	1.9	702,149	2.2	13.5
Nasopharynx	86,691	0.6	1.2	50,831	0.6	0.7	228,698	0.7	4.4
Other pharynx	142,387	1.0	1.9	96,105	1.2	1.3	309,991	1.0	6.0
Oesophagus	455,784	3.2	5.9	400,169	4.9	5.0	464,063	1.4	8.9
Stomach	951,594	6.8	12.1	723,073	8.8	8.9	1,538,127	4.7	29.6
Colorectum	1,360,602	9.7	17.2	693,933	8.5	8.4	3,543,582	10.9	68.2
Liver	782,451	5.6	10.1	745,533	9.1	9.5	633,170	2.0	12.2
Gallbladder	178,101	1.3	2.2	142,823	1.7	1.7	205,646	0.6	4.0
Pancreas	337,872	2.4	4.2	330,391	4.0	4.1	211,544	0.7	4.1
Larynx	156,877	1.1	2.1	83,376	1.0	1.1	441,675	1.4	8.5
Lung	1,824,701	13.0	23.1	1,589,925	19.4	19.7	1,893,078	5.8	36.5
Melanoma of skin	232,130	1.7	3.0	55,488	0.7	0.7	869,754	2.7	16.8
Kaposi sarcoma	44,247	0.3	0.6	26,974	0.3	0.3	80,395	0.2	1.5
Breast	1,671,149	11.9	43.1	521,907	6.4	12.9	6,232,108	19.2	239.9
Cervix uteri	527,624	3.8	14.0	265,672	3.2	6.8	1,547,161	4.8	59.6
Corpus uteri	319,605	2.3	8.3	76,160	0.9	1.8	1,216,504	3.7	46.8
Ovary	238,719	1.7	6.1	151,917	1.9	3.8	586,624	1.8	22.6
Prostate	1,094,916	7.8	30.7	307,481	3.7	7.8	3,857,500	11.9	148.6
Testis	55,266	0.4	1.5	10,351	0.1	0.3	214,666	0.7	8.3
Kidney	337,860	2.4	4.4	143,406	1.7	1.8	906,746	2.8	17.5
Bladder	429,793	3.1	5.3	165,084	2.0	1.9	1,319,749	4.1	25.4
Brain, nervous system	256,213	1.8	3.4	189,382	2.3	2.5	342,914	1.1	6.6
Thyroid	298,102	2.1	4.0	39,771	0.5	0.5	1,206,075	3.7	23.2
Hodgkin lymphoma	65,950	0.5	0.9	25,469	0.3	0.3	188,538	0.6	3.6
Non-Hodgkin lymphoma	385,741	2.7	5.1	199,670	2.4	2.5	832,843	2.6	16.0
Multiple myeloma	114,251	0.8	1.5	80,019	1.0	1.0	229,468	0.7	4.4
Leukaemia	351,965	2.5	4.7	265,471	3.2	3.4	500,934	1.5	9.6
All cancers excl. non-melanoma skin cancer	14,067,894	100.0	182.0	8,201,575	100.0	102.4	32,455,179	100.0	625.0

Incidence and mortality data for all ages. 5-year prevalence for adult population only. ASR (W) and proportions per 100,000.

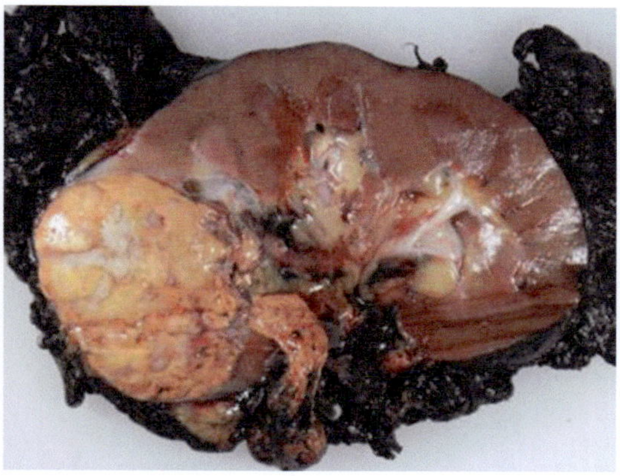

Fig. 13.1 Represents clear cell renal cell carcinoma (ccRCC). Golden color (lower left) is due to intracellular lipid accumulation while white areas are foci of Sarcomatoid differentiation [68]

clinical and genetic factors [6, 7]. Major risk factors include cigarette smoking, alcohol use, over use of pain relievers containing phenacetin, hypertension and obesity (increased body weight being directly proportional to RCC incidence) [8–11]. Some of the occupational and environmental factors are (extended exposure to cadmium, asbestos, petroleum products, ionizing radiations, and acetaminophen abuse). Clinically the patients with acquired cystic kidney disease (ACKD) and hepatitis C appear to have an increased risk of developing RCC masses [4]. Some autosomal dominant, inherited RCC syndromes caused by mutations (such as missense, nonsense, frameshifts, insertion, deletion etc.) in the germline are: Von Hippel-Lindau disease (VHL), hereditary leiomyomatosis RCC (HLRCC), Birt-Hogg-Dubé (BHD) syndrome, hereditary papillary RCC (HPRC) syndrome [4].

Recent advent in molecular techniques (gene sequencing, FISH, qRT-PCR and microarrays) and the advancement in translational research have directed more studies in search for early diagnosis and prognosis in kidney cancer, and develop more targeted therapies and personalized patient care. In this chapter, we have focused on recent studies undertaken in quest for potential kidney cancer biomarkers using non-invasive to minimal invasive methods. We have also discussed the challenges associated with these molecular markers (MMs) and the kidney cancer disease.

13.2 Classification of Renal Cancer

Due to kidney heterogeneity, renal carcinomas are classified on the basis of tissue histology and type of kidney cells getting affected. Pathologists have identified as many as 20 different types of kidney cancer cells. Kidney cancers can be of many types (Table 13.2).

13.2.1 Renal Cell Carcinoma (RCC)

In 85–90% cases the patient suffers from RCC, in which the cancer develops in the proximal renal tubules. According to the 2004 WHO classification, several histological RCC subtypes are recognized. The most frequent histological subtypes include: (a) clear cell renal cell carcinomas (ccRCC), (b) papillary renal cell carcinomas (pRCC), and (c) chromophobe renal cell carcinomas (crRCC). These three subtypes together represent more than 90% of all RCCs, while there are still other types of rare RCCs, such as medullary, Xp11 translocation, renal mucinous and spindle cell carcinoma etc., that can be identified in a very small population (Fig. 13.2) [12, 13].

13.2.1.1 Clear Cell Renal Cell Carcinomas (ccRCC)

About 70% of kidney cancers are ccRCCs and originates in the proximal tissue of the kidney. The ccRCC is a renal cortical tumor typically characterized by malignant epithelial cells with clear cytoplasm and a compact-alveolar (nested) or acinar growth pattern interspersed with intricate, arborizing vasculature. A variable proportion of cells with granular eosinophilic cytoplasm may be present. The ccRCCs can range from slow to fast growing tumors.

13.2.1.2 Papillary Kidney Cancer (pRCC)

The pRCC represents 15–20% of RCC. Based on histology pRCC is divided into 2 main subtypes, called type 1 and type 2 (Fig. 13.2). Currently little is known about the genetic basis of non-hereditary (sporadic) pRCC and patients receive

Table 13.2 Main histological subtypes of RCC—epidemiology, histology and imaging characteristics [12]

Subtype	Incidence	Origin, histology	Patients' age	Signal/density pattern	Biological behaviour	Post-contrast hemodynamic pattern	Associations and predisposition
Clear cell	75%	Proximal nepron, tubular epithelium	>50 years	Heterogeneous density/signal	Aggressive, according to the stage, Furhman grade and sarcomatoid transformation	Hypervascular	Von Hippel-Lindau (25–45%), tuberous sclerosis (2%)
Papillary	10%	Distal nephron, tubular epithelium	>50 years	Low T2 signal, hypodense	Aggressive, according to the stage, Furhman grade and sarcomatoid transformation	Hypovascular	Hereditary papillary RCC
Chromophobe	5%	Distal nephron, intercalated cells of the distal tubules	>50 years	Hypodense, intermediate signal intensity	Low mortality (10%)	Hypovascular	Birt-Hogg-Dubé syndrome (in association with oncocytomas)
Cystic-solid	1–4%	Similar to renal clear cell carcinoma, without solid nodules	Fourth and fifth decades of life	High T2 signal intensity, fluid density	Indolent, without metastases	Septal and solid portions enhancement	Predominance in men
Collecting ducts (Bellini)	1%	Collecting tubules	>50 years	Low T2 signal, heterogeneous	Very aggressive, mortality: 70% in 2 years	Hypovascular	Subtle predominance in men
Medullary	1%	Distal nephron	Second and third decades of life	Heterogeneous, infiltrating	Extremelly aggressive	Hypovascular	Associated with sickle cell disease
Xp11 translocation	Rare	Distal/proximal nephron, may be similar to papillary or clear cell carcinoma	Children (early childhood)	Hypodense, intermediate T2 signal intensity	Indolent	Hypovascular	TFE3 gene involved in the tumor genesis
Mucinous tubular and spindle cell	Rare	Distal nephron, tubular cells	Fourth and fifth decades of life	Subtle T2 hypersignal, central scar may be observed	Slow-growing, rare metastases	Hypovascular	Predominance in women
Associated with neuroblastoma	Rare	Proximal tubular epithelium	Adolescence (mean 13 years)	Hypodense, intermediate T2 signal intensity	Indolent	Hypovascular	Previous history of neuroblastoma
Non classified	4–6%	Variable	Variable	Variable	High mortality	Variable	–

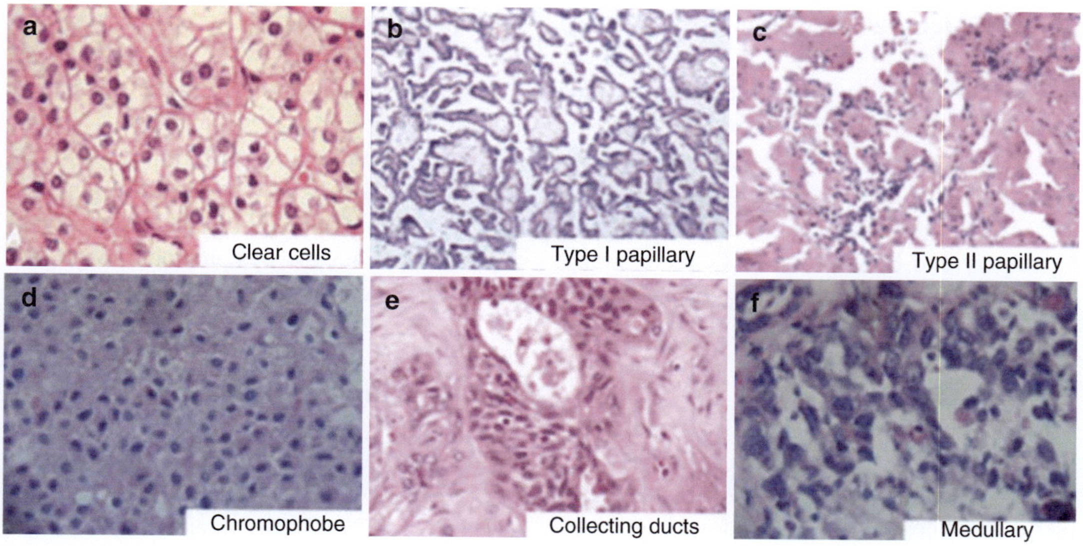

Fig. 13.2 Histology of the most common RCC subtypes. (**a**) Clear cell RCC—cells with lipid-rich ample cytoplasm, hence the name of the neoplasm. (**b**) Type 1 Papillary RCC—small basophilic cells with scarce cytoplasm, organized in a spindle-shaped pattern, in a single layer of cells surrounding the basal membrane. (**c**) Type 2 Papillary RCC—cells organized in a spindle-shaped pattern with papillae covered by cells with abundant eosinophilic granular cytoplasm with prominent nucleoli. (**d**) Chromophobe RCC—large pale cells with reticulated cytoplasm and perinuclear halos. (**e**) Collecting duct RCC—histology shows an irregular, infiltrating cells arrangement in the collecting duct walls, showing remarkable desmoplasia. (**f**) Medullary RCC—it originates in the distal nephron, also with an irregular cell arrangement, remarkable pleomorphism and hyperchromatic nuclei [12]

treatment simply based on disease stage. The course of treatment is in the same way as ccRCC. However, many treatments are recommend through clinical trials since treatment with targeted therapy is often not as successful for people with papillary kidney cancer as it is for people with ccRCC.

13.2.1.3 Chromophobe (chRCC)

Chromophobe kidney cancer is a malignant tumor that accounts for 5% of all RCCs, are mostly sporadic and detected incidental. *TP53* and *PTEN* are tumor suppressor genes that normally regulate cell growth and apoptosis (programmed cell death) and are frequently mutated in chRCC renal cell carcinoma. This is another rare cancer that may form indolent tumors and run in families as part of a rare genetic disorder called Birt-Hogg-Dubé (BHD) syndrome. Currently very little is known about the genetic basis of sporadic chRCC. Gene expression data suggest that chRCC originates from distal regions of the kidney while clear cell renal cell carcinoma arises in the proximal tissue of the kidney.

13.2.2 Urothelial Carcinoma (UCC)

UCC is also called transitional cell carcinoma and accounts for remaining 10–15% cases where the cancer starts in renal pelvis, area of the kidney where urine collects before moving to the bladder. Renal pelvis opens into ureter (tube that carries urine from the kidney to the bladder) and the urine is excreted out of the body through a tube called the urethra. Cancers of the renal pelvis and ureter are similar to bladder cancers rather than kidney cancers and this type of cancer starts in the cells that line the inside of the renal pelvis, ureter and bladder.

13.2.3 Sarcomatoid

Sarcoma of the kidney is rare but aggressive kind of tumor. This develops in the soft part of the tissue such as the thin layer of the connective tissue surrounding the kidney, called the capsule or the surrounding fat. Sarcomas are mostly removed by surgery and have the tendency of returning. Therefore, the following surgery or chemotherapy may be recommended.

13.2.4 Wilms Tumor

These tumors are mostly seen in children and rarely in adults. Wilms tumor is treated differently from kidney cancer in adults. This type of tumor is more likely to be successfully treated with radiation therapy and chemotherapy than the other types of kidney cancer when combined with surgery, which has resulted in a different approach to the treatment.

13.2.5 Lymphoma

Lymphoma may lead to bilateral kidney enlargement, associated with infected and enlarged lymph nodes (lymphadenopathy) in other parts of the body, including the neck, chest, and abdominal cavity. In rare cases, kidney lymphoma can appear as a lone tumor mass in the kidney and may include enlarged regional lymph nodes. If lymphoma is suspected, a biopsy is done and chemotherapy is recommended instead of surgery.

13.2.6 Oncocytoma

This is a slow-growing benign growth of kidney that rarely, if ever, spreads. Oncocytoma is the tumor of the oncocyte cells; epithelial cells characterized by excessive amount of mitochondria. Oncocytoma are usually asymptomatic and are often discovered incidentally.

13.2.7 Angiomyolipoma

Angiomyolipoma is a benign tumor that is usually less likely to grow and spread. It is generally best treated with surgery or, if it is small, active surveillance. Epithelioid is an aggressive form of angiomyolipoma that in some instance can spread to nearby lymph nodes or organs such as the liver.

13.3 Renal Cancer Stages

Histological staging system most often used for kidney cancer is the American Joint Committee on Cancer (AJCC) **TNM** system. The TNM system is based on three key pieces of information where T stands for **tumor** size, N represents if the cancer has spread to near by lymph **nodes** and M represents if the cancer has **metastasized** to other organs, such as lungs, bones and brain (See Table 13.1). The other cancer staging system is the numbered system divided from stage zero to stage four (Tables 13.3 and 13.4) [14].

The stage of cancer helps decide the course of treatment; if a local treatment such as surgery or radiotherapy is appropriate to treat cancer confined to one place or if they need treatment that circulates throughout the body; in cases where cancer has spread to the other parts of the body, such as chemotherapy, hormone therapy, immunotherapy and targeted cancer drugs. Conventional, staging is a process used to determine the extent of the malignancy and staging may sometimes include the grading of the cancer. This describes how similar a cancer cell is to a normal cell. If uncertain that the cancer has metastasized, cancer cells in the lymph nodes near the cancer are tested. Seeing cancer cells in these nodes is a sign that the cancer has begun to spread. This is often called as having "positive lymph nodes". It demonstrates that the cancer cells have dispersed and got trapped in the lymph nodes, but it isn't always possible to tell if they have gone anywhere else.

Table 13.3 TNM classification for renal cell carcinoma [14]

Primary tumors (T)	
TX	Primary tumor cannot be assessed
T0	No evidence of primary tumor
T1	Tumor ≤7 cm in greatest dimension, limited to the kidney
T1a	Tumor ≤4 cm in greatest dimension, limited to the kidney
T1b	Tumor >4 cm but ≤7 cm in greatest dimension, limited to the kidney
T2	Tumor >7 cm in greatest dimension, limited to the kidney
T2a	Tumor >7 cm but ≤10 cm in greatest dimension, limited to the kidney
T2b	Tumor >10 cm, limited to the kidney
T3	Tumor extends into major veins or perinephric tissues but not into the ipsilateral adrenal gland and not beyond the Gerota fascia
T3a	Tumor grossly extends into the renal vein or its segmental (muscle-containing) branches, or tumor invades perirenal and/or renal sinus fat but not beyond the Gerota fascia
T3b	Tumor grossly extends into the vena cava below the diaphragm
T3c	Tumor grossly extends into the vena cava above the diaphragm or invades the wall of the vena cava
T4	Tumor invades beyond the Gerota fascia (including contiguous extension into the ipsilateral adrenal gland)
Regional lymph node (N)	
NX	Regional lymph nodes cannot be assessed
N0	No regional lymph node metastasis
N1	Metastasis in regional lymph node(s)
Distant metastasis (M)	
M0	No distant metastasis
M1	Distant metastasis

Table 13.4 Anatomic stage/prognostic groups [14]

Stage	T	N	M
I	T1	N0	M0
II	T2	N0	M0
III	T1–2	N1	M0
T3	N0 or N1	M0	
IV	T4	Any N	M0
Any T	Any N	M1	

13.4 Genetic Aberrations in Renal Cancer

In 95% cases RCC is sporadic with an average onset age of 61 years; characterized by alterations, such as mutations, hypermethylation, and loss of heterozygocity (LOH) of von-Hippel-Linau (*VHL*) tumor suppressor gene located on chromosome 3p but rarely by mutation in hereditary kidney cancer genes, such as c-MET and FH [13]. The remaining 5% of RCC cases are familial and associated with inherited mutations majorly in VHL causing VHL syndrome or is linked to HLRCC, BDH and HPCR syndrome. Patients with familial RCC show kidney cyst and multiple bilateral ccRCC at an average age of 37 years [13]. In ccRCC, loss of *VHL* function leads to the accumulation of hypoxia-inducible factor alpha subunits (HIF-1α–3α). HIF-α is a transcription factor, which otherwise is hydroxylated by prolyl-hydroxylase and is recognized for proteasomal degradation by VHL protein (pVHL) that is a part of an E3-ubiquitin ligase complex. HIF-α subunit translocates to the nucleus and heterodimerize with their binding partner aryl hydrocarbon receptor nuclear translocator (ARNT) also called HIF-1β to transcriptionally regulate target genes containing hypoxia response elements. Association of HIF-α/β leads to downstream upregulation of hypoxia-regulated genes that has a well-established relevance to the pathogenesis of acute and chronic kidney diseases (Fig. 13.3). Among others these include many of the proangiogenic genes, such as vascular endothelial growth factor (VEGF), erythropoietin, and carbonic anhydrase 9 (CA9). Upregulation of VEGF and other angiogenic genes allow tumor cells to form new blood vessels and extend their size and metastasize. Identification of VHL as the resulting phenotype of angiogenesis, lead to the successful clinical development of the first target of ccRCC, particularly using VEGF and mammalian target of rapamycin (mTOR) pathway inhibitors [15].

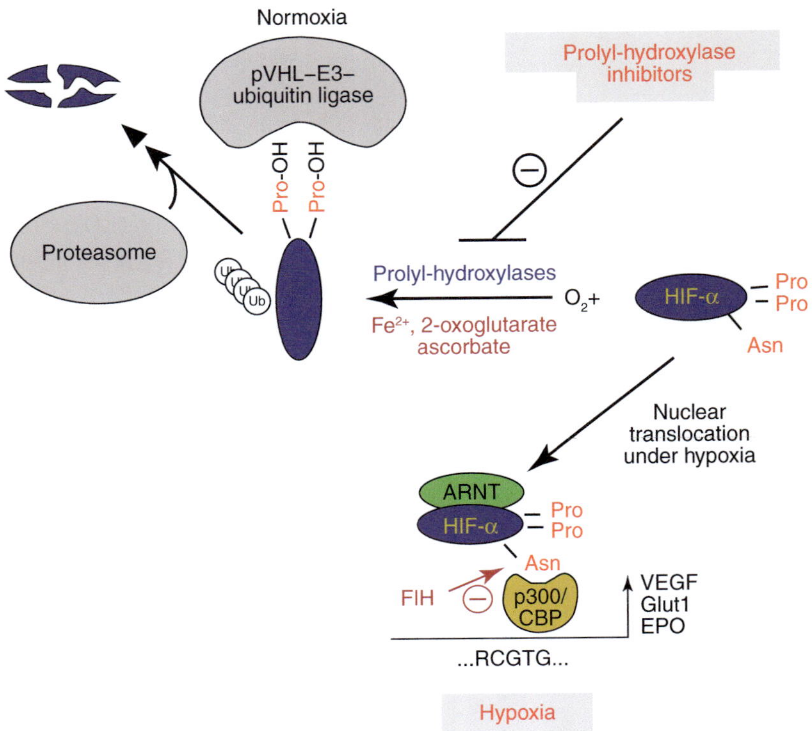

Fig. 13.3 The pVHL–E3-ubiquitin ligase targets hydroxylated HIF-*α* for proteasomal degradation. Under normoxia, hydroxylation of HIF-*α* subunits by prolyl-hydroxylases is required for binding to the pVHL–E3-ubiquitin ligase complex. After polyubiquitination, HIF-*α* is degraded by the proteasome. During hypoxia or when prolyl-hydroxylases are inhibited pharmacologically, or in the absence of functional pVHL irrespective of oxygen tension, HIF*α* subunits are not degraded and translocate to the nucleus where they bind to the HIF-*β* subunit ARNT. HIF-*α*/ARNT heterodimers then bind to HIF-DNA consensus-binding sites resulting in increased transcription of HIF-target genes, for example, *EPO, VEGF*, and *glucose transporter-1*. Factor-inhibiting-HIF (FIH) is an asparagine hydroxylase that modulates cofactor recruitment to the HIF transcriptional complex via asparagine hydroxylation of the HIF-*α* carboxy-terminal transactivation domain. Also shown is the core sequence (RCGTG) of a hypoxia-responsive element (HRE). *Pro* proline, *Asn* asparagine [15]

Type 1 hereditary papillary RCC (HPRC) is a genetic condition associated with a trisomy on chromosome 3q, 7, 12, 16, 17 and 20, along with the loss of chromosome Y in men. Even in the absence of prominent papillae, the chromosomal alterations on these chromosomes should confirm pRCC. Similarly in cases with prominent manifestation of papillae but no genetic modifications on these genes must not be considered as pRCC [16–18]. Missense point mutation in the tyrosine kinase (TK) domain of *MET* (also called hepatocyte growth factor *HGFR*) proto-oncogenes, which is a cell surface receptor for the ligand hepatocyte growth factor (HGF), and both of which are located on human chromosome 7 has been associated with sporadic and germline activating missense point mutations causing HPRC. HGF/c-Met signaling is involved in cell survival, motility and proliferation signaling that are altered in pRCC (Fig. 13.4) [13, 16, 17, 19].

Individuals with hereditary leiomyomatosis RCC (HLRCC) syndrome are at an increased risk of developing aggressive type 2 inherited pRCC. HLRCC is an autosomal dominant condition caused by germline mutation in *fumarate hydratase* (*FH*), an enzyme involved in tricarboxylic acid (TCA/Krebs) cycle. People with HLRCC syndrome are also at increased risk of developing cutaneous lesions and multiple uterine leiomyomas (fibroids) [18, 20].

Incidence rate of sporadic chRCC is much lower than any other kind of RCC. Genetic chRCC

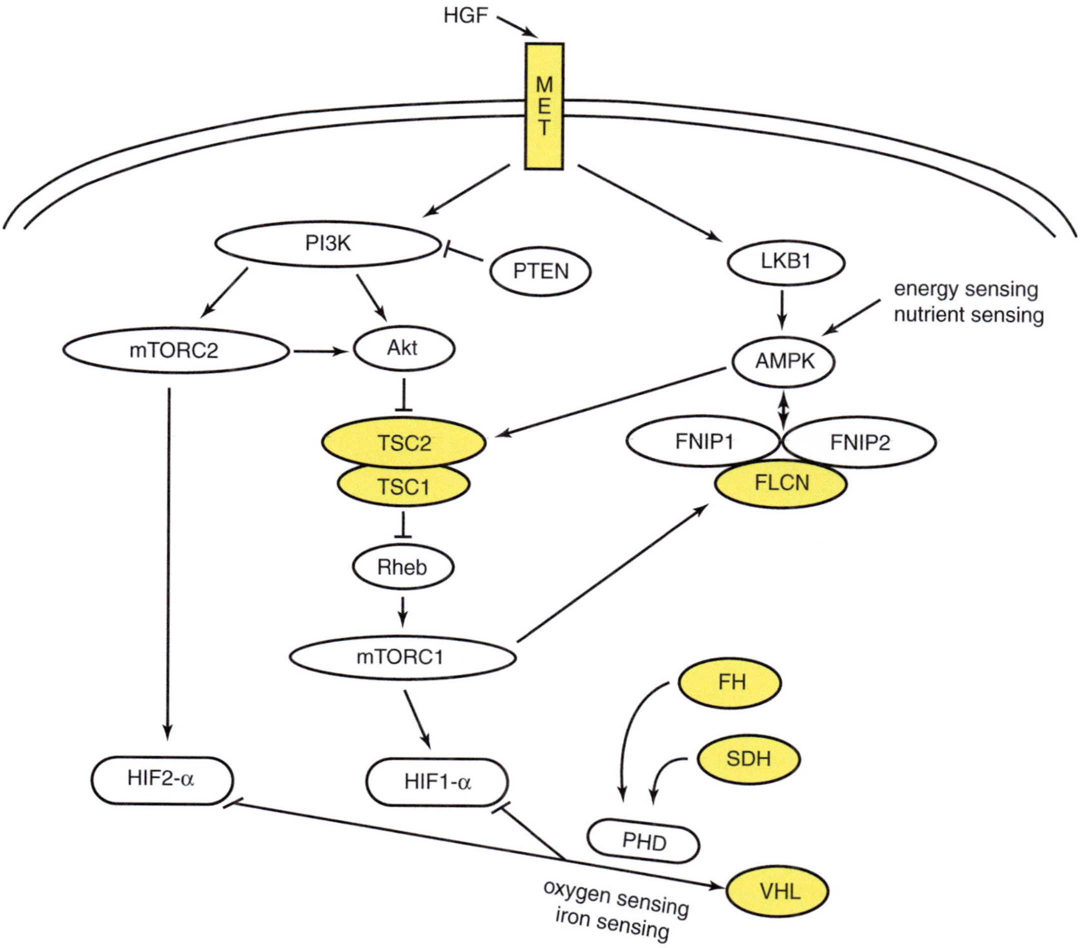

Fig. 13.4 The genetic basis of kidney cancer: a metabolic disease [18]

is caused by the mutation of *TP53* (codes for protein p53) and *PTEN* (**P**hosphatase and **Ten**sin homolog deleted on chromosome Ten), tumor suppressor genes normally responsible for DNA synthesis/repair, cell growth and apoptosis (programmed cell death). Birt-Hogg-Dubé (BHD) syndrome, an autosomal dominant condition caused by mutations in *Folliculin* (*FLCN*, a tumor suppressor gene) and characterized by benign skin tumors and pneumothorax, confers an increased risk of familial chRCC [21, 22].

Some epigenetics factors are also involved in causing RCC. The best-studied epigenetic alteration in RCC is hypermethylation of the DNA. These alterations can also accumulate other histone and nonhistone related alterations in the chromatin (such as acetylation/deacetylation, phosphorylation, ubiquitination, and methylation) [23]. Hypermethylation of promoter or enhancer CpG regions can result in the inactivation of important tumor suppressor genes (such as VHL and p53) whereas hypomethylation of genomic DNA has been associated with chromosomal instability and tumorigenesis [15, 24].

13.5 Molecular Biomarkers for Renal Cancer

In certain cases cancer can be detected earlier then the others but most of the kidney cancer findings are very incidental since there are no early symptoms specific to RCC. Based on life style, some routine tests may be suggested to find overall health of an individual such as urinalysis and complete blood count but these are not the screening tests for kidney cancer detection. Conventional, TNM stage and the Fuhrman nuclear grade renal cancer staging methods are primarily based on tissue histology. Even though immunohistochemistry (IHC) in combination with imaging and blood chemistry tests have been highly promising, it is semi-quantitative and highly dependent on a range of variables, such as, type and time of fixation, choice of antibody, inconsistency in specimen handling and technical procedures, and variability in the interpretation of the data. A particular challenge in treating RCC is the heterogeneity of disease, since a renal mass may range from benign to indolent, to metastatic stage. Another important challenges of cancer research are predicting the invasiveness and metastatic potential of cancer at an early stage. A marker or subset of markers that would correlate with such behavior would be of significant value for RCC prognosis [25]. The diagnostic and prognostic potential of various clinical, pathological, radiographic, serological, cytogenetic, epigenetic and molecular markers has been studied in RCC [26].

With the advancement and integration in transcriptomics, proteomics and metabolomics, researchers have quantified a wide range of chemical fingerprints left behind by various diseases and compared them to the controls. These quantifiable changes which specifically relate to a disease are called biomarkers and has the potential to guide individualized care of RCC patients and assist in future directions for the development of novel RCC biomarkers and treatments. The idea of reflecting health in biofluid existed from ancient times but has gained interest in recent years. More researchers are trying to map the altered changes associated with specific diseases and their stage using non-invasive methods. Biomarkers in RCC may be based on: (1) the source of the marker (tissue, serum or urine based), (2) the clinicopathological significance/biochemical structure (histological type of RCC, progression, survival, response to therapy, hypoxia inducible pathway, proliferation, cell cycle regulation, cell adhesion, immunogens, apoptosis, enzymes, and CD based, proteinaceous, glycoprotein and DNA based markers) and (3) diagnosis vs. prognosis. [25, 26] Unfortunately, there is no clinically proven biomarker for RCC diagnosis (i.e., detection of a disease state), prediction and prognosis (i.e., prediction of clinical response to a therapy/follow-up), since most of these biomarkers have low specificity to RCC and seem to change in other malignancies as well. Although, most of the statistical data is based on small sample size and relatively short follow-up, some molecules showed promising results to be used as a biomarker in future. Some of the possible biomarkers detected non-invasively in urine and serum are described below (Tables 13.5 and 13.6).

Table 13.5 Potential urinary biomarkers in RCC [4]

Marker	Author (year)	RCC versus CG
NMP-22	Kaya et al. (2005)	↑
	Ozer et al. (2002)	↑
	Huang et al. (2000)	↑
NGAL	Di Carlo (2013)	↑
	Morrissey et al. (2011)	↑
KIM-1	Morrissey et al. (2011)	↑
MMPs	di Carlo (2012)	↑
AQP-1	Morrissey and Kharasch (2013)	↑
AQP-1	Morrissey et al. (2014)	↑
PLIN2	Morrissey and Kharasch (2013)	↑
PLIN2	Morrissey et al. (2014)	↑

RCC renal cell carcinoma, *CG* control group, *NMP-22* nuclear matrix protein-22, *KIM-1* kidney injury molecule-1, *MMP* matrix metalloproteinases, *AQP-1* aquaporin-1, *PLIN2* Perilipin 2

Table 13.6 Potential serum biomarkers in RCC [4]

Marker	Author (year)	RCC (number)	HC (number)	RCC versus HC	Stage	Grade
TRAF-1	Rajandram et al. (2014)	15	15	↑		
Hsp27	White et al. (2014)	54	36	↑		
SAA	Mittal et al. (2012)	422			↑	
	Fischer et al. (2012)	115	24	↑		
hsCRP	de Martino et al. (2013)	41			↑	↑
	Steffens et al. (2012)	1.161			↑	
GGT	Hofbauer et al. (2014)	921			↑	↑
TRAIL	Toiyama et al. (2013)	84	52	↓		
M-65	Yildiz et al. (2013)	39	39	↑		
Ab anti-PHD3	Tanaka et al. (2011)	22	26	↑		
CA IX	Takacova et al. (2013)	74			↑	
TuM2-PK	Nisman et al. (2010)	116	20	↑	↑	↑
TK1	Nisman et al. (2010)	116	20	↑	↑	
20S proteasome	de Martino et al. (2012)	113	15	↑		
OPN	Papworth et al. (2013)	269			↑	

RCC renal cell carcinoma, *HC* healthy control, *No* number, *TRAF-1* tumor necrosis factor receptor-associated Factor-1, *Hsp27* heat shock protein 1, *GGT* Gamma-glutamyl transferase, *M65* intact form of CK18, *TRAIL* tumor necrosis RCC: renal cell carcinoma, *HC* healthy control, *No* number, *TRAF-1* tumor necrosis factor receptor-associated Factor-1, *Hsp27* heat shock protein 1, *GGT* Gamma-glutamyl transferase, *M65* intact form of CK18, *TRAIL* tumor necrosis factor-related apoptosis inducing ligand, *CA IX* carbonic anhydrase IX, *hsCRP* high sensitivity C-reactive protein, *SAA* serum amyloid A, *OPN*: osteopontin, *anti-PHD3 Ab* anti-hypoxia-inducible factor prolyl hydroxylase-3 antibody, *TuM2-PK* pyruvate kinase type M2, *TK1* thymidine kinase 1

13.6 Molecular Markers in Urine

Detection of tumor-specific molecular biomarkers in the excretory products of the kidney is highly desirable since urine contains metabolic signatures of many biochemical pathways and its collection is noninvasive. However, there is limitation such as many fold dilution of the protein compared to serum samples. Additionally, presence of proteases, differences in protein concentrations due to hydration, and the potential contamination of urine with seminal and vaginal fluids (Table 13.5).

Nuclear Matrix Protein (NMP-22) is an internal membrane protein that forms a part of the nuclear framework and is known to be involved in DNA replication, transcription and gene expression. Several studies showed a significant increase in NMP-22 protein in urine samples of RCC patients compared to patients with kidney stones and simple renal cysts used as control. Also other studies reported increased NMP-22 levels in preoperative urine samples of RCC patients compared to subjects with benign renal conditions. NMP-22 is the only Federal Drug Administration (FDA) approved screening marker since urinary NMP-22 is know to be specific for transitional cell carcinoma. Screening kits are available from various manufacturers, such as Biocompare and Alere to measure serum, plasma and urinary NMP-22 protein is based on the principle to quantify proteins using ELISA [25].

Neutrophil gelatinase-associated lipocalin (NGAL), also called lipocalin 2 is a small extracellular protein of 25 kDa, expressed in the epithelial cells of the kidney and considered to be a transporter of hydrophobic ligands and kidney development. NGAL binds covalently to matrix metalloproteinase-9 (MMP-9), a zinc-containing endopeptidase with a major role in proteolytic degradation of all types of extracellular matrix

(ECM) components, and are directly and indirectly involved in tumor growth and invasiveness. MMP-9/NGAL complex protects circulating MMP-9 from proteolytic degradation and thus promote tumorigenicity. NGAL and MMP-9/NGAL complex is a tubular injury marker and showed increased expression in serum ELISA of cRCC and pRCC patients but exhibit lower expression levels in oncocytoma and urothelial carcinoma [4, 27]. In spite, showing increased levels in ccRCC there was no correlation with disease type, size, grade and stage in either study [4, 25–27].

Kidney injury molecule (KIM-1) is a nonspecific urinary marker for tubular cell injury and subsequently shows an increased expression in many kidney injuries due to the damage caused to proximal tubular epithelial cells. Urinary KIM-1 protein and RNA can be detected using ELISA, immunostaining, western blot and qRT-PCR, but has limited its specificity as a diagnostic marker [4, 28, 29].

Aquaporin-1 (AQP-1) is a water channel protein localized in the apical membrane of the proximal tubules and has the potential to increase the migration and metastatic potential of tumor cells. Adipocyte differentiation-related protein perilipin 2 (PLIN 2), also called adipophilin (ADFP) adds up to the prominent pathologic features of ccRCC and macrophages and accounts for accumulated glycogen granules. While most of the previous urinary markers did not show huge specificity to kidney cancer diagnosis, Western Blot urine concentration of AQP-1 and ADFP, were significantly higher in ccRCC and pRCC patients compared to control patients undergoing nonnephrectomy surgery, patients with oncocytoma and a group of healthy volunteers and reduced significantly in postoperative cancer patients but were unchanged in control group after non nephrectomy surgery [4, 30].

13.7 Molecular Markers in Serum

Tumor necrosis factor receptor-associated factor-1 (TRAF-1) is an adaptor protein involved in the regulation of cell survival, proliferation, differentiation, and stress responses. Two independent studies using tissue microarrays and IHC in RCC patients showed highly expressed TRAF-1 protein in the proximal tubular epithelium of normal kidney that significantly reduced in ccRCC tissue. On contrary, the same study also reported an increased expression of serum TRAF-1 in RCC compared to normal patients. Increased serum TRAF-1 in RCC has a potential to be a useful non-invasive indicator of RCC development [31, 32].

13.8 Inflammatory Proteins

Under disease state, oxidative stress called hypoxia represents one of the main environmental stress conditions and promotes tumor initiation and progression by upregulating the expression of stress proteins, such as (heat shock protein 27) Hsp27. Hsp27 plays an important role as a molecular chaperon in protein folding and unfolding and has been found to be hyperphosphorylated in many cancer types. Studied have reported an increased expression of Hsp27 in both serum and urine samples of high-grade RCC patients [4].

Gamma-glutamyl transferase (GGT) is an enzyme involved in glutathione metabolism and is known to increase in human malignancies, due to inflammation produced in liver, kidney and bile ducts. GGT has been reported to be a prognostic marker for RCC patient care, as its levels were directly correlated to tumor staging and grading as measured by Roche/Hitachi analyser and Olympus 5400 analyzer, along with colorimetric assays [33].

13.9 Molecules Involved in Apoptosis

A balance between apoptotic and anti-apoptotic genes decide cells future. Apoptosis is essential to discard the outdated, unused proteins and other molecules. Tumorigenesis requires alterations in physiological apoptotic mechanism, by promoting abnormal activity of anti-apoptotic proteins or by inhibition or suppression of proapoptotic mediators. A major proapoptotic mediator reported to promote extrinsic apoptosis particularly in RCC cell lines using qRT-PCR is tumor necrosis factor-related apoptosis inducing ligand (TRAIL) [34]. Another author revealed a strong decrease in serum TRAIL in pre-surgery RCC patients compared to controls [4, 35]. Cytokeratins (CK) are apoptotic-derived products released into the blood and can be measured in RCC patients one such factor is M65. In an ELISA study, serum M65 levels were elevated in patients with metastatic RCC. The author also concluded that serum M65 levels could be predictive of progression-free survival (PSF) in RCC patients with a cutoff of 313.6 U/L [36].

13.10 Molecules Related to Tumor Microenvironment

Sporadic/genetic mutations, and epigenetics alter tumor microenvironment, in which components like fibroblasts and macrophages release growth factors, cytokines, and angiogenic factors to allow tumor progression. Hypoxia is one such environmental factor that characterizes the microenvironment of tumors cells in general and in RCC. In most RCCs, *VHL* is mutated that promote accumulation of HIF-α, leading to downstream upregulation of hypoxia-regulated genes that has a well-established relevance to the pathogenesis of acute and chronic kidney diseases. Among others these include many of the proangiogenic genes, such as vascular endothelial growth factor (VEGF), erythropoietin, and carbonic anhydrase 9 (CA9) [15]. Along with VHL protein, hypoxia-inducible factor prolyl hydroxylase-3 (PHD3) is involved in HIF-α degradation [4, 37]. Increased Serum PHD3 levels were observed in patients with RCC, which declined after surgery in ELISA assay [4, 38]. Hypoxia also promotes the expression of enzymes, such as carbonic anhydrase IX (CA IX) that increase in both serum and tissue of patients with ccRCC, as determined by IHC, ELISA, Western blot and RT-PCR [4, 39].

Serum tissue factor (TF) is a transmembrane protein responsible to trigger coagulation pathways and was upregulated by several-fold in ccRCC patients. The post-operative ELISA results showed a threefold reduction in the serum TF levels of ccRCC patients and these reduced serum TF levels were comparative to control group of patients with benign diseases [40].

13.11 Molecular Techniques to Detect Renal Cancer Biomarkers

Some of the techniques used to detect MMs are: (a) immunoassays such as enzyme-linked immunosorbent assay (ELISA), flow cytometry (FACs), Western blot, immunonephelometry, radioimmunoassay (RIA), and co-immunoprecipitation (Co-IP) and pull-down assay, (b) gene expression assays such as microarray, quantitative polymerase chain reaction (qRT-PCR), fluorescence in-situ hybridization (FISH) and next-generation DNA sequencing (NGS), (c) histology techniques such as IHC and tissue microarray, and d) other high-throughput or molecular techniques such as liquid chromatography-mass spectrometry (LC-MS), surface-enhanced laser desorption/ionization time-of-flight mass spectrometry (SELDI-TOF MS), microRNAs and liquid biopsy (Fig. 13.5).

13.11.1 Immunoassays

Immunoassays are based on the interaction between antibody and antigen (Ag) and can be measured by labeling either Ag or Ab with enzymes, fluorescence, radioisotopes and DNA reporters or unlabeled Ag-Ab complex detected by surface plasmon resonance. Some of the immunoassays used routinely on blood and urine samples are ELISA.

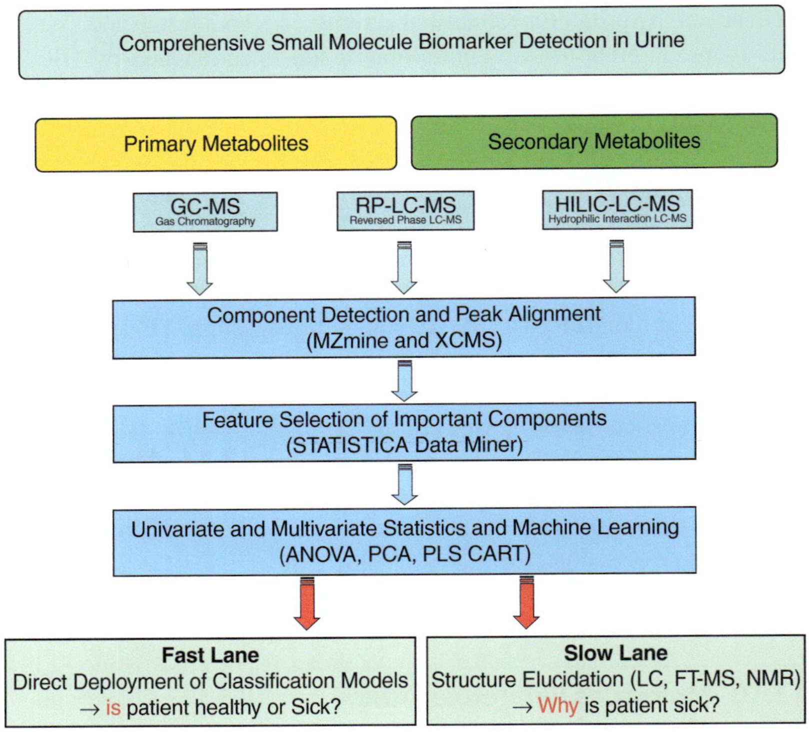

Fig. 13.5 Algorithm describing the metabolomic approaches for biomarker identification using complementary analytical techniques covering the whole metabolome or small molecule space [58]

13.11.2 Microarray and Quantitative Real-Time Polymerase Chain Reaction (qRT-PCR)

Microarray is a high-throughput assay, which can analyze and compare the expression of thousands of genes on a single chip. In most of the cases the microarray results are verified using qRT-PCR. In a study using genome-wide expression array, a panel of 661 inflammation related genes were analyzed in 93 patients tumor and adjacent normal tissue and association with recurrence and survival was validated in 258 tumors using qRT-PCR. Results suggest an upregulation of *GADD45G*, and *CARD9*, *CIITA* and *NCF2* to be prognostic marker for recurrence and death, respectively in patients with ccRCC [41].

13.11.3 Fluorescence In-Situ Hybridization (FISH)

It is a molecular cytogenetic technique that exploits the binding of fluorescent DNA/RNA probes to a particular region of chromosome or mRNA and miRNA of interest with high degree of sequence complementarity. FISH can detect genetic abnormalities in touch imprint tissue smears and help subtype RCCs accurately [42]. Several studies demonstrated TFE3 break-apart fluorescence in situ hybridization (FISH) assay to be better over TFE3 immunostaining to confirm Xp11 translocation, which has exceptionally high prevalence in children. TFE3-FISH helps diagnose the genetic defects even in the formalin fixed tissue that is usually not appropriate for analysis by karyotyping or RT-qPCR [43, 44].

13.11.4 Next Generation Sequencing (NGS)

NGS is a high-throughput technique that can identify the nucleotide sequence of the fragmented DNA or the target DNA by creating amplicon library. NGS consists of four steps: (a) library preparation, (b) clustering, (c) sequencing, and (d) data analysis. RNA sequencing has been able to distinguish TFE3 translocation RCC (TFE3 tRCC) from other RCCs [45]. Tumor tissue and circulating tumor DNA (ctDNA) studies using NGS are frequently used to diagnose genomic alterations and help guide therapy, especially in metastatic RCC [46].

13.11.5 Immunohistochemistry (IHC) and Tissue Microarray (TMA)

Molecular markers released in biofluids can give a good estimate of the occurrence of the disease but results from proteomic and gene expression profiling needs to be evaluated in the tumor tissue by the tissue analysis technique such as IHC. IHC allows detection and localization of the antibody directly onto the tissue [47]. Another high-throughput technique that can detect hundreds to thousands of cancerous tissues on a single slide is tissue microarrays (TMAs). In TMAs, a large number of tissues can be placed in parallel and analyzed for various RCC tissue biomarkers, such as PAX-8 and PAX-2 that have been investigated as markers for RCC. PAX-8 and PAX-2 are a group of paired box gene family of transcription factors responsible for renal and thyroid organogenesis [48]. PAX-8 has been detected in the renal epithelial cells of the renal tubules and the Bowman's capsule. PAX-8 is demonstrated to be a specific marker for primary and metastatic RCC (mRCC) [48]. Specificity and sensitivity of PAX-8 was excellent in distinguishing RCCs and ovarian cancers from other malignancies. Unlike other investigated markers including vimentin, cytokeratin, CK-7, CD10, CAIX and PAX-2; PAX-8 has >90% reliability in distinguishing RCC from UCC [49].

Cytokeratins and vimentin are important cytoskeletal proteins in the mesenchyme, which can distinguish ccRCC and pRCC from chRCC and oncocytomas. CK7 can differentiate pRCC from ccRCC [44, 46, 48]. CD117 (c-kit), is a tyrosine kinase receptor involved in cell signal transduction pathways by phosphorylating the downstream molecules in apoptosis, cell differentiation, proliferation, chemotaxis and cell adhesion [50]. CD117 has high specificity and sensitivity to chRCC and thus can differentiate it from oncocytomas [51]. While most of the other cytokeratin stains are of limited utility in renal tumors, a recent study has shown 34βE12 to be useful for identifying clear cell papillary RCC (ccpRCC) and can best in distinguishing ccpRCC from ccRCC, particularly when the morphology is equivocal [52]. Cathepsin K is a cysteine protease and plays an important part in the function of microphthalmia-associated transcription factor (MITF) transcription. Cathepsin K has proved to be a useful marker for angiomyolipoma and translocation RCC. Due to its role in MITF transcription, it also shows positivity in Xp11 translocation RCC, as translocation RCCs involves transcription factor binding to IGHM enhancer (TFE3 or TFEB) genes, which are members of the microphthalmia (MITF)/TFE family. The MITF/TFE is a family of transcription factors emerging as global regulators of cancer cell survival and energy metabolism, both through the promotion of lysosomal genes as well as newly characterized targets, such as oxidative metabolism and the oxidative stress response [53, 54]. Research surrounding MITF/TFE family indicates that these transcription factors are promising therapeutic targets and biomarkers for cancers that thrive in stressful niches [54].

Some of the other IHC markers useful in differential diagnosis of renal tumors in conjunction with other stains are CA-IX, α-methylacyl coenzyme A racemase (AMACR), CD10 and epithelial membrane antigen (EMA). In instance of poor morphology, a transmembrane protein called CA-IX can identify ccRCC since it is specifically positive in ccRCC and typically negative in all other RCC types [53]. AMACR is a mitochondrial enzyme that is normally expressed in proximal renal tubules. It is helpful in identifying pRCC and ccpRCC, as it is positive in these two entities, and typically negative in other RCC subtypes. CD10 is a cell-surface glycoprotein that is helpful in identifying ccRCC and pRCC. Immunohistochemical staining for CA IX, CK7, AMACR and TFE3 comprises a concise panel for distinguishing RCC with papillary and clear pattern [55]. In comparison to individual analysis, immunohistochemistry, FISH and RT-PCR in combination can show high incidence of Xp11 translocation RCC [56].

13.11.6 Mass Spectrometry (MS)

Examination of the urine samples using high-resolution two-dimensional PAGE (2D-PAGE) and by liquid chromatography/tandem mass spectrometry (LC-MS) has identified hundreds of proteins [57–59] (Fig. 13.5). In order to improve immunotherapeutic strategies for the treatment of diseases, several studies aimed at the role or inflammatory immune cells and cytokines in RCC tumorigenesis and metastasis. In liver, the cytokine stimulation leads to the production of specific proteins in RCC patients. Some of these acute phase proteins, such as serum interleukin-6 (IL-6), amyloid A (SAA) and C-reactive protein (CRP) were detected with high specificity in RCC serum using immunoassays and surface-enhanced laser desorption/ionization time-of-flight mass spectrometry (SELDI-TOF MS). Detection of SAA in RCC serum is an outstanding proteomic finding. SAA provide an opportunity to be used as diagnostic and follow-up biomarker in advanced RCC since it showed a higher sensitivity and greater increase than CRP, to the stimulation of inflammatory cytokines [60].

13.11.7 Micro RNAs (miRNA)

MicroRNAs are a class of ~22 nucleotide small non-coding RNA molecules that negatively regulate the expression of a wide variety of genes mainly through direct interaction with the 3′-untranslated regions (3′-UTR) of corresponding mRNA targets. Recent advances in the understanding of the role of miRNAs have lead to the findings of potential prognostic and diagnostic serum/plasma, urine and tissue miRNAs in RCC [61] (Ref 18/532). A recent study showed increased expression of miR-1233 in serum as a diagnostic implication in RCC [61]. Some of the miRNAs reported to be upregulated in RCC tissue are miR-7, 21, 23b and 155. While, some of the miRNAs downregulated in RCC tissue include miR-1/133a, 30c, 30d, 34a, 99a and 133b (Ref 33/533). In another study, serum miRNA was determined in 25 RCCs compared to 25 noncancer controls (training set) using TaqMan Low Density Array and validated in 107 RCCs and 107 noncancer controls using qRT-PCR. The results showed increased levels of miR-193a-3p, miR-362 and miR-572, and reduced levels of miR-28-5p and miR-378 in RCC patients. A panel of these five miR markers has the potential to diagnose early-stage in RCC [62]. Although an increased number of miRNAs were altered in RCC, there are no clinically approved miRNA in RCC diagnosis and prognosis. Therefore, large-scale studies are needed to fully explore the circulatory miRNA profile in RCC [63].

13.11.8 Long Non-coding RNA (LncRNA)

As the name suggests, long non-coding RNA (lncRNA) is a long-sequence of RNA transcribed from genomic regions, has a minimum length of 200 nucleotides with a limited protein-coding capacity. LncRNA participates in a large variety of biological processes including cancer biology and a new insight of lncRNA profiling has emphasized its function as oncogenes or tumor suppressor genes that can modulate a variety of biological function such as regulating cell proliferation, cell cycle, invasion and metastasis [64]. Microarray study of non-tumorous (NT) tissues compared to ccRCC tissue in six patients showed that downregulation of lncRNA was more common than upregulation. The qPCR results from the same study showed aberrant expression of four lncRNA—ENST00000456816, X91348, BC029135 and NR_024418 in 63 pairs of histologically matched normal renal tissue and ccRCC samples [65]. A recent study identified that the expression level of CYP4A22-2/3 can discriminate ccRCCs from normal kidney tissues [66]. Furthermore in the same study, lnc-ZNF180-2 expression levels were an independent predictor of progression-free survival, cancer-specific survival and overall survival in ccRCC patients and quantification of lnc-ZNF180-2 may be useful for the prediction of ccRCC patients outcome following nephrectomy [66]. LncRNA silencing or overexpression might be a viable therapeutic option to reduce the growth and/or metastatic potential of RCC [66]. Detailed study of lncRNA may serve as a new class of biomarkers in tumor prognosis, diagnosis and even serve in targeted gene therapy [64].

13.11.9 Liquid Biopsy

Establishing tumors genomic profile via tissue biopsy has limited implications due to the difficulty in sampling, sampling bias and risk to the patient. Blood based biomarkers (liquid biopsy) is advantageous in the initial detection, diagnosis and monitoring of renal cancer, since it is non-invasive and has limited to no risk to the patients. Circulating tumor cells (CTCs) are present in the peripheral blood of the patients with most type of advanced cancer but the sensitivity of CTCs in less advance cancer stages is questionable. A study demonstrated that only 27% of patients with metastatic RCC have detectable CTCs [67]. Circulating miRNA in the blood has gained interest as a potential marker for RCC in the past few years but their ability to predict response to therapy is uncertain. Circulating tumor DNA (ctDNA) is another unique component of the peripheral blood that has recently emerged as another promising biomarker. Levels of ctDNA reflect tumor load and increased levels can be found pre-malignancy. Gene alterations (such as hypermethylation and mutations) in ctDNA can easily be measured and used to guide therapy. In ctDNA qRT-PCR study, VHL mutation was detected in one of four RCC patients pre-operative and decreased to undetectable levels post-nephrectomy [53]. The ctDNA dynamics seem to correlate with the tumor burner; however, further optimized approach is needed to use them as a clinical marker.

13.12 Challenges

Kidney carcinoma is an aggressive disease. Some of the challenges in treating renal carcinomas are: kidney tissue heterogeneity and extremely incidental findings of RCC, most of the symptoms may appear in late stages or are due to the paraneoplastic syndrome. Till date renal cancer are diagnosed using tissue immunohistochemistry (IHC) and imaging such as computed tomography (CT) and ultrasounds (US). These tools have been successful in detecting advance stage of renal cancer but come with pitfalls: (a) advancements in imaging, staging and the treatments have led to a significant and progressive increase in relative 5-year survival rates for patients with RCC but has not been able to find complete cure [5], (b) adjuvant treatments such as chemotherapies and radiation therapies are not effective in RCC and RCCs has a high post-operative recurrence, (c) according to the national kidney foundation average life expectancy on dialysis is 5–10 years while some patients can live longer, only 35% of hemodialysis patients remain alive after 5 years of treatment, (d) for analysis, samples are collected using CT or US guided endoscopic biopsy or fine needle aspiration, which are invasive methods of collecting small tissues samples and may have risk to the patients, and (e) also the small tissue biopsies collected using fine needle aspiration are not the best samples for histological analysis or genetic studies.

On the technical front, IHC has its own drawbacks, such as the selection of right antibodies, antibody concentrations, tissue fixation, handling and imaging. Also it is difficult to extract DNA from tissue biopsy that has been fixed. This poor quality of DNA may not be informative in providing the correct status of the disease. One of the major drawback in RCC is, the cancer gets detected when it is in the advance stage or has metastasized to other organs such as bones and lungs and has no other treatments available other then radical nephrectomy or nephron-sparing surgery.

13.13 Conclusion

Non-invasive methods for detecting cancer markers sounds very lucrative but has its limitations since a single biomarkers is not enough to confirm the type and stage of renal carcinoma and instead present circumstances urgently demand for suitable MMs that can detect the disease and prevent its progression at early stages by using more targeted and personalized therapies. For more then a decade scientists have tried to find MMs specific to RCC and has detected several promising biomarkers; however, due to the technical limitations and small clinical trials there are still not many clinically approved biomarkers. To overcome these challenges more laboratory-based tests should be run in parallel to the above historical tests and larger clinical trials need to be done to test for already established MMs. While everyone is focused on finding novel biomarkers, more focus should be on establishing panels of MMs in biofluids and to detect particular renal carcinomas using least invasive methods.

References

1. Ferlay J, Soerjomataram I, Mea E. GLOBOCAN 2012 v1.0, cancer incidence and mortality worldwide: IARC CancerBase No. 11. Lyon: International Agency for Research on Cancer; 2013. p. 1.0.
2. Bray F, Ren JS, Masuyer E, Ferlay J. Global estimates of cancer prevalence for 27 sites in the adult population in 2008. Int J Cancer. 2013;132(5):1133–45.
3. Linehan W, et al. Molecular diagnosis and therapy of kidney cancer. Annu Rev Med. 2010;61:329–43.
4. Pastore AL, et al. Serum and urine biomarkers for human renal cell carcinoma. Dis Mark. 2015;2015:251403.
5. Leppert JT, Pantuck AJ, Figlin RA, Belldegrun AS. The role of molecular markers in the staging of renal cell carcinoma. BJU Int. 2007;99(5b):1208–11.
6. Audenet F, Yates D, Cancel-Tassin G, Cussenot O, Rouprêt M. Genetic pathways involved in carcinogenesis of clear cell renal cell carcinoma: genomics towards personalized medicine. BJU Int. 2012;109:1864–70.
7. Daniel CR, et al. Large prospective investigation of meat intake, related mutagens, and risk of renal cell carcinoma. Am J Clin Nutr. 2012;95(1):155–62.
8. T P, et al. Body size and risk of renal cell carcinoma in the European prospective investigation into cancer and nutrition (EPIC). Int J Cancer. 2006;118(3):728–38.
9. Xu Y, et al. The impact of smoking on survival in renal cell carcinoma: a systematic review and meta-analysis. Tumor Biol. 2014;35(7):6633–40.
10. Sanfilippo KM, et al. Hypertension and obesity and the risk of kidney cancer in 2 large cohorts of US men and women. Hypertension. 2014;63(5):934–41.
11. Hu J, et al. Renal cell carcinoma and occupational exposure to chemicals in Canada. Occup Med. 2002;52(3):157–64.
12. Muglia VF, Prando A. Renal cell carcinoma: histological classification and correlation with imaging findings. Radiol Bras. 2015;48(3):166–74.
13. Cairns P. Renal cell carcinoma. Cancer Biomark. 2011;9(1–6):461–73.
14. Sachdeva K. Renal cell carcinoma staging; 2017. https://www.cancer.org/cancer/kidney-cancer/detection-diagnosis-staging/staging.html.
15. Haase VH. The VHL/HIF oxygen-sensing pathway and its relevance to kidney disease. Kidney Int. 2006;69(8):1302–7.
16. Organ S, Tsao M. An overview of the c-MET signaling pathway. Ther Adv Med Oncol. 2011;3(1 Suppl):S7–S19.
17. L S, et al. Germline and somatic mutations in the tyrosine kinase domain of the *MET* proto-oncogene in papillary renal carcinomas. Nat Genet. 1997;16(1):68–73.
18. Linehan WM, Srinivasan R, Schmidt LS. The genetic basis of kidney cancer: a metabolic disease. Nat Rev Urol. 2010;5:277.
19. Linehan WM, Walther MM, Zbar B. The genetic basis of cancer of the kidney. J Urol. 2003; 170(6 Part 1):2163.
20. Menko FH, et al. Hereditary leiomyomatosis and renal cell cancer (HLRCC). Renal cancer risk, surveillance and treatment. Fam Cancer. 2014;13(4):637–44.
21. Schneider M, et al. Early onset renal cell carcinoma in an adolescent girl with germline *FLCN* exon 5 deletion. Fam Cancer. 2018;17(1):135–9. Cite as(1):135–9.
22. Pavlovich C, et al. Renal tumors in the Birt-Hogg-Dubé syndrome. Am J Surg Pathol. 2002;26(12):1542–52.
23. Ramakrishnan S, Ellis L, Pili R. Histone modifications: implications in renal cell carcinoma. Epigenomics. 2013;5(4):453–62.
24. Shenoy N, et al. Role of DNA methylation in renal cell carcinoma. J Hematol Oncol. 2015;8:88.
25. Tunuguntla HS, Jorda M. Diagnostic and prognostic molecular markers in renal cell carcinoma. J Urol. 2008;179(6):2096.
26. Eichelberg C, Junker K, Ljungberg B, Moch H. Diagnostic and prognostic molecular markers for renal cell carcinoma: a critical appraisal of the current state of research and clinical applicability. Eur Urol. 2009;55(4):851–63.
27. DI Carlo A. Evaluation of neutrophil gelatinase-associated lipocalin (NGAL), matrix metalloproteinase-9 (MMP-9) and their complex MMP-9/NGAL in sera and urine of patients with kidney tumors. Oncol Lett. 2013;5(5):1677–81.
28. Won KH, et al. Human kidney injury molecule-1 is a tissue and urinary tumor marker of renal cell carcinoma. J Am Soc Nephrol. 2005;16(4):1126–34.

29. Bonventre J. Kidney injury molecule-1 (KIM-1): a urinary biomarker and much more. Nephrol Dial Transplant. 2009;24(11):3265–8.
30. Jeremiah JM, Amy NL, Jingqin L, Evan DK. Urinary biomarkers for the early diagnosis of kidney cancer. Mayo Clin Proc. 2010;85(5):413–21.
31. Rajandram R, et al. Tumour necrosis factor receptor-associated factor-1 (TRAF-1) expression is increased in renal cell carcinoma patient serum but decreased in cancer tissue compared with normal: potential biomarker significance. Pathology. 2014;46(6):518–22.
32. Bennett NC, et al. Patient samples of renal cell carcinoma show reduced expression of TRAF1 compared with normal kidney and functional studies in vitro indicate TRAF1 promotes apoptosis: potential for targeted therapy. Pathology. 2012;44(5):453–9.
33. Hofbauer S, et al. Pretherapeutic gamma-glutamyltransferase is an independent prognostic factor for patients with renal cell carcinoma. Br J Cancer. 2014;111(8):1526–31.
34. Ramp U, et al. Apoptosis induction in renal cell carcinoma by TRAIL and γ-radiation is impaired by deficient caspase-9 cleavage. Br J Cancer. 2003;88(11):1800–7.
35. Déjosez M, et al. Sensitivity to TRAIL/APO-2L-mediated apoptosis in human renal cell carcinomas and its enhancement by topotecan. Cell Death Differ. 2000;7(11):1127–36.
36. I Y, et al. Serum M65 as a biomarker for metastatic renal cell carcinoma. Clin Genitourin Cancer. 2013;11(3):290–6.
37. Frew IJ, Moch H. A clearer view of the molecular complexity of clear cell renal cell carcinoma. Annu Rev Pathol Mech Dis. 2015;10(1):263–89.
38. Tanaka T, Kitamura H, Torigoe T, et al. Autoantibody against hypoxia-inducible factor prolyl hydroxylase-3 is a potential serological marker for renal cell carcinoma. J Cancer Res Clin Oncol. 2011;137(5):789–94.
39. Takacova M, et al. Carbonic anhydrase IX is a clinically significant tissue and serum biomarker associated with renal cell carcinoma. Oncol Lett. 2013;5(1):191–7.
40. Silva D, et al. Serum tissue factor as a biomarker for renal clear cell carcinoma. Int Braz J Urol. 2018;44(1):38–44.
41. Tan W, et al. Role of inflammatory related gene expression in clear cell renal cell carcinoma development and clinical outcomes. J Urol. 2011;186(5):2071–7.
42. Iqbal MA, Akhtar M, Al Dayel F, Ulmer C, Paterson MC. Use of fish analysis for diagnosis of renal cell carcinoma subtypes. Ann Saudi Med. 1999;19(6):495–500.
43. Kim S, et al. Usefulness of a break-apart FISH assay in the diagnosis of Xp11.2 translocation renal cell carcinoma. Virchows Arch. 2011;459(3):299–306.
44. Pradhan D, et al. Validation and utilization of a TFE3 break-apart FISH assay for Xp11.2 translocation renal cell carcinoma and alveolar soft part sarcoma. Diagn Pathol. 2015;10(1):179.
45. Pflueger D, et al. Identification of molecular tumor markers in renal cell carcinomas with TFE3 protein expression by RNA sequencing. Neoplasia. 2013;15(11):1231–40.
46. Hahn AW, et al. Correlation of genomic alterations assessed by next-generation sequencing (NGS) of tumor tissue DNA and circulating tumor DNA (ctDNA) in metastatic renal cell carcinoma (mRCC): potential clinical implications. Oncotarget. 2017;8(20):33614–20.
47. Di Napoli A, Signoretti S. Tissue biomarkers in renal cell carcinoma: issues and solutions. Cancer. 2009;115(10 Suppl):2290–7.
48. Barr ML, et al. PAX-8 expression in renal tumours and distant sites: a useful marker of primary and metastatic renal cell carcinoma? J Clin Pathol. 2014;68(1):12–7.
49. Knoepp S, Kunju LP, Roh MH. Utility of PAX8 and PAX2 immunohistochemistry in the identification of renal cell carcinoma in diagnostic cytology. Diagn Cytopathol. 2012;40(8):667–72.
50. Miettinen M, Lasota J. KIT (CD117): a review on expression in normal and neoplastic tissues, and mutations and their clinicopathologic correlation. Appl Immunohistochem Mol Morphol. 2005;13(3):205–20.
51. Ahmed EA, Youssif ME. Immunohistochemical study of c-KIT (CD117) expression in renal cell carcinoma. J Egypt Natl Canc Inst. 2009;21(2):121–32.
52. Martignoni G, et al. Validation of 34betaE12 immunoexpression in clear cell papillary renal cell carcinoma as a sensitive biomarker. Pathology. 2017;49(1): 10–8.
53. Farber N, et al. Renal cell carcinoma: the search for a reliable biomarker. Transl Cancer Res. 2017;6(3): 620–32.
54. Slade L, Pulinilkunnil T. The MiTF/TFE family of transcription factors: master regulators of organelle signaling, metabolism, and stress adaptation. Mol Cancer Res. 2017 15(12):1637–43.
55. Alshenawy HA. Immunohistochemical panel for differentiating renal cell carcinoma with clear and papillary features. Pathol Oncol Res. 2015;21(4): 893–9.
56. Lee HJ, et al. Combination of immunohistochemistry, FISH and RT-PCR shows high incidence of Xp11 translocation RCC: comparison of three different diagnostic methods. Oncotarget. 2017;8(19): 30756–65.
57. Kim K, et al. Urine metabolomics analysis for kidney cancer detection and biomarker discovery. Mol Cell Proteomics. 2009;8(3):558–70.
58. Kind T, Tolstikov V, Fiehn O, Weiss R. A comprehensive urinary metabolomic approach for identifying kidney cancer. Anal Biochem. 2007;363(2):185–95.
59. Rogers M, et al. Proteomic profiling of urinary proteins in renal cancer by surface enhanced laser desorption ionization and neural-network analysis. Cancer Res. 2003;63(20):6971–83.

60. Fischer K, Theil G, Hoda R, Fornara P. Serum amyloid a: a biomarker for renal cancer. Anticancer Res. 2012;32(5):1801–4.
61. Wulfken L, et al. MicroRNAs in renal cell carcinoma: diagnostic implications of serum miR-1233 levels. PLoS One. 2011;6(9):e25787.
62. Wang C, et al. A panel of five serum miRNAs as a potential diagnostic tool for early-stage renal cell carcinoma. Sci Rep. 2015;5(1):7610.
63. Li M, et al. MicroRNAs in renal cell carcinoma: a systematic review of clinical implications (review). Oncol Rep. 2015;33(4):1571–8.
64. Li M, Wang Y, Cheng L, Niu W, Zhao G, Raju JK, et al. Long non-coding RNAs in renal cell carcinoma: a systematic review and clinical implications. Oncotarget. 2017;8(29):48424–35.
65. Yu G, et al. LncRNAs expression signatures of renal clear cell carcinoma revealed by microarray. PLoS One. 2012;7(8):e42377.
66. Ellinger J, et al. The long non-coding RNA lnc-ZNF180–2 is a prognostic biomarker in patients with clear cell renal cell carcinoma. Am J Cancer Res. 2015;5(9):2799–807.
67. Ball MW, et al. Circulating tumor DNA as a marker of therapeutic response in patients with renal cell carcinoma: a pilot study. Clin Genitourin Cancer. 2016;14(5):e515–20.
68. Cohen RJ. Pathology of clear cell renal cell carcinoma; 2016. https://emedicine.medscape.com/article/1612043-overview.

Molecular Biomarkers and Urinary Bladder Cancer (UBC)

14

A. N. Srivastava, Kirti A. Gautam, and S. N. Sankhwar

14.1 Introduction

Urinary bladder cancer (UBC) is one of the most common cancers in the world. Majorly occur of these in developed countries, however in developing countries, the incidence is also increasing due to change in lifestyle. UBC is the seventh most common cancer all over the world in men and seventeenth in women [1]. In 2008, there were an estimated 386,300 new cases of UBC and approximately 150,200 deaths [1]. The incidence of UBC varies 14-fold internationally with higher occurrence in males as compared to females [2]. Within India, the age standardized incidence rate of UBC is 2.7 for men and 0.6 for women, respectively and according to the recent report of National Cancer Registry Programme in India, the highest incidence rate of UBC in men is found in Delhi (6.8%, 2008–2009) (Leading sites of cancer, Bangalore, 2013). The mortality rates have been stabilized in males and decreased in females of United States [3] and Europe [4] due to reduction in smoking prevalence and occupational exposures.

14.2 Risk Factors

The exact etiology of bladder cancer is unknown. A risk factor may change susceptibility of individual of getting UBC and may have different impact on the pathophysiology of UBC [5]. Therefore it is important to know about the potential risk factors so that a person may change his/her life style (i.e. avoidance of causative agents) and got routine checkups (i.e. screening) for expected carcinogen to reduce the chances of occurrence of UBC.

14.2.1 Demographical Risk Factors

14.2.1.1 Age, Gender and Ethnicity

The risk of being diagnosed with UBC increases substantially with age and the median age of diagnosis is 65–75 year. Other risk factors like smoking and occupational exposure can be controlled but person's age or family history cannot be changed. The incidence of UBC in women is lower up to four fold than men [6] while mortality is higher in women than men. Pelucchi et al. [7], hypothesized

A. N. Srivastava (✉)
Department of Pathology, Era University, Era's Lucknow Medical College and Hospital, Lucknow, India

K. A. Gautam
Department of Urology, King George's University, Lucknow, India

Department of Pediatric, GSVM Medical College, Kanpur, India

S. N. Sankhwar
Department of Urology, King George's University, Lucknow, India

K. K. Shukla et al. (eds.), *Molecular Diagnostics in Cancer Patients*,
https://doi.org/10.1007/978-981-13-5877-7_14

that the higher incidence of bladder cancer among men is mainly due to higher exposures to tobacco smoke and aromatic amines [7]. As found in other cancers, disparity in UBC incidence and survival vary among different ethnic groups [8]. Lower incidence and poor survival have been reported in blacks as compared with whites, this difference persists between them despite similar grade, stage and treatment [9]. Five-year disease-specific survival was 82.8% in whites compared with 70.2% in blacks, 80.7% in Hispanics, and 81.9% in Asian/Pacific Islanders [10].

14.2.2 Life Style Related Risk Factors

14.2.2.1 Smoking and Tobacco Chewing

Tobacco smoke, which contains aromatic amines and other carcinogens, is a well known bladder cancer risk factor [11]. Tobacco smoke alone is recognized for about half of UBC cases. Recently, a study on population attributed risk of UBC for tobacco smoke has been found 50–60% in men and 20–35% in women and a meta-analysis reported that ever smoker have a risk of 2.57 (95%CI 2.20–3.00) compared with never-smokers and it increases with the number of cigarettes smoked and the number of years one has smoked [7, 12]. According to U.S. Department of health and human services, tobacco smoke contains a number of carcinogens including polycyclic aromatic hydrocarbons (PAHs), N-nitrosamines, heterocyclic amines, aldehydes and aromatic amines, like β-naphthylamine, which are reported to cause UBC. International Agency for Research on Cancer (IARC) has also established smoking as a risk factor for bladder cancer [13]. Furthermore, cessation of smoking is associated with the reduced risk of UBC as reported in a pooled analysis of 11 case-control studies.

14.2.2.2 Dietary Factors

Dietary products like meat, vegetable oil, seafood (mostly bivalves) and tea contain PAHs (benzo[e]pyrene and benz[b]fluoranthene) which have been reported to be involved in causing UBC in European population [14]. Other than this, consumption of coffee and alcohol has been suggested to have no association with UBC risk although findings are not always consistence [15–17]. These inconsistent results may have occurred due to the presence of confounders [18]. In East Asian and Native American groups, bracken fern (*Pteridium aquillinum*) is consumed as a vegetable. Quercetin, kaempferol and ptaquiloside, present in this fern, have been found to be carcinogenic [19] as they cause esophageal cancer in humans and UBC or intestinal carcinoma in rats.

Saccharin has also been found to be carcinogenic due to presence of o-toluene sulphonamide that causes UBC in rats. Therefore, it was listed as carcinogen in 2000 in the US National Toxicology Program's Report on Carcinogens. However due to no clear evidence of its carcinogenic activity in humans, in December 2010 Environmental protection agency (EPA) stated that saccharin is no longer considered a potential hazard to human health.

14.2.3 Environmental Risk Factors

14.2.3.1 Occupational Risk

After smoking, the second most common risk factor for UBC is occupational exposure to carcinogens, which include aromatic amines (benzidine, 2-naphthylamine (2-NA) and 4-aminobiphenyl (4-ABP)), polycyclic aromatic hydrocarbons (PAHs), and chlorinated hydrocarbons. Industries that commonly use these chemicals include dye [20], rubber [21] and textile manufacturing. In 1895, Rehn et al., has first described occupational exposure as a risk factor of UBC among workers of European population in the aniline dye industry [22]. Later in 1938, Hueper et al., applied 2-NA to induce UBC in dog [23]. Further, the ban on industrial production of these aromatic amines reduces the incidence of occupational UBC worldwide [24]. In 2008, Clapp et al. documented a decrease in bladder cancer incidence among dye workers due to protective measures and elimination of exposure to specific aromatic amines [25].

14.2.4 Other Risk Factors

14.2.4.1 Medications

Certain drugs like cyclophosphamide, chloronaphazine and phenacetin are reported to induce UBC in human [26–28]. Chloronaphazine is a derivative of 2-NA and was classified as carcinogenic agent to humans by the International Agency for Research on Cancer (IARC) in 2010 and 2012 [29, 30]. Nitrate is used as food preservative and in the production of rubber, fertilizer, pesticides and cosmetics when combines with amino acid in stomach, results in the production of nitrosamines which are regarded as carcinogens [31]. Other than these, Chinese herbs called Mu Tong, that contains aritolochic acid (AA), have been found to increase the risk of UBC [32].

14.2.5 Genetic Risk Factor

Experimental studies dictate that genetic changes either in germ line genes or in somatic genetic alteration must occur for tumor initiation as well as propagation in later stages of tumor development. Studies using the Utah population [33] and the Swedish [34] family cancer databases found that subjects with familial history of UBC have a higher risk of developing UBC. Analysis of data from the latter found that familial risk increased with a history of bladder cancer among first-degree relatives (RR = 1.35; 95% CI: 0.97–1.79 and RR = 2.29; 95% CI: 1.46–3.29), among males and females, respectively. Crawford [35], found a significantly increased risk of bladder cancer among first-degree relatives of individuals who have bladder cancer, with an earlier age of disease onset; and the risk was even higher if they were smokers [35]. Genetic slow acetylator N-acetyltransferase-2 (NAT2) variant and glutathione S-transferase mu-1 (GSTM1)-null genotype are the recognized inherited genetic risk factors for UBC. These genetic risk factors are associated with UBC development but confer additional risk to exposure to carcinogens such as tobacco products.

Environmental carcinogenic substances like aromatic and heterocyclic amines require metabolic activation and result in the formation of electrophilic intermediates such as arylnitrenium ions from arylamines and the diol-epoxide from benzopyrene [36, 37]. These electrophilic intermediates react with DNA of urothelial cell, this results in the damage to the guanine residues and if remain unrepaired by DNA repair system then may lead to carcinogenesis [36, 38, 39]. Somatic genetic alterations observed in UBC tissues include activation of proto-oncogenes and inactivation of tumor suppressor genes. Mutations, non-random deletion or gain at multiple chromosomal sites and epigenetic alterations are causes of genetic heterogeneity of UBC.

14.3 Types and Clinical Features

Generally, UBC occurs in the inner most lining of urinary bladder i.e. epithelial cell or transitional cell hence called urothelial cell carcinoma (UCC) or transitional cell carcinoma (TCC) which stands for 90% of all primary bladder cancers [40]. Other 10% histopathological types are squamous cell carcinoma, adenocarcinoma and small cell carcinoma. Approximately, 70–80% of urothelial carcinomas are confined to the epithelium or are non-invasive, whereas the rest are muscle invasive carcinomas. According to the growth pattern, UBC are classified into different stages in TNM system, which includes information about primary tumor (T), nodal involvement (N), and metastasis (M) [41]. Primary tumors (T) are classified as non-invasive papillary carcinomas (Ta), infiltrative carcinomas that extended into lamina proporia and invade the sub-epithelial connective tissue (T1), muscle invasive carcinoma that extend to the muscular layer (T2+), or as superficial flat carcinoma *in situ* (CIS). Depending on the cytological grade of malignancy, UBC are subdivided into five different malignant grades namely, G1 (well differentiated), G2 (moderately differentiated), G3 (poorly differentiated), G4 (undifferentiated) and Gx (grade cannot be assessed) [42, 43]. According to the WHO 2004 classification, UBC papillary urothelial neoplasm of low malignant potential (TaG1) no longer carries the label of 'cancer' [44].

Low grade papillary Ta tumors (TaG1) almost never progress and patients with this disease seldom die due to the tumor. However, a 50–70% recurrence for TaG2 tumors is reported. Although a majority of patients with T1 cancer show good prognosis in response to Bacillus Calmette-Guerin (BCG) treatment, about one third of the patients do not respond to BCG and in such cases the cancer progresses to invade the muscle usually resulting in death [45]. Literature suggest that, 5 year survival rate is very low in the developing countries, such as India (39%) and Thailand (48%) [46] as compared to the developed countries, such as the United States (97%) [47] and Europe (72.4%) [48].

14.4 Diagnosis

Diagnosis of UBC is done by different conventional methods including—*Urine test* is performed to check for blood or cancer cells but presence of blood cells in urine does not confirm the bladder cancer. *Cystoscopy* is performed to observe cell structure inside the bladder. If any abnormal structure is found, a small piece of tissue is removed and sent to the lab to investigate whether cancer is present and what kind of cancer it is (stage and grade of cancer). Other imaging tests like intravenous pyelogram (IVP), retrograde pyelogram, computed tomography (CT) scan, magnetic resonance imaging (MRI), ultrasound, chest X-ray and bone scan can be performed to diagnose bladder cancer or to observed metastatic conditions.

14.5 Need for the Molecular Marker

Conventionally, clinical and pathologic parameters (cystoscopy, histopathology) are widely used for the diagnosis, assessment of the grade & stage of tumor and to predict clinical outcome of transitional cell carcinoma (TCC) of UBC. The prognostic ability of these parameters is limited because these methods are invasive, expensive and have complications after procedure. Furthermore, long survival rate and 50–70% recurrence rate demands aggressive surveillance that result UBC acquiring the highest cost per patients ($96,000–$187,000 at 2001 levels) [49]. After treatment cystoscopy and urine cytology are essential in every 3 months for first 3 years, every 6 months for next 1–3 years and annually thereafter. Cystoscopy is an invasive, expensive and associated with substantial patient discomfort and has different sensitivity while urine cytology has high specificity (90–96%) but poor sensitivity in examining low grade tumor and its accuracy is dependent on the pathologist's experience [50]. It is a well-established fact that early detection of most of the cancers improves survival rate, outcome and reduce the chances of recurrence.

Therefore, the biggest challenge in front of urologist and researchers is to develop relevant protocol that is cost effective, more sensitive and a non-invasive method for diagnosis. Molecular markers can give possible benefit of detection, surveillance and prognostication of disease as well as investigating the molecular profile of individual patient which can guide clinician into a new era of improving prediction of natural history of tumor and providing a more personalized and tailored intravesical and systemic treatment to that particular patient [51].

To date, numerous potential biomarkers in relation to UBC have been identified by various molecular and genetic studies. In addition, some urine based tumor bio-markers have also been developed. The Food and Drug Administration (FDA) has approved some of these makers test (like—bladder tumor antigen-stat (BTA-stat), bladder tumor antigen-TRAK (BTA-TRAK), fibrinogen-fibrin degradation (FDP), UroVysion, nuclear matrix protein 22 assay (NMP22) and Immunocyt) for routine check-up of UBC patients [52]. Unfortunately, none of the markers have shown significant sensitivity and specificity for the detection of the whole spectrum of bladder cancer diseases in routine clinical practice [53].

14.5.1 Molecular Pathogenesis of the UBC

In the process of cancer development, the central event is loss of genomic integrity which itself probably initiates from the alterations of genomic

DNA by exogenous or endogenous carcinogens. These genetic alterations occur in regulatory pathways that play a vital role in the control of normal cellular proliferation and differentiation [54]. The genetic alterations give the cell a growth advantage over the nearby cells and eventually result in progressive transformation of normal cell to cancerous cell. Over the past decades several molecules, biochemical substances and different tumor acquired capabilities of cancerous cells are disclosed through extensive research, which are used by possibly all type of cancers in the multistep process of tumorigenesis. Sustained replication (to be immortal), neo-angiogenesis, inflammation and chronic proliferation are induced positively during cancer development and progression while the other processes like resisted apoptosis, growth suppressors signaling and enabled growth promoting signaling processes are hampered [55]. Cancerous cell also have a tendency to evade from immune system and growth suppressor mechanisms. By acquiring these properties, cancerous cells have a tendency to metastasize during the advance stages. Thus, these hallmarks are acquired by possibly most if not all cancers, through various mechanistic strategies (Table 14.1). Several biomolecules involved in an inter-relationship pattern towards the processes of carcinogenesis have been discovered and can be used as biomarker for the screening purposes.

The advance molecular biomarker approaches are used for the detection of most of the biological molecule present in blood, tissue or any other body fluids for the purpose of diagnosis of certain diseases. Molecular biomarkers are used routinely in the clinical management of several cancers such as prostate, colon, breast, ovarian and pancreatic cancer but there is a lack of management decisions in UBC that could allow prospective assessment of risk for individual patients.

Table 14.1 Hall-marks of carcinogenesis

Properties	Cancer hallmarks
Induced process	Replication Sustaining proliferative signaling (continue to replicate) Angiogenesis Inflammation
Hampered process	Resisting cell death (apoptosis) Signals that stop cell growth and proliferation
Evade from	Growth suppressors Immune system
Activation of	Invasion and metastasis

14.5.2 Genetic Molecular Markers Investigated Till Now

Genetic biomarkers measure alterations in chromosomes or DNA within cellular level. Since, DNA encodes for proteins that are needed for normal physiology and cellular structure. Therefore, alteration at DNA or chromosomal level, if not repaired, could lead to tumor development. These alterations may be because of insertion, deletion, single nucleotide polymorphism (SNP) and short tandem repeats (STR) in DNA [56]. Exposure to carcinogenic compounds like aromatic amines or polycyclic aromatic hydrocarbons (PAHs) can cause mutations in gene. Prolonged exposure to carcinogens may lead to accumulation of mutations in somatic and germ cells that eventually lead to cancer development. Potential genetic bio-markers can be used as a probable tool for the early screening for tumors, for personalized therapy and identification of group of people those are at higher risk of developing cancer. In addition, these genetic biomarkers can also be used for the prediction of outcome of cancer. In following sections genetic bio-markers in relation with UBC have been described.

14.5.2.1 Chromosomal Genetic Biomarkers

Cytogenetic studies have investigated various alterations in the structure and copy number of chromosomes in transitional cell carcinoma (TCC). **Loss of heterozygosity (LOH)** studies found that loss of 9q associated with different grades of UBC especially in primary events of carcinogenesis, however, loss of 17p, 3p, 13p, 18q or 10q is more frequently associated with high grade of UBC [57]. In early events of tumor formation deletion of 11p and 8p and gain of 8q and 1q has been observed [58], while loss of 17p which is detected in 60% of late events of UBC,

Table 14.2 Potential chromosomal marker associated with UBC

S. no.	Chromosomal marker	Grade and stage of UBC	Reference
1	LOH of 9q	Low grade and high grade	Knowles [57]
2	LOH of 17p, 3p, 13q, 18q, 10q	High grade and stage	Tsai et al. [61], Presti et al. [62]
3	Deletion of 11p and 8p	Low grade	Fadl-Elmula et al. [58]
4	Gain of 8q and1q	Low grade	Fadl-Elmula et al. [58]
5	Microsatellite instability	High grade	Sardi et al. [59]

suggested its role in cancer progression [58]. Many tumors also abide DNA replication errors (RER), these RER arise from the dysfunction of DNA mismatch repair genes and results in **microsatellite instability**. Usually, microsatellite alterations in UBC are associated with invasive cancer [59, 60]. However, this finding requires further verification by systematic studies based on large sample size. Thus, the search for microsatellite instability can only complement current diagnostic methods (Table 14.2).

14.5.2.2 DNA Molecular Markers

Molecular epidemiology based studies have revealed several genetic polymorphisms associated with the UBC, these polymorphisms predispose an individual towards the higher risk of developing UBC. Briefly summarized information about the role of these DNA molecular markers have been presented in the following sections.

14.5.2.3 Carcinogen Metabolism Genes and UBC Risk

Several environmental toxins (carcinogens) require activation and detoxification by drug-metabolizing enzymes. The dynamic equilibrium between the enzymes of activation and detoxification of these carcinogens is the basic requirement to find out the cell fate after exposure to carcinogens. Genetic polymorphisms in these genes differ from one individual to other in cancer susceptibility and can be used as marker for disease diagnosis. Phase I and phase II enzymes are involved in the process of activation and detoxification of carcinogens, respectively.

Cytochrome P-450 (CYPs), a phase I enzyme, commonly involved in activation of carcinogens which results in the accumulation of reactive intermediates, which are more toxic and may cause damage to DNA if not further detoxified by phase II enzymes. Various CYP alleles (CYP1A1, CYP1A2, CYP1B1, CYP2C19, CYP2D6, and CYP2E1) have been known to associate with altered activity or complete absence of enzyme activity [63–65]. Polymorphisms in these drug-metabolism genes are associated with the risk of UBC. CYP1A1 is an important gene and involved in activation of polycyclic aromatic hydrocarbons (PAHs) and aromatic amines. A strong relationship has been attributed among polymorphic genes, cigarette smoke and an increased risk of UBC [65, 66].

There are several phase II enzymes encoded by corresponding genes that have been thoroughly examined in relation with UBC. Below the findings related to UBC risk and DNA polymorphisms of phase II enzymes have been summarized.

There are substantial activities of **glutathione S-transferases (GSTs)** in urinary bladder epithelium and usually they are involved in detoxification of carcinogenic compounds by the conjugation of soluble glutathione to electrophilic centers on a variety of substrates and are important line of defense in protection of cellular components against reactive species. These enzymes play a vital role in defense of DNA from oxidative damage. Genetic polymorphisms of GSTs genes predispose an individual towards the risk of UBC [67, 68]. **Glutathione S-transferases M1 (GSTM1)** gene has highest activities with most electrophiles and products of oxidative stress. [69] Among GST genes, GSTM1 is thoroughly examined gene for their association with UBC risk. Null-genotype of GSTM1 is mostly present in human population, with major ethnic differences. The frequency of GTSM1 null-genotype in normal healthy individuals is approximately 67% in Australians, 50% in Caucasians, 22% in Nigerians and 33%

in Indian [70, 71]. The null-genotype of GSTM1 has statistically significant increased risk of UBC [72]. However, some researcher did not find the same results [73, 74]. **Glutathione S-transferases T1 (GSTT1)** gene have a major role in biotransformation of a number of drugs and industry related chemicals. Prevalence of the null-genotype is 10–65% that varies among different ethnic groups [75]. The approximate frequency of GSTT1 null-genotype in normal healthy Indian population is 18.4% [70]. The GSTT1 null-genotype is marginally related with increased risk of UBC. The Caucasian population is at higher risk of UBC, while Asian population is not [76–78]. A significant higher UBC risk is observed when individuals carry both GSTM1 and GSTT1 null genotypes [79, 91]. **Glutathione S-transferases P1 (GSTP1)** enzyme plays a key role in the detoxification of cigarette smoke carcinogens, such as benzo[a] pyrene diol epoxide [69]. An A → G substitution at position 313 (rs1695) in the GSTP1 gene, results in an Ile → Val change at codon 105 (exon 5) (Isoleusine 105 Valaine) [80]. The amino acid substitution due to SNP affects the kinetic properties of the enzymes and results in reduced detoxification capacity [80]. In healthy Caucasians, the frequencies of the heterozygous and rare homozygous allele are 39.4 and 9.1%, respectively [81]. Genetic polymorphism of **Glutathione S-transferases A1 (GSTA1)** results two variant alleles, GSTA1*A and GSTA1*B and associated with a statistically significant decreased protein expression. **Glutathione S-transferases M3 (GSTM3)** gene contains two alleles, A and B. The GSTM3*B allele has a three base pair deletion in intron 6 that subsequently affects GSTM3 expression [82].

N-acetyltransferases (NATs) are cytosolic enzymes involve in activation and detoxification of carcinogens [83]. Aromatic amines are believed to be the most common urothelial carcinogens that are metabolized by two distinct NATs, NAT1 and NAT2 [84]. Genes encoding NAT1 and NAT2 are extremely polymorphic and their genetic variations result in rapid or slow acetylator phenotype. Polymorphisms leading to rapid acetylation by NAT1 enzyme and slow acetylation by NAT2 enzyme are the possible risk factors for UBC [85]. These polymorphisms also cause inter-individual differences in bio-transformation of heterocyclic and aromatic amine carcinogens. Since aromatic amines that are present in cigarette smoke are a major risk factor for bladder cancer and are metabolized by NAT enzymes therefore, the polymorphisms of the NAT genes have significant roles in predisposing the individuals towards the risk of UBC [86].

N-acetyltransferase1 (NAT1) has a marginal role of NAT1 gene polymorphisms and risk of UBC. However a significant increased risk has been found in smokers and in individuals who are exposed to benzidine [87, 88]. The **N-acetyltransferase2 (NAT2)** involves in acetylation of aromatic amines and hydrazine drugs, thus it affects therapeutic efficacy and toxicity [89]. NAT1 and NAT2 catalyze detoxification reactions; however, NAT2 has a three- to fourfold higher affinity than NAT1 for urinary bladder carcinogens such as 4-aminobiphenyl (ABP) and β-naphthylamine (BNA) [83]. NAT2 gene is polymorphic and the lack of two functional alleles results in reduced enzyme activity, giving the slow acetylation phenotype. Individuals with any two mutant alleles (out of NAT2*5, NAT2*6 and NAT2*7) were considered as slow acetylators and with NAT2*4 as rapid acetylators. There is a strong relationship between NAT2 polymorphisms and risk of UBC.

The joint effect of NAT1 and NAT2 genotypes has also been investigated in some studies. Taylor et al. [90], observed that UBC risk from smoking exposure is high in those who inherit NAT2 slow alleles in combination with one or two copies of the NAT1*10 allele [90]. Hung et al. [91], observed a significant increased risk when NAT1 slow and NAT2 slow genotypes were combined [91]. In a recent meta-analysis the authors found a joint effect of NAT1 rapid genotypes, NAT2 slow genotypes and smoking as factor for increasing cancer risk [92].

Other phase II enzyme actively involved in carcinogen metabolism is **soluble sulfotransferases (SULT).** SULT1A1 is expressed by SULT gene and primarily involved in phenolic xenobiotic compound removal from the body. Genetic polymorphism in SULT1A1 results in a decreased activity and lower stability of enzyme. Persons carrying variant allele have a statistically significant role against the UBC risk [91, 93]. **UDP-glucuronosyltransferase (UGT)** gene encodes for enzyme that plays a vital role in the detoxification and removal of endogenous and exogenous carcinogens and this response is primarily catalyzed by the UGT1A and UGT2B enzymes [94]. UGT genetic polymorphisms affect the capability of enzyme and therefore are associated with an increased risk of UBC [95]. **Myeloperoxidase (MPO)** gene encodes for enzyme that is involved in activation of procarcinogen found in tobacco smoke, such as benzo[a] pyrene [96]. The variant A allele is associated with reduced mRNA expression [97]. **Catechol-omethyltransferase (COMT)** involved in the protection of DNA from oxidative damage by methylation of various endogenous and exogenous substances, preventing quinine formation and redox cycling [98]. A G-to-A allele transition results to a lower COMT enzyme activity [99]. **Manganese superoxide dismutase (MnSOD)** catalyzes the dismutation of anion superoxide into hydrogen peroxide and oxygen [94]. The activity of MnSOD can be induced in the presence of excessive free radical and cigarette smoke; therefore, it plays a key role in protecting cells from oxidative stress [100, 101]. A polymorphism in MnSOD is associated with protein structure change leading to defective mitochondrial localization of the protein. MnSOD variant genotype significantly increased the risk of UBC about twofold [91].

Glutathione peroxidase1 (GPX1) gene encodes for a selenium-dependent enzyme that involves in the detoxification of hydrogen peroxide and a wide range of organic peroxides [102]. The polymorphic variant allele is less responsive than the common allele during stimulation of the GPX1 enzyme by in vitro selenium supplementation and it increases that risk of UBC [103]. **Alcohol dehydrogenase type3 (ADH3)** gene catalyzes the oxidation of ethanol to acetaldehyde [104]. Genetic polymorphisms result altered kinetic properties of enzyme. Gamma1 and gamma2 are two different alleles of ADH3 and moderate drinkers with the "high-risk" (gamma1 gamma1) genotype appeared to have a threefold higher risk of UBC as compared to moderate drinkers with a "low-risk"(gamma1 gamma2 or gamma2 gamma2) genotype [104].

14.5.2.4 Cytokine Genes and UBC Risk

Cytokines have a significant role in cancer development. Cytokines plays the role of inflammatory mediator during cell damage, infection and oxidative stress and inflammation is observed as a "secret killer", as well as inflammatory components are present in the microenvironment of most neoplastic tissue, including some in which a direct relationship with inflammation has not yet been proven [105]. Therefore, by targeting gene responsible for inflammation, diagnostic and prognostic markers can be designed. Well studied cytokines in relation with UBC risk has been summarized.

Interleukine-6 (IL-6) is a pleiotropic and multifunctional cytokine, particularly involved in immune inflammatory response. It plays a key role in the initiation of different intracellular pathways like JAK/STAT, MAPK, PI3K that concomitantly activate expression of other genes resulting in enduring inflammation and cancer development [106]. IL-6 is known to possess both pro-inflammatory and anti-inflammatory effects [107]. In the urinary bladder, IL-6 may transform urothelial cell and provide selective growth advantage to urothelial cancerous cells. In vitro examination demonstrates that urothelial malignant cells secrete a large amount of IL-6 as compared to normal urothelium and treatment with anti-IL-6 antibody and antisense oligonucleotide was found to exert anti-tumor effect [108]. IL-6 is also involved in cancer cell differentiation, tumor growth and change in the microenvironment of tissue. Immuno-histochemistry studies reveal that IL-6 immuno-positivity was seen in 80% of the cases and IL-6 has been suggested to be a prognostic marker and a target for anti-cancer therapy [109]. IL-6-174 G → C variation affects gene transcription and the level of

IL-6 protein [110]. **Interleukine-4 (IL-4)** is an anti-inflammatory cytokine by virtue of its ability to suppress genes of pro-inflammatory cytokines. IL-4 is chiefly produced by activated CD4+ T cell, mast cell and basophils. IL-4 plays a key role in surveillance and elimination of transformed cells by Th2 development, eliminating extracellular pathogens and inhibiting Th1 [111]. Population based studies observed that genetic variation of IL-4 is associated with UBC risk [112–114].

Transforming growth factor-β (TGF- β) gene encodes for a signal transduction protein that normally controls cellular homeostasis in normal cell and early stages of cancer; however, in late stages, the pathway is believed to help in tumor proliferation and metastasis. There are three isoforms of TGF-β: TGF-β1, TGF-β2, and TGF-β3; each of them being encoded by distinct genes. TGF-β1 harbors many genetic variations that influence TGF-β1 protein expression [115]. TGF-β1 is a potent inhibitor of proliferation in epithelial cells and act as tumor suppressor, it controls cell proliferation by reducing the ability if cell to enter S-phase [116], while loss of this response associates with continuous expression of TGF-β by cancerous cells which assists aggressive progression of cancer [117, 118]. Since TGF-β1 plays dual roles in cellular processes, its expression and association with different carcinomas has been found depending on cellular content and tumor stage. Cancerous cells become resistant to inhibitory effect of TGF-β1 through mutations or inactivation of TGF-β1 receptors. In the late stages of cancer, TGF-β1 makes the microenvironment like angiogenesis, evasion of apoptosis and proliferation that favors the progression and metastases of cancer [119–121]. Polymorphisms in the TGF-β1 result significant association with the risk of UBC [122–124].

Tumor necrosis factor alpha (TNF-α) gene is the primary mediator of inflammation, host defense and tissue homeostasis/cellular organization. Depending on its concentration and duration of cell exposed, TNF-α have beneficial or harmful consequences including destruction of blood vessels and cell-mediated killing of certain tumors as well as acting as a tumor promoter [125]. An individual's resistance ability in response to these risk factors may be changed due to variation in genetic composition of TNF-α [126]. TNF-α has also been linked to all steps involved in tumorigenesis, including cellular transformation, promotion, survival, proliferation, invasion, angiogenesis, and metastasis [126]. Tumor cells secrete their own TNF-α in autocrine manner which further enhance the expression of other growth factors like epidermal growth factor receptor (EGFR) [127]. The discovery of functional regulatory polymorphisms of TNF-α gene and its receptors have led to a conceptual breakthrough in our understanding of the genetic control of inflammation and its other functions [128]. The connection between TNF-α gene polymorphisms and UBC is controversial [129–131].

Peroxisome proliferator-activated receptors (PPARs) gene is a ligand-activated intracellular transcription factors and have a significant role in cellular differentiation, development and metabolism [132]. There are three known types of PPARs; alpha (α), beta (β) and gamma (γ). A remarkable attention has been given to PPARgamma for its important role in anti-inflammatory response. Genetic polymorphism in the coding region of PPARgamma affects PPARgamma's receptor activity [133]. PPARgamma expression in human bladder tumor (BT) is statistically high as well as correlation between PPARgamma expression and progression of UBC is also found [134]. In addition, agonists of PPARgamma have been used as promising therapeutic target [135].

Cyclooxygenase-2 (COX-2) gene also known as prostaglandin-endoperoxide synthase (PTGS) has a fundamental role in inflammatory response. COX-2 serves as a mediator of acute and chronic response to inflammation and involved in cellular repair and proliferation [136]. Therefore, pharmaceutical inhibition of COX-2 provides aid from pain and inflammation. Genetic variations of COX-2 result in aberrant expression of COX-2 that has been found to be associated with carcinogenesis [137]. Genetic polymorphisms of COX-2 have also a significant association with UBC in smokers [138, 139].

Several DNA genetic markers have association with UBC. Genetic alterations in non-invasive UBC and muscle-invasive UBC of urinary bladder caused by different genes that act separately or mutually in the pathogenesis and progression of UBC. Focusing on genes of vital pathway of tumor-suppressor genes, tumor-promoter genes, cell cycle regulation and cell-signaling can predict nature of tumor.

Fibroblast growth factors (FGFs) play crucial role in cell homeostasis and in pathological process. Mutation in **fibroblast growth factors receptor (FGFR-3)** results in its over-expression and has strong association with low-grade non-muscle invasive TCCs. On the other hand, high grade and higher stage TCC are associated with decreasing expression of FGFR-3. Hence this molecular marker can give important prognostic information for non-muscle invasive UBC [140]. Furthermore, inhibition of FGFR using TKI258 an FGFR3 inhibitor, has a cytotoxic role on cancerous urothelial cells, hence targeting these pathways are currently being studied in clinical trials as potential treatments for UBC (www.clinicaltrials.gov NCT00790426) [141].

Cyclin D1 and Cyclin E has a vital role in cell-cycle regulation and critical target of proliferation signals in G1-phase. Alteration in their expression associated with progression of cancer. Cyclin D1 protein is found in higher levels in non-invasive UBC compared to muscle-invasive UBC and patients with over-expressed cyclin D1 have a significantly lower survival rate compared to patients having a lower expression of cyclin D1, [142]. While elevated level of cyclin E shorten the G1 phase and induces tumor development. Therefore both have clinical value as a prognostic marker and potential therapeutic target [143] (Table 14.3).

TP53 gene located on short arm of chromosome 17 has a key role of tumor suppressor via cell cycle regulation and apoptosis [146]. Mutation in TP53 gene has strong association with high stage and high grade of UBC and nearly 50% of muscle invasive UBC show this mutation. Few studies have investigated its association with progression of UBC [146–148] although, a well-designed meta-analysis of 117 studies observed that there is insufficient evidence to conclude that TP53 is a good prognostic marker [149]. Recent clinical trial also found no association of TP53 mutation with recurrence rate in UBC patients [150]. However, TP53 mutation increases with tumor grade and stage while FGFR-3 mutation increases with tumor grade and stage [151]. TP53 also regulate expression of **p21** gene which plays a crucial role in cell proliferation, DNA replication and DNA repair. **Retinoblastoma (RB)** gene located on long arm of chromosome13 is also a tumor suppressor gene which has a central role in apoptosis and cell growth regulation [152]. Deletion or mutations of this gene have a correlation with higher stage, grade and poor prognosis [152].

Tumor promoter gene like vascular endothelial growth factor (VEGF) and epidermal growth factor receptor (EGFRs) plays an important role in carcinogenesis. VEGF promote angiogenesis that is a crucial step in carcinogenesis. VEGF expression is associated with high grade and stage of UBC and the presence of high level of VEGF in later stage of cancer can predict tumor metastasis [153, 154]. Clinical trials are in progress to investigate the therapeutic role of VEGF. Suramin is a strong inhibitor of angiogenic factors used against VEGF in preventing angiogenesis. **Epidermal growth factor receptor (EGFR)** related to tyrosine kinase growth factor receptor have role in cell signaling, growth and differentiation [153]. Over-expression of this genetic marker strongly associated with high

Table 14.3 Potential DNA genetic markers of non-invasive UBC

S. no.	Non-muscle invasive UBC (Low grade)	Location	Prospective prognostic value	Reference
1	FGFR3	4p16.3	Low grade, low stage	[140]
2	Cyclin D1	11q13	Low grade, low stage, recurrence	[143, 144]
3	Cyclin E	19q12	Low stage survival	[145]

grade and stage of UBC [154]. Currently, EGFR targeted treatment is being investigated for UBC in several trials (CALBG-90102, NCT00088946, NCT00380029). Therefore, VEGF and EGFR markers have a great interest to provide an idea about drugs that could help fight with UBC.

Survivin is located on short arm of chromosome 17, has important role in normal cell division and inhibition of apoptosis [155]. It is majorly expressed by embryonic and fetal tissues and minimally by normal human tissues. However, pathologically survivin is exclusively extracted from malignant tissues and is a marker of grave prognosis [155]. Therefore it is hugely investigated in various cancers including UBC. It can easily measure in urine of UBC patients. A systematic review observing the role of urinary survivin in the UBC diagnosis found that the pooled sensitivity and specificity of the urinary survivin tests were 95% CI 0.772 (0.745–0.797) and 95% CI 0.918 (0.899–0.934), respectively [156]. It also reported that urinary survivin had better sensitivity than urinary cytology for diagnosing bladder cancer [156].

Another relevant marker, **Cytokeratin-20 (CK-20)** is normally present in the umbrella cells of the urothelium. The expression of the CK-20 in deeper cells layers is associated with recurrence, aggressiveness and progression of UBC [157]. CK-20 expression in the urine can predict the invasiveness of UBC [152] (Table 14.4).

14.5.2.5 Epigenetic Molecular Markers

Epigenetics is the study of inherited reversible changes in gene function or other cell phenotypes that occur without any alteration in DNA sequence. Epigenetic changes in DNA alter expression of related genes via silencing of tumor suppressor genes due to alteration of DNA methylation that consequently results in carcinogenesis [159]. In recent studies DNA hypermethylation is frequently investigated and widely linked to pathogenesis and aggressiveness of various cancers including UBC [160]. In UBC patients hypermethylation of CpG islands around the promoter region results in decreased expression of tumor-suppressor genes RUNX3, RASSFIA, p16, RARβ AND E-cadherin [161]. Among these tumor-suppressor genes RUNX3 is mainly interesting because methylation of its promoter region confers 100-fold increased risk of UBC [162]. Therefore, epigenetic drugs such as DNA methylase inhibitor or histone deacetylase inhibitors which can restore the activity of suppressed gene are chiefly area of interest.

14.6 Conclusion

The use of molecular markers has facilitated the development of novel and more accurate diagnostic, prognostic, and therapeutic strategies. However, advance research in cancer genomics results overabundance of molecular biomarkers

Table 14.4 Potential genetic markers of muscle-invasive UBC

S. no.	Muscle invasive UBC/ carcinoma *in situ*	Location	Prospective prognostic value	Reference
1	RB	13q14.2	High stage, prognosis, recurrence, survival, progression	[163]
2	P53	17p13.1	High stage, prognosis, recurrence, survival, progression	[149, 150]
3	P21	6p21.2	High stage, progression	[164]
4	P27	12p13.1	High grade, survival	[158]
5	EGFRs	7p12	High grade and stage	[154]
6	VEGF	Chromosome 6	High grade and stage	[153, 154]
7	CK20	Chromosome 17	Recurrence, progression	[152, 157]
8	Survivin	Chromosome 17	Prognosis	[156]

but there is also a need to elucidate crosstalk between the markers of different pathways. Prospective trials are still needed, however, to objectively establish the true benefit of these markers in prognostic and therapeutic field.

References

1. Ferlay J, Shin HR, Bray F, Forman D, Mathers C, Parkin DM. Cancer incidence and mortality worldwide: GLOBOCAN 2008 v2.0. Lyon: International Agency for Research; 2010. Report No.: IARC CancerBase No. 10.
2. Jemal A, Bray F, Center MM, et al. Global cancer statistics. CA Cancer J Clin. 2011;61:69.
3. Edwards BK, Ward E, Kohler BA, et al. Annual report to the nation on the status of cancer, 1975-2006, featuring colorectal cancer trends and impact of interventions (risk factors, screening, and treatment) to reduce future rates. Cancer. 2010;116:544–73.
4. Karim-Kos HE, de Vries E, Soerjomataram I, et al. Recent trends of cancer in Europe: a combined approach of incidence, survival and mortality for 17 cancer sites since the 1990s. Eur J Cancer. 2008;44:1345–89.
5. Burger M, Catto JW, Dalbagni G, et al. Epidemiology and risk factors of urothelial bladder cancer. Eur Urol. 2013;63:234–41.
6. Fajkovic H, Halpern JA, Cha EK, et al. Impact of gender on bladder cancer incidence, staging, and prognosis. World J Urol. 2011;29:457–63.
7. Pelucchi C, Bosetti C, Negri E, et al. Mechanisms of disease: the epidemiology of bladder cancer. Nat Clin Pract Urol. 2006;3:327–40.
8. Madeb R, Messing EM. Gender, racial and age differences in bladder cancer incidence and mortality. Urol Oncol. 2004;22:86–92.
9. Underwood W 3rd, Dunn RL, Williams C, et al. Gender and geographic influence on the racial disparity in bladder cancer mortality in the US. J Am Coll Surg. 2006;202:284–90.
10. Yee DS, Ishill NM, Lowrance WT, et al. Ethnic differences in bladder cancer survival. Urology. 2011;78:544–9.
11. Vineis P, Simonato L. Proportion of lung and bladder cancers in males resulting from occupation: a systematic approach. Arch Environ Health. 1991;46:6–15.
12. Zeegers MP, Tan FE, Dorant E, et al. The impact of characteristics of cigarette smoking on urinary tract cancer risk: a meta-analysis of epidemiologic studies. Cancer. 2000;89:630–9.
13. Murata M, Tamura A, Tada M, et al. Mechanism of oxidative DNA damage induced by carcinogenic 4-aminobiphenyl. Free Radic Biol Med. 2001;30:765–73.
14. Fontcuberta M, Arqués JF, Martínez M, et al. Polycyclic aromatic hydrocarbons in food samples collected in Barcelona, Spain. J Food Prot. 2006;69:2024–8.
15. Jacobsen BK, Bjelke E, Kvåle G, et al. Coffee drinking, mortality, and cancer incidence: results from a Norwegian prospective study. J Natl Cancer Inst. 1986;76:823–31.
16. Pelucchi C, Galeone C, Tramacere I, et al. Alcohol drinking and bladder cancer risk: a meta-analysis. Ann Oncol. 2012;23:1586–93.
17. Zeegers MP, Tan FE, Verhagen AP, et al. Elevated risk of cancer of the urinary tract for alcohol drinkers: a metaanalysis. Cancer Causes Control. 1999;10:445–51.
18. Pelucchi C, La Vecchia C. Alcohol, coffee, and bladder cancer risk: a review of epidemiological studies. Eur J Cancer Prev. 2009;18:62–8.
19. Takanashi H, Also S, Hirono I, et al. Carcinogenicity test of Quercetin and kaempferol in rats by oral administration. J Food Saf. 1983;5(2):55–60.
20. Jankovic S, Radosavljevic V. Risk factors for bladder cancer. Tumori. 2007;93(1):4–12.
21. Howe GR, Burch JD, Miller AB, et al. Tobacco use, occupation, coffee, various nutrients and bladder cancer. J Natl Cancer Inst. 1980;64:701–13.
22. Rehn L. Bladder tumors in Fuchsine-workers. Married Dtsch Gesellsch Chir. 1895;24:240–52.
23. Hueper WC, Wiley FH, Wolfe HD. Experimental production of bladder tumors in dogs by administration of ß-naphthylamine. J Ind Hyg Tox. 1938;20:46–84.
24. Wallace DMA. Occupational urothelial cancer. Br J Urol. 1988;61:175–82.
25. Clapp RW, Jacob MM, Loechler EL. Environmental and occupational causes of cancer: new evidence 2005-2007. Rev Environ Health. 2008;23(1):1–37.
26. Angervall L, Bengtsson U, Zetterlund CG, et al. Renal pelvic carcinoma in a Swedish district with abuse of a phenacetin-containing drug. Br J Urol. 1969;41:401–5.
27. Knight A, Askling J, Granath F, et al. Urinary bladder cancer in Wegener's granulomatosis: risks and relation to cyclophosphamide. Ann Rheum Dis. 2004;63:1307–11.
28. Laursen B. Cancer of the bladder in patients treated with chlornaphazine. Br Med J. 1970;3:684–5.
29. IARC. Aromatic amines, organic dyes, and related exposures. IARC Monogr Eval Carcinog Risks Hum. 2010;99:1–658.
30. IARC. Chemical agents and related occupations. IARC Monogr Eval Carcinog Risks Hum. 2012;100(Pt-F):9-562.
31. Bartsch H, Ohshima H, Pignatelli B, et al. Endogenously formed N-nitroso compounds and nitrosating agents in human cancer etiology. Pharmacogenetics. 1992;2:272–7.

32. Arlt VM, Stiborova M, Schmeiser HH. Aristolochic acid as a probable human cancer hazard in herbal remedies: a review. Mutagenesis. 2002;17:265–77.
33. Goldgar DE, Easton DF, Cannon-Albright LA, et al. Systematic population-based assessment of cancer risk in first-degree relatives of cancer probands. J Natl Cancer Inst. 1994;86(21):1600–8.
34. Plna K, Hemminki K. Familial bladder cancer in the National Swedish Family Cancer Database. J Urol. 2001;166:2129–33.
35. Crawford JM. The origins of bladder cancer. Lab Investig. 2008;88(7):686–93.
36. Hail M, Grover PL. Polycyclic aromatic hydrocarbons: metabolism, activation, and tumour initiation. In: Cooper CS, Grover PL, editors. Chemical carcinogenesis and mutagenesis. 1st ed. Berlin: Springer; 1990. p. 327–72.
37. Shields PG, Harris CC. Principles of carcinogenesis: chemical. In: DeVita VT, Hellman S, Rosenberg SA, editors. Cancer: principles and practice of oncology. Chapt 11. 4th ed. Philadelphia: Lippincott; 1993. p. 200–12.
38. Kadlubar FF. DNA adducts of carcinogenic aromatic amines. IARC Sci Pub. 1994;125:199–216.
39. Robbins JR, Yang L-NL, Anderson BG, et al. Photogenerated arylnitrenium ions. Reactions of N-tertbutyl 1(2-acetyl 1±4-substituted) phenyl nitrenium ions with alcohols and water studied by laser flash photolysis. J Am Chem Soc. 1995;117:6544–52.
40. Longe J. Gale encyclopedia of cancer: a guide to cancer and its treatments, vol. 137. Detroit: Thomson Gale; 2005.
41. Hall RR, Prout GR. Staging of bladder cancer: is the tumor, node, metastasis system adequate? Semin Oncol. 1990;17:517–23.
42. Malmstrom PU, Wijkstrom H, Thordtenson A, et al. Recurrence, progression and survival in bladder cancer: a retrospective analysis of 232 patients with greater than or equal to 5-year follow-up. Scand J Urol Nephrol. 1987;21:185–95.
43. Mostofi FKDC, Sesterhnn IA. Histological typing of urinary bladder tumors. Geneva: WHO; 1999.
44. Montironi R, Lopez-Beltran A. The 2004 WHO classification of bladder tumors: a summary and commentary. Int J Surg Pathol. 2005;13:143–53.
45. Larsson P, Wijkstrom H, Thorstenson A, et al. A population based study of 53 patients with newly detected urinary bladder neoplasms followed during 5 years. Scand J Urol Nephrol. 2003;37: 195–201.
46. Sankaranarayanan R, Swaminathan R, Brenner H, et al. Cancer survival in Africa, Asia, and Central America: a population-based study. Lancet Oncol. 2010;11(2):165–73.
47. Altekruse SF, Kosary CL, Krapcho M, et al., editors. SEER cancer statistics review; 1975 2007. Bethesda: National Cancer Institute. http://seer.cancer.gov/csr/1975_2007/ [based on November 2009 SEER data submission, posted to the SEER web site 2010].
48. Sant M, Allemani C, Santaquilani M, et al. EUROCARE working group: survival of cancer patients diagnosed in 1995–1999. Results and commentary. Eur J Cancer. 2009;45(6):931–91.
49. Smith ZL, Guzzo TJ. Urinary markers of bladder cancer. F1000Prime Rep. 2013;5:5–21.
50. Kim WJ, Bae SC. Molecular biomarkers in urothelial bladder cancer. Cancer Sci. 2008;99(4):646–52.
51. Shariat SF, Karam JA, Lerner SP. Molecular markers in bladder cancer. Curr Opin Urol. 2008;18(1):1–8.
52. Lokeshwar VB, Habuchi T, Grossman HB, et al. Bladder tumor markers beyond cytology: International Consensus Panel on bladder tumor markers. Urology. 2005;66:35–63.
53. Van RBW, Van DPHG, Van DKTH. Urine markers for bladder cancer surveillance: a systematic review. Eur Urol. 2005;47:736–48.
54. Hanahan D, Weinberg RA. The hallmarks of cancer. Cell. 2000;100:57–70.
55. Hanahan D, Weinberg RA. The hallmarks of cancer: the next generation. Cell. 2011;144(5):646–74.
56. Botstein D, Risch N. Discovering genotype underlying human phenotype: past successes for mendelian disease, future approaches for complex disease. Nat Genet. 2003;33(Suppl):228–37.
57. Knowles MA. What we could do now: molecular pathology of bladder cancer. Mol Pathol. 2001;54:215–21.
58. Fadl-Elmula I, Kytola S, Pan Y, et al. Characterization of chromosomal abnormalities in uroepithelial carcinomas by G-banding, spectral karyotyping and FISH analysis. Int J Cancer. 2001;92:824–31.
59. Sardi I, Bartoletti R, Occhini I, et al. Microsatellite alterations in superficial and locally advanced transitional cell carcinoma of the bladder. Oncol Rep. 1999;6:901–5.
60. Thibodeau SN, Bren G, Schaid D. Microsatellite instability in cancer of the proximal colon. Science. 1993;260:816–9.
61. Tsai YC, Nichols PW, Hiti AL, et al. Allelic losses of chromosomes 9, 11, and 17 in human bladder cancer. Cancer Res. 1990;50:44–7.
62. Presti JC Jr, Reuter VE, Galan T, et al. Molecular genetic alterations in superficial and locally advanced human bladder cancer. Cancer Res. 1991;51:5405–9.
63. Altayli E, et al. CYP1A2, CYP2D6, GSTM1, GSTP1, and GSTT1 gene polymorphisms in patients with bladder cancer in a Turkish population. Int Urol Nephrol. 2009;41(2):259–66.
64. Pavanello S, et al. CYP1A2 polymorphisms, occupational and environmental exposures and risk of bladder cancer. Eur J Epidemiol. 2010;25(7): 491–500.
65. Tian Z, et al. Role of CYP1A2 1F polymorphism in cancer risk: evidence from a meta-analysis of 46 case-control studies. Gene. 2013;524(2): 168–74.
66. Tao L, et al. Cytochrome P4501A2 phenotype and bladder cancer risk: the Shanghai bladder cancer study. Int J Cancer. 2012;130(5):1174–83.

67. Brockmoller J, Cascorbi I, Henning S, et al. Molecular genetics of cancer susceptibility. Pharmacology. 2000;61:212–27.
68. Strange RC, Fryer AA. The glutathione S-transferases: influence of polymorphism on cancer susceptibility. In: Vineis P, Malats N, Lang M, d'Errico A, Caporaso N, Cuzick J, Boffetta P, editors. Metabolic polymorphisms and susceptibility to cancer. Lyon: IARC; 1999. p. 231–49.
69. Hayes JD, Pulford DJ. The glutathione S-transferase supergene family: regulation of GST and the contribution of the isoenzymes to cancer chemo-protection and drug resistance. Crit Rev Biochem Mol Biol. 1995;30:445–600.
70. Mishra DK, Kumar A, Srivastava DSL, et al. Allelic variation of GSTT1, GSTM1 and GSTP1 genes in north Indian population. Asian Pac J Cancer Prev. 2004;5:362–5.
71. Smith CM, Kelsey KT, Wiencke JK, et al. Inherited glutathione S-transferase deficiency is a risk factor for pulmonary asbestosis. Cancer Epidemiol Biomark Prev. 1994;3:471–7.
72. Shao J, Gu M, Zhang Z, et al. Genetic variants of the cytochrome P450 and glutathione S-transferase associated risk of bladder cancer in a south-eastern Chinese population. Int J Urol. 2008;15:216–21.
73. Grando JP, Kuasne H, Losi-Guembarovski R, et al. Association between polymorphisms in the biometabolism gene CYP1A1, GSTM1, GSTT1 and GSTP1 in bladder cancer. Clin Exp Med. 2009;9:21–8.
74. McGrath M, Michaud D, De Vivo I. Polymorphisms in GSTT1, GSTM1, NAT1 and NAT2 genes and bladder cancer risk in men and women. BMC Cancer. 2006;6:239.
75. Nelson HH, Wiencke JK, Christiani DC, et al. Ethnic differences in the prevalence of the homozygous deleted genotype of glutathione S-transferase q. Carcinogenesis. 1995;16:1243–5.
76. Brockmoller J, Cascorbi I, Kerb R, et al. Combined analysis of inherited polymorphisms in Arylamine N-acetyltransferase 2, glutathione S-transferases M1 and T1, microsomal epoxide hydrolase, and cytochrome P450 enzymes as modulators of bladder cancer risk. Cancer Res. 1996;56:3915–25.
77. Moore LE, Wiencke JK, Bates MN, et al. Investigation of genetic polymorphisms and smoking in a bladder cancer case- control study in Argentina. Cancer Lett. 2004;211:199–207.
78. Sanyal S, Festa F, Sakano S, et al. Polymorphisms in DNA repair and metabolic genes in bladder cancer. Carcinogenesis. 2004;25:729–34.
79. Srivastava DS, Kumar A, Mittal RD, et al. NAT2 gene polymorphism in bladder cancer: a study from north India. Int J Hum Genet. 2004;4:201–5.
80. Ali-Osmam F, Akande O, Antoun G, et al. Molecular cloning, characterization and expression in Escherichia coli of full length cDNAs of three human glutathione S-transferase pi gene variants. Evidence for different catalytic activity of the encoded protiens. J Biol Chem. 1997;272:10004–12.
81. Wu K, Wang X, Xie Z, et al. Glutathione S-transferase P1 gene polymorphism and bladder cancer susceptibility: an updated analysis. Mol Biol Rep. 2013;40:687–95.
82. Inskip A, Elexperu-Camiruaga J, Buxton N, et al. Identification of polymorphism at the glutathione S-transferase, GSTM3 locus: evidence for linkage with GSTM1*A. Biochem J. 1995;312:713–6.
83. Hein DW, Doll MA, Rustan TD, et al. Metabolic activation and deactivation of arylamine carcinogens by recombinant human NAT1 and polymorphic Mat2 acetyltransferases. Carcinogenesis. 1993;14:1633–8.
84. Hein DW, Doll MA, Fretland AJ, et al. Molecular genetics and epidemiology of the NAT1 and NAT2 acetylation polymorphisms. Cancer Epidemiol Biomark Prev. 2000;9:29–42.
85. Jian G, Liang D, Wang Y, et al. Effects of N-acetly transferase 1 and 2 polymorphisms on bladder cancer risk in Caucasians. Mutat Res. 2005;581:97–104.
86. Franekova M, Halasova E, Bukovska E, et al. Gene polymorphisms in bladder cancer. Urol Oncol. 2008;26(1):1–8.
87. Carreon T, Ruder AM, Schulte PA, et al. NAT2 slow acetylation and bladder cancer in workers exposed to benzidine. Int J Cancer. 2006;118:161–8.
88. Hsieh FI, Pu YS, Chern HD, et al. Genetic polymorphisms on M-acetyltransferase 1 and 2 and risk of cigarette smoking-related bladder cancer. Br J Cancer. 1999;81:537–41.
89. Weber WW, Hein DW. N-acetylation pharmacogenetics. Pharmacol Rev. 1985;37:25–79.
90. Taylor JA, Umbach DM, Stephens E, et al. The role of N-acetylation polymorphisms in smoking-associated bladder cancer: evidence of a gene-gene-exposure three-way interaction. Cancer Res. 1998;58(16):3603–10.
91. Hung RJ, Boffetta P, Brennan P, et al. Genetic polymorphism of MPO, COMT, MnSOD, NQO1, interaction with environmental exposures and bladder cancer risk. Carcinogenesis. 2004;25:973–8.
92. Sanderson S, Salanti G, Higgins J. Joint effects of the N-acetyltransferase 1 and 2 (NAT1 and NAT2) genes and smoking on bladder carcinogenesis: a literature-based systematic HuGE review and evidence synthesis. Am J Epidemiol. 2007;166(7):741–51.
93. Zheng L, Wang Y, Schabath MB, et al. Sulfotransferase 1A1 (SULT1A1) polymorphism and bladder cancer risk: a case-control study. Cancer Lett. 2003;202:61–9.
94. Hu DG, Mackenzie PI, McKinnon RA, et al. Genetic polymorphisms of human UDP-glucuronosyltransferase (UGT) genes and cancer risk. Drug Metab Rev. 2016;48:47–69.
95. Lin GF, Guo WC, Chen JG, et al. An association of UDPglucuronosyltransferase 2B7 C802T (His268Tyr) polymorphism with bladder cancer in benzidine-exposed workers in China. Toxicol Sci. 2005;85:502–6.
96. Kadlubar FF, Butler MA, Kaderlik KR, et al. Polymorphisms for aromatic amine metabolism

in humans: relevance for human carcinogenesis. Environ Health Perspect. 1992;98:69–74.
97. Piedrafita FJ, Molander RB, Vansant G, et al. An Alu element in the myeloperoxidase promoter contains a composite SP1-thyroid hormone-retinoic acid response element. J Biol Chem. 1996;271:14412–20.
98. Zhu BT. Catechol-O-methyltransferase (COMT)-mediated methylation metabolism of endogenous bioactive catechols and modulation by endobitics and xenobiotics: importance in pathophysiology and pathogenesis. Curr Drug Metab. 2002;3:321–49.
99. Lotta T, Vidgren J, Tilgmann C, et al. Kinetics of human soluble and membrane-bound catechol O-methyltransferase: a revised mechanism and description of the thermolabile variant of the enzyme. Biochemistry. 1995;34:4202–10.
100. McCord JM. Superoxide dismutase in aging and disease: an overview. Methods Enzymol. 2002;349:331–41.
101. Rosenblum JS, Gilula NB, Lerner RA. On signal sequence polymorphisms and diseases of distribution. Proc Natl Acad Sci U S A. 1996;93:4471–3.
102. Chada S, Whitney C, Newburger PE. Posttranscriptional regulation of glutathione peroxidase gene expression by selenium in the HL-60 human myeloid cell line. Blood. 1989;74:2535–41.
103. Hu YJ, Diamond AM. Role of glutathione peroxidase 1 in breast cancer: loss of heterozygosity and allelic differences in the response to selenium. Cancer Res. 2003;63:3347–51.
104. van Dijk B, van Houwelingen KP, Witjes JA, et al. Alcohol dehydrogenase type 3 (ADH3) and the risk of bladder cancer. Eur Urol. 2001;40:509–14.
105. Zhu Z, Shen Z, Xu C. Inflammatory pathways as promising targets to increase chemotherapy response in bladder cancer. Mediat Inflamm. 2012;2012:1–11.
106. Tawara K, Jorcyk C, Oxford JT. Clinical significance of interleukin (IL)-6 in cancer metastasis to bone: potential of anti-IL-6 therapies. Cancer Manag Res. 2011;3:177–89.
107. Scheller J, Chalaris A, Schmidt-Arras D, et al. The pro- and anti inflammatory properties of the cytokine interleukin-6. Biochim Biophys Acta. 2011;1813:878–88.
108. Li CG, Li ML, Shu XH, et al. Antitumor effects of recombinant human interleukin-6 on mouse bladder carcinoma through Fas-mediated apoptosis. Cancer Chemother Pharmacol. 2010;66(5):981–6.
109. Naik DS, Sharma S, Ray A, et al. Epidermal growth factor receptor expression in urinary bladder cancer. Indian J Urol. 2011;27:208–14.
110. Fishman D, Faulds G, Jeffery R, et al. The effect of novel polymorphisms in the interleukin-6 (IL-6) gene on IL-6 transcription and plasma IL-6 levels, and an association with systemic-onset juvenile chronic arthritis. J Clin Invest. 1998;102:1369–76.
111. Muller-Hermelink N, Braumuller H, Pichler B, et al. TNFR1 signalling and IFN-gamma signalling determine whether T cells induce tumor dormancy or promote multistage carcinogenesis. Cancer Cell. 2008;13:507–18.
112. Chu H, Ma L, Wang M, et al. The polymorphisms of IL-4, IL-4R and IL-13 genes and bladder cancer risk in a Chinese population: a case-control study. Mol Biol Rep. 2012;395:5349–57.
113. Gaur P, Mittal M, Mohanti B, Das S. Functional variants of IL4 and IL6 genes and risk of tobacco-related oral carcinoma in high-risk Asian Indians. Oral Dis. 2011;17:720–6.
114. Gomes M, Coelho A, Araujo A, Teixeira AL, Catarino R, Medeiros R. Influence of functional genetic polymorphism (-590C/T) in non-small cell lung cancer (NSCLC) development: the paradoxal role of IL-4. Gene. 2012;504:111–5.
115. Watanable Y, Kinoshita A, Yamada T, et al. A catalog of 106 single-nucleotide polymorphisms (SNPs) and 11 other types of variations in genes for transforming growth factor-beta1 (TGF-beta1) and its signaling pathway. J Hum Genet. 2002;47:478–83.
116. Alexandrow MG, Moses HL. Transforming growth factor β and cell cycle regulation. Cancer Res. 1995;55:1452–7.
117. Massague J. Receptors for the TGF-β family. Cell. 1992;69:1067–70.
118. Parsons R, Myeroff LL, Liu B, et al. Microsatellite instability and mutations of the transforming growth factor β type II receptor gene in colorectal cancer. Cancer Res. 1995;55:5548–50.
119. Ding Z, Wu CJ, Chu GC, et al. SMAD4-dependent barrier constrains prostate cancer growth and metastatic progression. Nature. 2011;470:269–73.
120. Kubiczkova L, Sedlarikova L, Hajek R, et al. TGF-β—an excellent servant but a bad master. J Transl Med. 2012;10:183.
121. Noordhuis MG, Fehrmann RS, Wisman GB, et al. Involvement of the TGF-β and β-catenin pathways in pelvic lymph node metastasis in early-stage cervical cancer. Clin Cancer Res. 2011;17(6):1317–30.
122. Gautam KA, Singh P, Sankhwar SN, et al. c.29C>T polymorphism in the transforming growth factor-β1 (TGFB1) gene correlates with increased risk of urinary bladder cancer. Cytokine. 2015;75(2):344–8.
123. Joshi NN, Kale MD, Hake SS, et al. Transforming growth factor β signaling pathway associated gene polymorphisms may explain lower breast cancer risk in western Indian women. PLoS One. 2011;6(8):e21866.
124. Wu GY, Lu Q, Hasenberg T, et al. Association between EGF, TGF-β1, TNF-α gene polymorphisms and cancer of the pancreatic head. Anticancer Res. 2010;30:5257–62.
125. Balkwill F. Tumor necrosis factor or tumor promoting factor? Cytokine Growth Factor Rev. 2002;13:135–41.
126. Sethi G, Sung B, Aggarwal B. TNF: a master switch for inflammation to cancer. Front Biosci. 2008;13:5094–107.
127. Schmiegel W, Roeder C, Schmielau J, et al. Tumor necrosis factor alpha induces the expression of transforming growth factor alpha and the epidermal growth factor receptor. Proc Natl Acad Sci U S A. 1993;90:863–7.

128. McDermott MF. TNF and TNFR biology in health and disease. Cell Mol Biol. 2001;47:619–35.
129. Azmy IAK, Balasubramanian SP, Wilson AG, et al. Role of tumor necrosis factor gene polymorphisms (−308 and −238) in breast cancer susceptibility and severity. Breast Cancer Res. 2004;6:395–400.
130. Gupta R, Sharma SC, Das SN, et al. Association of TNF-alpha and TNFR1 promoters and 3'UTR region of TNFR2 gene polymorphisms with genetic susceptibility to tobacco-related oral carcinoma in Asian Indians. Oral Oncol. 2008;44:455–63.
131. Kohaar I, Tiwari P, Kumar R, et al. Association of single nucleotide polymorphisms (SNPs) in TNF-LTA locus with breast cancer risk in Indian population. Breast Cancer Res Treat. 2009;114:347–55.
132. Dunning KR, Anastasi MR, Zhang VJ, et al. Regulation of fatty acid oxidation in mouse cumulus-oocyte complexes during maturation and modulation by PPAR agonists. PLoS One. 2014;9(2):e87327.
133. Wang Y, Lerner S, Leibovici D, et al. Polymorphisms in the inflammatory genes IL-6, IL-8, TNF- alpha, NFKB1, and PPARG and bladder cancer risk. Proc Am Assoc Cancer Res Abstract. 2004;45:3979.
134. Yoshimura R, Matsuyama M, Segawa Y, et al. Expression of peroxisome proliferator-receptors (PPARs) in human urinary bladder carcinoma and growth inhibition by its agonists. Int J Cancer. 2003;104(5):597–602.
135. Mansure JJ, Nassim R, Kassouf W. Peroxisome proliferator-activated receptors gamma in bladder cancer: a promising therapeutic target. Cancer Biol Ther. 2009;8(7):6–15.
136. Vane JR, Bakhle YS, Botting R. Cyclooxygenases 1 and 2. Annu Rev Pharmacol Toxicol. 1998;38:493–501.
137. Tsujii M, Kawano S, Tsujii S, et al. Cyclooxygenase regulates angiogenesis induced by colon cancer cells. Cell. 1998;93:705–16.
138. Gangwar R, Mandhani A, Mittal RD. Functional polymorphisms of cyclooxygenase-2 (COX-2 gene) and risk of urinary bladder cancer in India. Surgery. 2011;149(1):126–34.
139. Kang S, Kim YB, Kim MH, et al. Polymorphism in the nuclear factor kappa-B binding promoter region of cyclooxygenase-2 is associated with an increased risk of bladder cancer. Cancer Lett. 2005;217:11–6.
140. Shariat SF, Chade DC, Karakiewicz PI, et al. Combination of multiple molecular markers can improve prognostication in patients with locally advanced and lymph node positive bladder Cancer. J Urol. 2010;183:68–75.
141. Lamont FR, Tomlinson DC, Cooper PA, et al. Small molecule FGF receptor inhibitors block FGFR-dependent urothelial carcinoma growth in vitro and in vivo. Br J Cancer. 2011;104:75–82.
142. Jirawatnotai S, Hu Y, Michowski W, et al. A function for cyclinD1 in DNA repair uncovered by protein interactome analyses in human cancers. Nature. 2011;474:230–4.
143. Kopparapu PK, Boorjian SA, Robinson BD, et al. Expression of cyclind1 and its association with disease characteristics in bladder cancer. Anticancer Res. 2013;33:5235–42.
144. Liukkonen T, Lipponen P, Raitanen M, et al. Evaluation of p21WAF1/CIP1 and cyclin D1 expression in the progression of superficial bladder cancer. Finbladder Group. Urol Res. 2000;28:285–92.
145. Kamai T, Takagi K, Asami H, et al. Decreasing of p27 (Kip1) and cyclin E protein levels is associated with progression from superficial into invasive bladder cancer. Br J Cancer. 2001;84:1242–51.
146. Salinas-Sánchez AS, Atienzar-Tobarra M, Lorenzo-Romero JG, et al. Sensitivity and specificity of p53 protein detection by immunohistochemistry in patients with urothelial bladder carcinoma. Urol Int. 2007;79:321–7.
147. Ecke TH, Sachs MD, Lenk SV, et al. TP53 gene mutations as an independent marker for urinary bladder cancer progression. Int J Mol Med. 2008;21:655–61.
148. Youssef RF, Mitra AP, Bartsch G, Jones PA, et al. Molecular targets and targeted therapies in bladder cancer management. World J Urol. 2009;27:9–20.
149. Malats N, Bustos A, Nascimento CM, et al. P53 as a prognostic marker for bladder cancer: a meta-analysis and review. Lancet Oncol. 2005;6:678–86.
150. Stadler WM, Lerner SP, Groshen S, et al. Phase III study of molecularly targeted adjuvant therapy in locally advanced urothelial cancer of the bladder based on p53 status. J Clin Oncol. 2011;29: 3443–9.
151. Cheng L, Zhang S, MacLennan GT, et al. Bladder cancer: translating molecular genetic insights into clinical practice. Hum Pathol. 2011;42(4):455–81.
152. Bryan RT, Zeegers MP, James ND, et al. Biomarkers in bladder cancer. BJU Int. 2000;105:608–13.
153. Villares GJ, Zigler M, Blehm K, et al. Targeting EGFR in bladder cancer. World J Urol. 2007;25:573–9.
154. Vrooman OP, Witjes JA. Molecular markers for detection, surveillance and prognostication of bladder cancer. Int J Urol. 2009;16:234–43.
155. Adida C, Crotty PL, McGrath J, et al. Developmentally regulated expression of the novel cancer anti-apoptosis gene survivin in human and mouse differentiation. Am J Pathol. 1998;152: 43–9.
156. Ku JH, Godoy G, Amiel GE, Lerner SP. Urine survivin as a diagnostic biomarker for bladder cancer: a systematic review. BJU Int. 2012;110:630–6.
157. Barbisan F, Santinelli A, Mazzucchelli R, et al. Strong immunohistochemical expression of fibroblast growth factor receptor 3, superficial staining pattern of cytokeratin 20, and low proliferative activity define those papillary urothelial neoplasms of low malignant potential that do not recur. Cancer. 2008;112:636–44.
158. Korkolopoulou P, Christodoulou P, Konstantinidou AE, et al. Cell cycle regulators in bladder cancer: a multivariate survival study with emphasis on p27Kip1. Hum Pathol. 2000;31:751–60.

159. Jones PA, Baylin SB. The fundamental role of epigenetic events in cancer. Nat Rev Genet. 2002;3:415–28.
160. Tozawa T, Tamura G, Honda T, et al. Promoter hypermethylation of DAPkinase is associated with poor survival in primary biliary tract carcinoma patients. Cancer Sci. 2004;95:736–40.
161. Catto JW, Azzouzi AR, Rehman I, et al. Promoter hypermethylation is associated with tumor location, stage, and subsequent progression in transitional cell carcinoma. J Clin Oncol 2005;23:2903–10
162. Kim WJ, Kim EJ, Jeong P, et al. RUNX3 inactivation by point mutations and aberrant DNA methylation in bladder tumors. Cancer Res. 2005;65:9347–54.
163. Bryan RT, Zeegers MP, Nicholas DJ, Wallace MA, et al. Biomarkers in bladder cancer. BJU Int 2010;105:608–13.
164. Stein JP, Ginsberg DA, Grossfeld GD, et al. Effect of p21WAF1/CIP1 expression on tumor progression in bladder cancer. J Natl Cancer Inst 1998;90(14):1072–9

15 Molecular Pathway and Fluorescence In Situ Hybridization Testing of ERBB2 (HER2) Gene Amplification in Invasive Ductal Carcinoma of Breast

Tomasz Jodlowski and K. H. Ramesh

15.1 Introduction

15.1.1 Breast Cancer Etiology and Detection

Breast cancer is the most common non-skin malignancy among women and is the second most common cause of cancer death. Average lifetime risk of developing breast cancer is 1 in 8 women (approximately 12%). In 2017, about 252,710 new cases of invasive breast cancer were diagnosed in women in the U.S., along with 63,410 new cases of non-invasive (in situ) breast cancer [1]. All women are considered to be at risk, but level of risk varies in the population. Lifetime risk of developing invasive breast cancer ranges from 3% (for women without risk factors) to >80% (for women with highly penetrant germline mutations).

T. Jodlowski
Department of Pathology, Montefiore Medical Center and Albert Einstein College of Medicine, Bronx, NY, USA
e-mail: tjodlows@montefiore.org

K. H. Ramesh (✉)
Clinical Cytogenetics and Genomics, Department of Pathology, Montefiore Medical Center and Albert Einstein College of Medicine, Bronx, NY, USA
e-mail: kramesh@montefiore.org

Most risk factors cannot be modified (e.g., age, gender, ethnicity, family history-BRCA1 and BRCA2 mutation carriers) or would be very difficult to modify (e.g., age at first pregnancy, age at menopause). Some risk factors that can be modified include: dietary habits, exercise, alcohol use or smoking, and environmental exposure to genotoxic agents such as radiation. Increasing age, female gender, race, and individuals including migrants living in well developed countries are all established risk factors for increased risk of breast cancer. For post-menopausal women, obesity is associated with an increased risk of breast cancer, particularly in those who do not use hormone therapy. However, a higher body mass index has been associated with a lower risk of breast cancer in premenopausal women. Increased exposure to estrogen such as early menarche or late menopause is a risk factor for developing breast cancer. Reproductive factors that increase breast cancer risk include: later age at the time of first pregnancy, absence of breastfeeding, and nulli-parity [2].

- Regular physical exercise appears to provide modest protection against breast cancer.
- Alcohol consumption is associated with an increased risk of breast cancer with a dose-response relationship.
- The relationship between cigarette smoking and breast cancer is complicated by the

K. K. Shukla et al. (eds.), *Molecular Diagnostics in Cancer Patients*,
https://doi.org/10.1007/978-981-13-5877-7_15

interaction of smoking with alcohol and endogenous hormonal influences; however, smoking is a risk factor.

- A diet rich in fruits and vegetables, fish, and olive oil may result in a lower risk of breast cancer; however, the influence of dietary fat and red meat is not clear.

Early detection of breast cancer and classification are important to maximize life expectancy by preventing potential metastasis and aggressive proliferation of an early tumor [3]. Among females between the ages of 20 and 59, breast cancer is estimated to constitute 28% of all new cancers [4] and is second to lung cancer in cancer related mortality [5].

As cancer cells evolve, the level of genetic instability will typically increase [6, 7]. This promotes a non-clonal population, or heterogeneity, of cancer cells with a range of spontaneous mutations conferring acquired traits and making treatment difficult [8]. Aggressive cancer cells in more advanced tumors can metastasize, or spread, leading to low survival rates of patients with metastatic breast cancer. These patients have a poor prognosis and an increased resistance to chemotherapy [9, 10].

15.1.2 Genetic Instability Leading to Aberrant Signaling and Carcinogenesis

The process of carcinogenesis begins in most cases with a single cell, and follows a Darwinian model of clonal expansion where favorable traits allow increased cell survival [11, 12]. This model was proposed as early as 1976 by Nowell, and states that tumor progression and acquired traits typically involve common regulatory pathways. These pathways can lead to tumor cell initiation caused by DNA damage. Such damage includes mutational events causing errors in the base pair sequences that occur during replication and are not corrected by DNA repair genes [7, 13, 14]. Mutational events can also be caused by acquired factors such as smoking [4, 15, 16], or epigenetic mechanisms such as the interruption of cytokinesis by non-genetic factors [17].

Alterations of gene copy numbers can occur when DNA is replicated. During replication when a DNA loop is formed, replication slippage can cause the DNA in this loop to be copied twice, or in the alternative scenario not copied at all. Such events ultimately lead to a duplication or loss of a gene copy [18]. Copy number changes of oncogenes or transcription factors can then lead to aberrant signaling within their pathways, which in some cases increases cell survival and preserves the gain or loss of function of a gene [19].

During excessive activation of growth signaling cascades caused by genetic instability, the tumor cells begin to proliferate, expand, and evolve [20–22]. Tumor suppressor genes function normally at cell division checkpoints as negative regulators of cell division and growth. These genes thus work to prevent tumorigenesis, where a loss of function will lead to cancer as seen with TP53 [23, 24]. Genes that have a role in tumorigenesis can be classified as proto-oncogenes [25, 26] that act as oncogenes when once mutated [27, 28], or tumor suppressor genes [29, 30]. Proto-oncogenes that normally promote regulated cell growth and division are genes with the potential to become oncogenic, and can lead to tumorigenesis, once mutated or overexpressed. Signals received by G-protein coupled receptors (GPCR) and receptor tyrosine kinases (RTK) with their respective receptors as well as their downstream signaling pathways are examples of oncogenes that induce tumorigenesis by mediating cell proliferation and cell growth. These alterations in gene activity affect cellular functions including decreasing apoptosis, or programmed cell death [31, 32], and driving inappropriate growth signal transduction [33].

Cellular proliferation can be caused by growth signal cascades involving extracellular signaling with the hormone estrogen [34]. Estrogen can initiate signal transduction mediated by the estrogen receptor which is a seven-transmembrane-helix receptor proteins (7TM), specifically a GPCR [35, 36]. When high levels of estrogen are present in the extracellular environment, the 7TM protein GPCR will remain active and its set of downstream G-proteins will remain active. A G-protein is any guanine nucleotide-binding protein that when bound to a guanosine diphosphate (GDP) is in its inactive state. When that GDP is swapped by a guanosine exchange factor (GEF) with a guanosine triphosphate (GTP) the G-protein and its related signaling cascades remain active.

The RAS oncogene subfamily of small G-proteins are monomeric and share similarities with other G-proteins in how their active state changes with GDP and GTP binding [37]. While RAS is active, it can bind to and activate the kinase domain on the signaling protein RAF. RAF can then phosphorylate and activate a mitogen activated protein kinase (MEK) that phosphorylates and activates extracellular signal-regulated kinases (ERKs) also known as mitogen activating protein kinases—MAPK [38]. The result of MAPK pathway activation varies and includes regulating gene expression via RAS phosphorylation and GTP exchange by SOS [39], cell differentiation of stem cells by various MAPK and PI3K pathway activation [40], and inducing apoptosis via MAPK and ERK pathways [41–43].

The transformation of GDP to GTP can also activate secondary messengers, particularly adenylate cyclase that converts adenosine triphosphate (ATP) into cyclic adenosine monophosphate—cAMP [44]. cAMP then activates protein kinase A—PKA [45]. There are many different proteins that can subsequently be activated by PKA due to its ability to phosphorylate serine and threonine residues [46]. When the activating ligand of the 7TM receptor is no longer bound, the G-proteins will reset GTP through hydrolysis into GDP [47] or by phosphorylation of the GPCR and β-arrestin binding, which facilitates signal termination [48].

In this example, the 7TM G-protein receptor-30—GPR30, which has an extracellular estrogen ligand binding domain [49, 50], responds to estrogen binding by activating secondary messengers, which ultimately will increase levels of the cell cycle regulatory proteins, Cyclin-D1 [51] and Cyclin-D2 [52] inducing passage from the G_1 to S phase in the cell cycle [53]. Oncogene forms of these cyclin regulatory proteins will induce passage of the cell cycle checkpoints by preventing inhibition of synthesis proteins.

Another way growth signal transduction activation can occur is with the single transmembrane spanning proteins that contain an extracellular signal binding domain and an intracellular RTK domain. An example of this is the epidermal growth factor family of receptors—EGFR [54, 55]. Upon ligand binding, two EGFRs form a homodimer to bind a single EGFR in their extracellular EGFR-binding domain. The binding causes a conformational change in each EGFR to cross-phosphorylate tyrosines in the tyrosine-rich carboxyl-terminal tails of each monomer through their tyrosine kinase domains [56]. The conformational change brings the C-terminal regions of the EGFRs together to form an SRC homology 2—SH2 domain, which allows other proteins such as the accessory protein growth factor receptor-bound protein 2—GRB-2 [57] to dock onto the SH2 domain and bind to the phosphotyrosine residues on the RTK. Structurally GRB-2 contains one SH2 and two SH3 domains, of which one SH2 is used in the binding of GRB-2 to an RTK through phosphotyrosine residues. This event subsequently recruits the protein SOS to bind GRB-2 through its remaining two SH3 domains onto a polyproline-rich polypeptide of SOS. The formation of the EGFR dimer and recruitment of GRB-2 and SOS forms a complex that activates a small G-protein–RAS, by having the complex replace GDP in RAS with GTP making SOS a GEF [58]. Activated RAS then triggers cell proliferation as described above.

Another hallmark of cancer besides promoting cell proliferation and cell growth is evading apoptosis (programmed cell death). One possible mechanism by which this can occur is genetic instability in members of the PI3K/AKT/mTOR pathways [59]. In these pathways, signal transduction can be driven by G-proteins or RTK activation of specific kinases. For example, phosphorylation of the 3′ position on the inositol ring of phosphatidylinositol (3,4)-bisphosphate—PIP2 by phosphatidylinositol-kinase—PI3K (known as phosphatidylinositol-4,5-bisphosphate 3 kinase). PIK3CA forms the active form: phosphatidylinositol (3,4,5)-triphosphate—PIP3 [60]. These phospholipids are attached to the plasma membrane by covalently bound isoprene lipids and face the cytoplasm, and can lead to signaling of many pathways, one of which requires binding of PIP3 to protein kinase B—AKT [61].

Positioning of AKT by PIP3 allows AKT to be phosphorylated by phosphoinositide-dependent kinase 1—PDPK1 or PDK1 [62–64]. Activation of the mammalian target of rapamycin complex by AKT occurs when PRAS40 is phosphorylated by AKT, which is bound to a regulatory associated protein of mTOR–RAPTOR [65]. These phosphorylation events elevate the activity levels of AKT, which promotes further phosphorylating events and the activation of various anti-apoptotic proteins like BCL-2, which is implicated in regulating pro-caspase and in apoptosis or programmed cell death [66–68]. Alternatively, genetic instability in the tumor suppressor gene phosphatase and tensin homolog—PTEN [69], which dephosphorylates PIP3, can cause down-regulation of AKT and limit mTOR activation by AKT phosphorylation [70, 71].

The effect of uncontrolled growth signaling is the continuous division of cells leading to excessive tumor burden. Genetic instability in proto-oncogenes such as HER2 [72, 73] will accelerate tumor growth, and loss of tumor suppressor genes such as tumor protein P21 or TP53 [74–76] that will perpetuate the cell line by dysregulating cell cycle checkpoints and activation of apoptosis. A loss of function in a tumor suppressor gene such as retinoblastoma protein (RB1) can override cell cycle progression by interfering with cell division checkpoints [77], further reinforcing up-regulated growth rates. Accelerated cell proliferation can also be maintained due to increasing cell survivability by the loss of PIP3 and dephosphorylation by PTEN to derail cell cycle progression [78], which is seen in some breast cancers [79].

Genetically unstable cells do not form a homogenous mass of cells with identical genetic aberrations, but rather expand clonally as a mixed population of cells that vary in genetic abnormalities [53, 54, 80]. A high level of genetic instability however can lead to apoptosis or limit tumor growth, which can be caused by genetic instability [81, 82] or by disrupting mitotic checkpoints as seen in transformed tetraploid cells [83]. For example, there are cases with viable polysomy of chromosomes: X, 4, 6, 10, 14, 17, and 21, which is found in over 50% of acute lymphoblastic leukemia patients with a hyperdiploid karyotype [84, 85].

Evolution of the tumor, and the rate of genetic change can be attributed to selective pressures present in the microenvironment, such as nutrient deficiency [86] and cell cycle arrest signaling, which occurs by adhesion binding between adjacent cells [87]. As a tumor evolves it can overcome these pressures and break through its basal configurations as a primary tumor, and spread or metastasize [88].

One example of a signaling cascade including cell boundary or contact signaling involves E-cadherin binding in the extracellular environment between adjacent cells [30]. Localized to the plasma membrane, E-cadherin is a single-pass transmembrane protein whose C-terminal domain on the cytoplasmic side interacts with various catenin proteins to regulate growth as seen in the ERK p70 pathway [89]. This interaction also regulates cell polarity determination such as in the E-Cadherin/Discs Large Homolog 5—DLG5 pathway [90], and cell organization/cell adhesion via cadherin interactions between cells [91]. Signal transduction of E-cadherin is mediated by catenin. For example, α-catenin links the adherens junctions to actin in the cytoskeleton [92] and to β-catenin, which is phosphorylated by transcription growth factor β—TGFβ to regulate cell orientation or coordination [93]. One signaling pathway that TGFβ is involved in, is the epithelial to mesenchymal transition pathway—EMT. This pathway has been observed in breast cancers as a way of cell signaling to de-differentiate into mesenchymal stem cells, and lose cell-to-cell adhesion properties, facilitating cell migration and metastasis [94, 95].

Cytokines are small proteins which are involved in signaling and can lead to an inflammatory response by inducing cytolytic effector cell production. This process eventually leads to the recruitment of B and T lymphocytes which can kill the cancer cell as a biological response [96]. For this response, cancer cells must be recognized through ligand or antigen recognition such as the natural killer activating transmembrane protein—NKG2D [97], whose extracellular ligand receptor is recognized by natural killer immune cells (Li et al. 2009; [98]). Similarly, B lymphocytes or T lymphocytes of the immune system can recognize melanoma-associated antigen 3—MAGE-A3 [99–101], a tumor antigen. Some tumor cells in response to transformation or tumorigenesis will aberrantly secrete various cytokines, such as anti-transforming growth factors or interleukins [102, 103], thus allowing targeting and subsequent destruction by natural killer cells. However, in mesenchymal stem cells, the lack of various immunogenic signaling or major histocompatibility complex molecules—MHC prevents or minimizes inflammation and lytic activity [104, 105]. This can ultimately result in distal secondary tumor formation [106] by cells capable of surviving outside the primary tumor.

15.1.3 Molecular Basis of HER2

The proto-oncogene ERBB2 (human epidermal growth factor receptor) codes for HER2, a transmembrane RTK [107, 108]. HER2 is an orphan receptor that is constitutively active without epitope binding as a proto-oncogene [109–112]. Amplification of HER2 will initiate growth factor signaling pathways without conformational changes or dimerization as seen in other EGFRs [113]. As an orphan receptor, HER2 shares structural similarities with EGFR although a ligand specific to HER2 has not yet been identified. Even in the absence of a ligand, HER2 promotes excessive growth signaling by repeatedly autophosphorylating as a homodimer [109, 110], or heterodimer with other EGFRs [111, 112, 114]. Heterodimer activation of HER2 occurs by dimerization with members of the EGFR family such as: EGFR [115, 116], HER1 [117], HER3 [118–120], and HER4 [121]. Amplification of HER2 (ERBB2) as a result of an increase in ERBB2 gene expression increases the upstream signaling pathways involved in growth, anti-apoptosis, and cell adhesion [122]. An increase in the HER2 receptors leads to an increase in HER2 activation, and amplification of the HER2 gene (ERBB2) which then leads to an increase of HER2 growth signaling pathways.

As with the EGFR family receptors, the tyrosine kinase domain of HER2 autophosphorylates upon dimerization of the HER2 cytoplasmic domain, which activates its downstream signaling cascade [109, 112].

The proto-oncogene phosphokinase PIK3CA pathway that is activated upstream by HER2 [123] regulates many pathways such as AKT and RHO (RAS family) pathways, and small GTPase activation leading to proliferation [124], a normally highly regulated process. Overexpression of HER2 disrupts and dysregulates such processes.

Amplification of HER2 is also a driver of metastasis, and is indicative of aggressive breast cancer in cases with IDC of breast [125]. Thus, the altered signaling pathways in breast cancers are diverse and can lead to selected traits based on the micro-environment created locally by the cancer cells, or due to treatment-related acquired resistance [126–128].

Many of the discussed signaling pathways result from RTK phosphorylation, such as in RHO activation of the RHO-associated coiled-coil containing kinase (ROCK). Activation of ROCK can lead to cell invasion or metastasis [129]. In one example, HER2 and protein tyrosine kinase 6—PTK6 mediate activating kinase ROCK by phosphorylating PIP2, which results in AKT/PIP3 activation leading to increased ROCK/RH0 activation [130, 131].

In some HER2 amplified cancers the transcription factor c-MYC is upregulated, also leading to proliferation [132] and anti-apoptotic signaling [133]. The increase of upstream activation caused by HER2 will increase transcription of MYC (chromosome locus: 8q24.1) and activate the AKT/mTOR complex pathways facilitating cell cycle progression. This signaling cascade has been linked to chemotherapy resistance [75, 76].

Cell adhesion or cadherin-catenin interactions are modulated by HER2 tyrosine kinase phosphorylation of α-catenin, which interacts with β-catenin and E-cadherin [134]. The effects of HER2 phosphorylation of this pathway reduces E-cadherin expression and can lead to a loss of contact inhibition leading to cell motility or metastasis [135, 136].

15.1.4 Composition of Mammary Gland and Definition of IDC and DCIS

The structure of mammary glands is tree-like, with a system of ducts and lobules nested in fatty tissue (Fig. 15.1). The mammary epithelium forms the ducts and lobules which are composed of two cell types, the inner cuboidal shaped secretory luminal cells and the outer basal myoepithelial cells [137].

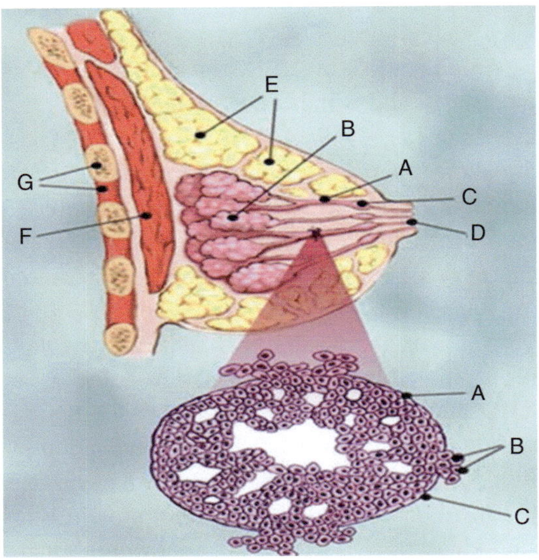

Fig. 15.1 Top: *A*—duct; *B*—lobules; *C*—Ampulla; *D*—lactiferous ducts; *E*—fatty tissue; *F*—pectoralis major muscle; *G* rib/spinal column. Bottom: *A*—normal duct cells; *B*—ductal cancer cells breaking through the basement membrane; *C*—basement membrane

The luminal cells are involved in secreting milk via smooth muscle contraction of the myoepithelial cells, which are responsible for the delivery of the milk [138, 139]. Evidence of progenitor mammary stem cells (MSC) in adults is observed during pregnancies when growth and development of secretory alveoli occurs. It has been widely speculated that a potential source of breast cancer is the MSCs, because these cells have properties of self-renewal [140] in addition to characteristics of EMT cells [141, 142]. Mammary cells that have gained the capacity to infiltrate the basal membrane are categorized as invasive ductal carcinoma also known as invasive carcinoma of no special type (ductal NST) or invasive carcinoma, not otherwise specified (ductal NOS). Historically many other names have been used for this form of breast cancer including scirrhous carcinoma, carcinoma simplex, and spheroidal cell carcinoma [143]. Infiltrating Ductal Carcinoma (Fig. 15.2a) was revised in 2003 [144, 145]. In contrast, ductal carcinoma in situ—DCIS (Fig. 15.2b) is determined when abnormal cells are found within the lining and the condition is not a definitive pre-IDC case [146, 147].

15.1.5 Breast Cancer Classification

The Cancer Genome Atlas Network (CGAN) and International Cancer Genome Consortium (ICGC) recognize three categories of breast

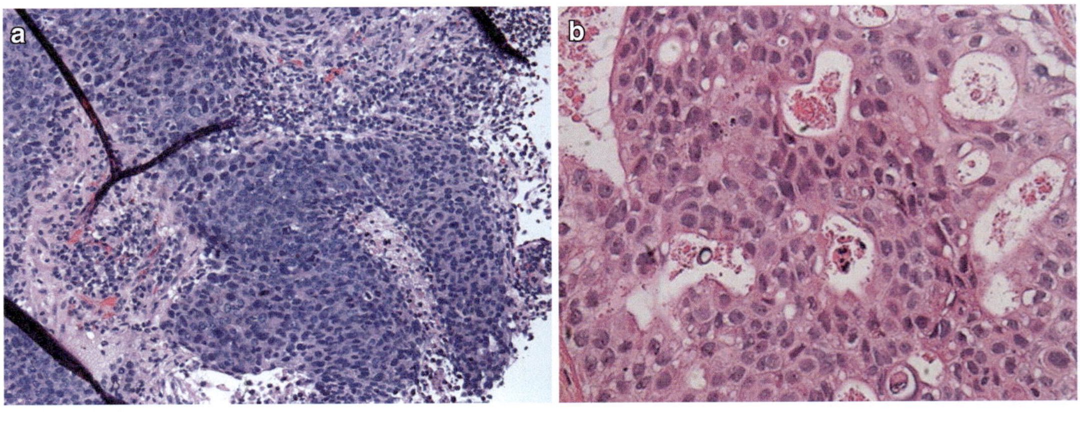

Fig. 15.2 (**a**) H&E stain: well differentiated infiltrating ductal carcinoma (IDC) with mitotic figures. (**b**) H&E Stain: ductal carcinoma in situ (DCIS), cribriform type, grade 2

cancer. The first category is the hormone positive or estrogen receptor (ER) and progesterone receptor (PR) positive group [148, 149]. The second category include the basal cell-like or Triple-Negative Breast Cancer Group (TNBC) which is negative for HER2 amplification and estrogen and progesterone receptor involvement. The third category is the HER2-amplified group [26]. In addition to these categories, the tissue subtype is important. Extensive gene profiling has classified breast tissue into various subtypes including luminal A and luminal B [150, 151], both of which are comprised of myoepithelial cells beneath the luminal cells. Subtype Claudin-low is typically in TNBC and comprised of epithelial-to-mesenchymal transition (EMT) mesenchymal cells [152]. The basal cell-like subtype is comprised of mesenchymal-to-epithelial transition (MET) epithelial cells [150, 151, 153].

Lastly, the HER2 amplified group has an effective antibody-based therapy determined by the status of HER2 gene copy number amplification [150, 151, 168, 169]. Carcinogenesis of mammary cells involving amplification of HER2 has been found to promote early progenitor cell tumor initiation [170] and is seen in aggressive tumors that undergo metastasis [126, 171]. Currently the treatment options are limited to those cases in which HER2 is amplified by FISH analysis or cases that score 3+ by IHC anlaysis [169, 172]. Early detection of HER2-positive breast cancer and subsequent treatment with adjuvant HER2 antibody-based therapy and chemotherapy have reduced death rates by up to 40% [170, 173–176]. The antibody-based therapy uses Herceptin®, a monoclonal antibody that targets the HER2 epitope, which prevents signaling by HER2 [3, 177].

15.1.6 Treatment of Breast Cancer

Once the tumor has been classified, a more specific and individualized treatment option can be used to target its specific oncogenic mechanisms. For ER-positive and negative for lymph node involvement breast cancers, the standard therapy is Tamoxifen, an endocrine-based chemotherapy. Tamoxifen competitively binds the ER, inhibiting transcription by secretory hormone antagonism [154–160]. The 7TM estrogen receptor when bound by the metabolic product of Tamoxifen, 4-hydroxytamoxifen, is an antagonist to ER growth pathway signaling; and this is achieved by recruiting repressors to ER growth factor signaling [161, 162].

TNBC is typically seen in individuals having a mutation of the tumor suppressor gene BRCA1 [163–165] or of African descent [166]. These subgroups of patients are negative for HER2 amplification, and negative for growth signaling, involving estrogen and progesterone hormones. There are limited treatment options other than chemotherapy-based treatments for patients harboring such mutations. These include local excision or radical mastectomy, along with cytotoxic-based chemotherapy [167].

15.1.7 HER2 Amplification in Breast Cancer

Amplification of HER2 is seen in approximately 10–30% of invasive breast cancers, and tends to have an aggressive phenotype and poor prognosis [109–112, 114, 122, 178, 179]. Several models of HER2 amplification exist: one model is based on the HER2 gene copy number, where repetitive segments of the gene is present in more than five copies per cell [3, 180–182]. Another model is based on chromosome 17 polysomy. ERBB2 (HER2) resides on chromosome 17; and the additional chromosome 17s—thus leading to HER2 amplification [158–160, 183, 184]. Finally, genetic heterogeneity (GH) can display HER2 amplification both at the gene locus and polysomy of chromosome 17 across the tumor population [53, 185, 186]. The tumor cell populations can differ either within the same tumor (intratumoral) or between a metastatic site and primary breast cancer site (inter-tumoral) in terms of the HER2 amplification status.

Breast cancers with HER2 amplification characteristically metastasize to tissues such as bone [171], brain [187, 188], and lungs [189, 190]. In the example of bone metastasis, the bone can become brittle due to the formation of lytic lesions within the bone as dense bone cells are being replaced with breast cancer cells [191–193]. One study by Meng et al. [194] describes circulating tumor cells that acquired HER2 amplification in relation to the non-amplified status of the primary tumor. Such metastatic activity and early progenitor cell initiation could be due to an expanding tumor population, where amplification of HER2 in cases of GH have the potential to evolve into aggressive breast cancers [195].

GH was once thought to be uncommon [196]; however, as extensive genetic profiling of cancers is being performed there exists increasing data suggesting that most tumors harbor many clones [197]. The data also suggest that tumor evolution is such that the initial tumor population with primary driver mutations might not be present in recurrent or metastasized cancers [198, 199].

GH in breast cancer can be considered in terms of the mammary gland composition, gene expression profiles, and Darwinian-based evolution. Luminal and basal cells within the mammary gland have different genetic profiles based on the subtype of breast cancer, i.e. basal types typically involve ER mutations [200] and luminal types typically involve TP53 mutations [158–160]. HER2 amplification is seen in either basal or luminal cells [201]. This could suggest that HER2-amplified tumors are not cell-type driven, but are driven by aberrant signaling that allows for increased cell survivability. The Darwinian clonal evolution model correlates well, when applied to HER2 amplification, as tumors can expand rapidly by genetic instability due to the number of HER2 tumorigenesis pathways that exist [202, 203]. As the tumor expands and evolves, the population of cells comprising the tumor can differ in their genetic profile based on the selective pressures of the tumor. Involvement of HER2 amplification expedites clonal expansion and survivability, which in cases of IDC of the breast is considered aggressive [204, 205]. Studies have shown that patients with aggressive tumors that are positive for amplification of HER2 have a poorer prognosis and decreased survival rates [206].

15.1.8 FISH Testing for HER2 Amplification

The present nomenclature for the HER2 gene is ERBB2 (erb-b2 receptor tyrosine kinase 2; HGNC: 3430, 2017), which is 42,512 kb in length and localized to the long arm of chromosome 17, at 17q12, mapping to the region 39,687,917-39,730,426 as of Ensembl release 89 ([207–209]; May 2017; http://www.ebi.ac.uk/; GRCh38:CM000679.2).

While IHC is used to detect the presence of protein localization in histology, FISH methodology is used in cytogenetics to detect gene rearrangements and copy number changes in genes or chromosomes. In classical cytogenetics, a tissue specimen is cultured and prepared for karyotype analysis by Giemsa staining (G-band) following protease treatment. A karyotype is generated using a computerized image analysis system, that enables photomicrography of metaphase spreads and subsequent classification of chromosomes. Such classifications are helpful in detecting numerical gains and losses, rearrangements (translocations, inversions), deletions, duplications, and other chromosomal abnormalities found in tumor cells. The drawback of karyotype analysis for breast cancer cases to detect HER2 copy number change is the relatively low resolution (>5 Mb; [208, 209]) and the specificity that is needed to detect single gene amplification. It is beyond the scope of karyotype analysis to establish a HER2 gene to centromere 17 ratio accurately, even with an observable form of amplification such as homogeneously staining regions (HSR) and double minutes—DMIN ([208, 209]).

In contrast, FISH analysis has a resolution as high as 150 kb; superior to karyotyping, and can establish gene-specific results far more quickly and precisely in tumor specimens. These features make it the ideal cytogenetic method for assessing amplifications associated with cancers. FISH analysis is considered the "gold standard" for the detection of HER2 amplification status in IDC breast cancer. For breast cancers that have an IHC score of 2+ (Table 15.2), FISH analysis is performed to assess the amplification status of the HER2 gene using DNA probes complimentary to the HER2 gene. FISH analysis allows accurate and rapid results that can be obtained in less than 6 h (DAKO, Denmark). These DNA probes are then visualized using fluorescent microscopy under 1000× magnification.

15.1.9 FISH Scoring Criteria: ASCO/CAP 2013 Guidelines

The scoring criteria based on ASCO/CAP guidelines for probes containing an internal control defines a tumor as positive for HER2 amplification when the average HER2 copy number is ≥6 signals per cell or with a ratio of HER2 to centromere 17 of ≥2 [169]. Internal controls in FISH are used to determine if the HER2 signal is present in multiple copies due to polysomy of chromosome 17, or if amplification is due to multiple copies of the gene alone.

Scoring HER2 FISH amplification by ratio is obtained by dividing the gene copy number by the centromere 17 copy number, where a ratio of 1.0 is equal to two copies of the HER2 gene (normal copy number in humans) for every two copies of centromere 17. Scoring FISH by copy number is based on the average number of copies of HER2 per cell, where the total HER2 copy number is divided by the total number of cells screened.

Cases are considered positive for amplification when the HER2/Centromere 17 ratio is ≥2.0 or ≥6.0 HER2 target signals per cell are identified (Table 15.1). A negative result by FISH is reported when the average HER2/Centromere 17 ratio is <2.0, and there are less than 4 copies of HER2 signals/cell.

Following the ASCO/CAP guidelines, FISH and IHC analyses will often give "equivocal" scores by FISH and IHC (Table 15.2). Such scores arise potentially due to screening only 20 cells by FISH analysis, and tumor sampling from tumors with focal areas consisting of just a few positive cells and IHC screening being subjective. Similarly, an equivocal result is reported when ≤10% of the tumor stains intensely by IHC or when ambiguously weak staining by IHC in

Table 15.1 2013-ASCO/CAP guidelines for reporting HER2 results as positive for amplification

Method	Positive for HER2 Amplification Guideline
IHC	IHC 3+ based on circumferential cell membrane staining that is complete and intense, and within greater than 10% of the tumor cells
FISH	A single-probe average of HER2 copies ≥6.0 signals/cell
	Dual-probe HER2/*CEP17* ratio ≥2.0 and HER2 copy number ≥4.0 signals/cell
	Dual-probe HER2/*CEP17* ratio ≥2.0 and HER2 copy number <4.0 signals/cell
	Dual-probe HER2/*CEP17* ratio <2.0 and HER2 copy number ≥6.0 signals/cell

Table 15.2 2013-ASCO/CAP guidelines for reporting HER2 results as equivocal for amplification

Method	Equivocal for HER2 Amplification Guideline
IHC	IHC 2+ Circumferential membrane staining that is incomplete and/or weak/moderate in staining within >10% of tumor cells or complete and circumferential membrane staining that is intense and within less than or equal to 10% of tumor cells[a]
FISH	Single-probe HER2 probe average copy number ≥4.0 signals/cell and <6.0 signals/cell[a]
	Dual-probe HER2/*CEP17* ratio <2.0 and a HER2 copy number of ≥4.0 signals/cell and <6.0 signals/cell
	GENETIC HETEROGENEITY (GH) More than 5%, but less than 50% of the screened tumor cells have HER2/Centromere 17 signal ratio of ≥2.0 and/or ≥6 copies of HER2 gene per cell

[a]Scoring Criteria revised by ASCO/CAP—2018 Scoring Guideline [172]

>10% of the tumor is seen*. Although the results are not clearly positive, there is ample reason to support the presence of suspicious cells due to the aggressive nature of IDC of breast that are seen in such "equivocal" cases [172, 210, 211].

The results from these methods for detecting HER2 amplification are critical for determining treatment options regulated by the United States Food and Drug Administration (FDA). When assessments from IHC are reported as equivocal (2+), the patient does not qualify for HER2 antibody-based therapy according to FDA regulations [169]. When small areas stain intensely positive by IHC as seen by 400× magnification, then FISH testing is required to further assess the HER2 amplification status by screening 20 cells of the invasive ductal region (only) under 1000× magnification. The ductal region, being an observed point of invasion and metastasis or IDC, needs this cellular level of analysis by FISH with DNA probes for HER2. This raises the question that if IHC shows a few intensely staining focal invasive tumor areas and FISH demonstrates a few highly amplified cells within the same focal region, then should not these cases of genetic heterogeneity (GH) be designated as HER2 amplified? In such a situation, the ASCO/CAP guidelines of 2018 [172] for equivocal results (Table 15.2) no longer recommends repeating the FISH test on another specimen or a different block if available, or an alternative FISH test with a different set of probes localizing to chromosome 17 [169, 172]. It has been reported that, following these guidelines, GH occurs in up to 40% of invasive breast tumors [128, 212].

Alternative testing was recommended by the ASCO/CAP 2013 guidelines for cases which scored equivocal for HER2 by FISH with or without GH. Alternative testing was also recommended for indeterminate FISH results due to either analytical test failure caused by artifacts, or inadequate specimen handling [169]. However, cases having GH and cases that are indeterminate or those that have analytical test failure are by definition mutually exclusive, due to that fact that FISH results of IDC of breast cancer revealed that cells with HER2 amplification are not indeterminate nor have failed analytically.

15.1.10 Alternative FISH Testing (No Longer Required: 2018 ASCO/CAP ERBB2 Testing Update)

In cases with HER2 equivocal—FISH results: laboratories could test a different region of the invasive tumor, repeating the assay for detecting HER2 amplification. For cases resulting in equivocal with and without GH, alternative testing was performed using another probe as an alternative loci; and this test could be used to detect if the tumor harbored polysomy-17 or a true HER2 amplification. This involved using a probe localized to chromosome 17 that would be a control probe, replacing or in addition to a centromere 17 probe as the control that is used with HER2 as the target DNA probe.

Two candidate DNA probes used routinely for clinical testing were: RARA (17q21.2) and RAI1 (17p11.2), which were both locus specific DNA probes for chromosome 17 [213]. By FISH, the probe for RARA is a common oncology probe used to detect a rearrangement of the RARA region [214] which is the hallmark chromosome anomaly in acute promyelocytic leukemia (APL). The RARA probe is labeled with two fluorescent colors: spectrum orange, spanning the 3′ RARA, and spectrum green, spanning the 5′ RARA, creating a fusion signal in the chromosomal band 17q21.2. When a breakage occurs the signals separate due to a translocation event that breaks or occurs between the 3′ and 5′ region of the RARA locus. The RAI1 probe is a dual color probe comprised of the critical region for Miller-Dieker syndrome [215], a congenital microdeletion syndrome. Cytogenetically this is detected by observing only one copy of (RAI1) 17p11.2, which detects Miller-Dieker syndrome, or a loss of (PAFAH1B1) 17p13.3, which detects Smith-Magenis syndrome [216]. As an alternative FISH test performed on the same block that was reported as equivocal for HER2 amplification, these probes rule out polysomy of chromosome 17 and confirmed that HER2 gene amplification was an aberration of the HER2 gene copy number specifically.

15.1.11 Clinical Background of HER2 Amplification

The National Cancer Institute (NCI) and FDA have granted approval for treatment with Herceptin® for patients displaying positive HER2 overexpression by IHC or positive HER2 gene amplification by FISH analysis following the ASCO/CAP guidelines [169]. The FDA approved treatment options of HER2-amplified cancers include Lapatinib, a dual tyrosine kinase inhibitor that interrupts HER2 signaling [217]; Pertuzumab, an inhibitor of HER2 dimerization [218]; Trastuzumab (Herceptin®), which interferes with the cell surface HER2 binding site [219, 220], and Emtansine (DM1), which interferes with HER2/HER3 heterodimer formation by binding tubulin inside the cell [221].

With regard to tumors positive for GH as candidates for receiving FDA approved therapy, Herceptin® would be a strong choice as the directed mechanism involves interfering with the cell surface HER2 binding site [120]. Early detection of HER2 amplified breast cancer and subsequent treatment with HER2 antibody-based therapy and concurrently with adjuvant chemotherapy reduced death rates by up to 40% [170, 173–176].

Herceptin® is an antibody-based therapy which binds to an extracellular epitope on the HER2 receptor. When Herceptin® binds this epitope (Fig. 15.3), downstream signaling pathways are interrupted due to the uncoupling of the heterodimer/homodimer complex. Such uncoupling disables the RTK from functioning, ultimately leading to the inactivation of HER2 [120]. The binding of Herceptin® also elicits an antibody dependent cellular cytotoxicity (ADCC) by recruiting natural killer cells, the T lymphocytes [222–225], and macrophages [226, 227].

The potential treatment options for HER2 breast cancer are often systemic and multidisciplinary. When necessary, adjuvant chemotherapy and targeted antibody-based treatment are used to prevent local recurrence and metastasis [228]. These customized treatment options are based on the results of IHC and FISH, which is why it is of absolute importance to characterize tumor heterogeneity, and ultimately consider patients with GH+ tumor(s) to be eligible for treatment with Herceptin®.

When an initial biopsy displays IDC of the breast, analysis of the Estrogen (ER) and Progesterone (PR) hormone receptors in addition to HER2, is performed [169, 228, 229]. Patients will then have either definitive surgery or neoadjuvant chemotherapy prior to surgery [230]. Patients likely to receive neoadjuvant chemotherapy include those with high grade or poorly differentiated cancers [169]. Patients with well or moderately differentiated invasive cancers that are ER positive and HER2 negative usually go directly to surgery as they are unlikely to benefit from neoadjuvant chemotherapy [128].

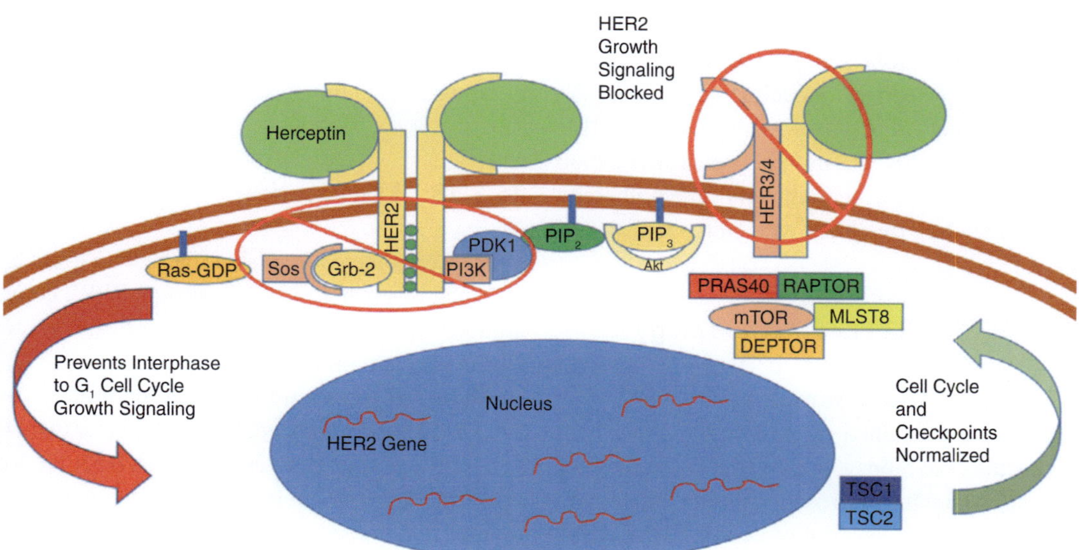

Fig. 15.3 HER2 signal transduction blocked using Herceptin®—the binding of HER2 with Herceptin® blocks HER2 family protein (e.g. EGFR, HER3, or HER4) dimerization and subsequent autophosphorylation. This stops the HER2 signal cascade by preventing downstream HER2 signaling pathways such as AKT/mTOR

The treatment of patients with HER2 amplification using adjuvant Herceptin® with chemotherapy have a higher response rate of about 50% vs. 32%, where only one therapy was used [173]. Cell proliferation was inhibited using murine monoclonal antibodies in vitro in a study by Slamon et al. [220], which determined the effectiveness of antibody therapy in reducing tumor growth.

The side effects observed from Herceptin® and chemotherapy include cardiomyopathy (5–30%) and less commonly, heart damage, heart failure, or stroke [173, 188]. Although side effects are seen in up to 30% of the patients treated as such, a positive response has been reported in up to 50% of those treated with adjuvant Herceptin® and chemotherapy [4, 173]. Thus, treating physicians must consider the potential outcomes of their patients with poor cardiac health prior to treatment with Herceptin®. Perez et al. [231] reported 53 patients in preclinical trials (NCCTG N9831, BCIRG 006, and BCIRG 005) with negative HER2-amplification who were treated with adjuvant Herceptin® and chemotherapy. In these cases, they recorded a disease-free state after 3 years and found a minimally significant rate of increased side effects ($p = 0.06$, $HR = 0.31$, 95% CI 0.11–0.91) post-treatment with concurrent Herceptin® and chemotherapy when compared to chemotherapy alone. As per the revised ASCO/CAP–HER2 scoring guideline of 2018, the authors report that cases with negative HER amplification or HER2 protein overexpression do not benefit from neo-adjuvant chemotherapy [172] including treatment with Herceptin®.

15.1.12 HER2 FISH Methodology

15.1.12.1 Tissue Sampling

Samples are obtained by post-surgical excision, by needle core biopsy, or from the excised tumor in cases where the macroscopic tumor has already been removed by surgical resection. These tissue samples are eventually used for histological, immune-histochemical, molecular analysis, and IDC of breast identification.

Tissue specimens are fixed in buffered-formalin for 6–72 h as per the ASCO/CAP guidelines. Fixed tissues are embedded in paraffin to generate a block. The formalin-fixed paraffin-embedded tissue (FFPE) block is sectioned at 4–6 μm thickness using a microtome onto sialanized microscope slides as per standard laboratory procedures.

The tumor sections are stained by hematoxylin and eosin (H&E), which can establish the diagnosis of IDC of breast based on cell morphology and differentiation. This is followed by an immunohistochemical (IHC) assay specific for ERBB2 to detect if cells are atypical by IHC for ERBB2. When screening for ERBB2 by IHC a score is assigned based on the intensity and completeness of staining as recommended by the American Society of Clinical Oncology and College of American Pathologists (ASCO/CAP; [169]). Cases scoring 2+ by IHC show an incomplete staining pattern or have areas of intense staining seen in ≤10% of the tumor area that is characteristic of IDCs. These IHC 2+ cases are classified as "equivocal", by the pathologist who then orders the reflex Fluorescence in situ hybridization (FISH) test to assess HER2 gene amplification status. ASCO/CAP 2018 HER2 Recommendation Committee has revised the definition of IHC 2+ (equivocal): as IDC of breast with "weak to moderate complete membrane staining seen in >10% of tumor cells in the invasive area [172].

15.1.13 FISH Scoring

HER2/Centromere 17 ratio less than 2.0 = Negative.

Equal or greater than 2.0 ratio or HER2 copy number equal or greater than 6 = Positive for HER2 gene amplification (Fig. 15.4).

Equivocal results are those that have an average HER2 copy number equal to or greater than 4 to 6 HER2 gene copies per cell with a HER2 ratio of less than 2.0. If equivocal, repeat screening is ordered and if results are still equivocal then testing with new specimen or alternate FISH testing with the same or new specimen is mandated. Alternate or repeat FISH testing on tumor

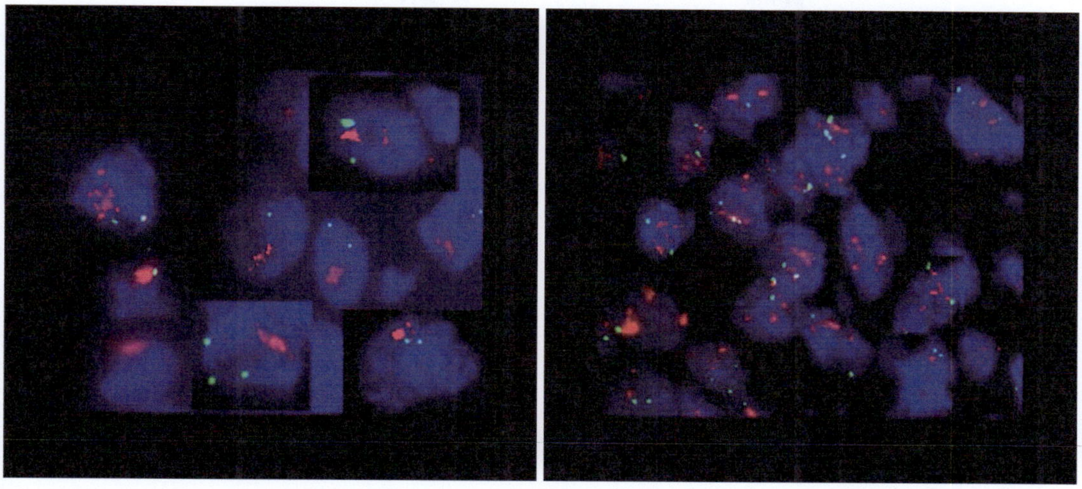

Fig. 15.4 Invasive ductal carcinoma of breast positive for HER2-amplification by FISH analysis. Red = HER2 gene, Green = Centromere 17 detected using PathVysion® fluorescent probes under 1000× total magnification. Images show negative for genetic heterogeneity and positive for amplification of HER2 by HER2 gene:centromere 17 ratio as per ASCO/CAP guidelines

sections from a different FFPE or the same FFPE used in the first HER2 FISH test with a different DNA probe other than the HER2 (17q12) DNA probe with Centromere 17 (control) DNA probe is no longer recommended as per the ASCO/CAP 2018 revised HER2 FISH testing scoring guidelines [172].

HER2 amplification scoring by FISH and IHC should follow the ASCO/CAP guidelines of 2013 and 2018 at the time of screening [169, 172]. The differences between the scoring criteria mandated by ASCO/CAP guidelines of 2007 and 2013 are outlined in Table 15.3.

HER2 Genetic Heterogeneity (GH): ≥5 to ≤50% of tumor cells in IDC with HER2/Centromere 17 ratio ≥2.0 and/or average of ≥6.0 HER2 copies per cell (Fig. 15.4). Specify if GH is present in clusters or scattered. This definition still holds good, and has not been addressed or changed in the revised ASCO/CAP 2018 revised HER2 FISH testing scoring guidelines.

Table 15.3 Comparison of 2007 and 2013 ASCO/CAP guidelines for FISH HER2 amplification status used in this study

Status	2007	2013
Positive	HER2/CEN17 ratio >2.2 or an average of >6 HER2/cell	Ratio ≥6.0 HER2/CEN17 Ratio ≥2.0 HER2/CEN17 and ≥4.0 average HER2/cell Ratio ≥2.0 HER2/CEN17 and <4.0 average HER2/cell Ratio <2.0 HER2/CEN17 and ≥6.0 average HER2/cell
Equivocal	HER2/CEN17 ratio 1.8–2.2 or an average of 4–6 HER2 copies/cell	Ratio ≥4.0 and <6.0 HER2/CEN17 Ratio <2.0 or ≥4.0 HER2/CEN17 and <6 average HER2/cell
Negative	HER2/CEN17 ratio <1.8 or an average of <4 HER2/cell	Ratio <2.0 HER2/CEN17 and <4.0 average HER2/cell Ratio <2.0 HER2/CEN17 and ≥6.0 average HER2/cell

HER2/CEN17 based on the total copies of HER2 DNA probe signals divided by the total copies of centromere 17 signals; HER2/cell is based on the average of HER2 DNA probe signals or copies per cell by dividing the HER2 DNA probe signals or copies by the total number of cells analyzed

15.1.14 FISH Analysis

To de-paraffinize the slides, they are baked overnight in a 60 °C oven, followed by three immersions in Citrisolv (Fisher Scientific, USA) and two rounds of dehydration in 100% ethanol, each for 5 min at room temperature (RT). After de-paraffinization, the samples are pretreated using paraffin pretreatment kit 2 following the manufacturers suggested protocol (Abbott Molecular, IL, USA).

A ThermoBrite® (Leica Biosystems, Germany) programmable hybridizer is used for co-hybridization of the FISH probe(s) using the PathVysion® HER2 probe (Abbott Laboratories, IL, USA) at full strength (Table 15.4; Figs. 15.5 and 15.6). Ten microliters of the DNA probe is applied directly onto the tumor tissue area, which is then covered with a 22 mm square coverslip. The Thermobrite® program settings used for hybridization are: denaturation at 76 °C for 5 min and annealing at 37 °C for 16 h.

Slides containing hybridized samples are placed in 2× SSC/0.3% NP40 at 72 °C for 2 min, followed by a second wash at RT for 2 min. Samples are air-dried and counterstained using DAPI (1000 ng/mL) and a coverslip is applied directly to the slide to complete specimen preparation for fluorescence microscopy analysis.

Table 15.4 Probe details for Abbott Molecular PathVysion® HER2 Probe Kit

Probe fluorophore color	Probe chromosome locus	Gene
Green: Excitation wavelength (497 nm)	17p11.1-q11.1 (D17Z1)	Centromere 17
Emission wavelength (524 nm)		
Orange: Excitation wavelength (559 nm)	17q11.2-12	Erbb-2 (HER2)
Emission wavelength (588 nm)		

15.1.15 Immunohistochemistry (IHC)

Immunohistochemistry (IHC) is performed with the DAKO (DAKO, Denmark) Herceptest™ kit usually in the surgical pathology laboratory. Screening of IHC samples should follow the ASCO guidelines (Tables 15.1 and 15.2; Fig. 15.7) for resulting IHC scores.

15.1.16 Microscopy

Note: the intensity of membrane staining in 2+ borderline image (C). Cases with equivocal HER2 results are reflex tested for HER2 amplification by FISH analysis with HER2/Centromere 17 DNA probes.

Fluorescence microscopy analysis can be performed using a Zeiss AxioPlan2 (Zeiss, Germany) microscope or any other microscope fitted with an X-Cite 120 light source (Excelitas, USA) and Chroma filter sets (Chroma Technology, VT, USA) appropriate for visualization of PathVysion fluorophores. Twenty interphase nuclei are scored by two readers from two different invasive ductal areas. HER2/centromere 17 ratio is calculated by dividing the total number of HER2 signals by the total number of centromere 17 signals; and the average HER2 copy number per cell is calculated by dividing the total number of HER2 signals by 20 cells.

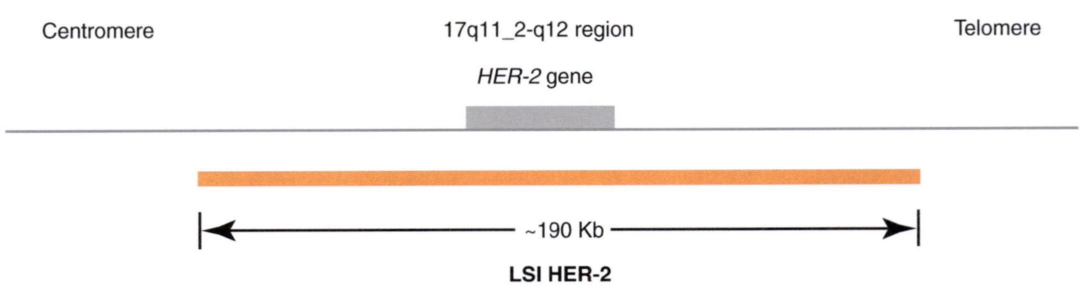

Fig. 15.5 HER2 Probe design (Abbott Molecular, IL, USA)

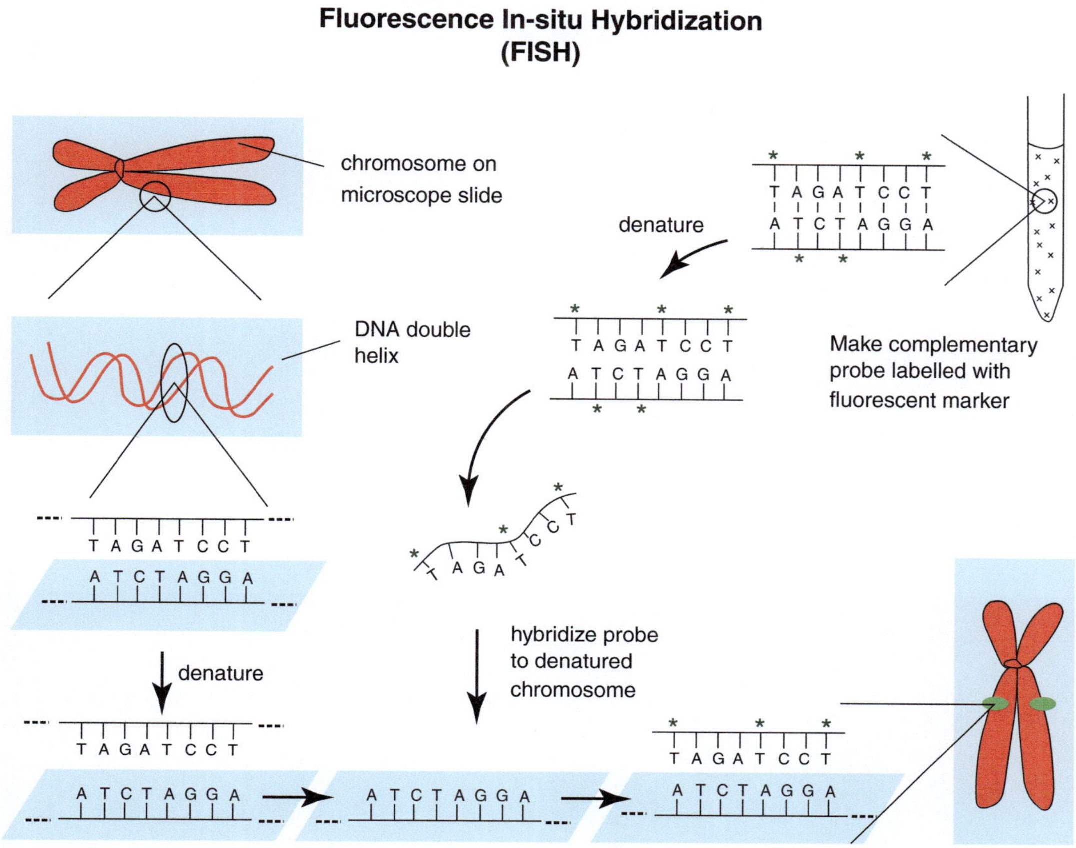

Fig. 15.6 Probe and target locus DNA denatured to single strand DNA and co-hybridized. If sequences are complementary there will be hybridization. Fluorophores enable visualization under UV Excitation

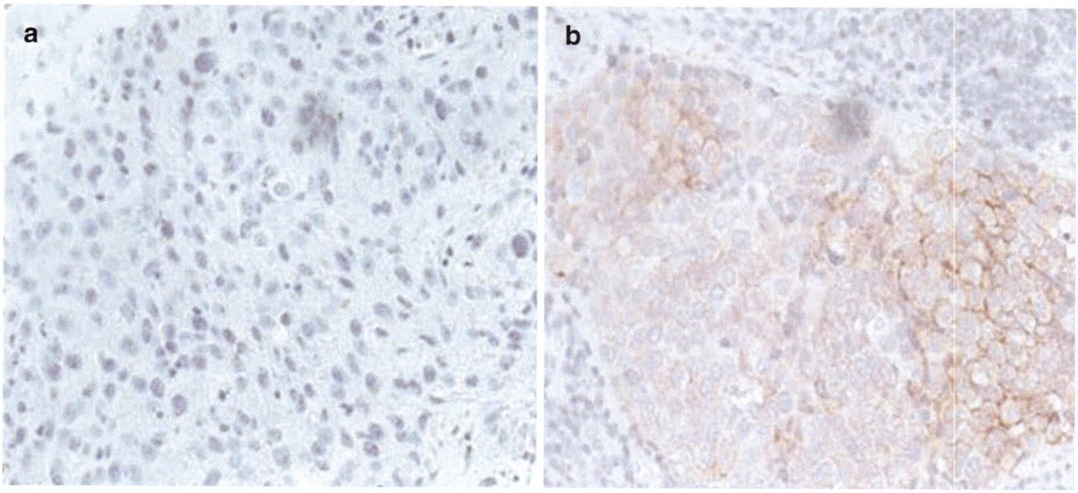

Fig. 15.7 IHC analysis results showing immunostaining grades with ratios 0 to 1+ are negative for HER2 membrane staining and 2+ are equivocal and 3+ are positive for HER2 membrane staining. (**a**) Score 0, normal by IHC, (**b**) Score 1+ normal by IHC, (**c**) Score 2+ equivocal by IHC, (**d**) Score 3+ abnormal

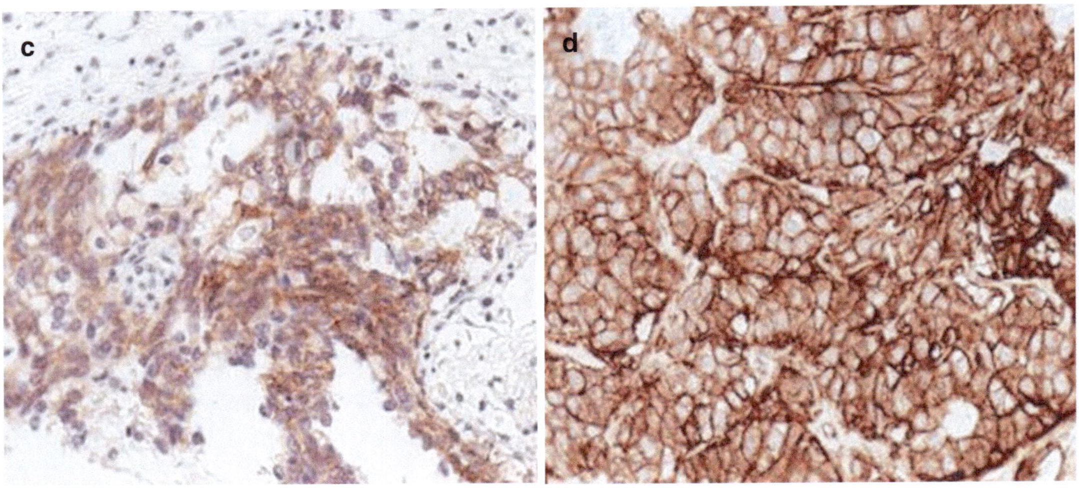

Fig. 15.7 (continued)

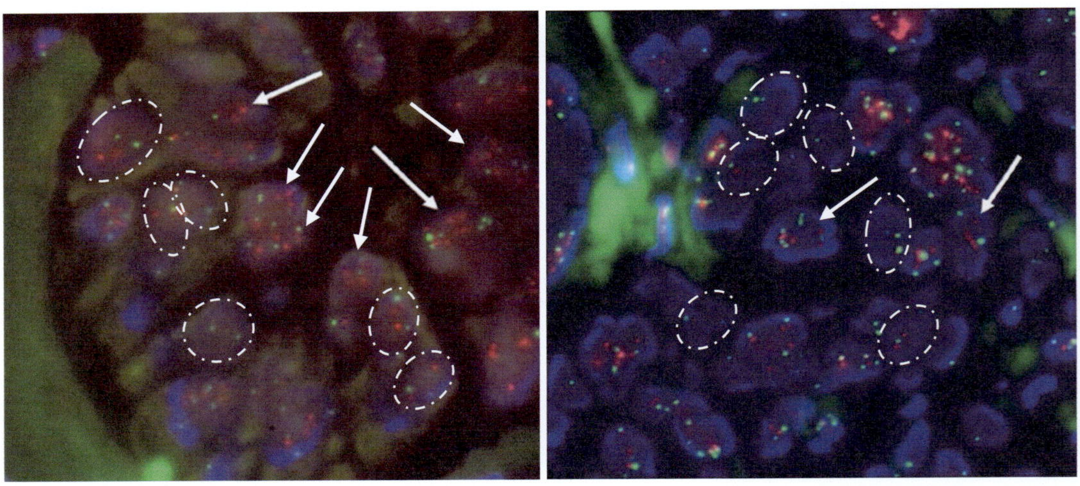

Fig. 15.8 GH+ Invasive Ductal Carcinoma with mixture of HER2 positive and HER2 negative cells—Arrows indicate cells with HER2 amplification under 1000× total magnification. Dotted circles outline normal cells. Red = HER2 gene, Green = Centromere 17 detected using PathVysion® fluorescent probes. Images show positive for genetic heterogeneity and negative for amplification by ASCO/CAP guidelines

Imaging of FISH analysis is performed using MetaSystems ISIS software (MetaSystems, MA, USA) or any other Image Analysis Software that is currently available in the market (Fig. 15.8).

A study of 2522 cases by Chang et al. [232] reported a 4% (24/666) rate of HER2 amplification in GH+ tumors. However, their rate of an "equivocal" score among GH+ tumors was 31.5% due to the overall HER2 ratio in cases with "equivocal" results being close to 2.2 [232]. One note should be made that a rate difference would likely be seen in the results published by Chang et al. [232] which would be attributed to ASCO/CAP guidelines used at the time of reporting (2007 versus 2013) as this would change the number of qualifying test results.

Human trials on newly diagnosed GH+/Amplification-negative cases have been carried out. The NSABP trial B-31 investigated adjuvant Herceptin® and chemotherapy, and found a benefit of disease-free survival in patients with normal HER2 copy number treated with antibody-based Herceptin® therapy [233]. Based on this evidence and ongoing clinical trials, the ASCO/CAP guidelines need to be revisited to establish the significance of reporting of GH+ IDC breast tumors by determining the efficacy of treatment in these patients.

Comparing our research data (unpublished data: Jodlowski T, Ramesh KH) from a total of 998 cases of GH+ and GH− tumors, the rates of HER2-negative results were similar; 67% of GH− tumors (Table 15.5) and 64% of GH+ tumors (Table 15.6) were HER2-negative. From our data, the HER2-cases reported that displayed GH totaled 77 (Table 15.6); this number represents the eligible patients over the course of 7 years who could have received potentially beneficial treatment of adjuvant chemotherapy in conjunction with Herceptin®, an additional 7.7% (77/998) of HER2-amplified patients.

Table 15.5 Distribution of the 878 HER2 GH-cases sorted by HER2 FISH amplification status using ASCO/CAP Scoring criteria

Criteria	N	%	Reported HER2 status
Positive: HER2 ratio <2 and ≥6 HER2 copies/cell average	198	22.5	Positive
Positive: HER2 ratio >2 and <4 HER2 copies/cell average	86	9.8	Positive
Negative: HER2 ratio <2 and <4 HER2 copies/cell average	594	67.7	Negative

Table 15.6 Distribution of the 120 HER2 GH+ cases sorted by HER2 FISH Amplification Status using ASCO/CAP Scoring criteria

Criteria	N	%	Reported HER2 status
Positive: HER2 ratio <2 and ≥6 HER2 copies/cell average	42	35.0	Positive
Positive: HER2 ratio >2 and <4 HER2 copies/cell average	1	0.8	Positive
Negative: HER2 ratio <2 and <4 HER2 copies/cell average	77	64.2	Negative

The use of Herceptin® demonstrates that antibody therapy can improve the quality of life, and life expectancy as well, especially in early treatment [127, 234]. Among the various antibody treatments for HER2+ IDC; Herceptin® decreased recurrence rates by about 50%, while increasing survival rates of patients with aggressive metastatic breast cancers that were positive for HER2 amplification [235]. Early detection of HER2+ breast cancer and subsequent treatment with adjuvant Herceptin® and chemotherapy reduced death rates by up to 40% [170, 173–176].

Following these examples, one can assume that tumorigenesis can be attenuated in these focally positive regions by inactivation of the HER2 signaling pathway using Herceptin® with adjuvant chemotherapy as treated in HER2 amplified tumors [120, 220]. This is supported because the cases submitted for FISH typically display IDC activity, where cells are found invading the ductal lining within the mammary tissue [236]. Antibody therapy would target these GH regions, as they overexpress HER2 at the cell surface.

In the microenvironment of mammary ducts, there are mammary stem cells that develop alveoli during pregnancy [237] in preparation for milk secretion. This suggests that mammary tissues are dynamic and heterogeneous, which can facilitate transformation and invasion when HER2 amplification is acquired among these cells, as there is evidence of HER2-induced EMT tumor evolution into a similar stem cell-like state [238]. These transformed cells are capable of metastasizing, and evading an immune response much like the mesenchymal stem cells native to the mammary gland [239, 240].

It is likely, that HER2 amplification is acquired during genetic instability events in HER2− tumors displaying IDC, following a Darwinian model of selection [241]. This suggests that these genetic instability events in GH+ tumors and microenvironment regions potentially select for HER2 amplification as early stages of an evolving HER2 amplified tumor [242, 243].

Identification by FISH of HER2 amplified cells nested in an IDC of the breast sample might be early stage identification of an evolving heterogeneous cancer, as the progenitor cell population for a metastatic tumor clone [126, 171]. Evidence suggesting that GH+ cases may be a snapshot of a precursor HER2 amplified cell population was described by Korkaya et al. [170], where circulating HER2 amplified cells were found as an acquired trait in relation to the primary tumor. Similarly, in another study by Meng et al. [194], secondary metastasized breast cancers were found positive for HER2 amplification while the primary tumor was negative for HER2 amplification.

15.1.17 Genetic Heterogeneity

HER2 genetic heterogeneity is defined as the presence of greater than 5% and less than 50% of tumor cells in IDC with a HER2/centromere 17 ratio of equal to or greater than 2.0, or 6.0 copies of the HER2 gene per tumor cell [169].

These GH+ and technically HER2-patients currently remain in the "grey zone". In such cases, conventional scoring by ACSO/CAP guidelines defines tumors as negative for HER2 amplification even for tumors comprised of cells that display the features of amplification by FISH. Treatment with adjuvant Herceptin® and chemotherapy in these patients with GH could potentially reduce HER2 activity, attenuating or preventing secondary tumor metastasis and proliferation [244].

15.1.18 FISH Scoring and Limitations

The data of interest for GH is a subset of clinical cases that scored mostly 2+ by IHC and were analyzed by FISH using 20 cells. Tumor sampling can lead to sampling bias based on the sectioned area submitted for testing or in cases where a needle core biopsy is used, further narrowing the capacity to screen a representation of the tumor by FISH. As tumors evolve, the composition of cells diversify, and tumor sampling in conjunction with various testing methodologies creates a snapshot of the current state of the tumor. Based on our findings, it would be beneficial to perform IHC or FISH testing on at least two or more (if possible) tumor regions or sections of the same block to better characterize GH and confirm or rule out HER2 amplification.

Another limitation by FISH is testing for polysomy in HER2 amplified cases [168, 245]. One study of HER2 breast cancer by Tse et al. [246] reported 58 of 130 cases that were originally classified as non-amplified and later found to be amplified by alternative testing. In the same study, 13 of 14 equivocal cases were found to be amplified using alternative blocks or sections.

Cases with polysomy of chromosome 17 by FISH comprise another facet of the complexity in determining amplification status. An increase in chromosome 17 copies is an alternative mechanism in which amplification of HER2 can occur [247]. Herceptin® treatment of patients found positive for polysomy 17 was seen to reduce overexpression by IHC and correlated with a positive response to therapy. Based on this, in cases with increased centromere 17 count, the HER2 copy number should be used to determine amplification status [248, 249]. In challenging cases where polysomy and copy number are equivocal, a repeat assessment on a new block [3] of the tumor or alternative probes localizing to chromosome 17 [250] should be used. Repeat FISH testing of "equivocal" HER2 FISH cases is no longer recommended as per the 2018 ASCO/CAP update for ERBB2 testing of IDC of breast [172].

As technology in clinical laboratories advance by use of state of the art techniques such as array comparative genomic hybridization—aCGH [251] or next-generation sequencing—NGS [252], a more in-depth analysis of relevant genes [253] can be made to better track and treat breast cancers. Sequencing of circulating tumor cells in plasma to stage tumor progression [254] and monitor chemotherapy resistance [255] is becoming increasingly available and popular [256]. As more data is collected and made available to physicians, a more personalized therapy [257, 258] can be provided based on serial monitoring and response to therapy.

15.1.19 Supporting HER2 Amplified Results in GH+ Cases

Our unpublished research data collected over the course of 7 years suggests that an update to the ASCO/CAP guidelines to include reporting GH (those where GH is seen in greater than 25% of cells) as positive for amplification would roughly equate to reporting an additional 8% of cases tested for HER2 by FISH (Table 15.6). This (8%) is a significant number considering that alternative treatment options available in lieu of Herceptin® are not as effective when treating patients suspected of HER2 amplification [259]. This especially holds true in TNBC cases, which respond very poorly to most treatment regimens. This recommendation would extend the available treatment options to those patients, based on literature review of treatment in cases of non-amplified HER2 status and the observed rates of GH. There are not many representative patients with GH+ scoring below IHC guidelines, and treatment may or may not benefit this small representative group of GH+ tumors [172, 260].

Ultimately, the risks of Herceptin® therapy need to be weighed against the benefits as cardiomyopathy is a serious risk factor in patients treated with Herceptin® [169]. Cardiac status monitoring prior to, during, and post Herceptin® treatment is the current standard of patient care which adds to the cost of Herceptin® treatment modality [176, 261]. Many patients positive with HER2+ IDC of breast fail to qualify for the benefits of Herceptin® treatment due to poor cardiac function or prior existing cardiac disease [262]. Non-amplified tumors of HER2 that have undergone only chemotherapy [263] have a lower pathological complete response rate than therapies directed toward HER2+ tumors [264], which indicates a lower effectiveness that could be due to treating an earlier stage or pre-amplified tumor.

The results are not clear in all cases, and studies on treatment with Herceptin® and adjuvant chemotherapy on HER2-negative tumors find either no additional benefit or some benefit [233] to relative disease-free survival. Patients with low level HER2 amplification or GH+ have been reported as having a shorter disease-free survival [265] and whether this shorter disease-free survival is due to not having Herceptin® therapy available or to other genetic factors that influence treatment outcomes is unknown.

Among the 998 cases in 7 years, a rate of 7.7% (77/998) of cases had GH+ and were reported as negative (Table 8). It is these GH+ cases that score negative for HER2 amplification that ultimately would benefit from a re-assessment by the ASCO/CAP Guideline Committee. It is also imperative to make public the outcomes of GH+ cases being treated with the FDA-approved treatment options for HER2 amplification to gather data on risk factors and disease-free survival which may influence ASCO/CAP guidelines.

15.2 Conclusion

Summary of HER2 ISH diagnostic criteria (ASCO/CAP, 2018)

HER2 positive	HER2 negative
Dual probe assay	
Group 1	Group 2 AND concurrent IHC 0-1 + or 2+
Group 2 AND concurrent IHC 3+	Group 3 AND concurrent IHC 0-1 +
Group 3 AND concurrent IHC 2+ or 3+	Group 4 AND concurrent IHC 0-1 + or 2+
Group 4 AND concurrent IHC 3+	Group 5

Group 1	Group 2	Group 3	Group 4	Group 5
Ratio ≥ 2.0	Ratio ≥ 2.0	Ratio < 2.0	Ratio < 2.0	Ratio < 2.0
≥4.0 signals/cell	<4.0 signals/cell	≥6.0 signals/cell	≥4.0 and <6.0 signals/cell	<4.0 signals/cell

Group 2

Comment: Evidence is limited on the efficacy of HER2-targeted therapy in the small subset of cases with a HER2/CEP17 ratio of >2.0 and an average HER2 copy number of <4.0 per cell. In the first generation of adjuvant Trastuzumab trials, patients in this subgroup who were randomly assigned to the Trastuzumab arm did not seem to derive an improvement in disease-free or overall survival, but there were too few such cases to draw definitive conclusions. IHC expression for

HER2 should be used to complement ISH and define HER2 status. If the IHC result is not 3+ positive, it is recommended that the specimen be considered HER2 negative because of the low HER2 copy number by ISH and the lack of protein overexpression.

Group 3

Comment: There are insufficient data on the efficacy of HER2-targeted therapy in cases with a HER2 ratio of <2.0 in the absence of protein overexpression because such patients were not eligible for the first generation of adjuvant Trastuzumab clinical trials. When concurrent IHC results are negative (0 or 1+), it is recommended that the specimen be considered HER2 negative.

Group 4

Comment: It is uncertain whether patients with an average of ≥4.0 and <6.0 HER2 signals per cell and a HER2/CEP17 ratio of, 2.0 benefit from HER2 targeted therapy in the absence of protein over expression (IHC 3+). If the specimen test result is close to the ISH ratio threshold for positive, there is a high likelihood that repeat testing will result in different results by chance alone. Therefore, when IHC results are not 3+positive, it is recommended that the sample be considered HER2 negative without additional testing on the same specimen.

The ASCO/CAP 2013 HER2 and IHC scoring guideline has been re-visited and revisions regarding IHC and FISH scoring criteria has been issued in June of 2018 [172] and is a mandated requirement to use this new scoring criteria to result HER2 FISH Analysis cases in the US as of January 2019. Some of the key changes include: IHC 2+ (equivocal) is defined as IDC of breast with "weak to moderate complete membrane staining seen in >10% of tumor cells in the invasive area" [172]. HER2 FISH results with ratio of ≥2.0 and HER2 copy number <4.0; and HER2 FISH results with ratio of ≤2.0 and HER2 copy number per cell ≥6.0 need to be re-scored by a second blind read after consultation with the pathologist and review of IHC slides. Results should be adjusted based on the results of the second blind read. Equivocal FISH results (HER2 ratio of <2.0 and copy number >4.0 to <6.0) has been eliminated. The definition of GH remains unchanged and has not been addressed in the revised guideline. For details on the ASCO/CAP 2018 revised ERBB2 status in breast cancer by IHC and FISH testing and Scoring Guidelines—readers are strongly encouraged to refer to the 2018 publication of Wolff et al. [172].

The efficacy of HER2-targeted therapy in GH+ cases must be established after review of the on-going world-wide clinical trials to ultimately validate treatment of GH+ cases with HER2 targeted therapies. This will have a significant impact on re-addressing the ASCO/CAP scoring guidelines for HER2 amplification in IDC of breast by IHC and FISH testing once again. Treatment options that are available to patients positive for HER2 amplification must also be made available to patients harboring GH+ (HER2 amplified) tumors. GH of the HER2 gene seen in greater than 25% of the tumor cells by FISH analysis should not be ignored!

References

1. Center for Disease Control [CDC]. Cancer Data and Statistics. 2017. https://www.cdc.gov/cancer/dcpc/data/index.htm.
2. Mulligan AM., O'Malley FP. The breast. Rubin's pathlogy. In: Strayer DS, editor. Clinico pathologic foundation of medicine, 7th edn. Philadelphia: Lippincott Williams & Wilkins. p. 1053–1078.
3. Wolff AC, Elizabeth M, Hammond H, Hayes DF, Dowsett M, Craig Alfred D, Karen KL, Badve S, Fitzgibbons PL, Francis G, Goldstein NS, Hayes M, Hicks DG, Lester S, Love R, Mangu PB, McShane L, Osborne KC, Paik S, Perlmutter J, Rhodes A, Sasano H, Schwartz JN, Sweep FC, Taube S, Torlakovic E, Valenstein P, Viale G, Visscher D, Wheeler T, Williams BR, Wittliff JL. American Society of Clinical Oncology/College of American Pathologists guideline recommendations for immunhistochemical testing of estrogen and progesterone receptors in breast cancer. Arch Pathol Lab Med. 2010;134:49–72.
4. Jemal A, Siegel R, Xu J, Ward E. Cancer statistics, 2010. CA Cancer J Clin. 2010;60(5):277–300.
5. DeSantis CE, Fedewa SA, Goding Sauer A, Kramer JL, Smith RA, Jemal A. Breast cancer statistics, 2015: convergence of incidence rates between black and white women. CA Cancer J Clin. 2016;66(1):31–42.
6. Abbas T, Keaton MA, Dutta A. Genomic instability in cancer. Cold Spring Harb Perspect Biol. 2013;5(3):a012914. https://doi.org/10.1101/cshperspect.a012914.

7. Negrini S, Gorgoulis VG, Halazonetis TD. Genomic instability—an evolving hallmark of cancer. Nat Rev Mol Cell Biol. 2010;11(3):220–8.
8. Martin SA, Hewish M, Lord CJ, Ashworth A. Genomic instability and the selection of treatments for cancer. J Pathol. 2010;220(2):281–9.
9. Chia SK, Speers CH, D'Yachkova Y, Kang A, Malfair-Taylor S, Barnett J, Coldman A, Gelmon KA, O'Reilly SE, Olivotto IA. The impact of new chemotherapeutic and hormone agents on survival in a population-based cohort of women with metastatic breast cancer. Cancer. 2007;110(5):973–9.
10. Ruiterkamp J, Ernst MF, de Munck L, van der Heiden-van der Loo M, Bastiaannet E, van de Poll-Franse LV, Bosscha K, Tjan-Heijnen VC, Voogd AC. Improved survival of patients with primary distant metastatic breast cancer in the period of 1995-2008. A nationwide population-based study in the Netherlands. Breast Cancer Res Treat. 2011;128(2):495–503.
11. Gerlinger M, Swanton C. How Darwinian models inform therapeutic failure initiated by clonal heterogeneity in cancer medicine. Br J Cancer. 2010;103(8):1139–43.
12. Marusyk A, Polyak K. Tumor heterogeneity: causes and consequences. Biochim Biophys Acta. 2010;1805(1):105.
13. Korona DA, LeCompte KG, Pursell ZF. The high fidelity and unique error signature of human DNA polymerase ε. Nucleic Acids Res. 2011;39(5):1763–73.
14. Nowell PC. The clonal evolution of tumor cell populations. Science. 1976;194(4260):23–8.
15. Mounawar M, Mukeria A, Le Calvez F, Hung RJ, Renard H, Cortot A, Bollart C, Zaridze D, Brennan P, Boffetta P, Brambilla E, Hainaut P. Patterns of EGFR, HER2, *TP53* and KRAS; mutations of p14 expression in non-small cell lung cancers in relation to smoking history. Cancer Res. 2007;67(12):5667.
16. Rexer BN, Arteaga CL. Intrinsic and acquired resistance to HER2-targeted therapies in HER2 gene-amplified breast cancer: mechanisms and clinical implications. Crit Rev Oncog. 2012;17(1):1–16.
17. Krajcovic M, Johnson NB, Sun Q, Normand G, Hoover N, Yao E, Richardson AL, King RW, Cibas ES, Schnitt SJ, Brugge JS, Overholtzer M. A non-genetic route to aneuploidy in human cancers. Nat Cell Biol. 2011;13(3):324–30.
18. Alexander JL, Beagan K, Orr-Weaver TL, McVey M. Multiple mechanisms contribute to double-strand break repair at rereplication forks in Drosophila follicle cells. Proc Natl Acad Sci U S A. 2016;113(48):13809–14.
19. Vassilev A, DePamphilis ML. Links between DNA replication, stem cells and cancer. Genes. 2017;8(2):45.
20. Corces-Zimmerman MR, Hong W-J, Weissman IL, Medeiros BC, Majeti R. Preleukemic mutations in human acute myeloid leukemia affect epigenetic regulators and persist in remission. Proc Natl Acad Sci. 2014;111(7):2548–53.
21. Hanahan D, Weinberg RA. The hallmarks of cancer. Cell. 2000;100(1):57–70.
22. Wu A, Zhang Q, Lambert G, Khin Z, Gatenby RA, Kim HJ, Pourmand N, Bussey K, Davies PC, Sturm JC, Austin RH. Ancient hot and cold genes and chemotherapy resistance emergence. Proc Natl Acad Sci U S A. 2015;112(33):10467–72.
23. Rhei E, Kang L, Bogomolniy F, Federici MG, Borgen PI, Boyd J. Mutation analysis of the putative tumor suppressor gene PTEN/MMAC1 in primary breast carcinomas. Cancer Res. 1997;57(17):3657–9.
24. Thor AD, Moore DH, Edgerton SM, Kawasaki ES, Reihsaus E, Lynch HT, Marcus JN, Schwartz L, Chen LC, Mayall BH, Smith HS. Accumulation of *TP53* tumor suppressor gene protein: an independent marker of prognosis in breast cancers. J Natl Cancer Inst. 1992;84(11):845–55.
25. Siegel PM, Dankort DL, Hardy WR, Muller WJ. Novel activating mutations in the neu proto-oncogene involved in induction of mammary tumors. Mol Cell Biol. 1994;14(11):7068–77.
26. Slamon D, Godolphin W, Jones L, Holt J, Wong S, Keith D, Levin W, Stuart S, Udove J, Ullrich A, Press M. Studies of the HER-2/neu proto-oncogene in human breast and ovarian cancer. Science. 1989;244(4905):707–12.
27. Halazonetis TD, Gorgoulis VG, Bartek J. An oncogene-induced DNA damage model for cancer development. Science. 2008;319(5868):1352–5.
28. Sarkisian CJ, Keister BA, Stairs DB, Boxer RB, Moody SE, Chodosh LA. Dose-dependent oncogene-induced senescence in vivo and its evasion during mammary tumorigenesis. Nat Cell Biol. 2007;9(5):493.
29. Jonkers J, Meuwissen R, van der Gulden H, Peterse H, van der Valk M, Berns A. Synergistic tumor suppressor activity of BRCA2 and *TP53* in a conditional mouse model for breast cancer. Nat Genet. 2001;29(4):418.
30. Berx G, Roy FV. The E-cadherin/catenin complex: an important gatekeeper in breast cancer tumorigenesis and malignant progression. Breast Cancer Res. 2001;3(5):289.
31. Teixeira C, Reed JC, Pratt MC. Estrogen promotes chemotherapeutic drug resistance by a mechanism involving Bcl-2 proto-oncogene expression in human breast cancer cells. Cancer Res. 1995;55(17):3902–7.
32. Vanhaesebroeck B, Reed JC, De Valck D, Grooten J, Miyashita T, Tanaka S, Beyaert R, Van Roy F, Fiers W. Effect of bcl-2 proto-oncogene expression on cellular sensitivity to tumor necrosis factor-mediated cytotoxicity. Oncogene. 1993;8(4):1075–81.
33. Franke TF, Kaplan DR, Cantley LC, Toker A. Direct regulation of the Akt proto-oncogene product by phosphatidylinositol-3, 4-bisphosphate. Science. 1997;275(5300):665–8.
34. Carmeci C, Thompson DA, Ring HZ, Francke U, Weigel RJ. Identification of a gene (GPR30) with homology to the G-protein-coupled receptor super-

family associated with estrogen receptor expression in breast cancer. Genomics. 1997;45(3):607–17.
35. Dastmalchi S, Church WB, Morris MB. Modelling the structures of G protein-coupled receptors aided by three-dimensional validation. BMC Bioinformatics. 2008;9(Suppl 1):S14.
36. Hibert MF, Trumpp-Kallmeyer S, Bruinvels A, Hoflack J. Three-dimensional models of neurotransmitter G-binding protein-coupled receptors. Mol Pharmacol. 1991;40(1):8–15.
37. Milburn MV, Tong L, deVos AM, Brunger A, Yamaizumi Z, Nishimura S, Kim SH. Molecular switch for signal transduction: structural differences between active and inactive forms of protooncogenic ras proteins. Science. 1990;247(4945):939–45.
38. Picard D, Bunone G, Liu JW, Donzé O. Steroid-independent activation of steroid receptors in mammalian and yeast cells and in breast cancer. Biochem Soc Trans. 1997;25(2):597–602.
39. Takai Y, Sasaki T, Matozaki T. Small GTP-binding proteins. Physiol Rev. 2001;81(1):153.
40. Harding A, Cortez-Toledo E, Magner NL, Beegle JR, Coleal-Bergum DP, Hao D, Wang A, Nolta JA, Zhou P. Highly efficient differentiation of endothelial cells from pluripotent stem cells requires the MAPK and the PI3K pathways. Stem Cells. 2017;35(4):909–19.
41. El-Ashry D, Miller DL, Kharbanda S, Lippman ME, Kern FG. Constitutive Raf-1 kinase activity in breast cancer cells induces both estrogen-independent growth and apoptosis. Oncogene. 1997;15(4):423–35.
42. Huang W, Alessandrini A, Crews CM, Erikson RL. Raf-1 forms a stable complex with Mek1 and activates Mek1 by serine phosphorylation. Proc Natl Acad Sci. 1993;90(23):10947–51.
43. Huang Y, Burns DJ, Rich BE, MacNeil IA, Dandapat A, Soltani SM, Myhre S, Sullivan BF, Lange CA, Furcht LT, Laing LG. Development of a test that measures real-time HER2 signaling function in live breast cancer cell lines and primary cells. BMC Cancer. 2017;17(1):199.
44. Kivi R, Solovjova K, Haljasorg T, Arukuusk P, Jarv J. Allosteric effect of adenosine triphosphate on peptide recognition by 3′5′-cyclic adenosine monophosphate dependent protein kinase catalytic subunits. Protein J. 2016;35(6):459–66.
45. Fernandez A, Cavadore JC, Demaille J, Lamb N. Implications for cAMP-dependent protein kinase in the maintenance of the interphase state. Prog Cell Cycle Res. 1995;1:241–53.
46. Kim C, Xuong NH, Taylor SS. Crystal structure of a complex between the catalytic and regulatory (RIalpha) subunits of PKA. Science. 2005;307(5710):690–6.
47. Rudack T, Xia F, Schlitter J, Kötting C, Gerwert K. The role of magnesium for geometry and charge in GTP hydrolysis, revealed by quantum mechanics/molecular mechanics simulations. Biophys J. 2012;103(2):293–302.
48. Gurevich VV, Song X, Vishnivetskiy SA, Gurevich EV. Enhanced phosphorylation-independent arrestins and gene therapy. Handb Exp Pharmacol. 2014;219:133–52.
49. Palczewski K, Kumasaka T, Hori T, Behnke CA, Motoshima H, Fox BA, Le Trong I, Teller DC, Okada T, Stenkamp RE, Yamamoto M, Miyano M. Crystal structure of rhodopsin: a G protein-coupled receptor. Science. 2000;289(5480):739–45.
50. Prossnitz ER, Arterburn JB, Sklar LA. GPR30: a G protein-coupled receptor for estrogen. Mol Cell Endocrinol. 2007;265–266:138–42.
51. Resnitzky D, Gossen M, Bujard H, Reed SI. Acceleration of the G_1/S phase transition by expression of cyclins D1 and E with an inducible system. Mol Cell Biol. 1994;14(3):1669–79.
52. Kanda N, Watanabe S. 17beta-estradiol stimulates the growth of human keratinocytes by inducing cyclin D_2 expression. J Invest Dermatol. 2004;123(2):319–28.
53. Stahl P, Seeschaaf C, Lebok P, Kutup A, Bockhorn M, Izbicki JR, Bokemeyer C, Simon R, Sauter G, Marx AH. Heterogeneity of amplification of HER2, EGFR, CCND1 and MYC in gastric cancer. BMC Gastroenterol. 2015;15:7.
54. Cantley LC, Auger KR, Carpenter C, Duckworth B, Graziani A, Kapeller R, Soltoff S. Oncogenes and signal transduction. Cell. 1991;64(2):281–302.
55. Danielsen AJ, Maihle NJ. Ligand-independent oncogenic transformation by the EGF receptor requires kinase domain catalytic activity. Exp Cell Res. 2002;275(1):9–16.
56. Burgess AW, Cho HS, Eigenbrot C, Ferguson KM, Garrett TP, Leahy DJ, Lemmon MA, Sliwkowski MX, Ward CW, Yokoyama S. An open-and-shut case? Recent insights into the activation of EGF/ErbB receptors. Mol Cell. 2003;12(3):541–52.
57. Boerner JL, Danielsen AJ, Lovejoy CA, Wang Z, Juneja SC, Faupel-Badger JM, Darce JR, Maihle NJ. Grb2 regulation of the actin-based cytoskeleton is required for ligand-independent EGF receptor-mediated oncogenesis. Oncogene. 2003;22(43):6679–89.
58. Nakamura Y, Hibino K, Yanagida T, Sako Y. Switching of the positive feedback for RAS activation by a concerted function of SOS membrane association domains. Biophys Physicobiol. 2016;13:1–11.
59. Mao Y, Xi L, Li Q, Cai Z, Lai Y, Zhang X, Yu C. Regulation of cell apoptosis and proliferation in pancreatic cancer through PI3K/Akt pathway via Polo-like kinase 1. Oncol Rep. 2016;36(1):49–56.
60. Leevers SJ, Vanhaesebroeck B, Waterfield MD. Signalling through phosphoinositide 3-kinases: the lipids take centre stage. Curr Opin Cell Biol. 1999;11(2):219–25.
61. Didichenko SA, Tilton B, Hemmings BA, Ballmer-Hofer K, Thelen M. Constitutive activation of protein kinase B and phosphorylation of p47phox by a membrane-targeted phosphoinositide 3-kinase. Curr Biol. 1996;6(10):1271–8.
62. Andjelkovic M, Alessi DR, Meier R, Fernandez A, Lamb NJ, Frech M, Cron P, Cohen P, Lucocq JM,

Hemmings BA. Role of translocation in the activation and function of protein kinase B. J Biol Chem. 1997;272(50):31515–24.

63. Di Blasio L, Gagliardi PA, Puliafito A, Primo L. Serine/threonine kinase 3-phosphoinositide-dependent protein kinase-1 (PDK1) as a key regulator of cell migration and cancer dissemination. Cancers (Basel). 2017;9(3).
64. Scott PH, Brunn GJ, Kohn AD, Roth RA, Lawrence JC Jr. Evidence of insulin-stimulated phosphorylation and activation of the mammalian target of rapamycin mediated by a protein kinase B signaling pathway. Proc Natl Acad Sci U S A. 1998;95(13):7772–7.
65. Ebner M, Sinkovics B, Szczygiel M, Ribeiro DW, Yudushkin I. Localization of mTORC2 activity inside cells. J Cell Biol. 2017;216(2):343–53.
66. Chang F, Lee JT, Navolanic PM, Steelman LS, Shelton JG, Blalock WL, Franklin RA, McCubrey JA. Involvement of PI3K/Akt pathway in cell cycle progression, apoptosis, and neoplastic transformation: a target for cancer chemotherapy. Leukemia. 2003;17(3):590–603.
67. Singh RP, Emery AN, Al-Rubeai M. Enhancement of survivability of mammalian cells by overexpression of the apoptosis-suppressor gene bcl-2. Biotechnol Bioeng. 1996;52(1):166–75.
68. Slupianek A, Nieborowska-Skorska M, Hoser G, Morrione A, Majewski M, Xue L, Morris SW, Wasik MA, Skorski T. Role of phosphatidylinositol 3-kinase-Akt pathway in nucleophosmin/anaplastic lymphoma kinase-mediated lymphomagenesis. Cancer Res. 2001;61(5):2194–9.
69. Lu Y, Lin YZ, LaPushin R, Cuevas B, Fang X, Yu SX, Davies MA, Khan H, Furui T, Mao M, Zinner R, Hung MC, Steck P, Siminovitch K, Mills GB. The PTEN/MMAC1/TEP tumor suppressor gene decreases cell growth and induces apoptosis and anoikis in breast cancer cells. Oncogene. 1999;18:7034–45.
70. Costoya JA, Finidori J, Moutoussamy S, Searis R, Devesa J, Arce VM. Activation of growth hormone receptor delivers an antiapoptotic signal: evidence for a role of Akt in this pathway. Endocrinology. 1999;140(12):5937–43.
71. Haas-Kogan D, Shalev N, Wong M, Mills G, Yount G, Stokoe D. Protein kinase B (PKB/Akt) activity is elevated in glioblastoma cells due to mutation of the tumor suppressor PTEN/MMAC. Curr Biol. 1998;8(21):1195–8.
72. Nass SJ, Herman JG, Gabrielson E, Iversen PW, Parl FF, Davidson NE, Graff JR. Aberrant methylation of the estrogen receptor and E-cadherin 5′ CpG islands increases with malignant progression in human breast cancer. Cancer Res. 2000;60(16):4346–8.
73. Oka H, Shiozaki H, Kobayashi K, Inoue M, Tahara H, Kobayashi T, Takatsuka Y, Matsuyoshi N, Hirano S, Takeichi M, Mori T. Expression of E-cadherin cell adhesion molecules in human breast cancer tissues and its relationship to metastasis. Cancer Res. 1993;53(7):1696–701.
74. Bartek J, Iggo R, Gannon J, Land DP. Genetic and immunocytochemical analysis of mutant *TP53* in human breast cancer. Oncogene. 1990;5(6):893–9.
75. Zhang M, Zhuang G, Sun X, Shen Y, Wang W, Li Q, Di W. TP53 mutation-mediated genomic instability induces the evolution of chemoresistance and recurrence in epithelial ovarian cancer. Diagn Pathol. 2017;12(1):16.
76. Zhang X, Ai Z, Chen J, Yi J, Liu Z, Zhao H, Wei H. Glycometabolic adaptation mediates the insensitivity of drug-resistant K562/ADM leukaemia cells to adriamycin via the AKT-mTOR/c-Myc signalling pathway. Mol Med Rep. 2017;15(4):1869–76.
77. Merten L, Agaimy A, Moskalev EA, Giedl J, Kayser C, Geddert H, Schaefer IM, Cameron S, Werner M, Strobel P, Hartmann A, Haller F. Inactivating mutations of RB1 and *TP53* correlate with sarcomatous histomorphology and metastasis/recurrence in gastrointestinal stromal tumors. Am J Clin Pathol. 2016;146(6):718–26.
78. Myers MP, Stolarov JP, Eng C, Li J, Wang SI, Wigler MH, Parsons R, Tonks NK. P-TEN, the tumor suppressor from human chromosome 10q23, is a dual-specificity phosphatase. Proc Natl Acad Sci. 1997;94(17):9052–7.
79. Davis NM, Sokolosky M, Stadelman K, Abrams SL, Libra M, Candido S, Nicoletti F, Polesel J, Maestro R, D'Assoro A, Drobot L, Rakus D, Gizak A, Laidler P, Dulińska-Litewka J, Basecke J, Mijatovic S, Maksimovic-Ivanic D, Montalto G, Cervello M, Fitzgerald TL, Demidenko ZN, Martelli AM, Cocco L, Steelman LS, McCubrey JA. Deregulation of the EGFR/PI3K/PTEN/Akt/mTORC1 pathway in breast cancer: possibilities for therapeutic intervention. Oncotarget. 2014;5(13):4603–50.
80. Ashworth A, Lord CJ, Reis-Filho JS. Genetic interactions in cancer progression and treatment. Cell. 2011;145(1):30–8.
81. Birkbak NJ, Eklund AC, Li Q, McClelland SE, Endesfelder D, Tan P, Tan IB, Richardson AL, Szallasi Z, Swanton C. Paradoxical relationship between chromosomal instability and survival outcome in cancer. Cancer Res. 2011;71(10):3447–52.
82. Stoecklein NH, Hosch SB, Bezler M, Stern F, Hartmann CH, Vay C, Siegmund A, Scheunemann P, Schurr P, Knoefel WT, Verde PE, Reichelt U, Erbersdobler A, Grau R, Ullrich A, Izbicki JR, Klein CA. Direct genetic analysis of single disseminated cancer cells for prediction of outcome and therapy selection in esophageal cancer. Cancer Cell. 2008;13(5):441–53.
83. Kops GJ, Foltz DR, Cleveland DW. Lethality to human cancer cells through massive chromosome loss by inhibition of the mitotic checkpoint. Proc Natl Acad Sci U S A. 2004;101(23):8699–704.
84. Heim S, Mitelman F. Cancer cytogenetics: chromosomal and molecular genetic aberrations of tumor cells. New York: Wiley; 2015.
85. Mrózek K, Harper DP, Aplan PD. Cytogenetics and molecular genetics of acute lymphoblastic leukemia. Hematol Oncol Clin North Am. 2009;23(5):991–1010.

86. Casey SC, Vaccari M, Al-Mulla F, Al-Temaimi R, Amedei A, Barcellos-Hoff MH, Brown DG, Chapellier M, Christopher J, Curran CS, Forte S, Hamid RA, Heneberg P, Koch DC, Krishnakumar PK, Laconi E, Maguer-Satta V, Marongiu F, Memeo L, Mondello C, Raju J, Roman J, Roy R, Ryan EP, Ryeom S, Salem HK, Scovassi A, Singh N, Soucek L, Vermeulen L, Whitfield JR, Woodrick J, Colacci AM, Bisson WH, Felsher DW. The effect of environmental chemicals on the tumor microenvironment. Carcinogenesis. 2015;36(Suppl 1):S160–83.
87. Kagawa Y, Matsumoto S, Kamioka Y, Mimori K, Naito Y, Ishii T, Okuzaki D, Nishida N, Maeda S, Naito A, Kikuta J, Nishikawa K, Nishimura J, Haraguchi N, Takemasa I, Mizushima T, Ikeda M, Yamamoto H, Sekimoto M, Ishii H, Doki Y, Matsuda M, Kikuchi A, Mori M, Ishii M. Cell cycle-dependent Rho GTPase activity dynamically regulates cancer cell motility and invasion in vivo. PLoS One. 2013;8(12):e83629.
88. Sawyer E, Roylance R, Petridis C, Brook MN, Nowinski S, Papouli E, Fletcher O, Pinder S, Hanby A, Kohut K, Gorman P, Caneppele M, Peto J, dos Santos Silva I, Johnson N, Swann R, Dwek M, Perkins K-A, Gillett C, Houlston R, Ross G, De Ieso P, Southey MC, Hopper JL, Provenzano E, Apicella C, Wesseling J, Cornelissen S, Keeman R, Fasching PA, Jud SM, Ekici AB, Beckmann MW, Kerin MJ, Marme F, Schneeweiss A, Sohn C, Burwinkel B, Guénel P, Truong T, Laurent-Puig P, Kerbrat P, Bojesen SE, Nordestgaard BG, Nielsen SF, Flyger H, Milne RL, Perez JIA, Menéndez P, Benitez J, Brenner H, Dieffenbach AK, Arndt V, Stegmaier C, Meindl A, Lichtner P, Schmutzler RK, Lochmann M, Brauch H, Fischer H-P, Ko Y-D, GENICA Network, Nevanlinna H, Muranen TA, Aittomäki K, Blomqvist C, Bogdanova NV, Dörk T, Lindblom A, Margolin S, Mannermaa A, Kataja V, Kosma V-M, Hartikainen JM, Chenevix-Trench G, Investigators K, Lambrechts D, Weltens C, Van Limbergen E, Hatse S, Chang-Claude J, Rudolph A, Seibold P, Flesch-Janys D, Radice P, Peterlongo P, Bonanni B, Volorio S, Giles GG, Severi G, Baglietto L, McLean CA, Haiman CA, Henderson BE, Schumacher F, Le Marchand L, Simard J, Goldberg MS, Labrèche F, Dumont M, Kristensen V, Winqvist R, Pylkäs K, Jukkola-Vuorinen A, Kauppila S, Andrulis IL, Knight JA, Glendon G, Mulligan AM, Devillee P, Tollenaar RA, Seynaeve CM, Kriege M, Figueroa J, Chanock SJ, Sherman ME, Hooning MJ, Hollestelle A, van den Ouweland AMW, van Deurzen CHM, Li J, Czene K, Humphreys K, Cox A, Cross SS, Reed MWR, Shah M, Jakubowska A, Lubinski J, Jaworska-Bieniek K, Durda K, Swerdlow A, Ashworth A, Orr N, Schoemaker M, Couch FJ, Hallberg E, González-Neira A, Pita G, Alonso MR, Tessier DC, Vincent D, Bacot F, Bolla MK, Wang Q, Dennis J, Michailidou K, Dunning AM, Hall P, Easton D, Pharoah P, Schmidt MK, Tomlinson I, Garcia-Closas M. Genetic predisposition to in situ and invasive lobular carcinoma of the breast. PLoS Genet. 2014;10(4):e1004285. https://doi.org/10.1371/journal.pgen.1004285.
89. Fujiki K, Inamura H, Miyayama T, Matsuoka M. Involvement of Notch1 signaling in malignant progression of A549 cells subjected to prolonged cadmium exposure. J Biol Chem. 2017;292:7942–53.
90. Liu J, Li J, Li P, Wang Y, Liang Z, Jiang Y, Li J, Feng C, Wang R, Chen H, Zhou C, Zhang J, Yang J, Liu P. Loss of DLG5 promotes breast cancer malignancy by inhibiting the Hippo signaling pathway. Sci Rep. 2017;7:42125.
91. Priest AV, Shafraz O, Sivasankar S. Biophysical basis of cadherin mediated cell-cell adhesion. Exp Cell Res. 2017;358(1):10–3.
92. Yonemura S, Itoh M, Nagafuchi A, Tsukita S. Cell-to-cell adherens junction formation and actin filament organization: similarities and differences between non-polarized fibroblasts and polarized epithelial cells. J Cell Sci. 1995;108(Pt 1):127–42.
93. Adams CL, Chen Y-T, Smith SJ, James Nelson W. Mechanisms of epithelial cell–cell adhesion and cell compaction revealed by high-resolution tracking of E-cadherin– green fluorescent protein. J Cell Biol. 1998;142(4):1105–19.
94. Bendris N, Lemmers B, Blanchard JM. Cell cycle, cytoskeleton dynamics and beyond: the many functions of cyclins and CDK inhibitors. Cell Cycle. 2015;14(12):1786–98.
95. Giordano A, Gao H, Anfossi S, Cohen E, Mego M, Lee B-N, Tin S, De Laurentiis M, Parker CA, Alvarez RH, Valero V, Ueno NT, De Placido S, Mani SA, Esteva FJ, Cristofanilli M, Reuben JM. Epithelial-mesenchymal transition and stem cell markers in patients with HER2-positive metastatic breast cancer. Mol Cancer Ther. 2012;11(11):2526–34.
96. Terunuma H, Deng X, Dewan Z, Fujimoto S, Yamamoto N. Potential role of NK cells in the induction of immune responses: implications for NK cell–based immunotherapy for cancers and viral infections. Int Rev Immunol. 2008;27(3):93–110.
97. Deng W, Gowen BG, Zhang L, Wang L, Lau S, Iannello A, Xu J, Rovis TL, Xiong N, Raulet DH. Antitumor immunity. A shed NKG2D ligand that promotes natural killer cell activation and tumor rejection. Science. 2015;348(6230):136–9.
98. Morgado S, Sanchez-Correa B, Casado JG, Duran E, Gayoso I, Labella F, et al. NK cell recognition and killing of melanoma cells is controlled by multiple activating receptor-ligand interactions. J Innate Immun. 2011;3(4):365–73.
99. Boon T, Coulie PG, Van den Eynde B. Tumor antigens recognized by T cells. Immunol Today. 1997;18(6):267–8.
100. Garcia-Lora A, Algarra I, Garrido F. MHC class I antigens, immune surveillance, and tumor immune escape. J Cell Physiol. 2003;195(3):346–55.
101. Sadanaga N, Nagashima H, Mashino K, Tahara K, Yamaguchi H, Ohta M, Fujie T, Tanaka F, Inoue

H, Takesako K, Akiyoshi T, Mori M. Dendritic cell vaccination with MAGE peptide is a novel therapeutic approach for gastrointestinal carcinomas. Clin Cancer Res. 2001;7(8):2277.
102. Arteaga CL, Hurd SD, Winnier AR, Johnson MD, Fendly BM, Forbes JT. Anti-transforming growth factor (TGF)-beta antibodies inhibit breast cancer cell tumorigenicity and increase mouse spleen natural killer cell activity. Implications for a possible role of tumor cell/host TGF-beta interactions in human breast cancer progression. J Clin Investig. 1993;92(6):2569–76.
103. Landskron G, De la Fuente M, Thuwajit P, Thuwajit C, Hermoso MA. Chronic inflammation and cytokines in the tumor microenvironment. J Immunol Res. 2014: Article ID 149185, 19 pages, 2014. https://doi.org/10.1155/2014/149185.
104. Rasmusson I, Ringden O, Sundberg B, Le Blanc K. Mesenchymal stem cells inhibit the formation of cytotoxic T lymphocytes, but not activated cytotoxic T lymphocytes or natural killer cells. Transplantation. 2003;76(8):1208–13.
105. Ryan JM, Barry FP, Murphy JM, Mahon BP. Mesenchymal stem cells avoid allogeneic rejection. J Inflam (Lond). 2005;2:8.
106. Ganguly KK, Pal S, Moulik S, Chatterjee A. Integrins and metastasis. Cell Adh Migr. 2013;7(3):251–61.
107. Bose R, Kavuri SM, Searleman AC, Shen W, Shen D, Koboldt DC, Monsey J, Goel N, Aronson AB, Li S, Ma CX, Ding L, Mardis ER, Ellis MJ. Activating HER2 mutations in HER2 gene amplification negative breast cancer. Cancer Discov. 2013;3(2):224–37.
108. Navolanic PM, Steelman LS, McCubrey JA. EGFR family signaling and its association with breast cancer development and resistance to chemotherapy (Review). Int J Oncol. 2003;22(2):237–52.
109. Garrett TP, McKern NM, Lou M, Elleman TC, Adams TE, Lovrecz GO, Kofler M, Jorissen RN, Nice EC, Burgess AW, Ward CW. The crystal structure of a truncated Erbb2 ectodomain reveals an active conformation, poised to interact with other Erbb receptors. Mol Cell. 2003;11(2):495–505.
110. Peles E, Bacus SS, Koski RA, Lu HS, Wen D, Ogden SG, Levy RB, Yarden Y. Isolation of the NeuHER-2 stimulatory ligand: a 44 kd glycoprotein that induces differentiation of mammary tumor cells. Cell. 1992;69(1):205–16.
111. Shih AJ, Telesco SE, Choi SH, Lemmon MA, Radhakrishnan R. Molecular dynamics analysis of conserved hydrophobic and hydrophilic bond-interaction networks in ErbB family kinases. Biochem J. 2011;436(2):241–51.
112. Sliwkowski MX. Ready to partner. Nat Struct Biol. 2003;10(3):158–9.
113. Cho HS, Mason K, Ramyar KX, Stanley AM, Gabelli SB, Denney DW Jr, Leahy DJ. Structure of the extracellular region of HER2 alone and in complex with the Herceptin® Fab. Nature. 2003;421(6924):756–60.
114. Huang C-Y, Chen J-Y, Kuo C-H, Pai P-Y, Ho T-J, Chen T-S, Tsai F-J, Padma VV, Kuo W-W, Huang C-Y. Mitochondrial ROS-induced ERK1/2 activation and HSF2-mediated AT1R upregulation are required for doxorubicin-induced cardiotoxicity. J Cell Physiol. 2018;233(1):463–75.
115. Cohen BD, Kiener PA, Green JM, Foy L, Fell HP, Zhang K. The relationship between human epidermal growth-like factor receptor expressioin and cellular transformation NIH3T3 cells. J Biol Chem. 1996;271:30897–903.
116. Milanezi F, Carvalho S, Schmitt FC. EGFR/HER2 in breast cancer: a biological approach for molecular diagnosis and therapy. Expert Rev Mol Diagn. 2008;8(4):417–34.
117. Elseginy SA, Lazaro G, Nawwar GA, Amin KM, Hiscox S, Brancale A. Computer-aided identification of novel anticancer compounds with a possible dual HER1/HER2 inhibition mechanism. Bioorg Med Chem Lett. 2015;25(4):758–62.
118. Galdy S, Lamarca A, McNamara MG, Hubner RA, Cella CA, Fazio N, Valle JW. HER2/HER3 pathway in biliary tract malignancies; systematic review and meta-analysis: a potential therapeutic target? Cancer Metastasis Rev. 2016;36(1):141–57.
119. Garrett JT, Olivares MG, Rinehart C, Granja-Ingram ND, Sánchez V, Chakrabarty A, Manning HC. Transcriptional and posttranslational up-regulation of HER3 (ErbB3) compensates for inhibition of the HER2 tyrosine kinase. Proc Natl Acad Sci. 2011;108(12):5021–6.
120. Junttila TT, Akita RW, Parsons K, Fields C, Lewis Phillips GD, Friedman LS, Sampath D, Sliwkowski MX. Ligand-independent HER2/HER3/PI3K complex is disrupted by trastuzumab and is effectively inhibited by the PI3K inhibitor GDC-0941. Cancer Cell. 2009;15(5):429–40.
121. Portier BP, Minca EC, Wang Z, Lanigan C, Gruver AM, Downs-Kelly E, Budd GT, Tubbs RR. HER4 expression status correlates with improved outcome in both neoadjuvant and adjuvant trastuzumab treated invasive breast carcinoma. Oncotarget. 2013;4(10):1662–72.
122. Bergamaschi A, Kim YH, Wang P, Sørlie T, Hernandez-Boussard T, Lonning PE, et al. Distinct patterns of DNA copy number alteration are associated with different clinicopathological features and gene-expression subtypes of breast cancer. Genes Chromosomes Cancer. 2006;45(11):1033–40.
123. Black JD, Lopez S, Cocco E, Bellone S, Altwerger G, Schwab CL, English DP, Bonazzoli E, Predolini F, Ferrari F, Ratner E, Silasi D-A, Azodi M, Schwartz PE, Santin AD. PIK3CA oncogenic mutations represent a major mechanism of resistance to trastuzumab in HER2/neu overexpressing uterine serous carcinomas. Br J Cancer. 2015;113(7):1020–6.
124. Dancey JE. Therapeutic targets: MTOR and related pathways. Cancer Biol Ther. 2006;5(9):1065–73.
125. Menard S, Fortis S, Castiglioni F, Agresti R, Balsari A. HER2 as a prognostic factor in breast cancer. Oncology. 2001;61(Suppl 2):67–72.
126. Freudenberg JA, Wang Q, Katsumata M, Drebin J, Nagatomo I, Greene MI. The role of HER2 in early

breast cancer metastasis and the origins of resistance to HER2-targeted therapies. Exp Mol Pathol. 2009;87(1):1–11.
127. Gajria D, Chandarlapaty S. HER2-amplified breast cancer: mechanisms of trastuzumab resistance and novel targeted therapies. Expert Rev Anticancer Ther. 2011;11(2):263–75.
128. Partridge AH, Pagani O, Abulkhair O, Aebi S, Amant F, Azim HA Jr, Costa A, Delaloge S, Freilich G, Gentilini OD, Harbeck N, Kelly CM, Loibl S, Meirow D, Peccatori F, Kaufmann B, Cardoso F. First international consensus guidelines for breast cancer in young women (BCY1). Breast. 2014;23(3):209–20.
129. Murakami E, Nakanishi Y, Hirotani Y, Ohni S, Tang X, Masuda S, Enomoto K, Sakurai K, Amano S, Yamada T, Nemoto N. Roles of Ras homolog A in invasive ductal breast carcinoma. Acta Histochem Cytochem. 2016;49(5):131–40.
130. Falkenberg N, Anastasov N, HoFig I, Bashkueva K, Lindner K, Hofler H, Rosemann M, Aubele M. Additive impact of HER2-/PTK6-RNAi on interactions with HER3 or IGF-1R leads to reduced breast cancer progression in vivo. Mol Oncol. 2015;9(1):282–94.
131. Gupta P, Srivastava SK. Inhibition of HER2-integrin signaling by Cucurbitacin B leads to in vitro and in vivo breast tumor growth suppression. Oncotarget. 2014;5(7):1812–28.
132. Watson PH, Pon RT, Shiu RPC. Inhibition of c-myc expression by phosphorothioate antisense oligonucleotide identifies a critical role for c-myc in the growth of human breast cancer. Cancer Res. 1991;51(15):3996–4000.
133. Nair R, Roden DL, Teo WS, McFarland A, Junankar S, Ye S, Nguyen A, Yang J, Nikolic I, Hui M, Morey A, Shah J, Pfefferle AD, Usary J, Selinger C, Baker LA, Armstrong N, Cowley MJ, Naylor MJ, Ormandy CJ, Lakhani SR, Herschkowitz JI, Perou CM, Kaplan W, O'Toole SA, Swarbrick A. c-Myc and HER2 cooperate to drive a stem-like phenotype with poor prognosis in breast cancer. Oncogene. 2014;33(30):3992–4002.
134. Caca K, Kolligs FT, Ji X, Hayes M, Qian J, Yahanda A, Rimm DL, Costa J, Fearon ER. Beta- and gamma-catenin mutations, but not E-cadherin inactivation, underlie T-cell factor/lymphoid enhancer factor transcriptional deregulation in gastric and pancreatic cancer. Cell Growth Differ. 1999;10(6):369–76.
135. De Leeuw WJ, Berx G, Vos CB, Peterse JL, Van de Vijver MJ, Litvinov S, Van Roy F, Cornelisse CJ, Cleton-Jansen AM. Simultaneous loss of E-cadherin and catenins in invasive lobular breast cancer and lobular carcinoma in situ. J Pathol. 1997;183(4):404–11.
136. Vos CB, Cleton-Jansen AM, Berx G, de Leeuw WJ, ter Haar NT, van Roy F, Cornelisse CJ, Peterse JL, van de Vijver MJ. E-cadherin inactivation in lobular carcinoma in situ of the breast: an early event in tumorigenesis. Br J Cancer. 1997;76(9):1131–3.
137. Shehata M, Teschendorff A, Sharp G, Novcic N, Russell IA, Avril S, Prater M, Eirew P, Caldas C, Watson CJ, Stingl J. Phenotypic and functional characterisation of the luminal cell hierarchy of the mammary gland. Breast Cancer Res. 2012;14(5):R134.
138. Macias H, Hinck L. Mammary gland development. Wiley Interdiscip Rev Dev Biol. 2012;1(4):533–57.
139. Visvader JE, Stingl J. Mammary stem cells and the differentiation hierarchy: current status and perspectives. Genes Dev. 2014;28(11):1143–58.
140. Asselin-Labat ML, Vaillant F, Sheridan JM, Pal B, Wu D, Simpson ER, Yasuda H, Smyth GK, Martin TJ, Lindeman GJ, Visvader JE. Control of mammary stem cell function by steroid hormone signalling. Nature. 2010;465(7299):798–802.
141. Mani SA, Guo W, Liao MJ, Eaton EN, Ayyanan A, Zhou AY, Brooks M, Reinhard F, Zhang CC, Shipitsin M, Campbell LL, Polyak K, Brisken C, Yang J, Weinberg RA. The epithelial-mesenchymal transition generates cells with properties of stem cells. Cell. 2008;133(4):704–15.
142. Tiede B, Kang Y. From milk to malignancy: the role of mammary stem cells in development, pregnancy and breast cancer. Cell Res. 2011;21(2):245–57.
143. Lakhani SL, Ellis IO, Schnitt SJ, Tan PH, Van de Vijver MJ, editors. WHO classification of tumours of the breast. 4th ed. Lyon: IARC; 2012. p. 33–8.
144. Adachi Y, Ishiguro J, Kotani H, Hisada T, Ichikawa M, Gondo N, Yoshimura A, Kondo N, Hattori M, Sawaki M, Fujita T, Kikumori T, Yatabe Y, Kodera Y, Iwata H. Comparison of clinical outcomes between luminal invasive ductal carcinoma and luminal invasive lobular carcinoma. BMC Cancer. 2016;16:248.
145. Tavassoli FA, Devilee P, editors. WHO classification of tumours of the breast and female genital organs. 3rd ed. Lyon: IARC; 2003.
146. Agosto-Arroyo E, Isayeva T, Wei S, Almeida JS, Harada S. Differential gene expression in ductal carcinoma in situ of the breast based on ERBB2 status. Cancer Control. 2017;24(1):102–10.
147. Han K, Nofech-Mozes S, Narod S, Hanna W, Vesprini D, Saskin R, Taylor C, Kong I, Paszat L, Rakovitch E. Expression of HER2neu in ductal carcinoma in situ is associated with local recurrence. Clin Oncol (R Coll Radiol). 2012;24(3):183–9.
148. Paik S, Shak S, Tang G, Kim C, Baker J, Cronin M, Baehner FL, Walker MG, Watson D, Park T, Hiller W, Fisher ER, Wickerham DL, Bryant J, Wolmark N. A multigene assay to predict recurrence of tamoxifen-treated, node-negative breast cancer. N Engl J Med. 2004;351(27):2817–26.
149. Van 't Veer LJ, Dai H, van de Vijver MJ, He YD, Hart AAM, Mao M, Peterse HL, van der Kooy K, Marton MJ, Witteveen AT, Schreiber GJ, Kerkhoven RM, Roberts C, Linsley PS, Bernards R, Friend SH. Gene expression profiling predicts clinical outcome of breast cancer. Nature. 2002;415(6871):530–6.
150. Perou CM, Sorlie T, Eisen MB, van de Rijn M, Jeffrey SS, Rees CA, Pollack JR, Ross DT, Johnsen H, Akslen LA, Fluge O, Pergamenschikov A, Williams

C, Zhu SX, Lonning PE, Borresen-Dale A-L, Brown PO, Botstein D. Molecular portraits of human breast tumours. Nature. 2000;406(6797):747–52.

151. Sørlie T, Perou CM, Tibshirani R, Aas T, Geisler S, Johnsen H, Hastie T, Eisen MB, van de Rijn M, Jeffrey SS, Thorsen T, Quist H, Matese JC, Brown PO, Botstein D, Lønning PE, Børresen-Dale A-L. Gene expression patterns of breast carcinomas distinguish tumor subclasses with clinical implications. Proc Natl Acad Sci. 2001;98(19):10869–74.
152. Prat A, Perou CM. Deconstructing the molecular portraits of breast cancer. Mol Oncol. 2011;5(1):5–23.
153. Lim E, Vaillant F, Wu D, Forrest NC, Pal B, Hart AH, Asselin-Labat M-L, Gyorki DE, Ward T, Partanen A, Feleppa F, Huschtscha LI, Thorne HJ, Fox SB, Yan M, French JD, Brown MA, Smyth GK, Visvader JE, Lindeman GJ. Aberrant luminal progenitors as the candidate target population for basal tumor development in BRCA1 mutation carriers. Nat Med. 2009;15(8):907–13.
154. Fisher B, Costantino J, Redmond C, Poisson R, Bowman D, Couture J, Dimitrov N, Wolmark N, Wickerham L, Fisher E, Margolese R, Robidoux A, Shibata H, Terz J, Paterson A, Feldman M, Farrar W, Evans J, Lickley L, Ketner M, et al. A randomized clinical trial evaluating tamoxifen in the treatment of patients with node-negative breast cancer who have estrogen-receptor-positive tumors. N Engl J Med. 1989;320:479–84.
155. Fisher B, Dignam J, Wolmark N, DeCillis A, Emir B, Wickerham D, Bryant J, Dimitrov N, Abramson N, Atkins J, Shibata H, Deschenes L, Margolese R. Tamoxifen and chemotherapy for lymph node-negative, estrogen receptor-positive breast cancer. J Natl Cancer Inst. 1989;89:1673–82.
156. Butts A, Martin JA, DiDone L, Bradley EK, Mutz M, Krysan DJ. Structure-activity relationships for the antifungal activity of selective estrogen receptor antagonists related to tamoxifen. PLoS One. 2015;10(5):e0125927.
157. Fisher B, Jeong JH, Bryant J, Anderson S, Dignam J, Fisher ER, Wolmark N. Treatment of lymph-node-negative, oestrogen-receptor-positive breast cancer: long-term findings from National Surgical Adjuvant Breast and Bowel Project randomised clinical trials. Lancet. 2004;364:858–68.
158. Liu C-Y, Hung M-H, Wang D-S, Chu P-Y, Su J-C, Teng T-H, Huang C-T, Chao T-T, Wang C-Y, Shiau C-W, Tseng L-M, Chen K-F. Tamoxifen induces apoptosis through cancerous inhibitor of protein phosphatase 2A–dependent phospho-Akt inactivation in estrogen receptor–negative human breast cancer cells. Breast Cancer Res. 2014;16:431.
159. Liu JC, Voisin V, Wang S, Wang DY, Jones RA, Datti A, Uehling D, Al-awar R, Egan SE, Bader GD, Tsao M, Mak TW, Zacksenhaus E. Combined deletion of Pten and *TP53* in mammary epithelium accelerates triple-negative breast cancer with dependency on eEF2K. EMBO Mol Med. 2014;6(12):1542–60.
160. Liu Y, Ma L, Liu D, Yang Z, Yang C, Hu Z, Chen W, Yang Z, Chen S, Zhang Z. Impact of polysomy 17 on HER2 testing of invasive breast cancer patients. Int J Clin Exp Pathol. 2014;7(1):163–73.
161. Desta Z, Ward BA, Soukhova NV, Flockhart DA. Comprehensive evaluation of tamoxifen sequential biotransformation by the human cytochrome P450 system in vitro: prominent roles for CYP3A and CYP2D6. J Pharmacol Exp Ther. 2004;310(3):1062–75.
162. Wang DY, Fulthorpe R, Liss SN, Edwards EA. Identification of estrogen-responsive genes by complementary deoxyribonucleic acid microarray and characterization of a novel early estrogen-induced gene: EEIG1. Mol Endocrinol. 2004;18(2):402–11.
163. Foulkes WD, Stefansson IM, Chappuis PO, Begin LR, Goffin JR, Wong N, Trudel M, Akslen LA. Germline BRCA1 mutations and a basal epithelial phenotype in breast cancer. J Natl Cancer Inst. 2003;95(19):1482–5.
164. Miki Y, Swensen J, Shattuck-Eidens D, Futreal PA, Harshman K, Tavtigian S, Liu Q, Cochran C, Bennett LM, Ding W. A strong candidate for the breast and ovarian cancer susceptibility gene BRCA1. Science. 1994;266(5182):66–71.
165. Sørlie T, Tibshirani R, Parker J, Hastie T, Marron JS, Nobel A, Deng S, Johnsen H, Pesich R, Geisler S, Demeter J, Perou CM, Lønning PE, Brown PO, Børresen-Dale A-L, Botstein D. Repeated observation of breast tumor subtypes in independent gene expression data sets. Proc Natl Acad Sci U S A. 2003;100(14):8418–23.
166. Carey LA, Perou CM, Livasy CA, Dressler LG, Cowan D, Conway K, Karaca G, Troester MA, Tse CK, Edmiston S, Deming SL, Geradts J, Cheang MC, Nielsen TO, Moorman PG, Earp HS, Millikan RC. Race, breast cancer subtypes, and survival in the Carolina Breast Cancer Study. JAMA. 2006;295(21):2492–502.
167. Joyce DP, Murphy D, Lowery AJ, Curran C, Barry K, Malone C, McLaughlin R, Kerin MJ. Prospective comparison of outcome after treatment for triple-negative and non-triple-negative breast cancer. Surgeon. 2017;15(5):272–7.
168. Hanna WM, Rüschoff J, Bilous M, Coudry RA, Dowsett M, Osamura RY, Penault-Llorca F, Van De Vijver M, Viale G. HER2 in situ hybridization in breast cancer: clinical implications of polysomy 17 and genetic heterogeneity. Mod Pathol. 2014;27:4–18.
169. Wolff AC, Hammond MEH, Hicks DG, Dowsett M, McShane LM, Allison KH, Allred DC, Bartlett JMS, Bilous M, Fitzgibbons P, Hanna W, Jenkins RB, Mangu PB, Paik S, Perez EA, Press MF, Spears PA, Vance GH, Viale G, Hayes DF. Recommendations for human epidermal growth factor receptor 2 testing in breast cancer: American Society of Clinical Oncology/College of American Pathologists clinical practice guideline update. Arch Pathol Lab Med. 2014;138(2):241–56.
170. Korkaya H, Paulson A, Iovino F, Wicha MS. HER2 regulates the mammary stem/progenitor cell popula-

tion driving tumorigenesis and invasion. Oncogene. 2008;27(47):6120–30.
171. Briasoulis E, Karavasilis V, Kostadima L, Ignatiadis M, Fountzilas G, Pavlidis N. Metastatic breast carcinoma confined to bone. Cancer. 2004;101(7):1524–8.
172. Wolff AC, Hale EM, Hammon KH, Allison KH, Harvey BE, Mangu PB, Bartlett JMS, Bilous M, Ellis IO, Fitzgibbons P, Wedad H, Jenkins RB, Press MF, Spears PA, Vance GH, Viale G, McShane LM, Dowsett M. Human epidermal growth factor 2 testing in breast cancer. American Society of Clinical Oncology/College of American Pathologists Clinical Practice Guideline focussed update. Arch Pathol Lab Med. 2018. https://doi.org/10.5858/arpa.2018-0902-SA.
173. Joensuu H, Kellokumpu-Lehtinen P-L, Bono P, Alanko T, Kataja V, Asola R, Utriainen T, Kokko R, Hemminki A, Tarkkanen M, Turpeenniemi-Hujanen T, Jyrkkiö S, Flander M, Helle L, Ingalsuo S, Johansson K, Jääskeläinen A-S, Pajunen M, Rauhala M, Kaleva-Kerola J, Salminen T, Leinonen M, Elomaa I, Isola J. Adjuvant docetaxel or vinorelbine with or without trastuzumab for breast cancer. N Engl J Med. 2006;354(8):809–20.
174. Magnifico A, Albano L, Campaner S, Delia D, Castiglioni F, Gasparini P, Sozzi G, Fontanella E, Menard S, Tagliabue E. Tumor-initiating cells of HER2-positive carcinoma cell lines express the highest oncoprotein levels and are sensitive to trastuzumab. Clin Cancer Res. 2009;15(6):2010.
175. Piccart-Gebhart MJ, Procter M, Leyland-Jones B, Goldhirsch A, Untch M, Smith I, Gianni L, Baselga J, Bell R, Jackisch C, Cameron D, Dowsett M, Barrios CH, Steger G, Huang C-S, Andersson M, Inbar M, Lichinitser M, Láng I, Nitz U, Iwata H, Thomssen C, Lohrisch C, Suter TM, Rüschoff J, Sütő T, Greatorex V, Ward C, Straehle C, McFadden E, Dolci MS, Gelber RD. Trastuzumab after adjuvant chemotherapy in HER2-positive breast cancer. N Engl J Med. 2005;353(16):1659–72.
176. Romond EH, Perez EA, Bryant J, Suman VJ, Geyer CE, Davidson NE, Tan-Chiu E, Martino S, Paik S, Kaufman PA, Swain SM, Pisansky TM, Fehrenbacher L, Kutteh LA, Vogel VG, Visscher DW, Yothers G, Jenkins RB, Brown AM, Dakhil SR, Mamounas EP, Lingle WL, Klein PM, Ingle JN, Wolmark N. Trastuzumab plus adjuvant chemotherapy for operable HER2-positive breast cancer. N Engl J Med. 2005;353(16):1673–84.
177. Hurst S, Ryan AM, Ng C-K, McNally JM, Lorello LG, Finch GL, Leach MW, Ploch SA, Fohey JA, Smolarek TA. Comparative nonclinical assessments of the proposed biosimilar PF-05280014 and trastuzumab (Herceptin(®)). BioDrugs. 2014;28(5):451–9.
178. Kalinsky K, Jacks LM, Heguy A, Patil S, Drobnjak M, Bhanot UK, Hedvat CV, Traina TA, Solit D, Gerald W, Moynahan ME. PIK3CA mutation associates with improved outcome in breast cancer. Clin Cancer Res. 2009;15(16):5049–59.
179. Stenehjem DD, Yoo M, Unni SK, Singhal M, Bauer H, Saverno K, Quah C, Masaquel A, Brixner DI. Assessment of HER2 testing patterns, HER2+ disease, and the utilization of HER2-directed therapy in early breast cancer. Breast Cancer Targets Ther. 2014;6:169–77.
180. Abramson V, Arteaga CL. New strategies in HER2-overexpressing breast cancer: many combinations of targeted drugs available. Clin Cancer Res. 2011;17(5):952–8.
181. Albertson DG. Gene amplification in cancer. Trends Genet. 2006;22(8):447–55.
182. Duru N, Fan M, Candas D, Menaa C, Liu H-C, Nantajit D, Wen Y, Xiao K, Eldridge A, Chromy BA, Li S, Spitz DR, Lam KS, Wicha MS, Li JJ. HER2-associated radiation resistance of breast cancer stem cells isolated from HER2-negative breast cancer cells. Clin Cancer Res. 2012;18(24):6634–47.
183. Downs-Kelly E, Yoder BJ, Stoler M, Tubbs RR, Skacel M, Grogan T, Roche P, Hicks DG. The influence of polysomy 17 on HER2 gene and protein expression in adenocarcinoma of the breast: a fluorescent in situ hybridization, immunohistochemical, and isotopic mRNA in situ hybridization study. Am J Surg Pathol. 2005;29(9):1221–7.
184. Krishnamurti U, Hammers JL, Atem FD, Storto PD, Silverman JF. Poor prognostic significance of unamplified chromosome 17 polysomy in invasive breast carcinoma. Mod Pathol. 2009;22(8):1044–8.
185. Ng CK, Martelotto LG, Gauthier A, Wen H-C, Piscuoglio S, Lim RS, Cowell CF, Wilkerson PM, Wai P, Rodrigues DN, Arnould L, Geyer FC, Bromberg SE, Lacroix-Triki M, Penault-Llorca F, Giard S, Sastre-Garau X, Natrajan R, Norton L, Cottu PH, Weigelt B, Vincent-Salomon A, Reis-Filho JS. Intra-tumor genetic heterogeneity and alternative driver genetic alterations in breast cancers with heterogeneous HER2 gene amplification. Genome Biol. 2015;16(1):107.
186. Skibinski A, Kuperwasser C. The origin of breast tumor heterogeneity. Oncogene. 2015;34(42):5309–16.
187. Altundag K, Bondy ML, Mirza NQ, Kau S-W, Broglio K, Hortobagyi GN, Rivera E. Clinicopathologic characteristics and prognostic factors in 420 metastatic breast cancer patients with central nervous system metastasis. Cancer. 2007;110(12):2640–7.
188. Crivellari D, Pagani O, Veronesi A, Lombardi D, Nolè F, Thürlimann B, Hess D, Borner M, Bauer J, Martinelli G, Graffeo R, Sessa C, Goldhirsch A, International Breast Cancer Study Group. High incidence of central nervous system involvement in patients with metastatic or locally advanced breast cancer treated with epirubicin and docetaxel. Ann Oncol. 2001;12(3):353–6.
189. Giuliano AE, Hunt KK, Ballman KV, Beitsch PD, Whitworth PW, Blumencranz PW, Leitch AM, Saha S, McCall LM, Morrow M. Axillary dissection vs no axillary dissection in women with invasive breast cancer and sentinel node metastasis: a randomized clinical trial. JAMA. 2011;305(6):569–75.

190. Wang L, Wang S-L, Shen H-H, Niu F-T, Niu Y. Breast metastasis from lung cancer: a report of two cases and literature review. Cancer Biol Med. 2014;11(3):208–15.
191. Aitelhaj M, Lkhoyaali S, Rais G, Boutayeb S, Errihani H. First line chemotherapy plus trastuzumab in metastatic breast cancer HER2+—observational institutional study. Pan Afr Med J. 2016;24:324.
192. Chinni SR, Yamamoto H, Dong Z, Sabbota A, Bonfil RD, Cher ML. CXCL12/CXCR4 transactivates HER2 in lipid rafts of prostate cancer cells and promotes growth of metastatic deposits in bone. Mol Cancer Res. 2008;6(3):446–57.
193. Katz D, Aharoni D. Lytic lesions in breast cancer. N Engl J Med. 2004;351(27):2850.
194. Meng S, Tripathy D, Shete S, Ashfaq R, Haley B, Perkins S, Beitsch P, Khan A, Euhus D, Osborne C, Frenkel E, Hoover S, Leitch M, Clifford E, Vitetta E, Morrison L, Herlyn D, Terstappen LWMM, Fleming T, Fehm T, Tucker T, Lane N, Wang J, Uhr J. HER-2 gene amplification can be acquired as breast cancer progresses. Proc Natl Acad Sci U S A. 2004;101(25):9393–8.
195. Sukov WR, Miller DV, Dueck AC, Tenner KS, Jenkins RB, Kaufman PA, Davidson NE, Dakhil SR, Martino S, Roy V, Perez EA. Benefit of adjuvant trastuzumab in breast cancer patients with focal HER2 amplified clones: data from N9831 intergroup adjuvant trial. J Clin Oncol. 2009;27(15S):520.
196. Hanna W, Nofech-Mozes S, Kahn HJ. Intratumoral heterogeneity of HER2/neu in breast cancer—a rare event. Breast J. 2007;13(2):122–9.
197. Schmidt F, Efferth T. Tumor heterogeneity, single-cell sequencing, and drug resistance. Pharmaceuticals. 2016;9(2):33.
198. Makohon-Moore AP, Zhang M, Reiter JG, Bozic I, Allen B, Kundu D, Chatterjee K, Wong F, Jiao Y, Kohutek ZA, Hong J, Attiyeh M, Javier B, Wood LD, Hruban RH, Nowak MA, Papadopoulos N, Kinzler KW, Vogelstein B, Iacobuzio-Donahue CA. Limited heterogeneity of known driver gene mutations among the metastases of individual patients with pancreatic cancer. Nat Genet. 2017;49(3):358–66.
199. Pusztai L, Viale G, Kelly CM, Hudis CA. Estrogen and HER-2 receptor discordance between primary breast cancer and metastasis. Oncologist. 2010;15(11):1164–8.
200. Cancer Genome Atlas Network Koboldt D, Fulton R, McLellan M, Schmidt H, Kalicki-Veizer J, McMichael J. Comprehensive molecular portraits of human breast tumours. Nature. 2012;490(7418):61–70.
201. Guy CT, Webster MA, Schaller M, Parsons TJ, Cardiff RD, Muller WJ. Expression of the neu protooncogene in the mammary epithelium of transgenic mice induces metastatic disease. Proc Natl Acad Sci U S A. 1992;89(22):10578–82.
202. Lim E, Wu D, Pal B, Bouras T, Asselin-Labat ML, Vaillant F, Yagita H, Lindeman GJ, Smyth GK, Visvader JE. Transcriptome analyses of mouse and human mammary cell subpopulations reveal multiple conserved genes and pathways. Breast Cancer Res. 2010;12(2):R21.
203. Pfefferle AD, Herschkowitz JI, Usary J, Harrell JC, Spike BT, Adams JR, Torres-Arzayus MI, Brown M, Egan SE, Wahl GM, Rosen JM, Perou CM. Transcriptomic classification of genetically engineered mouse models of breast cancer identifies human subtype counterparts. Genome Biol. 2013;14(11):R125.
204. Ding J, Hu P, Chen J, Wu X, Cao Y. The importance of tissue confirmation of metastatic disease in patients with breast cancer: lesson from a brain metastasis case. Oncoscience. 2016;3(9–10):268–74.
205. von Minckwitz G, Darb-Esfahani S, Loibl S, Huober J, Tesch H, Solbach C, Holms F, Eidtmann H, Dietrich K, Just M, Clemens MR, Hanusch C, Schrader I, Henschen S, Hoffmann G, Tiemann K, Diebold K, Untch M, Denkert C. Responsiveness of adjacent ductal carcinoma in situ and changes in HER2 status after neoadjuvant chemotherapy/trastuzumab treatment in early breast cancer—results from the GeparQuattro study (GBG 40). Breast Cancer Res Treat. 2012;132(3):863–70.
206. Jarvinen TTM, Rantanen V, Barlund M, Borg A, Grenman S, Isola J. Amplification and deletion of topoisomerase IIa associate with ErbB-2 amplification and affect sensitivity to topoisomerase II inhibitor doxorubicin in breast cancer. Am J Pathol. 2000;156(3):839–47.
207. Gray KH, Yates B, Seal RL, Wright MW, Bruford EA. Genenames.org: the HGNC resource in 2015. Nucleic Acids Res. 2015;43(Database issue):D1079–85. https://doi.org/10.1093/nar/gku1071. PMID:25361968.
208. McGowan-Jordan J, Simons A, Schmid M. ISCN 2013: an International System for Human Cytogenomic Nomenclature 2013. Basel: S. Karger AG; 2013.
209. McGowan-Jordan J, Simons A, Schmid M. ISCN 2016: an International System for Human Cytogenomic Nomenclature 2016. Basel: S. Karger AG; 2016.
210. Ballard M, Jalikis F, Krings G, Schmidt RA, Chen YY, Rendi MH, Dintzis SM, Jensen KC, West RB, Sibley RK, Troxell ML, Allison KH. 'Non-classical' HER2 FISH results in breast cancer: a multi-institutional study. Mod Pathol. 2017;30(2):227–35.
211. Ohlschlegel C, Zahel K, Kradolfer D, Hell M, Jochum W. HER2 genetic heterogeneity in breast carcinoma. J Clin Pathol. 2011;64(12):1112–6.
212. Shafi H, Astvatsaturyan K, Chung F, Mirocha J, Schmidt M, Bose S. Clinicopathological significance of HER2/neu genetic heterogeneity in HER2/neu non-amplified invasive breast carcinomas and its concurrent axillary metastasis. J Clin Pathol. 2013;66(8):649–54.
213. Jang MH, Kim EJ, Kim HJ, Chung YR, Park SY. Assessment of HER2 status in invasive breast

cancers with increased centromere 17 copy number. Breast Cancer Res Treat. 2015;153(1):67–77.
214. Singh MK, Parihar M, Arora N, Mishra DK, Bhave SJ, Chandy M. Diagnosis of variant RARA translocation using standard dual-color dual-fusion PML/RARA FISH probes: an illustrative report. Hematol Oncol Stem Cell Ther. 2017.
215. Park CH, Kim HJ, Lee ST, Seo JM, Kim SH. Molecular characterization of near-complete trisomy 17p syndrome from inverted duplication in association with cryptic deletion of 17pter. Gene. 2014;537(2):343–7.
216. Cardoso C, Leventer RJ, Dowling JJ, Ward HL, Chung J, Petras KS, Roseberry JA, Weiss AM, Das S, Martin CL, Pilz DT, Dobyns WB, Ledbetter DH. Clinical and molecular basis of classical lissencephaly: mutations in the LIS1 gene (PAFAH1B1). Hum Mutat. 2002;19(1):4–15.
217. Burris HA. Dual kinase inhibition in the treatment of breast cancer: initial eperience with the EGFR/ErbB-2 inhibitor lapatinib. Oncologist. 2004;9(3):10–5.
218. Gelmon KA, Fumoleau P, Verma S, Wardley AM, Conte PF, Miles D, Miles L, Gianni L, McNally VA, Ross G, Baselga J. Results of a phase II trial of trastuzumab (H) and pertuzumab (P) in patients (pts) with HER2-positive metastatic breast cancer (MBC) who had progressed during trastuzumab therapy. J Clin Oncol. 2008;26:1026.
219. Diermeir S, Horvath G, Knuechel-Clarke R, Hofstaedter G, Szollosi J, Brockhoff G. Epidermal growth factor receptor coexpressionmodulates susceptibility to Herceptin® in HER2/neu overexpressing breast cancer cells via specific erbB-receptor interaction and activation. Exp Cell Res. 2005;304:604–19.
220. Slamon DJ, Leyland-Jones B, Shak S, Fuchs H, Paton V, Bajamonde A, Fleming T, Eiermann W, Wolter J, Pegram M, Baselga J, Norton L. Use of chemotherapy plus a monoclonal antibody against HER2 for metastatic breast cancer that overxpresses HER2. N Engl J Med. 2001;344(11):783–92.
221. Eroglu Z, Tagawa T, Somlo G. Human epidermal growth factor receptor family-targeted therapies in the treatment of HER2-overexpressing breast cancer. Oncologist. 2014;19(2):135–50.
222. Collins DM, O'Donovan N, McGowan PM, O'Sullivan F, Duffy MJ, Crown J. Trastuzumab induces antibody-dependent cell-mediated cytotoxicity (ADCC) in HER-2-non-amplified breast cancer cell lines. Ann Oncol. 2012;23(7):1788–95.
223. Gennari R, Menard S, Fagnoni F, Ponchio L, Scelsi M, Tagliabue E, Castiglioni F, Villani L, Magalotti C, Gibelli N, Oliviero B, Ballardini B, Da Prada G, Zambelli A, Costa A. Pilot study of the mechanism of action of preoperative trastuzumab in patients with primary operable breast tumors overexpressing HER2. Clin Cancer Res. 2004;10(17):5650–5.
224. Sliwkowski MX, Lofgren JA, Lewis GD, Hotaling TE, Fendly BM, Fox JA. Nonclinical studies addressing the mechanism of action of trastuzumab (Herceptin). Semin Oncol. 1999;26(4 Suppl 12):60–70.
225. Spiridon CI, Guinn S, Vitetta ES. A comparison of the in vitro and in vivo activities of IgG and F(ab′)2 fragments of a mixture of three monoclonal anti-Her-2 antibodies. Clin Cancer Res. 2004;10(10):3542–51.
226. Arnould L, Gelly M, Penault-Llorca F, Benoit L, Bonnetain F, Migeon C, Cabaret V, Fermeaux V, Bertheau P, Garnier J, Jeannin JF, Coudert B. Trastuzumab-based treatment of HER2-positive breast cancer: an antibody-dependent cellular cytotoxicity mechanism? Br J Cancer. 2006;94(2):259–67.
227. Varchetta S, Gibelli N, Oliviero B, Nardini E, Gennari R, Gatti G, Silva LS, Villani L, Tagliabue E, Menard S, Costa A, Fagnoni FF. Elements related to heterogeneity of antibody-dependent cell cytotoxicity in patients under trastuzumab therapy for primary operable breast cancer overexpressing HER2. Cancer Res. 2007;67(24):11991–9.
228. Hammond MEH, Hayes DF, Dowsett M, Allred DC, Hagerty KL, Badve S, Fitzgibbons PL, Francis G, Goldstein NS, Hayes M, Hicks DG, Lester S, Love R, Mangu PB, McShane L, Miller K, Osborne CK, Paik S, Perlmutter J, Rhodes A, Sasano H, Schwartz JN, Sweep FCG, Taube S, Torlakovic EE, Valenstein P, Viale G, Visscher D, Wheeler T, Williams RB, Wittliff JL, Wolff AC. American society of clinical oncology/College of american pathologists guideline recommendations for immunohistochemical testing of estrogen and progesterone receptors in breast cancer. J Clin Oncol. 2010;28(16):2784–95.
229. Westbrook K, Stearns V. Pharmacogenomics of breast cancer therapy: an update. Pharmacol Ther. 2013;139(1):1–11.
230. Cheng YC, Ueno NT. Improvement of survival and prospect of cure in patients with metastatic breast cancer. Breast Cancer. 2012;19(3):191–9. https://doi.org/10.1007/s12282-12011-10276-12283.
231. Perez EA, Press MF, Dueck AC, Jenkins RB, Kim C, Chen B, Villalobos I, Paik S, Buyse M, Wiktor AE, Meyer R, Finnigan M, Zujewski J, Shing M, Stern HM, Lingle WL, Reinholz MM, Slamon DJ. Immunohistochemistry and fluorescence in situ hybridization assessment of HER2 in clinical trials of adjuvant therapy for breast cancer (NCCTG N9831, BCIRG 006, and BCIRG 005). Breast Cancer Res Treat. 2013;138(1):99–108.
232. Chang MC, Malowany JI, Mazurkiewicz J, Wood M. Genetic heterogeneity in HER2/neu testing by fluorescence in situ hybridization: a study of 2522 cases. Mod Pathol. 2012;25(5):683–8.
233. Paik S, Kim C, Wolmark N. HER2 status and benefit from adjuvant trastuzumab in breast cancer. N Engl J Med. 2008;358:1409–11.
234. Goldhirsch A, Winer EP, Coates AS, Gelber RD, Piccart-Gebhart M, Thürlimann B, Senn HJ, Panel members, Albain KS, André F, Bergh J, Bonnefoi H, Bretel-Morales D, Burstein H, Cardoso F,

Castiglione-Gertsch M, Coates AS, Colleoni M, Costa A, Curigliano G, Davidson NE, Di Leo A, Ejlertsen B, Forbes JF, Gelber RD, Gnant M, Goldhirsch A, Goodwin P, Goss PE, Harris JR, Hayes DF, Hudis CA, Ingle JN, Jassem J, Jiang Z, Karlsson P, Loibl S, Morrow M, Namer M, Kent Osborne C, Partridge AH, Penault-Llorca F, Perou CM, Piccart-Gebhart MJ, Pritchard KI, Rutgers EJT, Sedlmayer F, Semiglazov V, Shao Z-M, Smith I, Thürlimann B, Toi M, Tutt A, Untch M, Viale G, Watanabe T, Wilcken N, Winer EP, Wood WC. Personalizing the treatment of women with early breast cancer: highlights of the St Gallen international expert consensus on the primary therapy of early breast cancer 2013. Ann Oncol. 2013;24(9):2206–23.

235. Baselga JPE, Pienkowski T, Bell R. Adjuvant trastuzumab: A milesone in the treatment of HER-2 positive early breast cancer. Oncologist. 2006;11(Suppl 1):4–12.
236. Park GE, Kim SH, Kim EJ, Kang BJ, Park MS. Histogram analysis of volume-based apparent diffusion coefficient in breast cancer. Acta Radiol. 2017;58(11):1294–302.
237. Oakes SR, Gallego-Ortega D, Ormandy CJ. The mammary cellular hierarchy and breast cancer. Cell Mol Life Sci. 2014;71(22):4301–24.
238. Bottai G, Diao L, Baggerly KA, Paladini L, Gyorffy B, Raschioni C, Pusztai L, Calin GA, Santarpia L. Integrated microRNA-mRNA profiling identifies oncostatin M as a marker of mesenchymal-like ER-negative/HER2-megative breast cancer. Int J Mol Sci. 2017;18(1):194.
239. Ingthorsson S, Andersen K, Hilmarsdottir B, Maelandsmo GM, Magnusson MK, Gudjonsson T. HER2 induced EMT and tumorigenicity in breast epithelial progenitor cells is inhibited by coexpression of EGFR. Oncogene. 2016;35(32):4244–55.
240. Ulaner GA, Hyman DM, Ross DS, Corben A, Chandarlapaty S, Goldfarb S, McArthur H, Erinjeri JP, Solomon SB, Kolb H, Lyashchenko SK, Lewis JS, Carrasquillo JA. Detection of HER2-positive metastases in patients with HER2-negative primary breast cancer using 89Zr-trastuzumab PET/CT. J Nucl Med. 2016;57(10):1523–8.
241. Lloyd MC, Cunningham JJ, Bui MM, Gillies RJ, Brown JS, Gatenby RA. Darwinian dynamics of intratumoral heterogeneity: not solely random mutations but also variable environmental selection forces. Cancer Res. 2016;76(11):3136–44.
242. Harper KL, Sosa MS, Entenberg D, Hosseini H, Cheung JF, Nobre R, Avivar-Valderas A, Nagi C, Girnius N, Davis RJ, Farias EF, Condeelis J, Klein CA, Aguirre-Ghiso JA. Mechanism of early dissemination and metastasis in HER2+ mammary cancer. Nature. 2016;540(7634):588–92.
243. Jordan NV, Bardia A, Wittner BS, Benes C, Ligorio M, Zheng Y, Yu M, Sundaresan TK, Licausi JA, Desai R, O'Keefe RM, Ebright RY, Boukhali M, Sil S, Onozato ML, Iafrate AJ, Kapur R, Sgroi D, Ting DT, Toner M, Ramaswamy S, Haas W, Maheswaran S, Haber DA. HER2 expression identifies dynamic functional states within circulating breast cancer cells. Nature. 2016;537(7618):102–6.
244. Molnar IA, Molnar BA, Vizkeleti L, Fekete K, Tamas J, Deak P, Szundi C, Szekely B, Moldvay J, Vari-Kakas S, Szasz MA, Acs B, Kulka J, Tokes AM. Breast carcinoma subtypes show different patterns of metastatic behavior. Virchows Arch. 2017;470(3):275–83.
245. Tsiambas E, Ragos V, Grapsa D, Kavantzas N, Karameris A, Stamatelopoulos A, Georgakopoulos G, Fotiades PP, Patsouris E, Syrigos K. Chromosomes 7/17 multiplication vs true polysomy: a crucial issue in lung and breast EGFR/HER2 dependent carcinoma cases. J BUON. 2016;21(3):752–3.
246. Tse CH, Hwang HC, Goldstein LC, Kandalaft PL, Wiley JC, Kussick SJ, Gown AM. Determining true HER2 gene status in breast cancers with polysomy by using alternative chromosome 17 reference genes: implications for anti-HER2 targeted therapy. J Clin Oncol. 2011;29(31):4168–74.
247. Geiersbach KB, Willmore-Payne C, Pasi AV, Paxton CN, Werner TL, Xu X, Wittwer CT, Gulbahce HE, Downs-Kelly E. Genomic copy number analysis of HER2-equivocal breast cancers. Am J Clin Pathol. 2016;146(4):439–47.
248. Marchio C, Lambros MB, Gugliotta P, Di Cantogno LV, Botta C, Pasini B, Tan DS, Mackay A, Fenwick K, Tamber N, Bussolati G, Ashworth A, Reis-Filho JS, Sapino A. Does chromosome 17 centromere copy number predict polysomy in breast cancer? A fluorescence in situ hybridization and microarray-based CGH analysis. J Pathol. 2009;219(1):16–24.
249. Varga Z, Tubbs RR, Wang Z, Sun Y, Noske A, Kradolfer D, Bosshard G, Jochum W, Moch H, Ohlschlegel C. Co-amplification of the HER2 gene and chromosome 17 centromere: a potential diagnostic pitfall in HER2 testing in breast cancer. Breast Cancer Res Treat. 2012;132(3):925–35.
250. Donaldson AR, Shetty S, Wang Z, Rivera CL, Portier BP, Budd GT, Downs-Kelly E, Lanigan CP, Calhoun BC. Impact of an alternative chromosome 17 probe and the 2013 American Society of Clinical Oncology and College of American Pathologists guidelines on fluorescence in situ hybridization for the determination of HER2 gene amplification in breast cancer. Cancer. 2017;123(12):2230–9.
251. Holstege H, Horlings HM, Velds A, Langerød A, Børresen-Dale A-L, van de Vijver MJ, Nederlof PM, Jonkers J. BRCA1-mutated and basal-like breast cancers have similar aCGH profiles and a high incidence of protein truncating *TP53* mutations. BMC Cancer. 2010;10:654.
252. Beltran H, Yelensky R, Frampton GM, Park K, Downing SR, MacDonald TY, Jarosz M, Lipson D, Tagawa ST, Nanus DM, Stephens PJ, Mosquera JM, Cronin MT, Rubin MA. Targeted next-generation sequencing of advanced prostate cancer identifies potential therapeutic targets and disease heterogeneity. Eur Urol. 2013;63(5):920–6.
253. Natrajan R, Mackay A, Lambros MB, Weigelt B, Wilkerson PM, Manie E, Grigoriadis A, A'Hern R, van

der Groep P, Kozarewa I, Popova T, Mariani O, Turaljic S, Furney SJ, Marais R, Rodruigues D-N, Flora AC, Wai P, Pawar V, McDade S, Carroll J, Stoppa-Lyonnet D, Green AR, Ellis IO, Swanton C, van Diest P, Delattre O, Lord CJ, Foulkes WD, Vincent-Salomon A, Ashworth A, Stern MH, Reis-Filho JS. A whole-genome massively parallel sequencing analysis of BRCA1 mutant oestrogen receptor negative and positive breast cancers. J Pathol. 2012;227(1):29–41.
254. Lu Y, Li S, Zhu S, Gong Y, Shi J, Xu L. Methylated DNA/RNA in body fluids as biomarkers for lung cancer. Biol Proced Online. 2017;19:2. https://doi.org/10.1186/s12575-017-0051-8.
255. Lee JH, Long GV, Boyd S, Lo S, Menzies AM, Tembe V, Guminski A, Jakrot V, Scolyer RA, Mann GJ, Kefford RF, Carlino MS, Rizos H. Circulating tumour DNA predicts response to anti-PD1 antibodies in metastatic melanoma. Ann Oncol 2017. 2017;28(5):1130–6.
256. Cheng F, Su L, Qian C. Circulating tumor DNA: a promising biomarker in the liquid biopsy of cancer. Oncotarget. 2016;7(30):48832–41.
257. Murtaza M, Dawson S, Tsui D, Gale D, Forshew T, Piskorz A, Parkinson C, Chin S, Kingsbury Z, Wong A, Marass F, Humphray S, Hadfield J, Bentley D, Chin T, Brenton J, Caldas C, Rosenfeld N. Non-invasive analysis of acquired resistance to cancer therapy by sequencing of plasma DNA. Nature. 2013;497(7447):108–12.
258. Swanton C. Intratumour heterogeneity: evolution through space and time. Cancer Res. 2012;72(19): 4875–82.
259. Ramesh KH. Significance of HER2 heterogeneity detected by fluorescence in situ hybridization analysis in invasive ductal breast carcinoma. Einstein IRB Approval # 2015;2014-4133.
260. Giacchetti S, Hamy AS, Delaloge S, Brain E, Berger F, Sigal-Zafrani B, Mathieu MC, Bertheau P, Guinebretiere JM, Saghatchian M, Lerebours F, Mazouni C, Tembo O, Espie M, Reyal F, Marty M, Asselain B, Pierga JY. Long-term outcome of the REMAGUS 02 trial, a multicenter randomised phase II trial in locally advanced breast cancer patients treated with neoadjuvant chemotherapy with or without celecoxib or trastuzumab according to HER2 status. Eur J Cancer. 2017;75:323–32.
261. Kim IH, Lee JE, Youn HJ, Song BJ, Chae BJ. Cardioprotective effect of dexrazoxane in patients with HER2-positive breast cancer who receive anthracycline based adjuvant chemotherapy followed by trastuzumab. J Breast Cancer. 2017;20(1):82–90.
262. Costa RB, Kurra G, Greenberg L, Geyer CE. Efficacy and cardiac safety of adjuvant trastuzumab-based chemotherapy regimens for HER2-positive early breast cancer. Ann Oncol. 2010;21(11):2153–60.
263. von Minckwitz G, Rezai M, Fasching PA, Huober J, Tesch H, Bauerfeind I, Hilfrich J, Eidtmann H, Gerber B, Hanusch C, Blohmer JU, Costa SD, Jackisch C, Paepke S, Schneeweiss A, Kummel S, Denkert C, Mehta K, Loibl S, Untch M. Survival after adding capecitabine and trastuzumab to neoadjuvant anthracycline-taxane-based chemotherapy for primary breast cancer (GBG 40--GeparQuattro). Ann Oncol. 2014;25(1):81–9.
264. Ejlertsen B. Adjuvant chemotherapy in early breast cancer. Dan Med J. 2016;63(5).
265. Seol H, Lee HJ, Choi Y, Lee HE, Kim YJ, Kim JH, Kang E, Kim SW, Park SY. Intratumoral heterogeneity of HER2 gene amplification in breast cancer: its clinicopathological significance. Mod Pathol. 2012;25(7):938–48.
266. Gianni L, Eiermann W, Semiglazov V, Manikhas A, Lluch A, Tjulandin S, Zambetti M, Vazquez F, Byakhow M, Lichinitser M, Angel Climent M, Ciruelos E, Ojeda B, Mansutti M, Bozhok A, Baronio R, Feyereislova A, Barton C, Valagussa P, Baselga J. Neoadjuvant chemotherapy with trastuzumab followed by adjuvant trastuzumab versus neoadjuvant chemotherapy alone, in patients with HER2-positive locally advanced breast cancer (the NOAH trial): a randomised controlled superiority trial with a parallel HER2-negative cohort. Lancet. 2010;375(9712):377–84.

Exploring Potential of RPPA Technique in Oral Cancer Biomarker Discovery Research

16

Neera Singh and Sanghamitra Pati

16.1 Introduction

Cancer is the major cause of morbidity and mortality worldwide, with nearly 14 million new cases and over eight million deaths reported in 2015. Globally, the most frequently diagnosed malignancies are lung, colorectal, and prostate cancers for men and lung, colorectal, and breast cancers for women [1]. In United States alone, an estimated 1.7 million new cancer cases were diagnosed in 2016, resulting in approximately 600,000 deaths (Siegul et al. 2016). The global cancer burden is likely to increase in both developed and developing countries, with a projected 22 million new cancer cases and 13 million cancer-related deaths occurring annually by 2030 [2]. Interestingly, according to American Cancer Society, cancer mortality rate in US has declined steadily over the past two decades. This could be partly achieved because of development of population-level screening tests that detect cancers in early stages and facilitate treatment before the disease becomes clinically evident. However, the trend is slightly reverse in many low-income and middle-income countries including India with more people dying of cancer as compared to the previous years. This increasing magnitude of cancer in developing countries is mainly because of increasing economic development leading to widespread industrialization and urbanization and changing lifestyle including smoking, obesity and sedentary lifestyle. Increased cancer mortality is also primarily because of delayed and inaccurate diagnosis of the disease and absence of a well-regulated cancer care health system in these countries.

16.2 Oral Cancer

Oral cancer is the sixth most common malignancy worldwide with high prevalence rate in developing countries [3]. The Indian subcontinent alone accounts for one-third of the world burden of this malignancy where approximately 83,000 new oral cancer cases are reported annually. The term, 'oral cancer' also known as oral squamous cell carcinoma (OSCC) include all the malignancies of the squamous epithelium of the oral cavity that includes tumor of lip, tongue, gingival, palate, floor of mouth and buccal mucosa. A high prevalence of oral cancer in India and other Asian countries is mainly due to popular use of tobacco in different forms (areca nut and betel quid chewing). Despite improvement in surgical techniques and adjuvant therapies, the

N. Singh
DBT-BioCARE Women Scientist, Institute of Life Sciences, Bhubaneswar, Odisha, India

S. Pati (✉)
Department of Health Research, Government of India, ICMR Regional Medical Research Centre, Bhubaneswar, Odisha, India
e-mail: dirrmrcb@icmr.org.in

K. K. Shukla et al. (eds.), *Molecular Diagnostics in Cancer Patients*,
https://doi.org/10.1007/978-981-13-5877-7_16

prognosis for OSCC patients remains poor with the lowest 5-year survival rate (<50%). Mortality rate for the past three and a half decades has remained significantly higher (over 50%) largely because of late diagnosis, metastasis, resistant to therapy and lack of biomarker for early diagnosis. OSCC can arise de novo but majority of OSCCs are believed to develop from pre-existing oral lesions (leukoplakias, erythroplakias, lichen planus, oral submucous fibrosis, epithelial hyperplasia and dysplasia) collectively known as 'Oral potentially malignant disorders' (OPMD). Erythroplakias are generally considered to have a higher tendency to undergo malignant transformation than leukoplakias (90% or more). Leukoplakias are most commonly observed oral lesions with a potential for malignant transformation to OSCC. However, the exact mechanism at the cellular level that leads to malignant transformation in leukoplakia is not very clear. Therefore, it is crucial to understand these molecular changes in premalignant lesions as to why not all tobacco users develop oral cancer and how some patients with leukoplakia does not show any sign of malignant transformation for a significant period.

OSCC is considered as a multi-factorial disease affected by various genetic alterations and environmental factors where conventional diagnostic methods alone will not be efficient enough to detect the disease at an early stage (Fig. 16.1) [4]. Conventional diagnosis of oral cancer involves detailed oral examination and the key prognostic factor in these patients is still the clinical stage of disease (TNM stage) at the time of intervention. As a treatment regime, along with chemotherapy and radiotherapy, surgery remains the best option for OSCC patients but it is not effective for late-stage metastatic tumors. Unfortunately, for the past two decades there is no significant improvement in the techniques or methods that could help in early detection of oral cancers. Therefore, an early diagnosis of OSCC is critical for survival with minimum impairment and deformity in oral cancer patients [5].

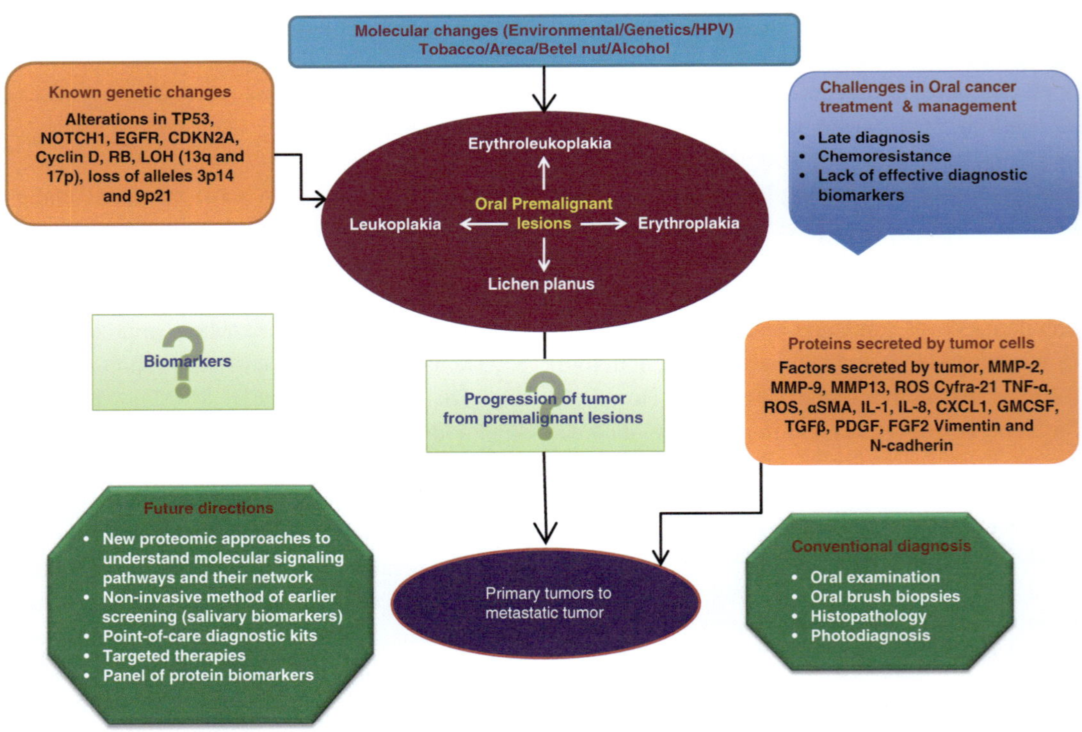

Fig. 16.1 A broad outline of molecular diagnostics in oral cancer

The chapter briefly provides overview of various molecular approaches used in cancer biomarker discovery. Further, the importance of proteomics in cancer diagnostics and biomarker discovery is discussed in details with special emphasis on application of protein microarrays in oral cancer.

16.3 Cancer Development and Importance of Biomarkers in Early Diagnosis

The best approach to prevent and control cancer is its early detection and treatment. In last few decades, due to increased cancer epidemics, a significant amount of research funding was fueled into cancer research. Since then a remarkable progress has been made towards understanding of various theories and mechanism involved in cancer development and treatment. Broadly, cancer is defined as a disease of uncontrolled growth and proliferation. However, the process of cancer development or carcinogenesis is an extremely complex process that involves a vast array of cellular pathways occurring both at genotype and phenotype levels. In a multistep process, cancer cell attains characteristics that enable them to divide uncontrollably with a metastatic potential. During the transformation of normal cells into malignant cells, cells become self-sufficient in growth signals and become insensitive to growth-inhibitory signals [6]. Cancer is essentially viewed as a genetic disease that evolve through accumulation of somatic mutations. Various genetic changes that occur during transformation of normal cells to malignant cells are mutations, deletions, gene amplification, gene rearrangements and translocations. Most of the genes altered in hereditary cancers include oncogenes, tumor suppressor genes and DNA repair genes. Increasing evidence suggest that cancer may also be triggered by aberrant epigenetic changes as histone modification and DNA methylation. The genetic alterations of cancer cells in majority of patients are associated with a specific type of cancer and such changes are manifested in the form of release of biochemical substances called tumor markers. Tumor markers are molecules produced by the tumor itself or by the host system in response to the tumor, which can be used as biomarkers to determine the risk of getting cancer, to detect and classify cancer or to predict therapeutic response [7]. Tumor marker not only comprises cancer-specific mutations but also change in gene expression or promoter methylation that can result in altered protein expression. The improved understanding of altered molecular mechanism of tumorigenesis revealed changes occurring in DNA, RNA, mRNA, miRNA and proteins within the cancer cells [8], which are easily detectable in tissues, and circulating fluids like saliva, urine and serum. Recent methods for cancer diagnosis combine these molecular changes and further translate them into clinical practice, which now forms the most successful approach in cancer detection and is termed as molecular diagnostics. Molecular diagnostics is thus, a collection of analytical tools used to assess an individual's health at the molecular level by detecting and analyzing biological molecules such as nucleic acids (DNA and RNA) and proteins. According to the National Cancer Institute, a biomarker is "a biological molecule found in blood, other body fluids, or tissues that is a sign of a normal or abnormal process, or of a condition or disease," such as cancer. A biomarker is a measurable indicator of physiological and pathological process that helps to differentiate a diseased state from the normal state. The underlying molecular changes occurring in the disease process can be reflected by differential genomic, proteomic, or metabolomic expressions.

16.3.1 Tumor Biomarkers

A tumor or cancer marker is any molecule produced by a tumor or by the host in response to a cancer cell that can be accurately measured and evaluated as an indicator of tumor development within the body. The tumor marker level should ideally reflect the extent (the stage) of the disease, indicating how quickly the cancer is likely to progress and aid in determining the prognosis (outlook). Tumor markers are classified into different categories such as

Table 16.1 Types of biomarkers in cancers

Type of biomarker	Use of the biomarker	Clinical objective
Prognostic biomarker e.g. PSA	Used for risk assessment	It is a clinical or biological characteristic that provides information on the likely course or outcome of the disease (disease recurrence, progression or death)
Diagnostic biomarker	Helps in the diagnosis, classification and screening of cancer	• Allow early detection of cancer for early treatment • Helps to distinguish the specific type of cancer
Predictive biomarker e.g. BRCA1, EGFR, Her2, ROS, BRAF	• Prognosis and prediction of treatment • Risk stratification • Personalized medicine	• Helps to estimate the likely outcome of the disease • Allows to predict the response of the patient to a targeted therapy • To evaluate the probability of occurrence or recurrence of cancer • To select the therapy with the highest probability of being effective in a particular patient
Therapeutic biomarker	Helps in monitoring treatment response	Used in measuring the efficacy and adverse drug events of a drug therapy

proteins, glycoproteins, oncofetal antigens, hormones, receptors, genetic markers, and RNA molecules. Based on the clinical application tumor biomarkers can be of four different types (Table 16.1). Kaplan and Pesce [9] suggested the following criteria for an ideal tumor marker:

1. An ideal tumor marker should be easily detectable and quantifiable in sample matrices such as serum, plasma, whole blood, urine, and tissue. It should be specific to the tumor being studied.
2. It should have a stoichiometric relationship between plasma levels of the marker and the associated tumor mass.
3. Tumor marker should have abnormal plasma level, urine level, or both in the presence of micro-metastases, that is, at a stage when no clinical or presently available diagnostic methods reveal their presence.
4. These marker should have plasma levels, urine levels, or both that are stable and not subjected to wild fluctuations.
5. They should predict a higher or lower risk for eventual development of recurrence.
6. Ideal tumor markers levels should change as the current status of the tumor changes over time.
7. They should precede and predict recurrences before they are clinically detectable.

16.3.2 Application of Tumor Markers

1. In screening and early detection of cancer.
2. In diagnosis of cancer and clinical staging of cancer.
3. Estimating tumor volume.
4. Tumor markers are used as prognostic indicators for disease progression.
5. Aid in evaluating the success of treatment and monitoring responses to therapy.
6. Use to predict/detect the recurrences.

16.4 Molecular Diagnostics in Cancer

Conventionally, clinical diagnosis of tumor is made by symptomatic assessments followed by histomorphological analysis of tumor samples (tissue biopsy, surgical specimens or cytology aspirate) by a pathologist. In recent years, the diagnosis of cancer has undergone a paradigm shift where it is no longer diagnosed based on histomorphological criteria. With increased understanding of significant molecular alterations (DNA, mRNAs, miRNAs and proteins) occurring in cancer, cancer diagnosis is becoming more reliable by using combined immunohistochemical and advanced molecular biology techniques. Revolution of “omics” in cancer diagnostics (Whole Genome sequencing,

Whole Exome sequencing, methylome, transcriptome (including the miRnome), microbiome, metabolome, proteome and topome) has led to the emergence of a completely new arena termed as "Molecular Oncodiagnostics" [7]. Molecular diagnosis serves as a powerful adjunct to histopathology and aid in quick and accurate tumor diagnosis, monitor disease progress, and response to therapy. There are three characteristic features of molecular diagnosis that confers advantage over conventional diagnostic methods. First, the sensitivity is high, so that small sample is sufficient for diagnosis. Second, the results are specific and reproducible and therefore objective, and third, data can be obtained faster using high throughput techniques. The advantages in sensitivity, objectivity and rapidity are of great significance for early clinical diagnosis of cancer.

Molecular diagnostics is now a rapidly evolving area of research in medicine, with new technologies being continually added. Moreover, with advances in chemistries and instrumentation, including automation, integration and throughput technologies such as real-time quantitative PCR, digital PCR, next-generation sequencing (NGS), mass spectrometry, microarray, bead-based suspension array, microfluidic chip, flow cytometry and electrically magnetic-controllable electrochemical biosensors, the detection of molecular markers in biological samples has simplified early and accurate diagnosis of various tumors. Further, application of molecular techniques yields a comprehensive detection panel of molecular alterations that provides a "molecular signature" specific for each tumor, which can be used as a template for personalized onco-pharmacogenomics.

16.5 Molecular Alterations (DNA/RNA/Proteins): What Is the Best Target?

One of the important goals for oncologists is to achieve early diagnosis and make accurate prognostic predictions of the disease. With the advancing technologies, it is now possible to rapidly identify molecular alterations in cancer with high sensitivity and reproducibility at all molecular levels (DNA, RNA and proteins). Use of genomic technologies like DNA micorarray has led to considerable progress in identifying a new 'molecular taxonomy' of cancer [10]. Nextgen sequencing has further provided insights into cancer genomics by uncovering large number of mutations thus generating a complex volume of information. Unfortunately, the major challenge is to decipher this information into clinical practice, as only a small fraction of the mutations detected are known to contribute to the tumor progression. Another limitations of genomic studies are that they cannot provide complete information of cellular, subcellular, and intercellular functions, in which proteins but not the genes govern the cellular functions. Moreover, there is no strict linear relationship between genes and the protein complement or "proteome" of a cell. In addition, many genes are pseudogenes that are no longer expressed in cells [11]. Though, cancer is well characterized by accumulation of genomic alterations, it is the protein pathways, network and their interactions that drive biological outcomes and information flow in a cell. The cellular proteome is a highly dynamic entity, that differ from cell to cell and is constantly changing. The nucleic acid content (DNA, mRNA, siRNA,) cannot provide direct information regarding the state of protein signaling pathways within a cell. It is the resultant encoded proteins that are the actual defective piece of machinery leading to alterations in cellular growth, survival or apoptosis [12]. Genomic profiling has not been quite successful in unraveling the complexity of cellular protein network, first, because gene transcript levels were not found to be significantly correlated with protein expression levels and second, RNA transcript levels provide very little understanding of cellular signaling network. Besides, rather than genes most therapeutic drugs target proteins like kinases and their substrates. The activation states of proteins and the signaling network they are involved in are constantly changing. Protein dynamics is more complex than genes due to various cellular mechanisms including alternative splicing and post-translational modifications of proteins (e.g., phosphorylation, glycosylation, acetylation, and proteolytic cleavage). Human proteome comprises more than 500,000 proteins isoforms derived from approximately 22,000 protein-coding genes. Thus, studying protein complement of the genome could be a befitting way to obtain more information on protein expression and protein modification in cells/tissues/organisms. Advancing proteomics technologies have allowed better understanding of proteins and their modifications, which may elucidate properties of cellular behavior not reflected by gene expression analysis. Proteomics applications can be successfully used to bridge the gap between genomic information and functional proteins in understanding tumor biology [13].

16.6 Application of Proteomics in Cancer Research

Advances in the field of genomics have been successfully utilized in cancer research. However, to complement the limitations of the genomics approach in cancer diagnostics, proteomics approach is gaining interest among researchers. Proteomics tools are considered one of the most dynamic and innovative tools that provide more elaborate information on functional state of disease as compared to other high-throughput approaches. There is no doubt that genomics technologies have significantly contributed towards identification of several genes related to cancers, but how they are regulated into functional proteomes remains poorly understood. Proteome is defined as the entire set of expressed proteins in a specific cell at a specific time. It is a complex and highly dynamic entity that changes with the physiological state of an organism and is ubiquitously affected in disease and disease response. Proteomics aims to study the dynamic protein products of the genome, including its structure, function, regulation and interactions, rather than focusing on the simple static DNA blueprint of a cell. It refers to a comprehensive and high-throughput approach to study proteins including detection, identification, measurement of protein concentration, detection and characterization of modifications, characterization of protein–protein interaction and regulation. Proteomics study fall into three different categories; expression proteomics, structural proteomics and functional proteomics. Expression or differential proteomics aims at measuring the up-regulation and down-regulation of protein levels. Structural proteomics deal with high-throughput characterization of three-dimensional structural of protein complexes. Where as functional proteomics aims at defining the biological function of the protein and involves analysis of protein activation, protein-protein interactions and activated pathway. Functional proteomics have wide clinical applications as it can be applied to serum, plasma, tissue and almost all body fluids including urine, cerebrospinal fluid, saliva, nipple fluid, ascites and pleural fluid. Proteomics technologies allow quantitative analysis of large numbers of proteins in complex protein mixtures and map the post-translational protein modifications under different circumstances. With the introduction of high-throughput proteomics technologies, researchers have identified cancer-related signatures between disease and healthy cohorts of patient [14], thus making cancer profiling a promising area for biomarker discovery. Protein biomarkers like CA125 and alpha-fetoprotein are successfully used in clinical practices for tumor diagnosis. Discovery of tumor protein biomarkers began in the last 15 years with the advent of high throughput proteomic technologies. Although, thousands of new potential cancer biomarkers have been reported in the literature, very few have been granted FDA approval. OVA1 is the first and the only FDA-cleared *in vitro* diagnostic multivariate index assay of proteomic biomarkers. It measures the levels of five different proteins in the serum: CA125, prealbumin, apolipoprotein A1, β_2-microglobulin and transferrin. With the exception of CA125, the other four proteins in the panel were discovered using SELDI-TOF-MS. US food and drug administration (FDA) has approved at least 19 protein biomarkers for cancer so far (Table 16.2) [15, 16].

Protein profiling is a promising methodology in proteomics that provide unique insights into biological events that leads to malignant transformation and widely applied in all cancers. It has greatly enhanced understanding of

Table 16.2 List of FDA-approved protein tumor markers currently used in clinical practice

Biomarker	Clinical use	Cancer type	Specimen	Methodology	Year first approved or cleared
PDL-1	Prognostic and predictive	Lung cancer	FFPE tissue	Immunohistochemistry	2015
BTA	Monitoring	Bladder	Urine	Immunoassay	
β-hGC	Staging	Testicum	Serum	Immunoassay	
EGFR	Therapy selection	Colorectal	Tissue	Immunohistochemistry	
Pro2PSA	Discriminating malignant from benign	Prostate	Serum	Immunoassay	2012
ROMA (HE4+CA-125)	Prediction of malignancy	Ovarian	Serum	Immunoassay	2011
OVA1 (multiple proteins)	Prediction of malignancy	Ovarian	Serum	Immunoassay	2009
HE4	Monitoring recurrence/progression of disease	Ovarian	Serum	Immunoassay	2008
Fibrin/fibrinogen degradation product	Monitoring progression of disease	Colorectal	Serum	Immunoassay	2008
AFP-L3%	Risk assessment for development of disease	Hepatocellular	Serum	HPLC, microfluidic capillary electrophoresis	2005
Circulating tumor cells (EpCAM, CD45, cytokeratins 8, 18+, 19+)	Prognosis	Breast	Whole blood	Immunomagnetic capture/ immune-fluorescence	2005
p63 protein	Aid in differential diagnosis	Prostate	FFPE tissue	Immunohistochemistry	2005
c-Kit	Diagnosis and therapy selection	Gastrointestinal	FFPE tissue	Immunohistochemistry	2004
CA19-9	Monitoring disease status	Pancreatic	Serum, plasma	Immunoassay	2002
Estrogen receptor (ER)	Prognosis, response to therapy	Breast	FFPE tissue	Immunohistochemistry	1999
Progesterone receptor (PR)	Prognosis, response to therapy	Breast	FFPE tissue	Immunohistochemistry	1999
HER-2/neu	Assessment for therapy	Breast	FFPE tissue	Immunohistochemistry	1998
CA-125	Monitoring disease progression, response to therapy	Ovarian	Serum, plasma	Immunoassay	1997
CA15-3	Monitoring disease response to therapy	Breast	Serum, plasma	Immunoassay	1997
CA 27-29	Monitoring disease response to therapy	Breast	Serum	Immunoassay	1997
Free PSA	Discriminating malignant from benign	Prostate	Serum	Immunoassay	1997
Thyroglobulin	Aid in monitoring	Thyroid	Serum, plasma	Immunoassay	1997
NMP22	Diagnosis and monitoring of disease	Bladder	Urine	Lateral flow immunoassay	1996
Alpha-fetoprotein (AFP)[b]	Staging	Testicular	Serum, plasma, amniotic fluid	Immunoassay	1992
Total PSA	Diagnosis and Monitoring	Prostate	Serum	Immunoassay	1986
CEA	Management and prognosis	Colorectal	Serum, plasma	Immunoassay	1985

cancer mechanisms and assisted in discovery of new biomarkers, making it possible to discriminate healthy and malignant cells more accurately. The power of proteomic techniques is not only limited to distinguishing the diseased state from the healthy state, but it also helps to resolve the tumor subtypes. The latter is especially important for the prediction the prognostic features of cancer and for determining the therapeutic strategy to be adopted.

16.6.1 Proteomics Technologies Used in Cancer Biomarker Discovery

High-throughput proteomics technologies combining with advanced bioinformatics are extensively used to monitor protein expression pattern of tumors and identify molecular signatures of diseases based on protein pathways and signaling cascades. Several proteomics techniques including two-dimensional polyacrylamide gel electrophoresis (2D-PAGE), surface enhanced laser desorption/ionisation time of flight (SELDI-ToF), protein arrays, isotope coded affinity tags (ICAT), iTRAQ and multidimensional protein identification technology (MudPIT) are widely implemented approaches in cancer research. High-throughput MS analysis of human plasma/serum/tissue proteomes is emerging as a powerful technique for identifying distinct protein profiles in cancer patients. MS-based proteomics biomarker study typically starts with a discovery platform, where differences in protein expression in small case-control cohorts are investigated in a semi-quantitative approach. In these discovery experiments, different proteomics platforms can be selected: a gel-based platform, a gel-free setup and an MS-imaging system. Apart from the requirement of sophisticated and expensive equipment and skilled expertise, the new candidate biomarkers discovered by MS-based discovery technique require extensive verification and validation. Mass spectrometry has its limitation in its ability to capture rare events, such as proteins or post-translational modifications, which are present in low levels in biological fluids. Further, MS-based proteome analysis is possible for only a limited number of proteins and also limited in accurately detecting low abundant proteins and the peptides with low abundant post-translational modifications.

Despite significant innovations in proteomic methods and technologies, the integration of new proteomic technologies in clinical laboratories is slow due to the costs associated with acquisition of new instruments, evaluation of biomarker specificity and sensitivity, and obtaining information on clinical validity of biomarkers in large populations [14]. Several diagnostics protein biomarkers approved by FDA are already in use in clinics, however, the methods used for their detection and evaluation are mostly old and well established techniques, such as serum protein electrophoresis, western blot, enzyme-linked immunoassays (ELISAs) and immuno-based assays. Application of immunoassays is often hindered by the lack of high-quality antibodies. Furthermore, ELISA assay allows detection of a single antigen, a drawback for the validation of biomarker panels. Also, the low-dynamic range and high cost of development of ELISA based assays indicate a moderate utility of this approach in large-scale validation studies.

In spite of remarkable progress in proteomic methods, including improved detection limits and sensitivity, these methods have not yet been established in routine clinical practice. The main technological limitations in biomarker research are still mainly related to sensitivity, accuracy, reproducibility and validation. The other limitations that prevent their integration into clinics are high cost of equipment, the need for highly trained personnel. The complexity of proteomics technologies in biomarker research increases further due to the current concept of cancer heterogeneity, sample variables and poor study designs. Using well-defined study designs, establishing robust validation assays and applying innovative tools or combinations of tools can minimize these challenges. To develop novel biomarkers, it is crucial to understand the molecular network underlying tumor formation and progression. Protein arrays provide a versatile and robust platform in cancer proteomics research because of their tremendous advantages of miniaturized features, high throughput, and sensitive detections.

16.6.2 Reverse Phase Protein Array

In recent years, numerous proteomic technologies have been developed for discovery of biomarkers to improve early diagnosis and better prognosis for cancer patients. Protein microarray is an automated, rapid, cost-effective, and highly sensitive technology that requires small quantities of samples and reagents.

Protein arrays are categorized in to two formats forward phase protein arrays (FFPA) and reverse phase protein arrays (RPPA) (Fig. 16.2). The former is also called analytic capture array, where as the latter is termed lysate array. In FFPA, antibodies are immobilized in each spot and each array is queried with a tumor sample that contains multiple protein lysates. Therefore, multiple protein expression and phosphorylation levels can be measured at the same time in a single array with a set of antibodies. In contrast, RPPA comprised of an immobilized cellular or protein-based lysate. RPPA represent a highly efficient and cost-effective descendent of miniaturized immunoassays. More than thousand patient samples with multiple protein lysates can be studied in parallel in a single array for each protein of interest using a validated antibody per array. Paweletz et al. first described RPPA in 2001 in a paper describing its application to cell signaling analysis of pre-malignant prostate lesions compared to normal epithelium and invasive carcinoma [18]. RPPA is suitable for profiling the expression and modification of signaling proteins in low abundance. Since, RPPA technology can be used to compare multiple protein samples in parallel, enabling high-throughput analyses in a large number of patient cohorts, it is ideally suited for biomarker discovery.

16.6.3 Advantages of RPPA over Conventional Proteomic Techniques

RPPA platform offers several unique advantages compared to other proteomics approaches and the technology is gradually making the transition to clinics. Table 16.3 briefly compares the pros and cons of major proteomic techniques.

1. First, RPPA is an inexpensive and highly automated platform that allows simultaneous analy-

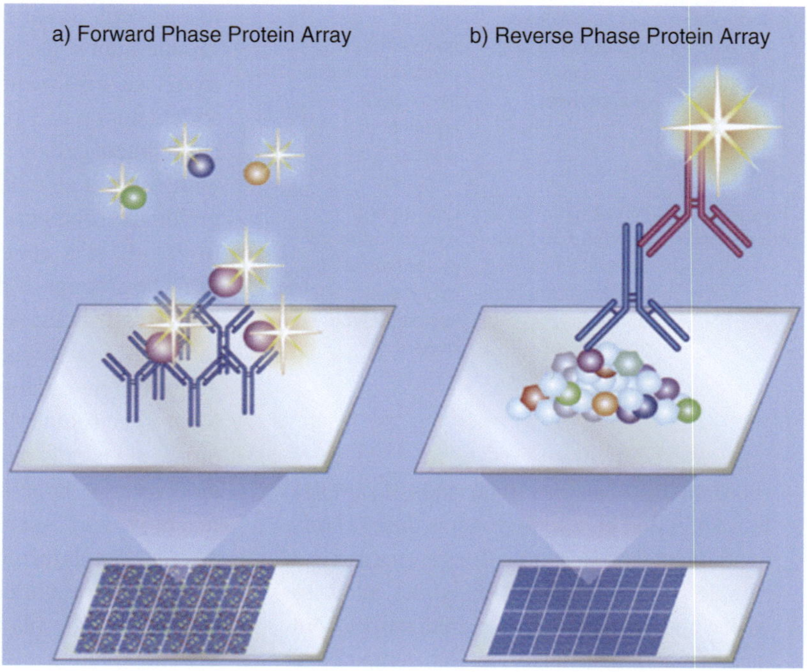

Fig. 16.2 Formats of protein array (Reproduced from [17])

Table 16.3 Advantages and limitations of common proteomic platforms

Proteomic technology	Advantages	Disadvantages
Western blot	Separation of proteins according to molecular weight	Work-intensive, high amounts of protein lysate required, low- or medium-throughput
IHC	Sensitivity, Cellular localization of protein of interest	Semi-quantitative, multiplexing, sensitivity often not sufficient to detect phosphorylated proteins, labor intensive
Immunoassays		
ELISA	Quantitative, very sensitive	High amount of lysate required, labor intensive
Mass spectrometry based techniques	*De novo* discovery platform, highly multiplex, protein isoforms can be distinguished, analysis of thousands of proteins, no protein binding reagent required	Complex sample preparation, poor analytical sensitivity compared to immunoassays, low-throughput
Forward protein array	Many analytes can be measured in parallel in a single sample, quantitative	Two highly specific antibodies are needed for every assay, high amounts of protein lysate required
Reverse protein array	Works with FFPE, multiplexing, low sample consumption, high sensitivity, detection of phosphoprotein available	One highly specific antibody is needed for every assay, special devices needed

sis of multiple samples (thousands of samples) for expression of several proteins under similar experimental conditions. Large numbers of samples spotted on the same slides allow for easier and more reliable normalization, comparison, and data analyses. As compared to mass spectrometry, RPPA offers more robust and accurate quantification as samples can be arrayed in serial dilutions. No other competing technology can quantitatively measure large numbers of low abundance proteins, such as phosphorylated signaling proteins in a single small amount of sample like RPPA does.

2. RPPA required a single highly specific primary antibody for each target protein as compared to ELISA that use two primary antibody against the same protein. Since the experimental conditions are consistent for each antibody, RPPA provides better reproducibility and sensitivity than other protein array techniques. Its quantitation, sensitivity, and multiplexing capacity largely exceed that of western blotting and immunohistochemistry.
3. Sample handling and preparations are straightforward and simple. RPPA can be used for both frozen and formalin-fixed and paraffin embedded (FFPE) tissue. RPPA enable large-scale sample screening for virtually all biological fluids (serum, urine, cerebrospinal fluid, or saliva). Rapid protein extraction and denaturation step prevents degradation and preserve proteins and phosphorylated proteins, which are often labile.
4. RPPA can perform robust quantification by using very small amount (nanograms) of samples such as biopsy specimens, tissues from laser capture microdissection and FACS-sorted minor cell populations (stem cells or cancer stem cells). To assay 200–300 proteins with varying abundance levels, 4–35 μg total protein is sufficient in a volume range from 20 to 35 μL at a concentration of 0.2–1.0 μg/μL. The amount of protein needed per spot is very small, at the level of nanograms, where for specific proteins; the detection is at picograms to femtograms levels per spot.
5. Mass spectrometry is a labor-intensive technique and is only available in specialized centers with a large-scale mass spectrometer machine and specially trained staff with advanced bioinformatics skills where as RPPA is a high throughput technique that entails a suite of robotic platforms for printing, staining and imaging and overall much less expen-

sive than the equivalent mass spectrometry equipment. Overall, RPPA is potentially much cheaper for large sample numbers than other immunoassay techniques and requires less sample and fewer reagents.

16.6.4 Overview of RPPA Methodology

RPPA technique can be applied to fresh, frozen or fixed tissues. It can be easily performed on cellular lysates obtained from laser capture microdissection, body fluids, cell culture and fine needle aspirates. The cellular lysate indicate the state of individual tissue cell populations from normal, malignant, or surrounding stroma. In RPPA, small (~μL) amounts of serially diluted protein lysate are transferred to 96- or 384 well microtiter plates and uniformly printed as individual spots onto a nitrocellulose-coated glass slide using a robotic arrayer (Fig. 16.3). As many as 6144 protein samples can be spotted onto standard glass slides using innovative pin spotting technology. The high protein binding capacity of the nitrocellulose allows immobilization of protein from dilute cell lysates (e.g. 0.25 mg/mL total protein). Using automated staining systems each slide is probed with a specific primary antibody (preferably monoclonal antibody) and a corresponding secondary antibody to detect expression of the target epitope. Signals are amplified using a Dako cytomation-catalyzed system (Dako) and visualized by DAB colorimetric reaction. Signal amplification is independent of the immobilized protein, permitting coupling of detection strategies with highly sensitive amplification chemistries (fluorescence, chemiluminescence and colorimetric). Slides were scanned, analyzed, and quantified using custom-

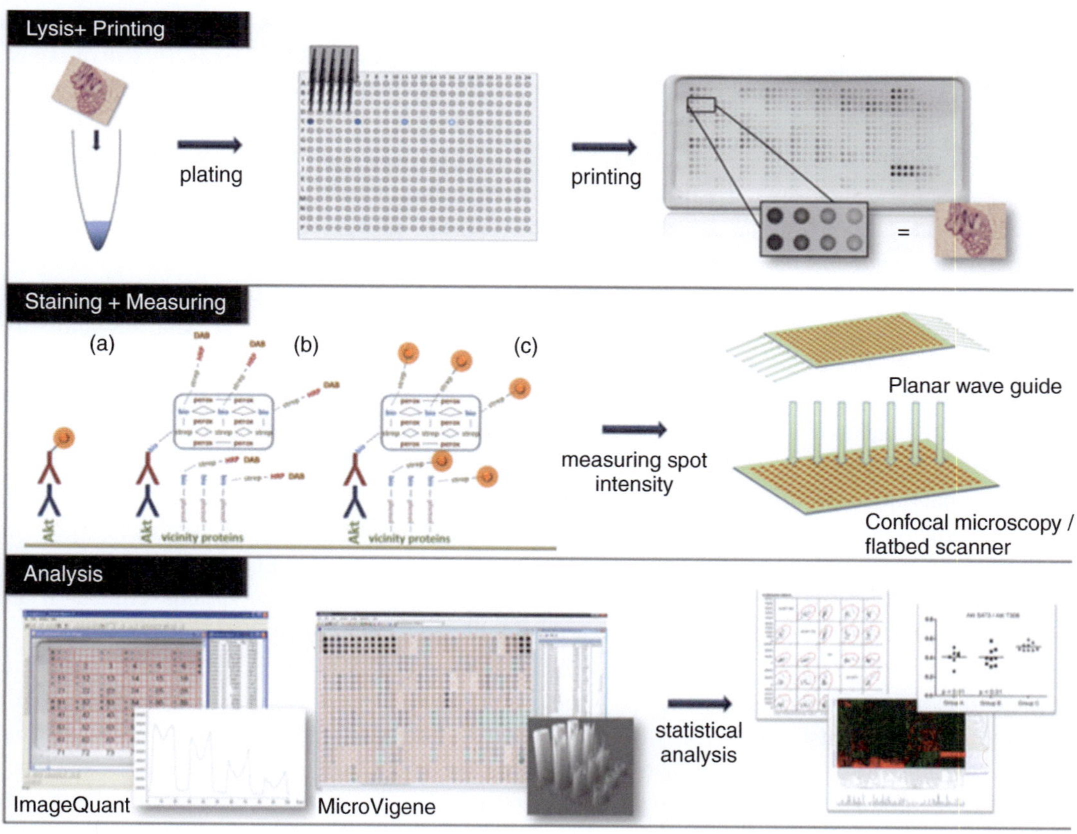

Fig. 16.3 Summary of the RPPA protocol from lysate preparation to data analysis (Reproduced from [19])

ized software Microvigene (VigeneTech Inc.). Besides, MicroVigene other programs suitable for RPPA data analysis are Array Pro (version 6.3, Media Cybernetics, Rockville, MD, USA), GenePix Pro (version 7.2.29, Molecular Devices, Sunnyvale, CA, USA), and Mapix (version 7.3.1, Innopsys, Carbonne, France). Multiplexing is achieved by batching samples, printing them on arrays, and analyzing tens to hundreds of samples under the same experimental conditions for any given analyte on a single array, thus providing direct quantifiable information on post-translational modifications across all samples.

16.6.5 Why RPPA Is a Promising Technique in Cancer Biomarker Discovery?

In last decade, RPPA has become a versatile and robust tool in cancer proteomics. RPPA is increasingly being used to determine deregulated signaling networks in different cancer tissues. The technology not only finds great application in biomarker discovery and validation but also used in personalized drug therapy and protein profiling and classification of various tumor types. The hypothesis that each patient's cancer has a unique set of specific molecular derangements is strongly supported by data generated by RPPAs. RPPA can efficiently monitor changes in protein phosphorylation over time, before and after the drug treatment, between normal and disease state, and between drug responders and non-responders [20]. With thousands of published articles, RPPAs is gaining popularity for profiling and comparing the functional state of cellular signaling pathways in several modalities, quantifying large numbers of samples on one array, under identical experimental conditions. It is also used to study intracellular signaling molecules within excised tumors, and compares them between patients and/or patients groups, or within the same patients before and after the drug treatment [21]. RPPA profiling of various protein and their pathways were investigated in different cancers like endometrial, lung, glioma, breast and prostate cancer. RPPA was successfully applied to validate clusterin as a blood biomarker of carcinogenesis and identified IGFBP2 as a candidate biomarker and therapeutic target of glioblastoma [19]. In a lung cancer study of 101 case-matched normal and tumor tissue samples, RPPA analysis of lung tumor tissues showed drastic abnormal expression of several molecules involved in DNA damage/repair, signal transductions, lipid metabolism, and cell proliferation. Further the increased expression of Stat5 was shown to have a favorable clinical outcome and therefore it has been proposed as a prognostic biomarker for lung cancer [12]. In another study, RPPA-based tumor profiling identified a protein biomarker signature consisting of caveolin-1, NDKA, RPS6, and Ki-67 with a high potential to determine the recurrence risk in patients with luminal breast cancer (with ER+ breast cancer) implying that it could potentially also be applied to predict a need for chemotherapy [22]. RPPA technology was successfully applied to discover a new phenotype of IHC and FISH HER2-negative breast cancer patients with levels of activated/phosphorylated HER2 as compared to IHC and FISH HER2-positive tumors [23]. RPPA platform has also been successfully utilized for biomarker discovery in colorectal cancer, colon cancer, breast carcinoma, prostate cancer, bladder cancer and non-small cell lung cancer. In ovarian cancer, RPPA helped in identifying autoantibody signatures in ovarian cancer and 15 proteins were identified as candidates for further study as tumor-associated antigens, 10 of which were reproducible in the cancer set [24, 25]. Thus, RPPA continue to evolve as a promising clinical research assay in personalized therapy, protein profiling and biomarker discovery and is currently being utilized in various clinical trials (Table 16.4).

Recently, the TheraLink HER family Assay, a RPPA-based diagnostic tool consisting of 14 HER2 family-related biomarkers for breast cancer, was introduced by Theranostics Health, Inc. (Rockville, MD) to identify tumors that are addicted to the function of cell surface receptors

Table 16.4 Clinical trial involving reverse phase protein microarray analysis (Reproduced from [19])

S. no.	Trial identifier	Acronym	Conditions	Study design	Phase
1	NCT01042379	I-SPY 2	Breast cancer	Open label, interventional	II
2	NCT01023477	PINC	Breast DCIS	Open-label; interventional	I/II
3	NCT01074814	Side-out	Metastatic breast cancer	Open-label; interventional	II/III
4	NCT00798655	N/A	Head and neck cancer	Open-label; interventional	II
5	NCT00952809	N/A	Lymphoma	Observational	NA
6	NCT00867334	NITMEC	Colorectal cancer	Open label; interventional	II/III

Table 16.5 Applications of protein microarray in cancer biomarker discovery

S. no.	Protein arrays	Studies	Commercial available array	Companies
1	Antibody microarray	Profiled MMPs/TIMPs signature in gastric garcinoma	ProtoArray Human Protein Microarrays	Thermo Fisher Scientific Inc.
2	Tissue microarray	Identified novel prognostically significant tumor	Proteome Profiler Antibody Arrays	R&D Systems, Inc.
3	Novel high-density custom protein microarrays (NAPPA)	Detected 119 antigens to autoantibodies in breast cancer	Protein Arrays	Cambridge Protein Arrays Ltd.
4	ProtoArray Human Protein Microarrays v4.0 & tissue microarray	Identified galectin-8, TARP and TRAP1 for biomarkers in prostate cancer	Protein Arrays	Applied Microarrays, Inc.
5	Protein microarray	Profiled biomarkers in bladder cancer, non-small lung cancer	PAK Protein Array Kits	GE Healthcare Companies
6	ProtoArrays	Discovered 15 potential tumour-associated antigens in ovarian cancer	Antibody microarray kit	Kinexus Bioinformatics Corporation
7	SELDI-TOF-MS protein microarrays	Identified serum biomarkers for lung cancer, renal cell carcinoma	Products for use with protein microarrays	SurModics, Inc.
8	SELDI-TOF-MS protein microarrays & CT scan	Distinguishes renal cell carcinoma from benign renal	Microarray tools	Grace Bio-Labs, Inc.
9	SELDI-TOF MS based ProteinChip arrays	Profiling for diagnostic and prognostic bladder cancer biomarkers	–	–

of HER2 family [26]. RPPA has thus become the preferred proteomic platform in precision medicine and is making transition to clinics. To accelerate the discovery of protein biomarkers in cancer, global RPPA community is now engaged in generating a worldwide database of high-quality antibodies with detailed information on validated antibodies and guidelines on antibody validation protocols that will help researchers to share and access latest updates.

These antibody databases named as Human Protein Atlas Project (www.proteinatlas.org/), Antibodypedia (http://www.antibodypedia.com/) and the Antibody Portal of the NCI (http://antibodies.cancer.gov). The existing validated antibody database covers a broad range of pathways involved in cancers, including proliferation, apoptosis, angiogenesis, and epithelial-mesenchymal-transition. Using available validated antibodies, researchers can quantify proteins of interest even if it is present in low abundance in both phosphorylated and unphosphorylated forms. Interestingly, protein microarray technology is now used alone or in combination with mass spectrometry for biomarker discovery in various cancers (Table 16.5). Commercially protein microarrays are now available in different formats for the researchers as mentioned in Table 16.5 [24, 25].

16.6.6 Outline of Unique Features and Advantages of RPPA

RPPA is basically a microscale dot-blot platform that enables the simultaneous quantification of protein expression in a large number of biological samples.

Unique characteristics of RPPA are:

1. Automated, high-throughput robotic instrumentation that can generate hundreds of arrays with very high content (up to thousands of independent samples printed on one array).
2. High sensitivity particularly when signal amplification systems (e.g., third-generation enzymatic reactions like streptavidin-mediated horseradish peroxidase deposition of biotinyl tyramide) are used.
3. Semi-quantitative/quantitative output allows direct comparison of the relative abundance of an analyte across hundreds of samples.
4. Utilization of microscopic quantities of sample. The technology is amply sensitive to detect femtograms of proteins in nanograms of starting material.
5. Sample handling and preparations are straightforward and simple. The sample preparation is similar to that used in western blotting, which is familiar to most laboratories.
6. Each patient sample can be spotted as a serial dilution series to ensure quantification with in linear range of detection.
7. Post-translation modifications of protein can be quantified.
8. Compatible with diverse range of biological specimens (cell lysates from cell lines, tissues and all body fluids).
9. Labeling of proteins with fluorescent dyes and mass tags not required thus minimizing technical variation in sample preparations.
10. RPPA has exceptional ability to quantify multiple phosphorylated proteins and probe pathway activity in very small amounts of tissue samples, make it a suitable platform for patient-tailored therapy or precision medicine.

16.7 Current Status of Biomarkers in Oral Cancer

Majority of OSCC arises de novo without prior visible changes in mucosa and are known to progress very fast from early to advance stage within a very short time, possibly few weeks hindering early diagnosis. The mechanism that leads to transformation of the premalignant lesions to OSCC is not yet clear. Oral carcinogenesis is a complex, multifactorial process that is believed to result from the progressive accumulation of genetic lesions after long-term betel-quid and tobacco exposure.

Oral cancers are characterized by a multitude of genetic events within signal transduction pathways governing normal cellular functions including cell division, differentiation and cell death. Common alterations for oral cancer are inactivation of TP53 (located at 17p13), gain of chromosomal material at 3q26 and 11q13, and losses at 3p21, 13q21 and 14q32. The putative tumor suppressor genes or oncogenes in these regions still need to be identified. Loss of chromosomal material (allelic losses) at 3p, 9q and 17p was frequently observed in a fairly high proportion of dysplastic lesions and therefore these alterations were projected as early markers of carcinogenesis. However, these early genetic changes do not necessarily correlate with the altered morphology of the tumor [4]. Apart from molecular and biochemical alterations, clinical changes occurring in the affected epithelial tissues, known as precancerous lesions (leukoplakia, oral submucos fibrosis, erythroplakia, lichen planus) are characterized by increased risk of malignant transformation into OSCC. Conventional techniques (histopathological analysis, optical diagnostics) are unable to predict malignant changes. Therefore, there is an increasing focus on developing sensitive molecular biomarkers capable of identifying the subset of premalignant lesions that are likely to progress to malignant lesions. In spite of the increasing innovations in proteomic techniques, biomarkers in oral cancer are still in the discovery phase and need further validation to be implemented in clinical practice. Several studies have investigated the use of salivary proteins as potential diagnostic markers for oral cancer. Most of these studies have used conventional proteomic techniques to identity single protein biomarkers, which lack sufficient sensitivity and specificity. The early detection of oral cancer thus warrants aggressive research in discovering non-invasive, highly sensitive and effective biomarkers.

16.7.1 Protein Biomarkers in Oral Cancer Tissues

The studies on proteome analysis of oral cancer tissues are limited. The first proteomic analysis of oral tongue carcinoma was only reported in the year 2004. With the development in high throughput proteomic technologies in last decade several studies focused on the differential protein expression in premalignant lesions and oral cancer. These differentially expressed proteins can be used as candidate biomarkers of OSCC. Several studies have identified differentially expressed proteins in oral cancer tissues for potential use as biomarkers (Table 16.6) [27]. The proteosome activator PA28 was studied for their expression and interactive networks correlated with oral malignancy. Proteasome activator complex PA28 'a' and 'b' were selected for further validation. They both exhibited a high expression level in cancer tissues (four to sixfold increase) when compared with the precancerous OLK tissues. In a recent study, aberrant expression of vimentin was observed in oral premalignant lesions (inflammatory lesions, leukoplakia, submucous fibrosis) and carcinomas using

Table 16.6 Potential tissue protein biomarker identified in OSCC

S. no.	Patients	Technique	Differentially expressed proteins	Number of proteins
1	Oral leukoplakia tissues (n = 6)	2D-ESI-Q-TOF MS/MS	PA28, a, b and g	85 proteins (52 upregulated, 33 downregulated)
2	Stage I and II (n = 5) Stage III and IV (n = 5)	2D SDS-PAGE-MS	Hsp90, HSPA5, HSPA8, Keratins (K1, K6A, K17), tubulin, cofilin-1, 14-3-3s, metabolic enzymes	68 proteins differentially expressed, 39 significantly altered
3	OSSC tissues and matched controls (n = 10)	2DE	AlphaB-crystallin, tropomyosin 2, myosin light chain 1, Hsp27, stratifin, thioredoxin-dependent peroxide reductase, flavin reductase, vimentin, rho-GDI2, GST-pi, MnSOD	41 proteins were overexpressed
4.	FFPE from normal squamous epithelium (n = 4), well differentiated (n = 4), and poorly differentiated (n = 4) HNSCC	Tandem MS and bioinformatics analysis	Cytokeratin 4, cytokeratin 16, vimentin, desmoplakin	115 protein identified
5.	FFPE tissue block of tongue SCC (n = 10)	2D converted analysis of LC and MS	TGM3, CK4, CK13, ANXA1	25,108 MS peaks
6.	Primary OSCC and matched control (n = 20)	iTRAQ analysis	TPT, ITGA6, CAB_{39} L	757 and 674 unique proteins
7.	OSCC (n = 144)	1 and 2DE, MS	Desmin, keratin 8, septin-2, ARP 2/3, CAP1, cofilin-1, CAPZA1, HSP90-a, tropomyosin a-3 isoform 4	223 differentially expressed proteins were found
8.	HNSCC and matched control (n = 8)	Protein labeling, 2D-DIGE and LS/MS	Keratin 4, cornulin	1000 common protein spots and 40 unique spots

immunofluorescence and western blot. The study showed a possible role of vimentin in early events of tobacco/areca nut-associated oral tumorigenesis [28]. During OSCC progression, deregulated keratin expression is known to be associated with impaired epithelial differentiation and organization. Keratin-76 expression was down regulated in human oral cancers. An immunohistochemical approach showed that with the disease progression, cyclin D1 expression significantly increases in OSCC patients. In another study, altered expression of β-Catenin and E-Cadherin in oral dysplasia and cancer was observed [29]. High levels of CD44 also showed a strong association to differentiate malignant from benign lesions. In a recent study, using mass spectrometry based comparative proteomic approach, novel signature proteins, ras-related protein Rab-2A isoform, RAB2A (4.6-fold), and peroxiredoxin-1, PRDX1 (2.2-fold) were identified that were not reported earlier in OSCC [30]. Expression of the cell cycle-associated proteins, p16, p27, pRb, p53 and Ki-67, was also investigated in cancerous and precancerous oral lesions by immunohistochemistry. Expression of pRb, p53 and Ki-67 significantly increased with tumor progression. The major drawback of most of these studies was the small sample size and often different studies collected tumor from different anatomic sites. Therefore, there is a need for large-scale validation in prospective, well-designed clinical studies in multicentric settings. Huang et al. investigated the GRP78 protein expression in cell lines and tissues from OSCC patients using the western blotting assay and immunohistochemistry. Immunohistochemical staining of clinical samples indicated that decreased GRP78 protein expression is significantly correlated with advance stage of tumor [31]. Few other proteins with potential role to be developed and validated as a marker of oral cancer risk and malignant transformation are Rho GTPase-activating protein 7, retinal dehydrogenase 1/prominin-1 (combined biomarkers), podoplanin, cortactin/focal adhesion kinase 1 (combined biomarkers) and catenin delta-1 [32]. Though, tumor tissues are the reliable sources for tumor biomarkers but obtaining sufficient and high quality tissue in adequate numbers is a major challenge. Human tissues are typically obtained from biopsies, surgeries and autopsies therefore tissues must be collected and processed according to standards that preserve the quality of the specimens. Owing to the challenges involved in discovery of tissue biomarkers, most researchers prefer noninvasive method (blood, saliva) of specimen collection.

16.7.2 Serum Protein Biomarkers in Oral Cancer

Serum is a complex fluid, with more than 10,000 diverse proteins many of which are secreted by cells during different physiological or pathological processes. Serum is considered as an excellent source for protein biomarker because it circulates through all the tissues. Serum/plasma proteomics is a simple, safe and minimally invasive approach for the discovery of protein biomarker for early detection and monitoring of various cancers. Unavailability of tissue samples present significant limitations in using comparative proteomic analysis of normal and cancerous tissues.

Several serum proteins with abnormal expression in other cancers were found to have a significant association with OSCC. For example, abnormal expression of serum P53 and VEGF protein earlier reported in breast cancer, colorectal cancer, pediatric neuroblastoma and gall bladder carcinoma, were found to be significantly higher in serum of oral cancer patients as compared to healthy controls. This could be because tumor P53 protein is known to play an important role in angiogenesis. The proteins from the intermediate filament (IF) family, in particular cytokeratins (CKs), have shown significant utility in cancer diagnostics. The most common cytokeratins tumor markers are tissue polypeptide antigen (TPA), tissue polypeptide specific antigen (TPS), and cytokeratin fragments 21-1 (Cyfra 21-1), which are being evaluated as serum markers for their clinical utility in various cancers. Some of these proteins significantly associated with OSCC in both serum and saliva of patients are Cyfra 21-1 (CK 19), TPA, CKs, (8, 18, 19), pro-inflammatory cytokines (interleukin-6 and TNFα), and anti-p53 antibodies. TPA was however reported to be a sensitive but a non-specific marker for OSCC. In a very recent study, scara 5 was identified as the potential marker for early diagnosis of OSCC. The down-regulation of scara5 expression was related with cell proliferation and invasion. Also, serum scara5 detection could clearly discriminate OSCC samples from normal samples with high sensitivity. Chai et al. discovered four serum protein biomarkers; gelsolin, fibronectin, angiotensinogen, and haptoglobin biomarkers for lymph-node metastasis in oral cancer [33]. Chronic inflammation is known to have a strong correlation with tumor development. C-reactive protein (CRP), an acute phase protein synthesized primarily in the liver, is a marker for inflammation and progression of many cancers. Mean CRP serum levels were elevated in patients with oral premalignant lesions as compared to controls. Elevated CRP serum levels in OSCC were also related with advance stage of tumors. Studies also revealed other potential serum protein biomarkers for OSCC, such as carcinoembryonic antigen (CEA), CA-50, CA19-9 and squamous cell carcinoma antigen (SCCA), and insulin-like growth factor binding protein 3. The involvement of big Endothelin-1 (ET-1) protein has been evaluated in tumor growth and progression in prostatic, ovarian, renal, pulmonary, colorectal, cervical, breast, lung, bladder, and endometrial cancer. Studies suggest that the serum levels of big ET-1 can also be used as an adjunctive serological marker for the diagnosis and prognosis of OSCC and in disease monitoring. However, prospective studies on larger number of patients are required for further validation. Gas6 protein is reportedly known to increase the metastatic capacity of OSCC cells. Gas6 levels are significantly increased in OSCC patients, in both serum and tumor tissues. Elevated serum Gas6 was related to late TNM stage and poorly differentiated oral tumors. Thus, high serum Gas6 level may predict nodal metastases, late cancer stage reflecting poor prognosis in OSCC patients and could be used as a diagnostic and prognostic biomarker in OSCC. Other differentially expressed host-specific proteins identified in serum of OSCC patients are leucine-rich a2-glycoprotein (LRG), alpha-1-B-glycoprotein (ABG), clusterin (CLU), PRO2044, haptoglobin (HAP), complement C3c (C3), proapolipoprotein A1 (proapo-A1), and retinol-binding protein 4 precursor (RBP4) [24, 25]. Proteomic studies that investigated the protein signatures associated with OSCC in serum of oral cancer patients are summarized in Table 16.7 [34]. Plasma proteomic analysis of OSCC patients in Taiwan (with 5 years history of betel nut chewig) identified at least 38 proteins including Fibrinogen chain, haptoglobin, eucine-rich alpha-2-glycoprotein and ribosomal protein S6 kinase alpha-3 (RSK2) that were not reported in earlier studies and were proposed to be associated with the progression and development of the disease. Tetranectin is identified as another potential biomarker for metastatic oral cancer. The serum level of tetranectin was significantly lower in OSCC patients compared to the healthy controls. Other candidate serum biomarkers identified in the same study are superoxide dismutase, ficolin 2, CD-5 antigen-like protein, RalA binding protein 1, plasma retinol-binding protein and transthyretin. However, further studies are required to validate these potential biomarkers for their clinical utility [35]. Serum/plasma proteomics is an attractive approach to discovery of disease biomarkers because testing of biomarkers in blood is simple and convenient. Compared to tissue biopsies, blood samples are easily accessible and therefore a large number of specimens can be enrolled for a clinical proteomic study. However, major obstacle to serum proteome analysis is the predominance of highly abundant proteins such as albumins, immunoglobulins, alpha-1-antitrypsin, haptoglobin, and their isoforms and fragments. The presence of higher abundance proteins interferes with the identification and quantification of lower abundance proteins thus lowering the sensitivity and specificity of the sample. Therefore, fractionation approaches to reducing the complexity of the plasma needs to be applied (electrophoresis, SELDI, and liquid chromatography).

Table 16.7 Potential protein biomarkers identified in serum of oral cancer patients

Samples	Method	Serum protein biomarkers
OSCC = 70, control = 63	ELISA	P53
Oral leukoplakia reticular = 13, Oral leukoplakia (atrophive erosive) = 13, control = 26	ELISA	TNF-α, sFas, and Bcl-2
OSCC = 57, control = 29	MALDI-TOF-MS	Fibrinogen α-chain
OSCC = 113, control = 0	ELISA	P53 antibodies
OSCC = 102, control = 38	ELISA	Galectin-1, 3, 7
OSCC = 30, control = 20	ELISA	IL-1α, IIL-6, IL-8, GM-CSF
OSCC = 34, control = 10	2DE and LC–MS/MS	Tetranectin
OSCC = 64, control = 31	ELISA	GDF-15
OSCC = 45, control = 45	ELISA	MMP-3
OSCC = 30, control = 10	Western blot	MDA and sialic acid
OSCC = 330	ELISA, western blot	MMP-11
OSCC = 98, Oral leukoplakia = 14, control = 24	ELISA	CCL2 and CCL3
OSCC = 70, control = 30	ELISA	VEGF
OSCC = 204, control = 212	ELISA	Anti MMP-7
OSCC = 27, Oral leukoplakia = 27	ELISA	EGF
OSCC = 40, control = 40	ELISA	Endothelin-1 (ET-1)
OSCC = 30, Oral leukoplakia = 20	ELISA	Collagenase-3, MMP-13
OSCC = 312	ELISA	CEA, SCC, CYFRA 21-1, and TPS
OSCC = 166, control = 120	MALDI-TOF MS	Glutathione S-transferase pi (GSTP1)
OSCC = 282	iTRAQ	Fibronectin, gelsolin, and angiotensinogen
OSCC = 450, control = 64	ELISA	TIMP-3
Metastases OSCC, n = 10 Lymph node metastases free:10, Control = 10	SDS-PAGE And LC-MS/MS with iTRAQ labeling	AOC3, APOD, C4B, C4A
OSCC = 10, Control = 10	Fluorescence 2D-DIGE-based proteomic	Fibrinogen chain, haptoglobin, leucine-rich alpha-2-glycoprotein and ribosomal protein S6 kinase alpha-3 (RSK2)

16.7.3 Protein Biomarkers for OSCC in Saliva

In routine clinical practice, oral examination and biopsies are the standard procedures used to determine the characteristics of mucosal lesions. Detection of cancerous lesion by biopsies is often associated with patient discomfort and may not provide accurate information because of limitations in selecting the right tissue and location while conducting the biopsies thus lacking enough sensitivity and specificity. The emerging field of salivary biomarkers offers great potentials to be used as a diagnostic fluid for earlier detection of OSCC. Saliva collection is minimally invasive, inexpensive and risk free with simple handling, transportation and storage. Whole saliva comprises of both salivary gland and serum-derived proteins, which can provide clues in oral and systemic diseases. There are more than 3000 proteins identified in saliva and the levels of many of these proteins are altered in malignant conditions. Saliva is preprogramed to respond to any change in molecular events in an oral cavity, probably that is the reason first biomarker for breast cancer, HER2/neu, was discovered in saliva. Tumor progression and metastasis indicates a change in protein expression levels of several proteins present in saliva, therefore it can be reliably used to monitor patients at cancer risk. For example, CA15-3 is a proteomic biomarker approved by US FDA for monitoring the metastasis of breast cancer. At least 20% of the salivary proteins are implicated in oral cancer.

Table 16.8 Salivary protein biomarkers identified in oral cancer

Group	Salivary protein biomarker for OSCC	Most promising biomarkers in saliva
Cytokines	IL-1α, IL1-β, IL6, IL-8, IL-10, IL-13, TNF α	MMP1, MMP3, MMP9, cytokines IL-6, IL-8, VEGF-A, TNF-α, transferrins, and fibroblast growth factors
Growth factors	TGF-β, VEGF, EGF, IGF-1, fibroblast growth factor	
Enzymes	α-amylase, catalase, LDH, telomerase	
Oxidative stress related molecules	Peroxidase, glutathione-S-transferase, superoxide dismutase, 8-hydroxy-2 deoxyguanosine, salivary carbonyls, 8-oxoguanine DNA glycosylase	
Plasma proteins	Transferrin, hemopexin, haptoglobulin, transthyretin	
Cytokeratins	Tissue polypeptide antigen, Cyfra21-1, Keratin 10, Keratin 36	
Serine protease inhibitors	Maspin, α-antitrypsin	
Complement proteins	Complement protein C3, C4d, CD59	
Matrix metalloproteinases (MMP)	MMP-1, MMP-2, MMP-3, MMP-9, MMP-10	
Cancer antigens	CA125, CEA, CA-50	
Other proteins	Defensin, Statherin, Endothelin-1, CD44, Mac-2 binding protein, Cyclin D1, 8-oxoguanine DNA glycosylase, phosphorylated Src, Ki-67 Profilin, Catalase, SA100A9, Zinc finger protein, Annexin 1, Peroxiredoxin 2 Tetranectin protein, Chemerin, truncated cytostatin SA-1, OAZ1, S100P, MRP-14, Salivary zinc finger, Hemopexin, P53 auntoantiboy, Rab-7, Moesin, Involucrin, Enolase1, Protein 510 peptide, Cofilin-1, Thioredoxin, Resistin, KNG1, ANA2, and HSPA5	

Since oral lesions are in direct contact of saliva, the biomarker discovery for OSCC in saliva appear to be more realistic than serum or plasma. Studies from different population suggest that more than 50 proteins in saliva have the potential to be used as diagnostic biomarkers for OSCC. The updated list of protein biomarkers identified in saliva from several studies in oral cancer patients is shown in Table 16.8 [36].

The most promising salivary protein markers detected in OSCC as reported by several studies carried out through different populations are interleukins (8, 6, 1β), matrix metalloproteinase (MMP 2, 9), transforming growth factor (TGF-1), Ki67, cyclin D1, intermediate filament protein (Cyfra 21.1), transferrin, α-amylase, tumor necrosis factor (TNF-α) and catalase. Interestingly, three well-known markers, cyfra-21-1, CA-125, tissue polypeptide antigen are found to be fourfold increased in the saliva of OSCC patients. Other informative protein biomarkers in saliva, which are significantly altered in OSCC patients as compared to healthy controls, are P53, cancer antigen (CA-125, CA-128), statherin, CD44, CD59, CEA and insulin growth factor. In a recent study, Wu et al. showed that salivary levels of nine proteins (SERPIND1, C6, FABP4, LPA, RETN, APOA2, C9, HPR, and EPHX1) were significantly elevated in the OSCC as compared to control and oral potentially malignant disorders (OPMD) group. Notably, these nine proteins were detected only in the saliva of the OSCC group but not in the other groups. Out of these nine proteins, RTEN was subjected to further verification in a large cohort (health, OSCC and OPMD) and the results suggested that the salivary levels of RTEN could be used for prognosis of oral cancer [37].

Techniques like 2D gel electrophoresis, ELISA, HPLC-laser induced fluorescence, MALDI-TOF and SELDI mass spectrometry were the most commonly used techniques for the analysis of these protein biomarkers. Most of these biomarker studies focused on single (or fewer) protein expression, which may not provide compelling evidence with respect to change in protein structure and function and other post-translational modifications occurring during

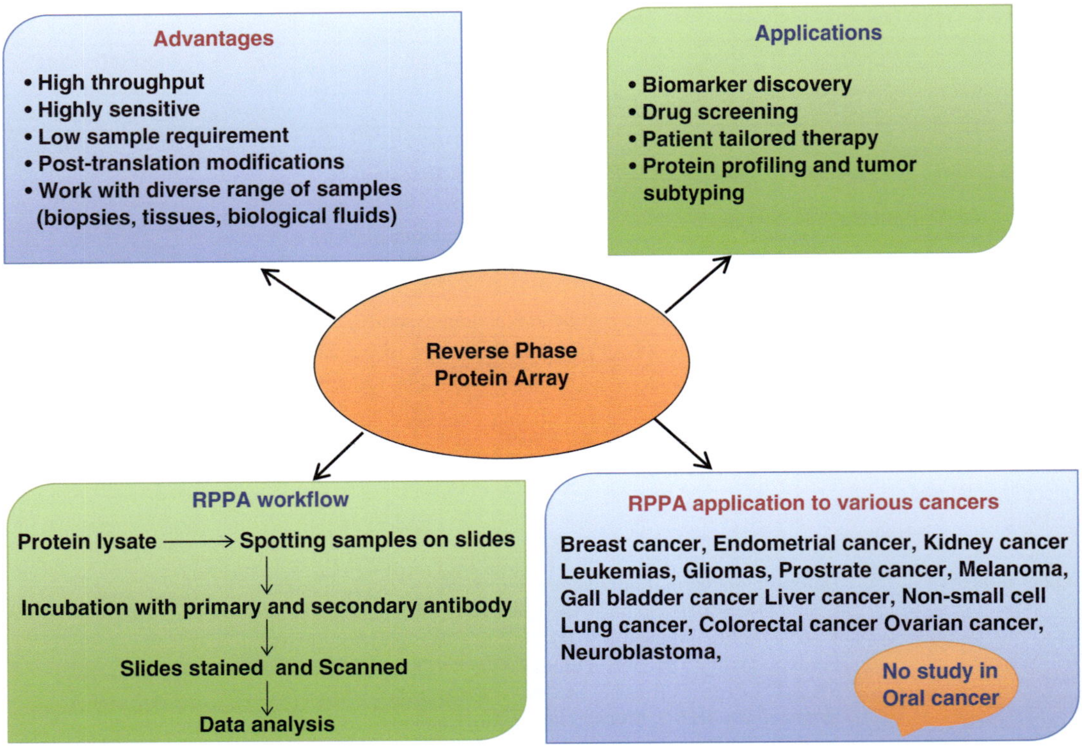

Fig. 16.4 RPPA overview in cancer research

progression of the disease. Probably like other cancers, alteration in signaling molecules are hard to predict with genomic and other conventional proteomic techniques like 2D, mass spectrometry etc. Most of these available studies lack a comprehensive analysis and as a result not a single effective and reliable biomarker is available for earlier detection of OSCC so far. Moreover, these techniques have certain limitations like large sample requirement, poor reproducibility and labor intensiveness, and cannot be easily automated thus limiting the biomarker discover to the lab.

RPPA holds a great potential in salivary proteomics and it can help to identify differential protein expression in both tissue and salivary fluids in a high-throughput manner and further validation by functional assays. RPPA technique has been successfully used to identify differentially expressed proteins in leukemia, prostate, breast and lung cancers in various studies carried out in United States. However, RPPA has not been applied to oral cancer in a single study so far, the reason being that not many oral cancer cases are reported in western population. To discover specific and accurate biomarkers for oral cancer, it is therefore crucial to apply RPPA technique on oral cancer tissues to gain insights of the mechanism of molecular pathways and signaling network involved in tumor development from premalignant lesions. The differentially expressed proteins as revealed by RPPA can be further explored in saliva as a non-invasive approach for early screening methods. Thus, RPPA can be used as a promising technique in oral cancer biomarker discovery owing to its unique features and advantages over established proteomic techniques as evident from its application in other cancers (Fig. 16.4).

16.7.4 Challenges in Salivary Biomarker Research

Salivary proteomics is a rapidly advancing discipline in oral cancer research to discover novel biomarkers for early detection of oral cancer. Undoubtedly, saliva is one of the most reliable tools for oral cancer diagnosis as it is easily accessible and noninvasive method compared to tissue biopsies. Furthermore, saliva collection is simple, cost effective, less time consuming and does not require any special collection device or special skill thus making salivary diagnostics a popular methodology for biomarker discovery. In last decade, more than 100 potential OSSS salivary biomarkers were reported in literature, yet no validated and definitive biomarker available for early detection of oral cancer. The major challenge in salivary biomarker research is the lack of standardization of saliva collection, processing and storage protocol (temperature and duration). There is huge discrepancy in saliva collection protocols particularly related to the timing of collection, whether it should be done prior to food or drink intake or use of oral hygiene products. Saliva is an extremely sensitive fluid, which is greatly affected by systemic, physiological, and biochemical changes in the oral cavity. Any variation in time of saliva collection, handling processing, and method of analysis can affect the biomarker analysis. For example, most researcher centrifuged the samples immediately after collection but degrees of centrifugal force and lengths of time varies greatly, such as 800 *g* for 10 min; 2000 *g* for 10 min; 2600 *g* for 15 min; 14,000 *g* for 20 min. Few investigators added proteinase inhibitors to the samples where as others did not add any inhibitors. Saliva sample storage temperature also varies from lab to lab, most researchers stored the saliva samples in −80 °C, others stored samples at −20 °C. There is no clear consensus on whether stimulated or unstimulated whole saliva should be used for proteomic biomarker analysis. Therefore, it is important to design a standardized and uniform protocol for saliva collection from all the patients and reduce the variation in collection time, method and storage. Most of the potential salivary biomarkers of oral cancer are salivary proteins, which are present in a very low concentration in saliva, thus necessitating use of high sensitivity methods and high-throughput technologies for accurate and uniform analysis.

Another hurdle in the salivary protein biomarker discovery is the variations in protein expression levels in different populations. Protein biomarkers identified in one population may not have significance in another population. For example, IL-8 was identified as a biomarker in the USA, India and Serbia but not in Japanese and Iranian population. Similarly, S100A9 was identified as a suitable OSCC biomarker in USA but not in China. Again, there were variations observed in same population by different investigators. The disparity in important biomarkers among different populations shows that biomarkers validated in one population may not have same predictive value in another population. Thus, discovery of biomarker is not really a concern but the issue lies in the preclinical verification and validation of these putative biomarkers. Nevertheless, proteomics technology like RPPA holds great potential in salivary biomarker diagnosis as specific protein signatures identified by various techniques in saliva can be used to develop a point-of-care diagnostics for earlier detection and screening of oral cancer.

16.8 Conclusion and Future Perspectives

Oral squamous cell carcinoma (OSCC) is one of the leading causes of cancer-related mortality worldwide. Due to lack of early detection methods, oral cancer is the most common malignancy after breast and cervical cancers in India. In complex disorders like cancer, genetic alterations do not always correlate with the disease causes. Changes in protein structure and expression levels play an important role in tumor development and progression. The multiple factors involved in the etiology of oral carcinogenesis alone cannot be identified by genomic, or transcriptome or single protein expression studies. Unfortunately, not even a single study was carried out using RPPA technique in oral cancer so far. The reason being this technology is still not so popular and only few labs in Europe and US have all the resources and set up of these arrays. Moreover, oral cancer is more prevalent in developing countries due to betel/tobacco chewing social habits and research in western countries is focused on other cancers like prostrate, lung colon and breast cancer.

High throughput proteomic approach like RPPA can help to identify and compare differential protein expression in premalignant and malignant lesions of patients to identify proteins involved in signaling network and molecular pathways involved in progression of oral cancer. These differentially expressed proteins can be explored in saliva to generate a "molecular signature" that can be developed as a non-invasive method for earlier detection. RPPA represents a rapidly emerging and advancing cost-effective technology that can quantitatively analyze large number of low-abundance signaling proteins/phosphoproteins from small amount clinical samples. Although, mass spectroscopy approaches hold great promise in biomarker discovery, but it cannot match the automation, sensitivity, and ability to deal with small amounts of material, or cost effectiveness of the RPPA platform. Additional efforts are needed to accelerate more widespread use of RPPA, in both areas of research and clinical practice. It is crucial to systematically link the discovery of a biomarker to the biology of the patient's tumor. Generating a list of activated proteins and pathways found in a diseased sample may not have any clinical impact if the biology of the tumor is not known. Understanding of the biological and biochemical effects of existing over-expressed and under expressed proteins in a patient's tumor will definitely improve the shortcomings of biomarker research. Recently, systematic cancer genomics projects including The Cancer Genome Atlas (TCGA) project have applied emerging genomic and proteomic technologies to the analysis of specific tumor types. TCGA's key objectives are to generate, quality control, merge, analyze, and interpret molecular profiles at the DNA, RNA, protein, and epigenetic levels for hundreds of clinical tumors from various tumor types and their subtypes. TCGA is currently an ongoing project to systematically profile more than 10,000 cancers of various histological subtypes, using all genomic, transcriptomic and miRNA and proteomic a platforms. TCGA dataset includes most extensive and recently published RPPA dataset of 3467 patient samples from eleven tumor subtypes generated by using 181 high-quality antibodies targeting 128 total proteins and 53 post translationally modified proteins. This chapter illustrates importance of proteomic approaches in biomarker discovery and further explores the potential role of high throughput technique, RPPA in providing insights into oral cancer biology.

References

1. Torre LA, Siegel RL, Ward EM, Jemal A. Global cancer incidence and mortality rates and trends—an update. Cancer Epidemiol Biomark Prev. 2016;25:16–27. https://doi.org/10.1158/1055-9965.EPI-15-0578.
2. Ferlay J, Soerjomataram I, Dikshit R, et al. Cancer incidence and mortality worldwide: sources, methods and major patterns in GLOBOCAN 2012. Int J Cancer. 2015;136:E359–86. https://doi.org/10.1002/ijc.29210.
3. Petersen PE. Oral cancer prevention and control—the approach of the World Health Organization. Oral Oncol. 2009;45:454–60. https://doi.org/10.1016/j.oraloncology.2008.05.023.
4. Fukuda M, Kusama K, Sakashita H. Molecular insights into the proliferation and progression mechanisms of the oral cancer: strategies for the effective and personalized therapy. Jpn Dent Sci Rev. 2012;48:23–41. https://doi.org/10.1016/j.jdsr.2011.08.001.
5. Mangalath U, Aslam S, Kooliyat AH, Khader A, Francis PG, Mikacha SK, et al. Recent trends in prevention of oral cancer. J Int Prev Commun Dent. 2014;4:S131–8. https://doi.org/10.4103/2231-0762.149018.
6. Hanahan D, Weinberg RA. Hallmarks of cancer: the next generation. Cell. 2011;144:646–74. https://doi.org/10.1016/j.cell.2011.02.013.
7. Sethi S, Ali S, Philip PA, Sarkar FH. Clinical advances in molecular biomarkers for cancer diagnosis and therapy. Int J Mol Sci. 2013;14:14771–84. https://doi.org/10.3390/ijms140714771.
8. Strimbu K, Tavel JA. What are biomarkers? Curr Opin HIV AIDS. 2010;5:463–6. https://doi.org/10.1097/COH.0b013e32833ed177.
9. William B, Ronald BH. Characteristics of the ideal tumor marker in Hollandfrei cancer medicine. 6th ed. Hamilton: BC, Decker; 2003.
10. Carr KM, Rosenblatt K, Petricoin EF, Liotta LA. Genomic and proteomic approaches for studying human cancer: prospects for true patient-tailored therapy. Hum Genomics. 2004;1:134–40. https://doi.org/10.1186/1479-7364-1-2-134.

11. Shruthi BS, Vinodhkumar P, Selvamani. Proteomics: a new perspective for cancer. Adv Biomed Res. 2016;5:67. https://doi.org/10.4103/2277-9175.180636.
12. Gallagher RI, Espina V. Reverse phase protein arrays: mapping the path towards personalized medicine. Mol Diagn Ther. 2014;18:619–30. https://doi.org/10.1007/s40291-014-0122-3.
13. Maes E, Mertens I, Valkenborg D, Pauwels P, Rolfo C, Baggerman G. Proteomics in cancer research: are we ready for clinical practice? Crit Rev Oncol Hematol. 2015;96:437–48. https://doi.org/10.1016/j.critrevonc.2015.07.006.
14. Hudler P, Kocevar N, Komel R. Proteomic approaches in biomarker discovery: new perspectives in cancer diagnostics. Sci World J. 2014;2014:260348. https://doi.org/10.1155/2014/260348.
15. Mordente A, Meucci E, Martorana GE, Silvestrini A. Cancer biomarkers discovery and validation: state of the art, problems and future perspectives. Adv Exp Med Biol. 2015;867:9–26. https://doi.org/10.1007/978-94-017-7215-0_2.
16. Parker CE, Borchers CH. Mass spectrometry based biomarker discovery, verification, and validation—quality assurance and control of protein biomarker assays. Mol Oncol. 2014;8:840–58. https://doi.org/10.1016/j.molonc.2014.03.006.
17. Masuda M, Yamada T. Signaling pathway profiling using reverse-phase protein array and its clinical applications. Expert Rev Proteomics. 2017;14:607–15. https://doi.org/10.1080/14789450.2017.1344101.
18. Paweletz CP, Charboneau L, Bichsel VE, Simone NL, Chen T, Gillespie JW, et al. Reverse phase protein microarrays which capture disease progression show activation of pro-survival pathways at the cancer invasion front. Oncogene. 2001;20:1981–9. https://doi.org/10.1038/sj.onc.1204265.
19. Mueller C, Liotta LA, Espina V. Reverse phase protein microarrays advance to use in clinical trials. Mol Oncol. 2010;4:461–81. https://doi.org/10.1016/j.molonc.2010.09.003.
20. Huang Y, Zhu H. Protein array-based approaches for biomarker discovery in cancer. Genomics Proteomics Bioinformatics. 2017;15:73–81. https://doi.org/10.1016/j.gpb.2017.03.001.
21. Tanase C, Albulescu R, Neagu M. Proteomic approaches for biomarker panels in cancer. J Immunoassay Immunochem. 2016;37:1–15. https://doi.org/10.1080/15321819.2015.1116009.
22. Wachter A, Bernhardt S, Beissbarth T, Korf U. Analysis of reverse phase protein array data: from experimental design towards targeted biomarker discovery. Microarrays. 2015;4:520–39. https://doi.org/10.3390/microarrays4040520.
23. Akbani R, Becker KF, Carragher N, Goldstein T, de Koning L, Korf U, et al. Realizing the promise of reverse phase protein arrays for clinical, translational, and basic research: a workshop report: the RPPA (Reverse Phase Protein Array) Society. Mol Cell Proteomics. 2014;13:1625–43. https://doi.org/10.1074/mcp.O113.034918.
24. Chen Y, Azman SN, Kerishnan JP, Zain RB, Chen YN, Wong Y-L, et al. Identification of host-immune response protein candidates in the sera of human oral squamous cell carcinoma patients. PLoS One. 2014;9:e109012. https://doi.org/10.1371/journal.pone.0109012.
25. Chen B, Liu Y, Shen Y, Xia Z, He G, Liang S. Protein microarrays in proteome-wide applications. J Proteomics Bioinform. 2014;S12:001. https://doi.org/10.4172/jpb.S12-001.
26. Creighton CJ, Huang S. Reverse phase protein arrays in signaling pathways: a data integration perspective. Drug Des Devel Ther. 2015;9:3519–27. https://doi.org/10.2147/DDDT.S38375.
27. Ni YH, Ding L, Hu QG, Hua ZC. Potential biomarkers for oral squamous cell carcinoma: proteomics discovery and clinical validation. Proteomics Clin Appl. 2015;9:86–97. https://doi.org/10.1002/prca.201400091.
28. Sawant S, Vaidya M, Chaukar D, Alam H, Dmello C, Gangadaran P, et al. Clinical significance of aberrant vimentin expression in oral premalignant lesions and carcinomas. Oral Dis. 2014;20(5):453–65. https://doi.org/10.1111/odi.12151.
29. Kaur J, Jacobs R, Huang Y, Salvo N, Politis C. Salivary biomarkers for oral cancer and pre-cancer screening: a review. Clin Oral Investig. 2018;22:633–40. https://doi.org/10.1007/s00784-018-2337-x.
30. Dey KK, Pal I, Bharti R, Dey G, Kumar BN, Rajput S, et al. Identification of RAB2A and PRDX1 as the potential biomarkers for oral squamous cell carcinoma using mass spectrometry-based comparative proteomic approach. Tumour Biol. 2015;36:9829–37. https://doi.org/10.1007/s13277-015-3758-7.
31. Huang TT, Chen JY, Tseng CE, Su YC, Ho HC, Lee MS, et al. Decreased GRP78 protein expression is a potential prognostic marker of oral squamous cell carcinoma in Taiwan. J Formos Med Assoc. 2010;109:326–37. doi: 10.1016/S0929-6646(10)60060-5.
32. Rivera C, Oliveira AK, Costa RAP, De Rossi T, Paes Leme AF. Prognostic biomarkers in oral squamous cell carcinoma: a systematic review. Oral Oncol. 2017;72:38–47.
33. Chai YD, Zhang L, Yang Y, Su T, Charugundla P, Ai J, et al. Discovery of potential serum protein biomarkers for lymph node metastasis in oral cancer. Head Neck. 2016;38:118–25. https://doi.org/10.1002/hed.23870.
34. Rai V, Mukherjee R, Ghosh AK, Routray A, Chakraborty C. "Omics" in oral cancer: new approaches for biomarker discovery. Arch Oral Biol. 2018;87:15–34. https://doi.org/10.1016/j.archoralbio.2017.12.003.
35. Arellano-Garcia ME, Li R, Liu X, Xie Y, Yan X, Loo JA, et al. Identification of tetranectin as a potential biomarker for metastatic oral cancer. Int J Mol Sci. 2010;11:3106–21. https://doi.org/10.3390/ijms11093106.
36. Bhattarai BP, Klongnoi B, Khovidhunkit SP, Wongsirichat, Natthamet. Protein biomarker in

saliva in oral squamous cell carcinoma. SWU Dent J. 2017;10:13. https://www.researchgate.net/publication/322832732_protein_biomarker_in_saliva_in_oral_squamous_cell_carcinoma. Accessed 20 Mar 2018.

37. Wu CC, Chu HW, Hsu CW, Chang KP, Liu HP. Saliva proteome profiling reveals potential salivary biomarkers for detection of oral cavity squamous cell carcinoma. Proteomics. 2015;15:3394–404. https://doi.org/10.1002/pmic.201500157.

Molecular Diagnostics in Liver Cancer

17

Anil Kumar Chauhan, Monika Bhardwaj, and Pankaj Kumar Chaturvedi

17.1 Introduction

Liver cancer is the third leading cause of cancer-related mortalities in the world [1], with hepatocellular carcinoma (HCC) [1] and intrahepatic cholangiocarcinoma (IHCC) [1] being the common forms of liver cancer. The incidence of liver cancer in men is particularly 2–4 times higher than in women [2]. Most of the liver cancer is diagnosed in well less developed nations primarily in East Asian and African countries [3, 4]. Every year more than 850,000 new cases of liver cancer are reported worldwide [5]. Underlying risks for the HCC occurrence and progression are influenced by etiology, activity, and stage of the underlying liver disease. Major risk factors for the development of HCC are distinct such as, cirrhosis (chronic liver damage caused by inflammation and fibrosis), hepatitis B virus (HBV) infection, hepatitis C virus (HCV) infection, alcohol abuse and metabolic syndrome [6]. Other cofactors which are well-characterized contributors to HCC are tobacco smoke inhalation and intake of aflatoxin B1 (a fungal carcinogen present in food supplies associated with mutations in the tumor suppressor gene TP53) [7–13].

A. K. Chauhan · M. Bhardwaj
Laboratory of Biochemistry and Cellular Engineering, Daegu Gyeongbuk Institute of Science and Technology, Daegu, Republic of Korea
e-mail: chauhananil48@dgist.ac.kr; monika03@dgist.ac.kr

P. K. Chaturvedi (✉)
Department of Radiation Oncology, Chungbuk National University Hospital,
Cheongju, Republic of Korea
e-mail: pankaj@chungbuk.ac.kr

17.2 Risk Factors Associated with Liver Cancer

Several epidemiological studies have demonstrated that chronic viral hepatitis, driven by HBV and HCV can lead to cirrhosis and/or HCC. HBV is a double-stranded, circular DNA molecule with eight genotypes (A to H). Among these, genotype C has been associated with the higher risk of HCC than genotypes A, B, and D [14]. There are various routes of the Hepatitis B transmission, for example, contaminated blood transfusions, intravenous injections, sexual contact and from mother to fetus [15]. Besides positive hepatitis B surface antigen (HBsAg), patients with positive hepatitis B core antibody (anti-HBc) who are HBsAg-negative also remain at risk for development of HCC. Antiviral treatment for hepatitis B has been associated with significant reduction of hepatocarcinogenicity of HBV.

HCV is a small, single-stranded RNA virus, which exhibits high genetic variability, which exhibits six different genotypes [16]. Around 80% of the patient infected with HCV progress to chronic hepatitis and ~20% among them may have chance of developing cirrhosis [17]. Cirrhotic patients are at the higher risk of

K. K. Shukla et al. (eds.), *Molecular Diagnostics in Cancer Patients*,
https://doi.org/10.1007/978-981-13-5877-7_17

developing HCC if they get the dual infection of HBV and HCV [18]. Patients who obtained a sustained viral response after treatment of HCV, are at significantly lower risk of HCC with a 54% reduction in mortality [19]. Besides that, alcohol consumption is considered as an important factor for HCC, which accounts for 40–50% of all HCC cases in Europe and the United States. The relation between alcohol and risk of liver cancer correlates with the heavy amount of alcohol consumed over a lifetime. The risk of liver cancer increases two- to four-times among persons drinking more than 60 g/day of ethanol [20].

17.2.1 Diabetes and Nonalcoholic Fatty Liver Disease

Obesity and diabetes mellitus are other key factors that are involved in the risk of liver cancer. The liver plays an essential role in the glucose metabolism which is directly affected by diabetes mellitus, that can lead to chronic hepatitis, fatty liver, liver failure, and cirrhosis [21, 22]. Diabetes mellitus has been significantly associated with about threefold increased risk of HCC. Pleiotropic effects of hyperinsulinemia play a role in carcinogenesis by regulating the anti-inflammatory cascade and cellular proliferation. Alongside diabetes mellitus, obesity-induced nonalcoholic fatty liver disease (NAFLD), steatosis, and cryptogenic cirrhosis may also lead to the development of HCC [23]. Majority of NAFLD induces HCC cases are observed in men, which may occur in the absence of cirrhosis. NAFLD-related tumors have an elevated level of des-γ-carboxy prothrombin (DCP) compared to α-fetoprotein (AFP) synthesis[elevated α-fetoprotein (AFP) synthesis is a hall mark for liver cancer] which is associated with HCV-related HCC [24, 25].

17.2.2 Other Factors

Sex may play a role in the development of HCC, which is found more often in males. Higher testosterone levels and intake of anabolic steroids have been linked to advanced hepatic fibrosis, hepatitis B carrier, and chronic hepatitis C infection compared to women [26]. Also, the higher amount of alcohol intake, cigarette smoking, and higher body mass index, makes the males more prone to viral hepatitis infection that increases the incidence of HCC [26].

Moreover, the food contaminated with certain mycotoxin, for example, aflatoxin B1 (AFB1) is also associated with the development of HCC. AFB1 is produced by Aspergillus species (molds) and is typically found ingrains, corn, peanuts, or soybeans stored in warm humid conditions. The duration and dose of AFB1 exposure is directly related to the risk of HCC [27]. Additionally, the synergistic effect of AFB1 on hepatitis B-and C-induced liver cancer tends to be more lethal compared with AFB1 exposure alone. So, the removal of AB1 exposure from environment may reduce the incidence of HCC occurrence [27].

Notwithstanding, some metabolic and genetic diseases like, Hemochromatosis, Wilson's disease, α-1 antitrypsin disease, tyrosinemia, glycogen-storage disease types I and II, and porphyrias are also associated with HCC. Thalassemia (iron overload) on the other hand has also been reported to have higher risk of HCV infection which eventually may contribute to the increased risk of primary liver cancer [28]. In addition, longer duration (>5 years) of exposure to oral contraceptives showed a significant increase in the risk of HCC [29].

17.3 Cellular Signaling Pathways Involved in Hepatocarcinogenesis

Being a complex process associated with genetic and epigenetic changes that are associated with initiation, development, and progression of hepatocarcinogenesis, liver cirrhosis is a predisposing condition for HCC. Emerging incidences of HCC have thrived the researchers with the hope to develop new therapeutic strategies by understanding the molecular, cellular and physiological mechanism of liver cancer. Activation of oncogenes and several other cellular events that regulates survival of cancerous cells by suppressing apoptosis and tumor suppressor genes have been well documented. Signal transduction pathways are being studied extensively to identify potential biomarkers and molecular targets of HCC. These pathways are briefly explained below:

17.3.1 Wnt/β-Catenin Pathway

First identified in *Drosophila melanogaster*, the Wnt signaling pathway is highly conserved and is deregulated in many cancers, including HCC. Wnt signaling participates in various evolutionary pathways that involve homeostasis, cell proliferation, differentiation, motility, and apoptosis [30]. The activation of Wnt pathway is generally observed after infection of HBV/HCV and liver cirrhosis leading to the development of HCC. In many cases, mutation of the proto-oncogeneβ-catenin or the inactivation of sliver-specific tumor suppressor gene adenomatous polyposis coli causes the activation of Wnt signaling [31].

Mutation in β-catenin promotes the up-regulation of frizzled-7 and dephosphorylation of β-catenin that prevent subsequent degradation. These mutations are related to the patients that were highly exposed to HCV infection and aflatoxin [32]. In addition, mutations in the negative regulators of Wnt pathway; Axin 1 and Axin 2 were also observed in HCC patients [33]. Therefore, targeted inactivation of Wnt/β-Catenin pathway could be a potential therapeutic target for HCC.

17.3.2 p53 Pathway

p53 is considered as 'guardian of the genome' which plays a critical role in cancer. In physiological conditions, p53 is expressed at low levels, which is up-regulated in response to intracellular and extracellular stress signals. In most of the human tumors, tumor suppressor TP53 gene is inactivated by a single point mutation that leads to subsequent defects in cell cycle arrest and apoptosis [34]. DNA-damaging agents and chemotherapeutic drugs activate p53 by phosphorylation of the transactivation domain and acetylation and phosphorylation of basic allosteric control region by ataxia telangiectasia mutated and related kinases [35].

p53 mutations and inactivation have been reported to play a critical role in HCC. In a clinical study of patients with HCC, a point mutation at the third base position of codon 249 has been found. The G → T and the G → C transversion were consistent with mutations caused by AFB1 in mutagenesis experiments. Moreover, in several other cancer cell lines, a mutational hotspot in codon 259 was also found [36]. The mutations in the codon 249 occur in HBsAg–seropositive carriers and the subsequent late events of these mutations are reflected as p53 DNA and protein mutation correlated to tumor stage [37]. Thus, the presence of mutated p53 in plasma of HCC patients serve as a biomarker for AFB1 exposure-related HCC.

Association of p53 mutations in hemochromatosis and Wilson disease is a notable effect of oxidative stress in liver carcinogenesis. G:C, T:A transversions at codon 249 as well as to C:T to A:T and C:G to T:A transversions at codon 250 alters the function of p53 gene [38]. Under oxidative stress, an elevated level of inducible nitric oxide synthase (iNOS) expression is observed which results in the development of cirrhosis and increased risk of HCC.

17.3.3 pRb Pathway

The tumor suppressor retinoblastoma protein (pRb1) controls cell cycle progression via repression of E2F transcription factor family of proteins and implement a major barrier to cancer development. pRb phosphorylation and G1/S cell cycle transition correlate the cyclin-dependent kinases (CDKs) phosphorylation [39]. Pediatric cancer retinoblastoma is caused by mutational inactivation of both *Rb1* alleles. Hereditary retinoblastoma has more tumor foci and early onset as it is produced by germline transmission of one mutational inactivated Rb1 allele and loss of the remaining wild-type allele in somatic retinal cells. In contrast, the occurrence of sporadic retinoblastoma requires inactivation of both *Rb1* alleles in somatic retinal cells, which delays their onset [40]. Previous studies on human tumor showed that DNA viruses, such as human papilloma viruses (HPV) results in parallel loss of pRb and lack of functional p53 [41].

Changes in the expression of CDK inhibitors such as $p16^{INK4A}$, $p21^{(WAF1/CIP1)}$, and $p27^{Kip1}$contributes to hepatocarcinogenesis. Inactivation of $p16^{INK4A}$ and reduced expression of $p21^{(WAF1/CIP1)}$, which is mainly associated with p53 gene mutation contributes to HCC [42]. The similarity in mechanism of disruption of pRb pathway was observed in various other cancers which suggests that pRb is an important target in cancer.

17.3.4 Ras Pathway

Small GTP-binding proteins known as human ras proteins (H-Ras, N-Ras, K-ras4A, and K-Ras4B) function as a molecular switch in various cellular physiological processes. Ras proteins interact with Raf-1(downstream serine/threonine kinase), that results in activation of MAPK kinases MEK1 and MEK2, to regulate cell growth, differentiation, proliferation, and apoptosis [43, 44]. Activation of Ras and expression of Ras pathway proteins such as p21 contributes to human HCC [45, 46]. Various chemicals such as N-nitrosomorpholine, bleomycin, 1-nitropyrene, and methyl (acetoxymethyl) nitrosamine causes single point mutation in codon 13 of H-ras, codon 12 of N-ras, and codon 61of K-ras that are commonly observed in HCC [47–53]. Members of the RASSF family of Ras inhibitors such as RASSF1A and NORE1A are inactivated in human HCC, which highlight the role of Ras pathway in liver cancer [54]. Suppression of Ras expression using antisense RNA and inhibition of kinases are successfully implemented in cell line and animal models of liver cancer [55, 56].

17.3.5 MAPK and JAK/STAT Pathway

The intracellular mitogen-activated protein kinase (MAPK) family consists of five subgroups; extracellular signal-regulated kinase protein homologs 1 and2 (ERK1/2), big MAPK-1 (BMK-1/ERK5), c-Jun N-terminal kinase homologs 1, 2, and 3 (JNK1/2/3), stress-activated protein kinase 2 (SAPK-2) homologs α, β, and δ (p38α/β/δ), and ERK6, also known as p38γ [57]. MAPKs executes diverse cellular functions ranging from cell proliferation to adhesion, and their activation depends upon phosphorylation of T and Y residues located in their activation loop [58, 59]. MAPK signaling pathway is being modulated at multiple steps by hepatitis proteins. Sprd protein (Sprouty-related protein with Ena/vasodilator-stimulated phosphoprotein homology-1 domain), an inhibitor of Ras/Raf-1/ERK pathway is highly deregulated in HCC, that results in enhanced secretion of matrix metalloproteinases 2 and 9 [60]. In human hepatoma Huh-7cells, HCV E2 protein assists in activation of MAPK pathway and promotes cell proliferation [61].

A family of transcription factors known as signal transducers and activators of transcription (STATs) has been reported to be ubiquitously activated in HCC. Activation of STATs has been mediated by a diverse range of cytokines, hormones, and growth factors, but primarily governed by tyrosine phosphorylation by Janus kinases (JAKs) [62, 63]. Activated STATs synthesize suppressor of cytokine signaling (SOCS) proteins, that are part of a negative feedback loop in JAK/STAT pathway. These proteins suppress over activation of cytokine-stimulated cells by binding with phosphorylated JAKs and their receptors, that attenuates cancer progression [63]. Deregulation of two other STAT inhibitors; SH2-containingproteins and inhibitor of activated STATs and inactivation of SSI-1, a JAK-binding protein has been reported in HCC [64]. Therefore, intervention in MAPKs and JAK/STAT signaling pathway could be a potential therapeutic target for treatment of HCC.

17.3.6 Others

The molecular dynamics of hepatocarcinogenesis can be influenced by various growth factors and other cellular pathways. For instance, several members of heat shock proteins (HSPs) family are key players in the occurrence of HCC. The decrease in serine phosphorylation HSP27 has been reported to be associated with the progression of HCC in clinical samples [65]. In addition, modulating the expression of inflammatory cytokines might play a critical role in monitoring HCC progression. For example, levels of Th2 cytokines are induced and Th1 cytokines decreased in liver metastases. Furthermore, vascular endothelial growth factor and fibroblast growth factor also play important roles in HCC development. The use of inhibitors against epidermal growth factor receptor and transforming growth factor β, helps to prevent the development of HCC in rat model [66, 67]. Induction of apoptosis by using RNA interference against anti-apoptotic myeloid cell leukemia-1 protein could be another target for HCC [68]. Alcohol metabolism, cellular transport, and ubiquitins are other additional physiological processes that regulate hepatocarcinogenesis [69].

17.4 Staging, Diagnosis, and Treatment of Liver Cancer

Early diagnosis for liver cancer plays a key role in determining the best treatment method for HCC. To circumvent such cases based on prognosis, patients diagnosed with HCC are categorized into groups. This stratification of patients (Staging system) can guide the clinicians in patient selection, choice of therapy, patient counseling and randomization for research protocols. Staging system helps to determine liver function, tumor stage and physical status of HCC patients [70]. There are two staging system in HCC i.e. clinical and pathological. Clinical staging includes Barcelona Clinic Liver Cancer Staging System (BCLC), Okuda Staging System, and Italian Program of the Liver Cancer score, on the other hand, American Joint Committee on Cancer, Japanese Integrated system, Liver Cancer Study Group of Japan, and Chinese University Prognostic Index are the pathological staging system. Among them, BCLC staging system is widely accepted for clinical trials and it outlines certain criteria to establish new drugs for HCC [71].

In HCC, cirrhotic livers exhibit increased hepatocyte proliferation that results in degenerative nodules. Ultrasonography (US) that detect nodules <1 cm are usually undefined and the patient must have a repeat US in 3–4 months. A radiologic investigation such as contrast-enhanced triple or quadriphasic multiphase computerized tomography (CT) scan for chest, abdomen and pelvis region or magnetic resonance imaging (MRI) must be conducted for patients who are diagnosed with nodules >1 cm [72]. MRI is a preferred diagnostic analyzer over CT scan for the evaluation of HCC due to its higher per-lesion sensitivity [73]. Moreover, US imaging sensitivity is variable which depends on the equipment and its operator. A bone scan is another vital tool to identify HCC staging and secondary diseases. Radiologic analysis helps to document certain tumor characteristics such as size, maximum diameter, and number of lesions, the location of tumors, vascular invasion, and extrahepatic disease [72]. If uncertainty persists in the diagnosis of HCC by radiologic test, a serum alpha(α)-fetoprotein (AFP) level >400 ng/mL can be used as an indicative prognostic value for HCC. The main function of AFP is to maintain the regulation of fatty acids in fetal and proliferating adult liver cells [74]. The main drawback of measuring serum AFP level is that it can be falsely raised in patients who have active hepatitis but no evidence of HCC. Moreover, elevated levels of AFP have been found in certain diseases such as acute hepatitis, cirrhosis, colitis, germ cell tumors, and intrahepatic cholangiocarcinoma [72, 74, 75].

In addition, another serum marker known as lens culinaris agglutinin-reactive fraction of α-fetoprotein (AFP-L3) expressed as a percentage of AFP has been found to be elevated in patients with HCC. AFP-L3 is associated with a more aggressive tumor, shorter doubling time, infiltrative growth pattern, vascular invasion, and intrahepatic metastasis [76]. Des-gamma-carboxy prothrombin (DCP) is another serum marker produced by malignant hepatocytes from an acquired posttranslational defect in vitamin K-dependent carboxylase system. DCP levels >125 mAU/mL is sensitive and specific for differentiating HCC from chronic hepatitis and cirrhosis [77]. The levels of DCP in blood serum are high in specificity but low at sensitivity [78].

The bitter truth of erroneous diagnosis for HCC that the patients have to pay a heavy price in the form of liver impairment and increased morbidity related to therapy. Unfortunately, there is no treatment available in present times that could improve the survival of patients diagnosed with the late stage of HCC. The best positive outcomes for treatments are achieved when patients are put on proper consistent surveillance for HCC at early stages and best treatment selection from various options. A multidisciplinary team of a hepatologist, a radiologist, a pathologist, a medical oncologist, an interventional radiologist, a transplant surgeon, and a hepatobiliary surgeon put their unique contributions to ensure optimal long-term outcomes for patients with HCC. Several treatment options available for treatment of HCC that can have a positive impact on survival are resection, liver transplantation (surgical approaches), transarterial chemoembolization, transarterial radiation, percutaneous local ablation, microwave ablation (nonsurgical approaches) and systemic therapy (sorafenib, an oral multitargeted tyrosine kinase inhibitor) [72, 79].

17.5 Molecular Diagnosis of Liver Cancer by Gene Expression Profile

More than decades ago, there has been a plethora of studies that documented about gene expression profiles in HCC (survival or recurrence) and other associated human liver diseases. The most promising way of molecular diagnosis in HCC and associated liver disease however is microarray-based gene profiling which usually is carried out by liver biopsy of normal and diseased liver that allows differentiating the gene responsible for HCC [80]. Patients with liver disease can avail the benefit of identification of therapeutic target by gene expression analysis.

17.5.1 Gene Expression Signature in Normal Liver

There are several gene variations that occur naturally because of the sophisticated gene expression patterns in human [81]. However, the liver is a multifunctional and metabolically active organ that encompasses a complex transcriptome profile second after to brain. Nearly, 25–40% of genes are expressed in this organ, whose function is still unknown [82]. Among them, few functional genes have been specifically characterized for liver cells or liver tissues. However, there are certain obstructions faced by clinicians and researchers during the comparative study between healthy and diseased human livers. Firstly, the complexity of transcriptomes can get double or even triple during disease which makes the situation less well understood [83]. Secondly, liver biopsy sample contained stellate cells, Kupffer cells, sinusoidal endothelial cells, blood cells, capillary material, cholangiocytes, and lymphocytes along with hepatocytes which make the liver samples heterogeneous [84]. Thirdly, there are chances of cell contamination during the microdissection of liver tumor specimens, which may partially deviate the expression signature [80, 85]. Fourthly, *in vitro* gene signature profiling can perturb which might influence the technique used to culture the cell [80, 85]. In normal liver tissue, ~50% of genes have been reported to be similarly expressed in DNA microarray study. Gene-Tag study which utilizes amplified fragment length polymorphism (AFLP)–based method of transcript imaging showed the presence and a >2.5-fold change inexpression level for at least one sample among four normal adult liver samples [86].

17.5.2 Gene Expression Signature in HCC

The BCLC staging system is based on tumor status, liver functional reserve, and health status and links staging with treatment strategy [87]. Patients at early, intermediate or terminal stages can survive up to 5 years, 14–20 months or 3 months respectively [88]. Gene expression profiling of HCC has classified the patients on the basis of stage of the disease, etiological agents, recurrence and survival that helps to deal with HCC patients [89–97].

Gene expression signature profiles for survival face certain limitations, as patients die from liver failure and tumor progression. Use of cancer-related death and selection of the cohort should be considered to minimize this limitation [96]. In a report, it was found that around 406 genes belonging to cell proliferation, apoptosis, ubiquitination, and histone modification were related to patient survival [97]. In another study, a 153-gene molecular signature relevant to metastatic HCC patients' survival was generated using a supervised machine-learning algorithm [91].

Several gene profiling studies have been employed to study the recurrence of HCC. Using high-density oligonucleotide microarrays, the 12-gene signature was identified for HCC recurrence in a study. Another PCR-based array study identified 20-gene expression signature on the platform of 3072 genes in HCC patients. On the other hand, metastases in the liver tumor can be predicted by pathological variables such as vascular invasion, poor histological differentiation, and satellites [94]. In patients with HCC, the expression of miR-26a and miR-26b was reduced that assist in activation of inflammatory signaling pathways (nuclear factor κB and interleukin-6). Patients with lower miR-26 also exhibit a better response to interferon therapy, but the overall survival rate is reported to be short [98]. Circulating tumor cells (CTCs) and circulating tumor microemboli (CTM) identification and counting helps to predict tumor stages, metastases and potential implications of therapeutic choices and clinical outcomes. However, a number of technical and methodologic drawbacks have limited the detection and interpretation of CTCs, due to their rare quantity (> 1/mL) [99]. This limitation can be circumvented by isolating the epithelial tumor cells (ISET) approach on the basis of their size. ISET is a simple and cheap technology that is broadly used in clinical oncology for cytopathological diagnosis of tumor cells and peripheral blood samples [100].

Many governing bodies have suggested a clear distinction between tissue biomarkers and serum biomarkers. However, between tissue and serum, serum biomarkers (AFP, DCP, and AFP-L3) tend to represent false positive results thus are not a confirmatory diagnosis of HCC. On the other hand, tissue markers seem to be reliable as they might differentiate the early HCC from those of the cirrhotic tissue, preneoplastic lesions and another type of neoplasms [101]. A number of research studies on the genomics of HCC have revealed heat shock protein 70 [102], glypican-3 [102], telomerase reverse transcriptase [93], serine/threonine kinase 15 [93], telomerase reverse transcriptase (TERT), topoisomerase 2A (TOP2A), and platelet-derived growth factor (PDGF) receptor alpha [103], and phospholipase A2 [93]as the principle markers for early HCC detection.

Antagonist-II (PIVKA-II) is another recent tumor growth protein marker that is brought by the deficiency of vitamin K. Patients who had no more than ten tumors, of at most 5 cm with PIVKA-II <400 mAU/mL have a 5-year survival rate of 68.5% [104–106]. Diagnosis of systemic inflammation including neutrophil-to-lymphocyte ratio (NLR) elevation is considered as a predictive marker of HCC recurrence [107]. A combination of elevated inflammatory serum marker C-reactive protein (CRP) >10 mg/L and lower albumin levels in HCC patients, represent an invasion of the vascular system, tumor growth, advanced stage and diminished recurrence-free rates of survival [108, 109].

Single-nucleotide polymorphism (SNP) array is a well appreciated and an evolving technology to study the genetic susceptibility to disease. SNP arrays provide a robust platform to define genome scale, somatic genetic changes in cancer. The use of 100K arrays helps in the completion of the large-scale analysis of various cancers [110]. Integrative genomic analysis approach (DNA microarray + SNP arrays) in molecular oncology research will help in identification of several novel oncogene and tumor suppressor genes that have not been previously participated in hepatocarcinogenesis [111].

17.6 Conclusion

The increasing trend of HCC has left a severe threat to the society, though; the recent advancements in the field of medicine have introduced some potential therapeutic approaches to combat the HCC. However, the poor diagnosis of HCC remains the major obstacle in the way of treatment strategies. The conventional diagnostic technique, for example, serum biomarkers have failed to predict the early stages of HCC resulting in poor treatment. Thus it is of the need to introduce some target specific HCC detection methods and molecular diagnosis seems to be the ideal methodology which not only could detect the early stage of HCC but may contribute to the development of targeted abolition of HCC.

References

1. Jemal A, et al. Global cancer statistics. CA Cancer J Clin. 2011;61:69–90.
2. Bosch FX, Ribes J, Díaz M, Cléries R. Primary liver cancer: worldwide incidence and trends. Gastroenterology. 2004;127(5 Suppl 1):S5–S16. Review.
3. Ferlay J, Soerjomataram I, Dikshit R, Eser S, Mathers C, Rebelo M, Parkin DM, Forman D, Bray F. Cancer incidence and mortality worldwide: sources, methods and major patterns in GLOBOCAN 2012. Int J Cancer. 2015;136(5):E359–86.
4. Yu J, Shen J, Sun TT, Zhang X, Wong N. Obesity, insulin resistance, NASH and hepatocellular carcinoma. Semin Cancer Biol. 2013;23:483–91.
5. Torre L, et al. Global cancer statistics, 2012. CA Cancer J Clin. 2015;65:87–108.
6. European Association for The Study of the Liver & European Organisation for Research and Treatment of Cancer. EASL–EORTC clinical practice guidelines: management of hepatocellular carcinoma. J Hepatol. 2012;56:908–43.
7. Liu J, Fan D. Hepatitis B in China. Lancet. 2007;369:1582–3.
8. Mohd Hanafiah K, Groeger J, Flaxman AD, Wiersma ST. Global epidemiology of hepatitis C virus infection: new estimates of age-specific antibody to HCV seroprevalence. Hepatology. 2013;57:1333–42.
9. Mohamoud YA, Mumtaz GR, Riome S, Miller D, Abu-Raddad LJ. The epidemiology of hepatitis C virus in Egypt: a systematic review and data synthesis. BMC Infect Dis. 2013;13:288.
10. El-Serag HB. Hepatocellular carcinoma. N Engl J Med. 2011;365:1118–27.
11. National Center for Health Statistics. Health, United States, 2014: with special feature on adults aged 55–64. Hyattsville: National Center for Health Statistics; 2015.
12. Omer RE, et al. Population-attributable risk of dietary aflatoxins and hepatitis B virus infection with respect to hepatocellular carcinoma. Nutr Cancer. 2004;48:15–21.
13. Laursen L. A preventable cancer. Nature. 2014;516:S2–3.
14. Bruix J, Sherman M. AASLD Practice Guidelines: management of hepatocellular carcinoma: an update. Hepatology. 2011;53(3):1020–2.
15. Ott JJ, Stevens GA, Groeger J, Wiersma ST. Global epidemiology of hepatitis B virus infection: new estimates of age-specific HBsAg seroprevalence and endemicity. Vaccine. 2012;30(12):2212–9.
16. Choo QL, Richman KH, Han JH, et al. Genetic organization and diversity of the hepatitis C virus. Proc Natl Acad Sci U S A. 1991;88(6):2451–5.
17. Asham EH, Kaseb A, Ghobrial RM. Management of hepatocellular carcinoma. Surg Clin North Am. 2013;93(6):1423–50.
18. Singal AK, Anand BS. Mechanisms of synergy between alcohol and hepatitis C virus. J Clin Gastroenterol. 2007;41(8):761–72.
19. Morgan RL, Baack B, Smith BD, Yartel A, Pitasi M, Falck-Ytter Y. Eradication of hepatitis C virus infection and the development of hepatocellular carcinoma: a meta-analysis of observational studies. Ann Intern Med. 2013;158(5):329–37.
20. Hassan MM, Hwang LY, Hatten CJ, et al. Risk factors for hepatocellular carcinoma: synergism of alcohol with viral hepatitis and diabetes mellitus. Hepatology. 2002;36(5):1206–13.
21. Gao C, Fang L, Zhao HC, Li JT, Yao SK. Potential role of diabetes mellitus in the progression of cirrhosis to hepatocellular carcinoma: a crosssectional case-control study from Chinese patients with HBV infection. Hepatobiliary Pancreat Dis Int. 2013;12(4):385–93.
22. Wang C, Wang X, Gong G, et al. Increased risk of hepatocellular carcinoma in patients with diabetes mellitus: a systematic review and meta-analysis of cohort studies. Int J Cancer. 2012;130(7):1639–48.
23. Reddy JK, Rao MS. Lipid metabolism and liver inflammation. Am J Physiol Gastrointest Liver Physiol. 2006;290:G852–8.
24. Wakai T, Shirai Y, Sakata J, Korita PV, Ajioka Y, Hatakeyama K. Surgical outcomes for hepatocellular carcinoma in nonalcoholic fatty liver disease. J Gastrointest Surg. 2011;15(8):1450–8.
25. Tokushige K, Hashimoto E, Yatsuji S, et al. Prospective study of hepatocellular carcinoma in nonalcoholic steatohepatitis in comparison with

hepatocellular carcinoma caused by chronic hepatitis C. J Gastroenterol. 2010;45(9):960–7.
26. White DL, Tavakoli-Tabasi S, Kuzniarek J, Pascua R, Ramsey DJ, El-Serag HB. Higher serum testosterone is associated with increased risk of advanced hepatitis C-related liver disease in males. Hepatology. 2012;55(3):759–68.
27. Chen JG, Egner PA, Ng D, et al. Reduced aflatoxin exposure presages decline in liver cancer mortality in an endemic region of China. Cancer Prev Res. 2013;6(10):1038–45.
28. Deugnier Y, Turlin B. Iron and hepatocellular carcinoma. J Gastroenterol Hepatol. 2001;16(5):491–4.
29. Gandini S, Botteri E, Iodice S, Boniol M, Lowenfels AR, Maisonneuve P. Tobacco smoking and cancer: a meta-analysis. Int J Cancer. 2008;122:155–64.
30. Nelson WJ, Nusse R. Convergence of Wnt, β-catenin, and cadherin pathways. Science. 2004;303:1483–7.
31. Herbst A, Kolligs FT. Wnt signaling as a therapeutic target for cancer. Methods Mol Biol. 2007;361:63–91.
32. Merle P, Kim M, Herrmann M, Gupte A, Lefrançois L, Califano S, et al. Oncogenic role of the frizzled-7/beta-catenin pathway in hepatocellular carcinoma. J Hepatol. 2005;43:854–62.
33. Taniguchi K, Roberts LR, Aderca IN, Dong X, Qian C, Murphy LM, et al. Mutational spectrum of beta-catenin, AXIN1, and AXIN2 in hepatocellular carcinomas and hepatoblastomas. Oncogene. 2002;21:4863–71.
34. Giaccia AJ, Kastan MB. The complexity of p53 modulation: emerging patterns from divergent signals. Genes Dev. 1998;12:2973–83.
35. Hsu IC, Metcalf RA, Sun T, Welsh JA, Wang NJ, Harris CC. Mutational hotspot in the p53 gene in human hepatocellular carcinomas. Nature. 1991;350:427–8.
36. Hsu I, Tokiwa T, Bennett W, Metcalf RA, Welsh JA, Sun T, et al. p53 gene mutation and integrated hepatitis B viral DNA sequences in human liver cancer cell lines. Carcinogenesis. 1993;14:987–92.
37. Hussain SP, Raja K, Amstad PA, Sawyer M, Trudel LJ, Wogan GN, et al. Increased p53 mutation load in nontumorous human liver of Wilson disease and hemochromatosis: oxyradical overload diseases. Proc Natl Acad Sci U S A. 2000;97:12770–5.
38. Goodrich DW. The retinoblastoma tumor-suppressor gene, the exception that proves the rule. Oncogene. 2006;25:5233–43.
39. Malumbres M, Barbacid M. To cycle or not to cycle: a critical decision in cancer. Nat Rev Cancer. 2001;1:222–31.
40. Weinberg RA. The retinoblastoma protein and cell cycle control. Cell. 1995;81:323–30.
41. Hsia CC, Di Bisceglie AM, Kleiner DE Jr, Farshid M, Tabor E. RB tumor suppressor gene expression in hepatocellular carcinomas from patients infected with the hepatitis B virus. J Med Virol. 1994;44:67–73.
42. Azechi H, Nishida N, Fukuda Y, Nishimura T, Minata M, Katsuma H, et al. Disruption of the p16/cyclin D1/retinoblastoma protein pathway in the majority of human hepatocellular carcinomas. Oncology. 2001;60:346–54.
43. Clark G, Quilliam LA, Hisaka MM, Der CJ. Differential antagonism of Ras biological activity by catalytic and Src homology domains of Ras GTPase activation protein. Proc Natl Acad Sci U S A. 1993;90:4887–97.
44. Jagirdar J, Nonomura A, Patil J, Thor A, Paronetto F. ras oncogene p21 expression in hepatocellular carcinoma. J Exp Pathol. 1989;4:37–46.
45. Nonomura A, Ohta G, Hayashi M, Izumi R, Watanabe K, Takayanagi N, et al. Immunohistochemical detection of ras oncogene p21 product in HEPATOLOGY, Vol. 48, No. 6, 2008 liver cirrhosis and hepatocellular carcinoma. Am J Gastroenterol. 1987;82:512–8.
46. Calvisi D, Ladu S, Gorden A, Farina M, Conner EA, Lee JS, et al. Ubiquitous activation of Ras and Jak/Stat pathways in human HCC. Gastroenterology. 2006;130:1117–28.
47. Challen C, Guo K, Collier JD, Cavanagh D, Bassendine MF. Infrequent point mutations in codons 12 and 61 of ras oncogenes in human hepatocellular carcinomas. J Hepatol. 1992;14:342–6.
48. Cerutti P, Hussain P, Pourzand C, Aguilar F. Mutagenesis of the H-ras protooncogene and the p53 tumor suppressor gene. Cancer Res. 1994;54:1934s–8s.
49. Baba M, Yamamoto R, Iishi H, Tatsuta M. Ha-ras mutations in N-nitrosomorpholine-induced lesions and inhibition of hepatocarcinogenesis by antisense sequences in rat liver. Int J Cancer. 1997;72:815–20.
50. Bai F, Nakanishi Y, Takayama K, Pei XH, Inoue K, Harada T, et al. Codon 64 of K-ras gene mutation pattern in hepatocellular carcinomas induced by bleomycin and 1-nitropyrene in A/J mice. Teratog Carcinog Mutagen. 2003:161–70.
51. Li H, Lee GH, Liu J, Nomura K, Ohtake K, Kitagawa T. Low frequency of ras activation in 2-acetylaminofluorene and 3'-methyl-4-(dimethylamino)azobenzene-induced rat hepatocellular carcinomas. Cancer Lett. 1991;56:17–24.
52. Watatani M, Perantoni AO, Reed CD, Enomoto T, Wenk ML, Rice JM. Infrequent activation of K-ras, H-ras, and other oncogenes in hepatocellular neoplasms initiated by methyl (acetoxymethyl) nitrosamine, a methylating agent, and promoted by phenobarbital in F344 rats. Cancer Res. 1989;79:1103–9.
53. Morrison DK, Cutler RE. The complexity of Raf-1 regulation. Curr Opin Cell Biol. 1997;9:174–9.
54. Liao Y, Tang ZY, Liu KD, Ye SL, Huang Z. Apoptosis of human BEL-7402 hepatocellular carcinoma cells released by antisense H-ras DNA—in vitro and in vivo studies. J Cancer Res Clin Oncol. 1997;123:25–33.

55. Liao Y, Tang ZY, Ye SL, Liu KD, Sun FX, Huang Z. Modulation of apoptosis, tumorigenesity and metastatic potential with antisense H-ras oligodeoxynucleotides in a high metastatic tumor model of hepatoma: LCI-D20. Hepatogastroenterology. 2000;47:365–70.
56. Grisham JW. Interspecies comparison of liver carcinogenesis: implications for cancer risk assessment. Carcinogenesis. 1997;18:59–81.
57. Yoon S, Seger R. The extracellular signal-regulated kinase: multiple substrates regulate diverse cellular functions. Growth Factors. 2006;24:21–44.
58. Wong CH, Cheng CY. Mitogen-activated protein kinases, adherens junction dynamics, and spermatogenesis: a review of recent data. Dev Biol. 2005;286:1–15.
59. Panteva M, Korkaya H, Jameel S. Hepatitis viruses and the MAPK pathway: is this a survival strategy? Virus Res. 2003;92:131–40.
60. Satoh T, Kaziro Y. Ras in signal transduction. Semin Cancer Biol. 1992;3:169–77.
61. Yoshida T, Hisamoto T, Akiba J, Koga H, Nakamura K, Tokunaga Y, et al. Spreds, inhibitors of the Ras/ERK signal transduction, are dysregulated in human hepatocellular carcinoma and linked to the malignant phenotype of tumors. Oncogene. 2006;25:6056–66.
62. Yoshikawa H, Matsubara K, Qian GS, Jackson P, Groopman JD, Manning JE, et al. SOCS-1, a negative regulator of the JAK/STAT pathway, is silenced by methylation in human hepatocellular carcinoma and shows growth-suppression activity. Nat Genet. 2001;28:29–35.
63. Wormald S, Hilton DJ. Inhibitors of cytokine signal transduction. J Biol Chem. 2004;279:821–4.
64. Nagai H, Kim YS, Konishi N, Baba M, Kubota T, Yoshimura A, et al. Combined hypermethylation and chromosome loss associated with inactivation of SSI-1/SOCS-1/JAB gene in human hepatocellular carcinomas. Cancer Lett. 2002;186:59–65.
65. Luk JM, Lam CT, Siu AF, Lam BY, Ng IO, Hu MY, et al. Proteomic profiling of hepatocellular carcinoma in Chinese cohort reveals heat-shock proteins (Hsp27, Hsp70, GRP78) up-regulation and their associated prognostic values. Proteomics. 2006;6:1049–57.
66. Breitkopf K, Haas S, Wiercinska E, Singer MV, Dooley S. Anti-TGF-beta strategies for the treatment of chronic liver disease. Alcohol Clin Exp Res. 2005;29:121S–31S.
67. Schulze-Bergkamen H, Fleischer B, Schuchmann M, Weber A, Weinmann A, Krammer PH, et al. Suppression of Mcl-1 via RNA interference sensitizes human hepatocellular carcinoma cells towards apoptosis induction. BMC Cancer. 2006;6:232.
68. Raghunand N, Gatenby RA, Gillies RJ. Microenvironmental and cellular consequences of altered blood flow in tumours. Br J Radiol. 2003;76:S11–22.
69. Aravalli RN, Steer CJ, Cressman EN. Molecular mechanisms of hepatocellular carcinoma. Hepatology. 2008;48(6):2047–63.
70. Nathan H, Pawlik TM. Staging of hepatocellular carcinoma. In: Masters KM, Vauthey J-N, editors. Hepatocellular carcinoma. Berlin: Springer. p. 69–80.
71. Bruix J, Sherman M, American Association for the Study of Liver Diseases. AASLD Practice Guideline: management of hepatocellular carcinoma: an update. Hepatology. 2011;53(2):1020–2.
72. Balogh J, Victor D 3rd, Asham EH, Burroughs SG, Boktour M, Saharia A, Li X, Ghobrial RM, Monsour HP Jr. Hepatocellular carcinoma: a review. J Hepatocell Carcinoma. 2016;3:41–53. eCollection 2016. Review.
73. Sangiovanni A, Manini MA, Iavarone M, et al. The diagnostic and economic impact of contrast imaging techniques in the diagnosis of small hepatocellular carcinoma in cirrhosis. Gut. 2010;59:638–44.
74. Di Bisceglie AM, Sterling RK, Chung RT, et al. Serum α-fetoprotein levels in patients with advanced hepatitis C: results from the HALT-C Trial. J Hepatol. 2005;43(3):434–41.
75. Masuzaki R, Omata M. Screening program in high-risk populations. In: Hepatocellular carcinoma. 2011. p. 55–68.
76. Khien VV, Mao HV, Chinh TT, et al. Clinical evaluation of lentil lectin-reactive alpha-fetoprotein-L3 in histology-proven hepatocellular carcinoma. Int J Biol Markers. 2001;16(2):105–11.
77. Marrero JA, Su GL, Wei W, et al. Des-γ carboxyprothrombin can differentiate hepatocellular carcinoma from nonmalignant chronic liver disease in American patients. Hepatology. 2003;37(5):1114–21.
78. Ishii M, Gama H, Chida N, et al. Simultaneous measurements of serumα-fetoprotein and protein induced by vitamin K absence for detecting hepatocellular carcinoma. South Tohoku District Study Group. Am J Gastroenterol. 2000;95(4):1036–40.
79. Forner RM, Rodriguez de Lope C, Bruix J. Current strategy for staging and treatment: the BCLC update and future prospects. Semin Liver Dis. 2010;30:61–74.
80. Lemmer ER, Friedman SL, Llovet JM. Molecular diagnosis of chronic liver disease and hepatocellular carcinoma: the potential of gene expression profiling. Semin Liver Dis. 2006;26(4):373–84. Review.
81. Morley M, Molony CM, Weber TM, et al. Genetic analysis of genome-wide variation in human gene expression. Nature. 2004;430:743–7.
82. Shackel NA, Gorrell MD, McCaughan GW. Gene array analysis and the liver. Hepatology. 2002;36:1313–25.
83. Velculescu VE, Madden SL, Zhang L, et al. Analysis of human transcriptomes. Nat Genet. 1999;23:387–8.
84. Kmiec Z. Cooperation of liver cells in health and disease. Adv Anat Embryol Cell Biol. 2001;161:III–XIII, 1–151.
85. Soukas A, Socci ND, Saatkamp BD, Novelli S, Friedman JM. Distinct transcriptional profiles of adipogenesis in vivo and in vitro. J Biol Chem. 2001;276:34167–74.

86. Wong LY, Hafeman A, Boyd VL, et al. Assessing gene expression variation in normal human tissues using GeneTag, a novel, global, sensitive profiling method. J Biotechnol. 2003;101:199–217.
87. Llovet JM, Bru C, Bruix J. Prognosis of hepatocellular carcinoma: the BCLC staging classification. Semin Liver Dis. 1999;19:329–38.
88. Llovet JM, Burroughs A, Bruix J. Hepatocellular carcinoma. Lancet. 2003;362:1907–17.
89. Okabe H, Satoh S, Kato T, et al. Genome-wide analysis of gene expression in human hepatocellular carcinomas using cDNA microarray: identification of genes involved in viral carcinogenesis and tumor progression. Cancer Res. 2001;61:2129–37.
90. Iizuka N, Oka M, Yamada-Okabe H, et al. Comparison of gene expression profiles between hepatitis B virus- and hepatitis C virus-infected hepatocellular carcinoma by oligonucleotide microarray data on the basis of a supervised learning method. Cancer Res. 2002;62:3939–44.
91. Ye QH, Qin LX, Forgues M, et al. Predicting hepatitis B virus-positive metastatic hepatocellular carcinomas using gene expression profiling and supervised machine learning. Nat Med. 2003;9:416–23.
92. Nam SW, Park JY, Ramasamy A, et al. Molecular changes from dysplastic nodule to hepatocellular carcinoma through gene expression profiling. Hepatology. 2005;42:809–18.
93. Smith MW, Yue ZN, Geiss GK, et al. Identification of novel tumor markers in hepatitis C virus-associated hepatocellular carcinoma. Cancer Res. 2003;63:859–64.
94. Iizuka N, Oka M, Yamada-Okabe H, et al. Oligonucleotide microarray for prediction of early intrahepatic recurrence of hepatocellular carcinoma after curative resection. Lancet. 2003;361:923–9.
95. Kurokawa Y, Matoba R, Takemasa I, et al. Molecular-based prediction of early recurrence in hepatocellular carcinoma. J Hepatol. 2004;41:284–91.
96. Lee JS, Chu IS, Heo J, et al. Classification and prediction of survival in hepatocellular carcinoma by gene expression profiling. Hepatology. 2004;40:667–76.
97. Lee JS, Heo J, Libbrecht L, et al. A novel prognostic subtype of human hepatocellular carcinoma derived from hepatic progenitor cells. Nat Med. 2006;12:410–6.
98. Ji J, Shi J, Budhu A, Yu Z, Forgues M, Roessler S, Ambs S, Chen Y, Meltzer PS, Croce CM, Qin LX, Man K, Lo CM, Lee J, Ng IO, Fan J, Tang ZY, Sun HC, Wang XW. MicroRNA expression, survival, and response to interferon in liver cancer. N Engl J Med. 2009;361(15):1437–47.
99. Vona G, Estepa L, Béroud C, Damotte D, Capron F, Nalpas B, Mineur A, Franco D, Lacour B, Pol S, Bréchot C, Paterlini-Bréchot P. Impact of cytomorphological detection of circulating tumor cells in patients with liver cancer. Hepatology. 2004;39(3):792–7.
100. Vona G, Sabile A, Louha M, Sitruk V, Romana S, Schütze K, Capron F, et al. Isolation by size of epithelial tumor cells: a new method for the immunomorphological and molecular characterization of circulating tumor cells. Am J Pathol. 2000;156:57–63.
101. Marrero JA, Lok AS. Newer markers for hepatocellular carcinoma. Gastroenterology. 2004; 127(Suppl 1):S113–9.
102. Chuma M, Sakamoto M, Yamazaki K, et al. Expression profiling in multistage hepatocarcinogenesis: identification of HSP70 as a molecular marker of early hepatocellular carcinoma. Hepatology. 2003;37:198–207.
103. Paradis V, Bieche I, Dargere D, et al. Molecular profiling of hepatocellular carcinomas (HCC) using a large-scale real time RT-PCR approach: determination of a molecular diagnostic index. Am J Pathol. 2003;163:733–41.
104. Proceedings of the fifth annual meeting of the Japanese Committee for the International Diagnostic Criteria in Psychiatry (JCIDCP). November 2, 1985, Kyoto. Abstracts. Jpn J Psychiatry Neurol. 1986;40:701–11. [PMID: 3599569].
105. Ito T, Takada Y, Ueda M, Haga H, Maetani Y, Oike F, Ogawa K, Sakamoto S, Ogura Y, Egawa H, Tanaka K, Uemoto S. Expansion of selection criteria for patients with hepatocellular carcinoma in living donor liver transplantation. Liver Transpl. 2007;13:1637–44. https://doi.org/10.1002/lt.21281. [PMID: 18044766].
106. Waller LP, Deshpande V, Pyrsopoulos N. Hepatocellular carcinoma: a comprehensive review. World J Hepatol. 2015;7(26):2648–63. https://doi.org/10.4254/wjh.v7.i26.2648. Review.
107. Yoshizumi T, Ikegami T, Yoshiya S, Motomura T, Mano Y, Muto J, Ikeda T, Soejima Y, Shirabe K, Maehara Y. Impact of tumor size, number of tumors and neutrophil-to-lymphocyte ratio in liver transplantation for recurrent hepatocellular carcinoma. Hepatol Res. 2013;43:709–16. https://doi.org/10.1111/hepr.12016. [PMID: 23190306].
108. Zheng LY, Yang LL, Li LR, Jing HR, Wang J, Wang QF, Wang Q. [Expressions of TNF-alpha, IL-6, CRP, and MCP-1 in phlegm-damp constitution population detected by multiplexed Luminex assay]. Zhongguo Zhongxiyi Jiehe Zazhi. 2013;33:920–3. [PMID:24063213].
109. Pinato DJ, Karamanakos G, Arizumi T, Adjogatse D, Kim YW, Stebbing J, Kudo M, Jang JW, Sharma R. Dynamic changes of the inflammation-based index predict mortality following chemoembolisation for hepatocellular carcinoma: a prospective study. Aliment Pharmacol Ther. 2014;40:1270–81. https://doi.org/10.1111/apt.12992. [PMID: 25327965].
110. Garraway LA, Widlund HR, Rubin MA, et al. Integrative genomic analyses identify MITF as a line age survival oncogene amplified in malignant melanoma. Nature. 2005;436:117–22.
111. Sachidanandam R, Weissman D, Schmidt SC, et al. A map of human genome sequence variation containing 1.42 million single nucleotide polymorphisms. Nature. 2001;409:928–33.

Molecular Diagnosis of Uterine Cancer

18

Rajani Rai, Iram Fatima, Katie Essel, and Vishal Chandra

18.1 Introduction

Cancer of the body of the uterus, also known as corpus uteri cancer, is the sixth most common cancer among women worldwide. In the developed world, uterine cancer is most common gynecologic malignancy in women with approximately 60,000 new cases per year accounting for 11,000 deaths per year in the United States. The disease frequently occurs in women's after menopause (>50 years) [1].

Risk factors include obesity, prolonged exposure to estrogen, an imbalance of estrogen due to early menarche (<12 year), late menopause, hormone replacement therapy (HRT) and infertility. Treatment for uterine cancer includes surgery, chemotherapy, and radiation and is guided by histology, grade, and stage as well as age, the presence of lymphovascular space invasion, and depth of invasion [2]. Uterine cancer is comprised of two subsets: endometrial adenocarcinoma and uterine sarcoma. *Endometrial cancer* arises from the endometrial lining of the uterus comprises over 95% of cases of uterine cancer. Uterine sarcomas arise from mesenchymal elements including the endometrial stroma and the uterine muscle; sarcomas are more aggressive and are associated with a poorer prognosis. Due to its increased prevalence, detailed information regarding molecular pathology is only available for endometrial cancer (Table 18.1).

R. Rai · K. Essel
Department of Obstetrics and Gynecology, University of Oklahoma Health Sciences Center, Oklahoma City, OK, USA
e-mail: Rajani-rai@ouhsc.edu; Kathleen-Essel@ouhsc.edu

I. Fatima
Department of Medicine, College of Medicine at UTHSC, UTHSC Center for Cancer Research, Memphis, TN, USA
e-mail: iram.fatima@unmc.edu

V. Chandra (✉)
Department of Obstetrics and Gynecology, University of Oklahoma Health Sciences Center, Oklahoma City, OK, USA
e-mail: Vishal-chandra@ouhsc.edu

18.2 Molecular Pathology of Endometrial Carcinoma and Its Pre-malignant Lesions

In 1983, Bokhman described a dualistic model of endometrial carcinoma based on the clinical and clinicopathologic correlations [3]. Type I endometrioid adenocarcinomas comprise approximately 80% of new cases of endometrial cancer, are low-grade and are associated with obesity, hormone-receptor positivity, and favorable prognosis when compared with type II endometrial cancer [4–6]. These have a hyperplastic back-

K. K. Shukla et al. (eds.), *Molecular Diagnostics in Cancer Patients*,
https://doi.org/10.1007/978-981-13-5877-7_18

Table 18.1 Risk factors for endometrial cancers

Risk factor	Relative risk
Atypical hyperplasia	29
Unopposed estrogen therapy	10–20
Tamoxifen	2.5–7
Estrogen-producing tumors	>5
Obesity	2–5
Polycystic ovary syndrome	4
Early Menarche	2.4
Increased parity	3
Nulliparity/infertility	2–3
Diabetes mellitus	2–3
Menstrual factors	1.5–3
Weight > 175 lb	2
Oral contraceptive pills	1

Francesmary Modugno, Roberta B. Ness, Chu Chen and Noel S. Weiss. Inflammation and Endometrial Cancer: A Hypothesis. Cancer Epidemiol Biomarkers Prev 2005;14(12). DOI: 10.1158/1055-9965. http://cebp.aacrjournals.org/content/14/12/2840
HYPERLINK "https://www.ncbi.nlm.nih.gov/pubmed/?term=Raglan%20O%5BAuthor%5D&cauthor=true&cauthor_uid=30387875" Raglan O, HYPERLINK "https://www.ncbi.nlm.nih.gov/pubmed/?term=Kalliala%20I%5BAuthor%5D&cauthor=true&cauthor_uid=30387875" Kalliala I, HYPERLINK "https://www.ncbi.nlm.nih.gov/pubmed/?term=Markozannes%20G%5BAuthor%5D&cauthor=true&cauthor_uid=30387875" Markozannes G, HYPERLINK "https://www.ncbi.nlm.nih.gov/pubmed/?term=Cividini%20S%5BAuthor%5D&cauthor=true&cauthor_uid=30387875" Cividini S, HYPERLINK "https://www.ncbi.nlm.nih.gov/pubmed/?term=Gunter%20MJ%5BAuthor%5D&cauthor=true&cauthor_uid=30387875" Gunter MJ, HYPERLINK "https://www.ncbi.nlm.nih.gov/pubmed/?term=Nautiyal%20J%5BAuthor%5D&cauthor=true&cauthor_uid=30387875" Nautiyal J, HYPERLINK "https://www.ncbi.nlm.nih.gov/pubmed/?term=Gabra%20H%5BAuthor%5D&cauthor=true&cauthor_uid=30387875" Gabra H, HYPERLINK "https://www.ncbi.nlm.nih.gov/pubmed/?term=Paraskevaidis%20E%5BAuthor%5D&cauthor=true&cauthor_uid=30387875" Paraskevaidis E, HYPERLINK "https://www.ncbi.nlm.nih.gov/pubmed/?term=Martin-Hirsch%20P%5BAuthor%5D&cauthor=true&cauthor_uid=30387875" Martin-Hirsch P, HYPERLINK "https://www.ncbi.nlm.nih.gov/pubmed/?term=Tsilidis%20KK%5BAuthor%5D&cauthor=true&cauthor_uid=30387875" Tsilidis KK, HYPERLINK "https://www.ncbi.nlm.nih.gov/pubmed/?term=Kyrgiou%20M%5BAuthor%5D&cauthor=true&cauthor_uid=30387875" Kyrgiou M. Risk Factors for Endometrial Cancer: An umbrella review of the literature. HYPERLINK "https://www.ncbi.nlm.nih.gov/pubmed/30387875" \o "International journal of cancer." Int J Cancer. 2018 Nov 2. doi: 10.1002/ijc.31961. PMID: 30387875. https://www.ncbi.nlm.nih.gov/pubmed/30387875

ground and show a strong association with high estrogen levels. Type I endometrial precancers are characterized *endometrial intraepithelial neoplasia*, reflecting their clonal origin, noninvasive growth, and risk of concurrent or incipient carcinoma. On the other hand, type II endometrial cancers encompass the remaining 10–20% of sporadic disease and include grade 3 endometrioid adenocarcinoma as well as serous, clear-cell, mucinous, and undifferentiated carcinoma [7]. They are more common in older, nonobese women and have worse outcome [4, 5]. *Type II endometrial cancer, endometrial* serous *carcinoma (ESC), typically arises* in a *background of atrophic or resting endometrium* and *usually* does not show a strong relation to high estrogen levels. Serous intraepithelial carcinoma (EIC) represents pre-invasive precursors for type II endometrial serous cancer. Endometrial glandular dysplasia (EmGD) is a recently described lesion with p53 alteration, BRCA mutations, overexpression of IMP-3, Nrf2 and a histology that is intermediate between normal and serous EIC [8].

Molecular genetic alterations have been extensively investigated in type I (endometrioid) and type II adenocarcinomas of the endometrium; their tumorigenesis follow separate pathways [9–11]. Type I endometrial cancers are associated with microsatellite instability (MSI), mutations of Phosphatase and Tensin Homolog (PTEN, a tumor suppressor gene), *K-ras (an oncogene)*, *β-catenin (CTNNB1)*, *phosphatidylinositol-4, 5-bisphosphate 3-kinase catalytic subunit alpha* (*PIK3CA*) and *phosphatidylinositol 3-kinase* (*PIK3*) genes. Furthermore, comparison of type and extent of genomic alterations between endometrioid type I endometrial cancer and EIN designates a greater accumulative mutational burden in the later, a feature considered one milestone in the definition of precancer [12]. The key molecular alterations in Type II cancers are P53 modifications and loss of heterozygosity (LOH), as well as abnormal function of p16, E-cadherin, and c-erb-B2 [13–15]. These molecular alterations

Table 18.2 Typical features of type I and type II endometrial cancers

	Type I	Type II
Percentage	70–80%	10–20%
Age	Pre- and peri-menopausal	Postmenopausal
Unopposed estrogen	Present	Absent
Other risk factor (obesity, diabetes, hyperlipidemia, hypertension)	Yes	No
Hyperplasia-precursor	Present	Absent
Hormone receptor	ER+, PR+	ER−, PR−
Tumor grade	Low	High
Histology	Well differentiated endometrioid adenocarcinoma	Poorly differentiated Serous or clear cell
Recurrence/Myometrial invasion	Local/minimal	Abdominal, lymphatic/deep
Stage at diagnosis	I or II	III or IV
Disease course/prognosis	Slow and stable/favorable	Aggressive/unfavorable
Molecular alterations	PTEN (%), MSI, MLH1, MSH6, K-ras, β-catenin, PIK3CA	HER2/neu, p53, LOH, Rb, p16, E-cadherine
5 year survival rate	85%	43%

HYPERLINK "https://www.ncbi.nlm.nih.gov/pubmed/?term=Binder%20PS%5BAuthor%5D&cauthor=true&cauthor_uid=24956294" Binder PS, HYPERLINK "https://www.ncbi.nlm.nih.gov/pubmed/?term=Mutch%20DG%5BAuthor%5D&cauthor=true&cauthor_uid=24956294" Mutch DG. Update on prognostic markers for endometrial cancer. HYPERLINK "https://www.ncbi.nlm.nih.gov/pubmed/24956294" \o "Women's health (London, England)." Womens Health (Lond). 2014 May;10(3):277-88. doi: 10.2217/whe.14.13. PMID: 24956294. https://www.ncbi.nlm.nih.gov/pubmed/24956294

Fatima, Iram. (2015). Recent Advances in Molecularly Targeted Therapies for Endometrial Cancer and their Future Clinical Implications. https://www.researchgate.net/publication/289882074_Recent_Advances_in_Molecularly_Targeted_Therapies_for_Endometrial_Cancer_and_their_Future_Clinical_Implications

are under investigation for the use of targeted therapy in clinical trials and one day may guide treatment for endometrial cancer regardless histopathologic subtype (Table 18.2).

18.3 Histopathology

Histopathological assessment of tumor grade and cell type is essential to the management of endometrial cancer, guiding the extent of surgery, and the use of radiation and chemotherapy. While definitions exist to guide the determination of tumor grade and cell type, there are significant challenges in the interpretation of the histopathology.

The grade of endometrioid adenocarcinoma is a critical prognostic factor in guiding the extent of surgery and subsequent treatment of early stage type I endometrial cancer. Under the 1988 International Federation of Gynecology and Obstetrics (FIGO) grading system, tumors are graded based on the percentage of solid non-squamous growth: grade 1, ≤5% solid growth; grade 2, 6–50% solid growth; grade 3, >50% solid growth. It is often difficult to distinguish between solid growth and areas of immature squamous metaplasia or compressed confluent glands. Additionally, quantification of the percentage of solid growth is somewhat arbitrary in cases that are near the diagnostic cut-points between grades. This results in significant interobserver variability in the grade assignment.

Assessment of cell type is critical in endometrial carcinoma. Early stage type I endometrioid tumors are often treated with adjuvant radiation, whereas similarly staged type II tumors are treated with adjuvant chemotherapy. Overall, there is moderate to excellent reproducibility of cell type diagnosis amongst endometrial carcinomas. The World Health Organization (WHO) defines endometrioid adenocarcinoma as a primary endometrial adenocarcinoma containing glands resembling those of normal endometrium, commonly amongst a background of atypical hyperplasia. Serous carcinoma exhibits a complex pattern of papillae with cellular budding, occasionally containing psammoma bodies, amongst an atrophic background. Clear cell adenocarcinoma consists of clear or hobnail cells arranged in solid tubulocystic or papillary patterns. Undifferentiated carcinomas lack any evidence of differentiation. Mixed tumors are regularly encountered.

Nevertheless, high-grade serous and endometrioid endometrial carcinomas can be difficult to subtype correctly, and intra-observer concordance among specialty pathologists is low. Some endometrioid carcinomas exhibit papillary growth or slit-like glandular spaces, while serous carcinomas can exhibit a predominantly or exclusively glandular architecture or areas of solid growth. Another controversy exists in the diagnosis of undifferentiated carcinoma versus grade 3 endometrioid adenocarcinoma or solid growth of serous carcinoma. The tumor cells of undifferentiated carcinoma are relatively uniform in size and can have a rhabdoid appearance, leading to a misinterpretation of carcinosarcoma. Another problem exists between the diagnosis of serous and clear cell carcinoma as there is morphological overlap between serous and clear cell carcinoma. Some studies reveal up to one-third of serous cancers have areas of clear cytoplasm.

18.4 Integrated Genomic Characterization by the TCGA Network and Endometrial Cancer Classification

The Cancer Genome Atlas (TCGA) network performed an integrated genomic, transcriptomic, and proteomic characterization of 373 patients with endometrial cancer (307 endometrioid and 66 serous) and they subsequently reclassified endometrial carcinomas into four categories based on MSI status, copy number clusters, and nucleotide substitution frequencies and patterns. Cluster 1 (POLE), the ultra-mutated group, consisted of tumors with very high mutation rates; this group had mutations in the exonuclease domain of POLE (catalytic subunit of DNA polymerase epsilon involved in DNA replication and repair). Cluster 2 consisted of hypermutated tumors with increased MSI, the majority of which were due to with promotor 1 hypermethylation. Cluster 3 (copy-number low) consisted of microsatellite stable (MSS) and had a lower mutation frequency; most of these tumors were endometrioid. Cluster 4 tumors had a low mutation frequency, but a high rate of somatic copy number alterations (SCNAs); this group contained most of the serous and mixed histology tumors with frequent TP53 mutations. At a median follow-up of 32 months, cluster 1 had a significantly longer progression-free survival (PFS), followed by cluster 2. Clusters 3 and 4 had significantly shorter PFS. The new POLE ultra-mutated category comprised approximately 10% of the endometrioid tumors. The TCGA molecular characterization data demonstrated approximately 25% of tumors classified as high-grade endometrioid are molecularly similar to uterine serous carcinomas, including frequent TP53 mutations and extensive SCNA. These similarities suggest that genomic-based classification may lead to improved management of these patients.

Molecular classification of endometrial cancer has proven to be reproducible and has demonstrated associations with clinical outcomes. The identified subgroups identify women who may have a risk of recurrence that is very different than what is recognized by traditional clinical risk group assessment. However, methodologies used for the TCGA study to identify the four genomic subgroups, including genome sequencing, were costly, complex and unsuitable for wider clinical application. Talhouk et al. demonstrated that molecular classification of endometrial cancers can be achieved using mismatch repair protein immunohistochemistry, POLE mutational analysis, and p53 immunohistochemistry as a surrogate for ‘copy-number’ status.

18.5 Symptoms, Screening and Diagnosis

Abnormal uterine bleeding (AUB) is the primary symptom of endometrial carcinoma and occurs in 90% of patients who are diagnosed with uterine cancer. All postmenopausal women who have vaginal bleeding should be evaluated for endometrial cancer. Pre- and perimenopausal women with menometrorrhagia also should be evaluated for endometrial cancer, particularly if they have other risk factors, such as anovulation or obesity [16]. Among women with postmenopausal bleeding, 3–20% are found to have endometrial carcinoma and an additional 5–15% have endometrial hyperplasia [17]. Due to its heralding symptom, the majority of patients with endometrial cancer are diagnosed at an early stage with 67% confined to primary site, 21% spread to regional organs and lymph nodes, and 8% diagnosed with distant metastases at initial diagnosis [18]. Advanced cases can be associated with abdominal pain, weight loss, anorexia, bloating, and a change in bowel or bladder habits. Approximately 5% of women are asymptomatic and are diagnosed after workup of abnormal cervical cytology. Currently, there is not an adequate screening test for uterine cancer in asymptomatic women.

Once a patient experiences AUB, ultrasound is utilized to evaluate the uterine cavity [2]. An endometrial stripe of ≤4 mm in a postmenopausal patient is associated with benign pathology (negative predictive value 99–100%) [19, 20]. Thus, postmenopausal women with AUB and an endometrial stripe >4 mm necessitate an endometrial biopsy either by a pipelle or fractional dilation and curettage (D&C). Measurement of the endometrial stripe is not predictive of pathology in women who are premenopausal. As such, any premenopausal woman with AUB and risk factors for endometrial cancer require endometrial sampling. While D&C is the preferred method for obtaining a tissue sample to rule out endometrial cancer, the Pipelle or the Vabra devices used for endometrial sampling are sensitive techniques for the detection of endometrial carcinoma (99.6 and 97.1%) and have shown to correlate well with D&C when analyzing final hysterectomy specimens [21]. The detailed management of endometrial cancer is represented in Fig. 18.1 (Table 18.3).

18.6 Molecular Marker for Endometrial Cancer Diagnosis

PTEN (Phosphatase and tensin homologue deleted from chromosome 10), a tumor suppressor that negatively regulates the PI3K-AKT signaling pathway, is the most frequently altered gene implicated in the pathogenesis of endometrial carcinoma [22]. Loss of PTEN function has been detected in 83% of endometrioid adenocarcinomas of the endometrium and in only less than 10% of non-endometrioid cancers of the endometrium [23–25]. Up to 80% of cases of endometrioid adenocarcinomas possess a loss of PTEN expression, predominantly due to mutations and, to a lesser extent, due to a loss of heterozygosity (LOH) [26]. Higher rates of PTEN gene mutations have been reported to coexist with MSI tumors (60–86%) when compared to tumors without MSI (24–35%) [14, 27]. PTEN mutations have also been well documented in endometrial hyperplasia suggesting that PTEN inactivation is an initiating event in endometrial carcinogenesis and is involved in the development of cytologic atypia in hyperplasia [28]. PTEN mutation and loss of PTEN expression is associated with endometrioid histology, early stage, and favorable prognosis [29, 30].

PTEN loss results in activation of Akt leading to enhanced mTOR activity. Thus, PTEN-negative cells are sensitive to mammalian target of rapamycin (mTOR) inhibitors [31]. The mTOR inhibitor, RAD001, was able to inhibit the progression of endometrial hyperplasia in the PTEN± murine knock-out mouse model through decreased cell proliferation and increased apoptosis. High-grade hyperplasia occurred in a significantly greater percentage of the untreated

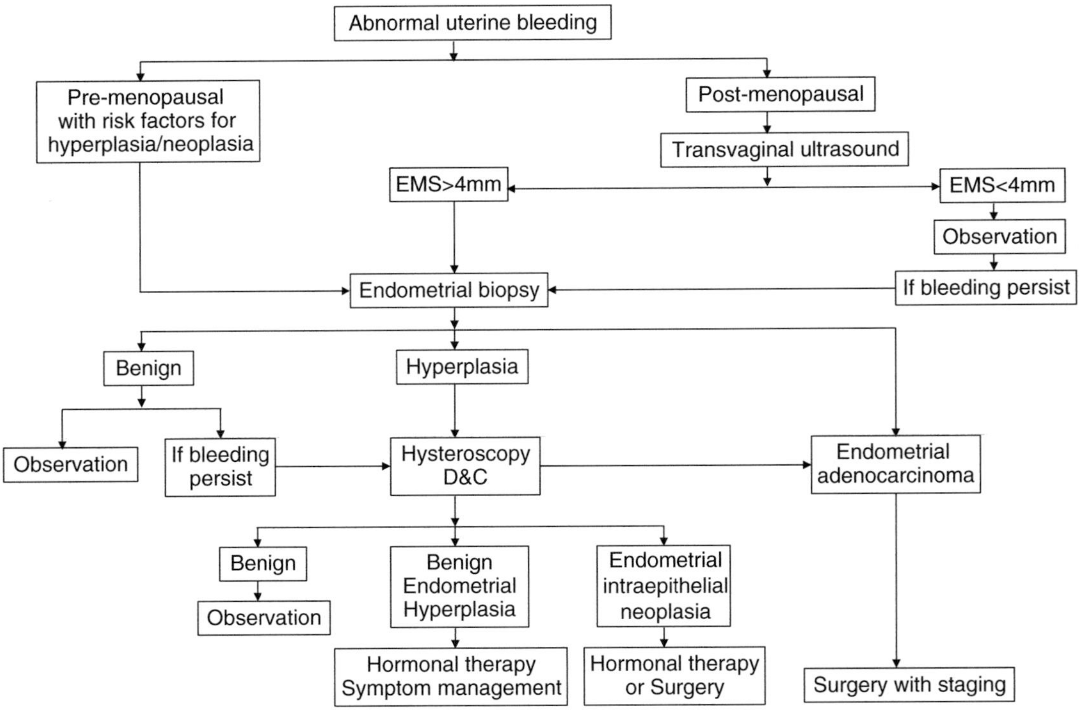

Fig. 18.1 Screening, diagnosis and clinical management of endometrial cancer

PTEN± mice (80%) compared with RAD001-treated PTEN± mice (20%) [32].

18.6.1 PIK3CA (Phosphatidylinositol-4, 5-Bisphosphate 3-Kinase)

In primary endometrial cancer lesions, *PIK3CA* is the second most commonly altered gene, with a frequency of 53%. PIK3CA mutation may lead to alteration of PI3K/AKT signaling in endometrioid cancer [33]. This alteration is more frequent in tumors that also have *PTEN* mutations [34]. Greater than 70% of all mutations affecting PIK3CA gene cluster at 3 "hotspot" codons in exon 9 (E542K, E545K) and in exon 20 (H1047R). These mutations promote cell growth and invasiveness [35]. PIK3CA mutations are associated with adverse clinicopathologic parameters such as high histological grade, myometrial invasion and stage [36, 37]. Nevertheless, PIK3CA mutations confer a survival advantage to patients with endometrioid adenocarcinoma of the endometrium [38].

18.6.2 RAS-RAF-MEK-ERK Signaling Pathway Marker

The K-ras gene encodes a small GTPase transductor protein called KRAS, which plays an important role in tumorigenesis and differentiation. Mutations of the K-ras proto-oncogene have been reported in 6–16% of atypical hyperplasia and 10–30% of endometrial carcinomas [24, 39–41]. Most of these mutation are reported as point mutations at codon 12 [41, 42]. Constitutive activating mutations in K-ras are more common in endometrial cancers showing MSI, suggesting that both events may occur simultaneously before clonal expansion [43]. During tumorigenesis, RAS is frequently activated conferring increased cell proliferation, transformation and cell survival. RAS effectors such as RASSF1A (RAS association domain family member 1) are anticipated to have an inhibitory growth signal which needs to be inactivated during tumorigenesis [13]. Currently, data regarding RASSF1A inactivation and K-RAS mutation in different tumors types is contradictory. In 2008, Pallare et al. revealed inactivation of RASSF1A by promoter hypermethylation may

Table 18.3 Symptoms, screening and diagnosis endometrial cancers

Clinical diagnosis	
History	• Things that affect hormone levels – Estrogen after menopause – Birth control pills – Tamoxifen – The number of menstrual cycles (over a lifetime) – Pregnancy – Obesity – Polycystic ovarian syndrome • Use of an intrauterine device • Age • Diet and exercise • Diabetes • Family history (having close relatives with endometrial or colorectal cancer) • Personal history of breast or ovarian cancer • Personal history of endometrial hyperplasia • Personal history of treatment with pelvic radiation therapy
Symptoms	• Postmenopausal bleeding • Abnormal uterine bleeding • An abnormal, watery or blood-tinged vaginal discharge • Pelvic pain
Pathological diagnosis	
Histological	• Endometrial biopsy • Hysteroscopy • Dilation and curettage (D&C)
Pathological diagnosis	
Serological	• Complete blood count • CA-125 blood test
Radiological diagnostic procedures	
Primary diagnosis	• Pelvic ultrasound • Transvaginal ultrasound (TVUS)
Metastasis diagnosis	• Chest x-ray • Computed tomography (CT)

contribute significantly to increased activity in the RAS-RAF-MEK-ERK pathway [44].

18.6.3 β-Catenin (CTNNB1)

β-catenin, a downstream transcriptional activator in the Wingless/Wnt signaling pathway, plays a critical role in cell differentiation, maintenance of epithelial cell-cell adhesion and normal tissue architecture. Mutations in β-catenin result in stabilization of proteins and lead to cytoplasmic and nuclear accumulation which ultimately participate in the signal transduction and transcriptional activation of genes involved in the development and progression of cancer [45]. *These* mutations are reported in up to 45% of endometrioid adenocarcinoma of the endometrium [46] and are independent of the presence of MSI, PTEN, or KRAS mutation. Amongst endometrioid tumors of all grades and stages, *CTNNB1* mutant tumors are associated with significantly higher rates of grade 1–2 disease, lower rates of deep myometrial invasion, and lower rates of lymphovascular space invasion as well as worse recurrence-free survival for grade 1–2 and stage I–II disease [47]. Increased levels of β-catenin expression is the characteristic feature of endometrioid adenocarcinoma of the endometrium (31–47%) while it is rare event in non-endometrioid carcinomas (0–3%) [48].

18.6.4 Vascular Endothelial Growth Factor (VEGF)

VEGF, a well-known angiogenic factor, is associated with poor prognosis. Elevated expression of VEGF is significantly associated with deep myometrial invasion, poor differentiation and lymph node metastasis in patients with endometrial cancer [49, 50]. Patients with metastases have higher serum levels of VEGF than those with localized disease [51].

18.6.5 Fibroblast Growth Factor (FGF) Signaling Pathway

The fibroblast growth factor receptor (FGFR) signaling pathway plays an important role in endometrial cancer by regulating tumor angiogenesis and metastasis [52]. Endometrial cancer cells with FGFR2 mutations are selectively sensitive to the pan-FGFR inhibitor, PD173074. FGFR2 mutations have been found in up to 16% of endometrial cancers, primarily those of endometrioid histology. Mutation status could potentially be used to identify patients who may benefit from more aggressive adjuvant radiation or chemotherapy after surgery [53]. Byron et al. demonstrated that FGFR2 mutations and PTEN loss of function mutations often coexist whereas FGFR mutations and K-ras mutations are mutually exclusive. These outcomes suggest that FGFR2 is a potential therapeutic target in endometrial cancer [13, 54].

18.6.6 TP53

The TP53, tumor suppressor gene, is the most commonly mutated gene in human cancers, and have been found to play important role in >50% of all human tumors by regulating cell cycle progression, DNA repair systems, and apoptosis [55]. *TP53* mutations were found in 15% of endometrioid adenocarcinomas, 88% of serous carcinomas, 91% of copy-number high, and 35% of POLE integrative genomic subtypes [56]. Thus, p53 mutation represents a useful diagnostic marker in distinguishing type 1 from 2 endometrial cancers [57]. Overexpression of TP53 is correlated with advanced stage, poor differentiation, deep myometrial invasion, lymph node metastases, high-grade and lower survival rates [40, 58].

18.6.7 p21 and p16

p21/WAF1 gene, a direct target of p53 gene, is an inhibitor of cyclin dependent kinases. Abu Backer et al. found that expression of p21/WAF1 is significantly associated with deep myometrial invasion and lymph node metastasis amongst patients with adenocarcinoma of the cervix [59]. *CDKN2A*/p16 is a tumor suppressor gene that functions as a cell cycle regulatory protein. P16 inactivation was observed in 40–45% of non-endometrioid endometrial carcinomas and 10% of endometrioid adenocarcinomas [4, 60]. Loss of p16 expression was observed in 14–74% of endometrial cancer; however, mutation, deletion and promoter methylation are recognized in only 2–6% of cases [61].

18.6.8 HER2/neu (ERBB2)

HER2/neu receptor, a transmembrane tyrosine kinase, is a member of the epidermal growth factor receptor family and regulates cell growth and differentiation. Activation results in uncontrolled cell proliferation. Amplification or overexpression of HER2/neu gene has been observed in numerous cancers including breast, ovarian, and endometrial cancers [62, 63]. HER2/neu is found to be upregulated in about 10–30% of all endometrial cancers, most frequently in serous carcinomas [64, 65]. HER-2/ERBB2-overexpression confers a poorer prognosis amongst patients with serous carcinoma [65, 66].

18.6.9 E-Cadherin

Loss of E-cadherin expression has been encountered in many types of human malignancies including breast, lung, prostate, and also endometrial carcinoma [23, 67]. Alterations in E-cadherin expression have been linked to defective cell—cell adhesiveness, resulting in invasion and metastasis. Several studies established that E-cadherin was mainly expressed in endometrioid carcinomas and less likely in non-endometrioid carcinomas [48, 67].

18.6.10 Epidermal Growth Factor Receptor (EGFR)

EGFR overexpression has been described in approximately 70% of endometrial stromal sarcomas [68] and 60–80% of all types of endometrial cancers [69]. EGFR overexpression is associated with advanced stage and poor prognosis [70, 71]. EGFR mutations have been found to predict therapeutic response to two major classes of EGFR-targeted therapies including: EGFR specific Tyrosine Kinase Inhibitors (TKIs) [gefitinib (Iressa, ZD1839), erlotinib (OSI-774), lapatinib (GW-572016) and imatinib (Gleevec; STI-571)] and anti-EGFR monoclonal antibody 'Monoclonal Antibodies (MoAbs)' [cetuximab (IMC-C225; Im-Clone Systems, New York, NY)] [72].

18.6.11 ER and PR

Estrogen and progesterone are steroid hormones that play a key role in the carcinogenesis of endometrioid adenocarcinoma. Estrogen promotes the development and growth of endometrioid adenocarcinoma, while progesterone inhibits growth and promotes differentiation [73]. In endometrial cancer, loss of progesterone receptor (PR) is associated with increased proliferation, poorer survival, and metastasis [74]. Estrogen receptor (ER-) and PR-positive tumors are associated with favorable prognostic factors including early age, early stage, and endometrioid subtype [75–77].

18.6.12 Ki-67

Ki-67, a marker of cellular proliferation, is increasingly being used in pre-surgical window studies in endometrial cancer as a primary outcome measure [78]. High expression of Ki-67 is more frequent in type II endometrial carcinoma, high-grade endometrial carcinoma and in invasive disease [79–81]. Ki-67 is inversely related to ER expression [77] and is significantly correlated with FIGO stage and histological grade [82].

18.6.13 Cox-2

Cyclooxygenase enzyme plays a key role in the conversion of arachidonic acid to prostaglandins (PG) and is often associated with inflammation and cancer. Loss of COX-2 compartmentalization in neoplastic epithelial cells is suggested as one of the molecular events underlying endometrial carcinogenesis [83]. COX-2 expression is highly prominent in endometrial cancer, particularly in patients with a low degree of differentiation, late stage, deep myometrial invasion, metastasis and shorter disease-free survival [84, 85]. Selective COX-2 inhibition is suggested as potential therapeutic option for COX-2 positive endometrial cancers.

18.6.14 DNA Ploidy

Aneuploidy, an abnormal number of chromosomes, is the most common genetic abnormality observed in cancer cells. Aneuploid tumors account for approximately 16–28% of endometrial cancers [40]. DNA ploidy is an independent prognostic marker for endometrial cancer and identifies high-risk patients who may have otherwise been classified as low-risk based on histopathological characteristics [86]. Recently Proctor et al., demonstrated that abnormal DNA ploidy correlates with poorer progression-free survival, lower BMI, higher grade and non-endometrioid histotypes [87]. Further, patients with aneuploidy tumors demonstrate higher recurrence rates and shorter disease-free intervals when compared to those with diploid tumors [88].

18.6.15 Serum Biomarker

Serum markers such as CA125, CA 19.9, CA 15.3, CA 72.4, CEA or HE4 and complete blood count and have been evaluated to monitor disease progression; however, results are inconclusive for endometrial cancer.

Cancer Antigen 125 or Carbohydrate Antigen 125 (CA125), is a mucin glycoprotein found upregulated in the blood stream of patients with deep myometrial invasion, extra uterine spread, positive peritoneal cytology, lymph node metastasis, recurrence, advanced stage, and reduced survival [89, 90].

Human epididymis protein 4 (HE4) has been found to be elevated in all stages of endometrial cancer and is potentially more sensitive in detecting early stage endometrial cancer as compared to CA125 [91, 92]. HE4 protein expression is associated with poorer prognosis [93]. Dong et al. suggests the combination of serum HE4 and CA125 represents an ideal marker for the diagnosis of endometrial [94].

18.6.16 Epigenetic Biomarkers for Endometrial Cancer Diagnosis

18.6.16.1 Microsatellite Instability (MSI)

Microsatellites are small repetitive nucleotide DNA sequences (1–5 base) dispersed throughout the genome. Microsatellite instability (MSI) is the state of genetic hypermutability due to dysfunction of DNA Mismatch Repair System (MMR). It is closely related to tumorigenicity of hereditary tumors, including Lynch syndrome and has been frequently observed in various human cancers [40, 95, 96].

MSI has been detected in 25–45% of sporadic endometrial carcinoma [97]. MSI-high is more common in endometrioid adenocarcinoma is associated with deep myometrial invasion and higher histologic grade [98]. MSI represents an important predictor of response to immune checkpoint inhibitors (anti-PD-1 antibody and anti-PD-L1 antibody) [95].

18.6.16.2 MiRNAs

MicroRNAs (miRNAs) are 20–25 nucleotide noncoding RNAs that regulate the function of their target gene by controlling their expression via inhibition of translation or initiation of RNA degradation. miRNA expression patterns are altered in endometrial adenocarcinoma compared to normal endometrium [99–101]. A growing body of evidence suggests that miRNA expression profiling of tumors can better predict diagnosis and cancer stage than traditional gene expression analyses and therefore holds great potential as a tool for classification and marker of prognosis in endometrial carcinoma [13, 102] (Table 18.4).

Table 18.4 MicroRNAs expressions in endometrial cancers

Up-regulated		Down-regulated	
mir-9	miR-34a	miR-10a	miR-15b
mir-101	miR-103	miR-20a	miR-30c
miR106a	miR-107	miR-31	miR-99b
miR-141	miR-182	miR-125a	miR-133
miR-183	miR-185	miR-141	miR-152
miR-200a	miR-200b	miR-155	miR-193
miR-200c	mir-203	miR-203	miR-204
mir-205	miR-210	miR-214	miR-221
miR-423	miR-429	miR-222	miR-193b
miR-449	miR-572	mir-410	miR-411
miR-650	miR-622	miR-424	miR-487b
miR-Let7c	mir-18a-3p	miR-Let7e	miR-17-5p

Lee TS, et al. Aberrant microRNA expression in endometrial carcinoma using formalin-fixed paraffin-embedded (FFPE) tissues. PLoS One. 2013;8(12):e81421. https://journals.plos.org/plosone/article?id=10.1371/journal.pone.0081421
Jurcevic S, Olsson B, Klinga-Levan K. MicroRNA expression in human endometrial adenocarcinoma. Cancer Cell Int. 2014;14(1):88. https://www.ncbi.nlm.nih.gov/pmc/articles/PMC4240838/
Widodo, Djati MS, Rifa'i M. Role of MicroRNAs in carcinogenesis that potential for biomarker of endometrial cancer. Ann Med Surg (Lond). 2016;7:9–13. https://www.ncbi.nlm.nih.gov/pubmed/27006767

Although, multiple biomarkers have been discussed for EC diagnosis however, till date none of these biomarkers have been established in clinical practice due to limited specificity and sensitivity. The sensitivity and specificity of currently used tumor markers can be improved if multiple tumor markers are measured. The combination of several tumor markers was not only more effective than the use of single markers, it is allowed them to accurately differentiate malignant from benign endometrial cancer. Serum levels of carcinoembryonic antigen (CEA), CA 125 and CA 15-3 were measured in 47 patients with endometrial cancer and 20 with endometrial hyperplasia. There was an increasing frequency of irregular levels of all markers in relation to a higher tumor stage (stage I: 36%; II: 66%; III: 100%). CA 15-3 was found associated with the prognostic factors of the disease. Moreover, CA 125 and CA 15-3 levels reflected the clinical course of the disease during chemotherapy and seemed to be useful for monitoring response to treatment [103].

18.7 Therapeutic Implications

Recent discoveries regarding the molecular signature of endometrial carcinoma has resulted in the discovery of biomarkers which may assist in the detection of cancer. In the era of personalized medicine, this information is being used for the development and use of targeted therapy. The Gynecologic Oncology Group (GOG) has conducted phase II trials for trastuzumab, bevacizumab, lapatinib, and gefitinib in the treatment of endometrial cancers.

18.7.1 HER2-Directed Agents

Human epidermal growth factor 2 (HER2) overexpression predicts patients with breast cancer who will respond to HER2-directed agents. Some data suggest that HER2 is a relevant target, especially in patients with uterine serous carcinomas. However, the role of HER2-directed therapy is investigational and patients should only be treated with these agents as part of a clinical trial.

Trastuzumab, a humanized monoclonal antibody targeting HER2 receptor, has resulted in improved survival in HER2-positive breast cancer patients. Two phase II trials of anti-HER2 therapy in recurrent endometrial cancer have been published. In GOG229D, women with recurrent or persistent endometrial cancer of all histologies (n = 30) were given single-agent lapatinib, a small molecule and a 4-anilinoquinazoline kinase inhibitors, resulting in one partial response (3.3%). Lapatinib is human epidermal growth factor receptor type 2 (HER2/ERBB2) and epidermal growth factor receptor (HER1/EGFR/ERBB1) tyrosine kinases inhibitor. In this study, HER2 expression was not a requirement. Subsequent analysis revealed only 8% of patients were HER2 positive [104]. In GOG181B, women with HER2-positive stage III-IV or recurrent endometrial cancer were treated with trastuzumab. Of the 33 women included in the trial, there were no objective tumor responses noted [105]. These trials suggest that single-agent therapies directed against HER2 have limited effect in endometrial cancer. The breast cancer experience reveals the presence of primary and acquired resistance to trastuzumab treatment amongst HER2-amplified breast cancers [106]. Different therapeutic interventions targeting resistance mechanisms have resulted in improved outcomes. In endometrial cancer, proposed strategies against anti-HER2 resistance mechanisms are largely untested, but mounting preclinical data suggest combination therapy targeting cancer cell simultaneously at multiple checkpoints in the HER2 signaling pathway may be a successful treatment approach in HER2-positive tumors [107].

18.7.2 Bevacizumab

Bevacizumab, a recombinant monoclonal antibody against vascular endothelial growth factor A (VEGF-A), appears to be an active agent in endometrial cancer. In GOG 229E, 53 women with recurrent or persistent endometrial cancer who had received up to two prior treatments for endometrial cancer were treated with bevacizumab as monotherapy until progression or prohibitive toxicity [108]. Treatment resulted in an objective response rate (ORR) of 15% with 36% progression-free at 6 months. Median PFS and OS were 4 and 11 months, respectively. There were no episodes of gastrointestinal perforation.

GOG 86P explored the role of bevacizumab as first-line treatment for advanced, metastatic, or recurrent endometrial cancer [109]. Of the 349 patients enrolled, more than 80% had received prior radiation therapy. Patients were randomized to receive carboplatin and paclitaxel plus bevacizumab (arm 1), carboplatin and paclitaxel plus temsirolimus (an mTOR inhibitor; arm 2), or carboplatin and ixebepilone plus bevacizumab (arm 3). When compared with a historical controls (using data from GOG 209), there was no difference in PFS. Median OS was improved in arm 1 (34 months versus 23 months), but was not different in arms 2 or 3 (median OS 25 months in both).

The Multicenter Italian Trials in Ovarian Cancer (MITO) Group END-2 trial further explored the role of bevacizumab as second-line treatment. In this study, 108 patients who had received ≤1 prior platinum-based regimens and progressed >6 months after completion of first-line therapy were treated with carboplatin plus paclitaxel and randomly assigned to treatment with or without bevacizumab [110]. Compared with carboplatin plus paclitaxel, the addition of bevacizumab resulted in a higher ORR (71.7% vs 54.3%), a significant improvement in PFS (median, 13 vs 8.7 months; HR 0.59, 95% CI 0.35–0.98), with no significant difference in OS.

These results suggest bevacizumab has activity in combination with chemotherapy for women with recurrent or metastatic endometrial cancer.

However, definitive data from phase III randomized trials are needed before adopting it as a standard treatment option.

18.7.3 Fibroblast Growth Factor Receptor (FGFR) Inhibitors

The fibroblast growth factor receptor (FGFR) pathway plays a role in angiogenesis as well as proliferation, differentiation, and survival during embryogenesis and adult tissue homeostasis has been implicated in a subset of endometrial cancers. *FGFR2* mutations have been identified in approximately 10–16% of endometrial cancers. Preclinical studies have demonstrated that inhibition of the FGFR pathway, alone or in combination with other signaling pathways or chemotherapy, results in antitumor activity in endometrial cancer models. Dutt et al. noted that inhibition of FGFR2 kinase activity in endometrial carcinoma cell lines bearing FGFR2 mutations inhibited transformation and survival [111]. Using the xenograft models, Konency et al. demonstrated the anti-cancerous activity of FGFR inhibitors (dovitinib and NVP-BGJ398) in FGFR2-mutated human endometrial cancer cells [112].

In the phase II study, GOG 229-I [113], patients with persistent or recurrent endometrial cancer who had received up to two prior cytotoxic regimens were treated with brivanib, a multi-targeted tyrosine kinase inhibitor with activity against VEGF and FGFR. Of the 43 evaluable patients, 8 patients had responses (18.6%) and 13 patients were progression free at 6 months. Median PFS and OS were 3.3 and 10.7 months, respectively. Brivanib was reasonably well tolerated, with nine patients (20.9%) experiencing grade 3 hypertension and one patient (2.3%) experiencing grade 4 confusion [113].

Vergote et al. [114] examined the efficacy of lenvatinib, an oral receptor tyrosine kinase inhibitor targeting VEGFR1-3, FGFR1-4, RET, KIT, and PDGFRβ. Patients (n = 133) with metastatic or unresectable endometrial cancer who had received up to two prior platinum-based treatments were given lenvatinib resulting in an ORR of 21.8%. Median PFS and OS were 5.4 months and 10.6 months respectively. Low BL Ang-2 level appeared to predict clinical benefit in a subset of patients (Clinical trial information: NCT01111461).

In a phase II study, Konecnyl et al. [115] explored the use of dovitinib as second-line therapy in patients with FGFR2 mutated or wild-type advanced and/or metastatic endometrial cancer. In the patients with FGFR2 mutations, 7/20 patients (35%) were progression free at 18 weeks. In the patients with FGFR2 wild-type, 5/20 (25%) were progression free at 18 weeks. FGFR2 status did not appear to affect the observed treatment effect. These data should be considered exploratory and additional studies are needed.

These results suggest that single-agent TKIs that target FGFR show efficacy in the advanced and/or recurrent endometrial cancer population. To date, all of the FGFR TKIs with clinical data are multitargeted and inhibit other signaling pathways beyond FGFR that may be critical for disease progression and/or tumor escape mechanisms. Future studies that stratify patients based on *FGFR2* mutations may provide further information to enable clinicians to make informed decisions and provide personalized care for their patients.

18.7.4 Metformin

Metformin, a biguanide drug widely used for the treatment of type II diabetes has emerged as a new adjunctive strategy for different cancer types, including endometrial cancer [116]. Metformin exerts its glucose-lowering effect primarily by suppressing hepatic gluconeogenesis and enhancing insulin suppression of endogenous glucose production and, to a lesser extent, by reducing intestinal glucose absorption [117]. Although the molecular mechanism of metformin has been well-studied in liver, muscle and fat, little is known about its effects on epithelial tissues, including the endometrium. It has been shown to reversibly inhibit mitochondrial complex I within cancer cells to reduce tumorigenesis [118]. Metformin is thought to behave as a novel mTOR inhibitor and has been shown to dramatically decrease proliferation in a number of different human cancer cell lines in vitro as well as in xenograft animal models of breast, prostate, and colon cancers. A recent study showed that Metformin significantly decreased proliferation in human endometrial cancer by inhibiting PI3K/AKT/mTOR signaling [119]. Furthermore, various epidemiological evidence suggests that metformin lowers all cancer risk and reduces cancer incidence and deaths among diabetic patients, including mortality from endometrial cancers [120].

GOG286B (NCT02065687) is a phase II/III trial evaluating the role of metformin in combination with the standard regimen, carboplatin and paclitaxel, in patients with advanced or recurrent endometrial cancer. In 2018, after review of interim analysis, the NRG recommended closure of the trial as metformin was unlikely to provide a benefit.

18.8 Conclusions

Advances in diagnostic imaging and pathologic techniques have improved our ability to diagnose uterine cancer. Nevertheless, our current technology does not allow us to predict whether or not a patient will develop endometrial cancer or the course of their disease. Identification of epigenetic mutations, miRNA abnormalities and other biomarkers has the potential to answer this age-old question. These methods will allow for a minimally invasive method of accurately identifying pathology. Multiple classifications of targeted therapy have been developed and studied as single agents as well as in combination with traditional cytotoxic agents. Continued investigation into the molecular pathways of endometrial cancer development and progression will enhance our knowledge of the disease process and will lead to the innovation of novel and superior therapeutic options for these patients.

References

1. Howlader N, Noone AM, Krapcho M, Miller D, Bishop K, Kosary CL, Yu M, Ruhl J, Tatalovich Z, Mariotto A, Lewis DR, Chen HS, Feuer EJ, Cronin KA, editors. SEER Cancer Statistics Review, 1975-2014. Bethesda: National Cancer Institute; 2017. https://seer.cancer.gov/csr/1975_2014/, based on November 2016 SEER data submission, posted to the SEER web site, April 2017. 1975–2014.
2. Micco M, et al. Imaging after treatment in uterine malignancies: spectrum of normal findings and most common complications. J Med Imaging Radiat Oncol. 2017;61(6):777–90.
3. Bokhman JV. Two pathogenetic types of endometrial carcinoma. Gynecol Oncol. 1983;15(1):10–7.
4. Liu FS. Molecular carcinogenesis of endometrial cancer. Taiwan J Obstet Gynecol. 2007;46(1):26–32.
5. Sherman ME, Bur ME, Kurman RJ. p53 in endometrial cancer and its putative precursors: evidence for diverse pathways of tumorigenesis. Hum Pathol. 1995;26(11):1268–74.
6. Sorosky JI. Endometrial cancer. Obstet Gynecol. 2008;111(2 Pt 1):436–47.
7. Felix AS, et al. Factors associated with Type I and Type II endometrial cancer. Cancer Causes Control. 2010;21(11):1851–6.
8. Fadare O, Zheng W. Endometrial Glandular Dysplasia (EmGD): morphologically and biologically distinctive putative precursor lesions of Type II endometrial cancers. Diagn Pathol. 2008;3:6.
9. Matias-Guiu X, et al. Molecular pathology of endometrial hyperplasia and carcinoma. Hum Pathol. 2001;32(6):569–77.
10. Lax SF, et al. The frequency of p53, K-ras mutations, and microsatellite instability differs in uterine endometrioid and serous carcinoma: evidence of distinct molecular genetic pathways. Cancer. 2000;88(4):814–24.
11. Llobet D, et al. Molecular pathology of endometrial carcinoma: practical aspects from the diagnostic and therapeutic viewpoints. J Clin Pathol. 2009;62(9):777–85.
12. Abushahin N, Pang S, Li J, Fadare O, Zheng W. Endometrial intraepithelial neoplasia. In: Intraepithelial neoplasia. 2012. 10.5772/30988.
13. Matias-Guiu X, Prat J. Molecular pathology of endometrial carcinoma. Histopathology. 2013;62(1):111–23.
14. Doll A, et al. Novel molecular profiles of endometrial cancer-new light through old windows. J Steroid Biochem Mol Biol. 2008;108(3–5):221–9.
15. Hecht JL, Mutter GL. Molecular and pathologic aspects of endometrial carcinogenesis. J Clin Oncol. 2006;24(29):4783–91.
16. Chen LM, McGonigle KF, Berek JS. Endometrial cancer: recent developments in evaluation and treat-

ment. Oncology (Williston Park). 1999;13(12):1665–70; discussion 1675–8, 1681–2
17. American College of Obstetricians and Gynecologists. ACOG practice bulletin, clinical management guidelines for obstetrician-gynecologists, number 65, August 2005: management of endometrial cancer. Obstet Gynecol. 2005;106(2):413–25.
18. Howlader N, Noone AM, Krapcho M, Miller D, Bishop K, Altekruse SF, Kosary CL, Yu M, Ruhl J, Tatalovich Z, Mariotto A, Lewis DR, Chen HS, Feuer EJ, Cronin KA, editors. SEER Cancer Statistics Review, 1975-2013. Bethesda: National Cancer Institute; 2016. https://seer.cancer.gov/csr/1975_2013/, based on November 2015 SEER data submission, posted to the SEER web site, April 2016. 1975–2013.
19. Braun MM, Overbeek-Wager EA, Grumbo RJ. Diagnosis and management of endometrial cancer. Am Fam Physician. 2016;93(6):468–74.
20. American College of Obstetricians and Gynecologists. ACOG Committee Opinion No. 440: the role of transvaginal ultrasonography in the evaluation of postmenopausal bleeding. Obstet Gynecol. 2009;114(2 Pt 1):409–11.
21. Dijkhuizen FP, et al. The accuracy of endometrial sampling in the diagnosis of patients with endometrial carcinoma and hyperplasia: a meta-analysis. Cancer. 2000;89(8):1765–72.
22. Gbelcova H, et al. PTEN sequence analysis in endometrial hyperplasia and endometrial carcinoma in Slovak women. Anal Cell Pathol (Amst). 2015;2015:746856.
23. Ellis PE, Ghaem-Maghami S. Molecular characteristics and risk factors in endometrial cancer: what are the treatment and preventative strategies? Int J Gynecol Cancer. 2010;20(7):1207–16.
24. Ahmed Q, et al. Gynecologic cancers: molecular updates. Clin Lab Med. 2013;33(4):911–25.
25. Lax SF. Molecular genetic pathways in various types of endometrial carcinoma: from a phenotypical to a molecular-based classification. Virchows Arch. 2004;444(3):213–23.
26. Simpkins SB, et al. PTEN mutations in endometrial cancers with 10q LOH: additional evidence for the involvement of multiple tumor suppressors. Gynecol Oncol. 1998;71(3):391–5.
27. Bilbao C, et al. The relationship between microsatellite instability and PTEN gene mutations in endometrial cancer. Int J Cancer. 2006;119(3):563–70.
28. Sun H, et al. Mutational analysis of the PTEN gene in endometrial carcinoma and hyperplasia. Am J Clin Pathol. 2001;115(1):32–8.
29. Akiyama-Abe A, et al. Loss of PTEN expression is an independent predictor of favourable survival in endometrial carcinomas. Br J Cancer. 2013;109(6):1703–10.
30. Risinger JI, et al. PTEN mutation in endometrial cancers is associated with favorable clinical and pathologic characteristics. Clin Cancer Res. 1998;4(12):3005–10.
31. Rajanbabu A. Molecular pathology and cytogenetics of endometrial carcinoma, carcinosarcoma, and uterine sarcomas. In: Rajaram S, Chitrathara K, Maheshwari A, editors. Uterine cancer: diagnosis and treatment. New Delhi: Springer; 2015. p. 13–23.
32. Oza AM, Elit L, Provencher D, Biagi JJ, Panasci L, Sederias J, Dancey JE, Tsao MS, Eisenhauer EA. A phase II study of temsirolimus (CCI-779) in patients with metastatic and/or locally advanced recurrent endometrial cancer previously treated with chemotherapy: NCIC CTG IND 160b. J Clin Oncol. 2008;26(15_suppl):5516.
33. Gao J, et al. Integrative analysis of complex cancer genomics and clinical profiles using the cBioPortal. Sci Signal. 2013;6(269):pl1.
34. Oda K, et al. High frequency of coexistent mutations of PIK3CA and PTEN genes in endometrial carcinoma. Cancer Res. 2005;65(23):10669–73.
35. Gymnopoulos M, Elsliger MA, Vogt PK. Rare cancer-specific mutations in PIK3CA show gain of function. Proc Natl Acad Sci U S A. 2007;104(13):5569–74.
36. Konopka B, et al. PIK3CA mutations and amplification in endometrioid endometrial carcinomas: relation to other genetic defects and clinicopathologic status of the tumors. Hum Pathol. 2011;42(11):1710–9.
37. Catasus L, et al. PIK3CA mutations in the kinase domain (exon 20) of uterine endometrial adenocarcinomas are associated with adverse prognostic parameters. Mod Pathol. 2008;21(2):131–9.
38. Lin DI. Improved survival associated with somatic PIK3CA mutations in copy-number low endometrioid endometrial adenocarcinoma. Oncol Lett. 2015;10(5):2743–8.
39. Enomoto T, et al. Alterations of the p53 tumor suppressor gene and its association with activation of the c-K-ras-2 protooncogene in premalignant and malignant lesions of the human uterine endometrium. Cancer Res. 1993;53(8):1883–8.
40. Zyla MM, et al. The significance of markers in the diagnosis of endometrial cancer. Prz Menopauzalny. 2016;15(3):176–85.
41. Dobrzycka B, et al. Mutations of the KRAS oncogene in endometrial hyperplasia and carcinoma. Folia Histochem Cytobiol. 2009;47(1):65–8.
42. Sammoud S, et al. Relationship between expression of ras p21 oncoprotein and mutation status of the K-ras gene in sporadic colorectal cancer patients in Tunisia. Appl Immunohistochem Mol Morphol. 2012;20(2):146–52.
43. Lagarda H, et al. K-ras mutations in endometrial carcinomas with microsatellite instability. J Pathol. 2001;193(2):193–9.
44. Pallares J, et al. Promoter hypermethylation and reduced expression of RASSF1A are frequent molecular alterations of endometrial carcinoma. Mod Pathol. 2008;21(6):691–9.
45. Norimatsu Y, et al. Diagnostic utility of phosphatase and tensin homolog, beta-catenin, and p53 for endo-

metrial carcinoma by thin-layer endometrial preparations. Cancer. 2008;114(3):155–64.
46. O'Hara AJ, Bell DW. The genomics and genetics of endometrial cancer. Adv Genomics Genet. 2012;2012(2):33–47.
47. Kurnit KC, et al. CTNNB1 (beta-catenin) mutation identifies low grade, early stage endometrial cancer patients at increased risk of recurrence. Mod Pathol. 2017;30(7):1032–41.
48. Moreno-Bueno G, et al. Abnormalities of the APC/beta-catenin pathway in endometrial cancer. Oncogene. 2002;21(52):7981–90.
49. Mahecha AM, Wang H. The influence of vascular endothelial growth factor-A and matrix metalloproteinase-2 and -9 in angiogenesis, metastasis, and prognosis of endometrial cancer. Onco Targets Ther. 2017;10:4617–24.
50. Topolovec Z, et al. Vascular endothelial growth factor and intratumoral microvessel density as prognostic factors in endometrial cancer. Coll Antropol. 2010;34(2):447–53.
51. Saarelainen SK, et al. Endoglin, VEGF, and its receptors in predicting metastases in endometrial carcinoma. Tumour Biol. 2014;35(5):4651–7.
52. Soufla G, Sifakis S, Spandidos DA. FGF2 transcript levels are positively correlated with EGF and IGF-1 in the malignant endometrium. Cancer Lett. 2008;259(2):146–55.
53. Winterhoff B, Konecny GE. Targeting fibroblast growth factor pathways in endometrial cancer. Curr Probl Cancer. 2017;41(1):37–47.
54. Byron SA, Pollock PM. FGFR2 as a molecular target in endometrial cancer. Future Oncol. 2009;5(1):27–32.
55. Rai R, et al. p53: its alteration and gallbladder cancer. Eur J Cancer Prev. 2011;20(2):77–85.
56. Schultheis AM, et al. TP53 mutational spectrum in endometrioid and serous endometrial cancers. Int J Gynecol Pathol. 2016;35(4):289–300.
57. Hayes MP, Ellenson LH. Molecular alterations in uterine serous carcinoma. Gynecol Oncol. 2010;116(2):286–9.
58. Kohler MF, et al. p53 overexpression in advanced-stage endometrial adenocarcinoma. Am J Obstet Gynecol. 1996;175(5):1246–52.
59. Abu Backer FM, Nik Mustapha NR, Othman NH. Clinicopathological comparison of adenocarcinoma of cervix and endometrium using cell cycle markers: P16ink4a, P21waf1, and p27Kip1 on 132 cancers. Infect Dis Obstet Gynecol. 2011;2011:857851.
60. Salvesen HB, Das S, Akslen LA. Loss of nuclear p16 protein expression is not associated with promoter methylation but defines a subgroup of aggressive endometrial carcinomas with poor prognosis. Clin Cancer Res. 2000;6(1):153–9.
61. Banno K, et al. Biomarkers in endometrial cancer: possible clinical applications (Review). Oncol Lett. 2012;3(6):1175–80.
62. Villella JA, et al. HER-2/neu overexpression in uterine papillary serous cancers and its possible therapeutic implications. Int J Gynecol Cancer. 2006;16(5):1897–902.
63. Roses RE, et al. HER-2/neu overexpression as a predictor for the transition from in situ to invasive breast cancer. Cancer Epidemiol Biomarkers Prev. 2009;18(5):1386–9.
64. Williams JA Jr, et al. Fluorescence in situ hybridization analysis of HER-2/neu, c-myc, and p53 in endometrial cancer. Exp Mol Pathol. 1999;67(3):135–43.
65. Morrison C, et al. HER-2 is an independent prognostic factor in endometrial cancer: association with outcome in a large cohort of surgically staged patients. J Clin Oncol. 2006;24(15):2376–85.
66. Diaz-Montes TP, et al. Clinical significance of Her-2/neu overexpression in uterine serous carcinoma. Gynecol Oncol. 2006;100(1):139–44.
67. Sakuragi N, et al. Decreased E-cadherin expression in endometrial carcinoma is associated with tumor dedifferentiation and deep myometrial invasion. Gynecol Oncol. 1994;53(2):183–9.
68. Moinfar F, Azodi M, Tavassoli FA. Uterine sarcomas. Pathology. 2007;39(1):55–71.
69. Bansal N, Yendluri V, Wenham RM. The molecular biology of endometrial cancers and the implications for pathogenesis, classification, and targeted therapies. Cancer Control. 2009;16(1):8–13.
70. Holcomb K, et al. E-cadherin expression in endometrioid, papillary serous, and clear cell carcinoma of the endometrium. Obstet Gynecol. 2002;100(6):1290–5.
71. Leslie KK, et al. A phase II evaluation of gefitinib in the treatment of persistent or recurrent endometrial cancer: a Gynecologic Oncology Group study. Gynecol Oncol. 2013;129(3):486–94.
72. Tsikouras P, et al. Endometrial cancer: molecular and therapeutic aspects. Eur J Obstet Gynecol Reprod Biol. 2013;169(1):1–9.
73. Decruze SB, Green JA. Hormone therapy in advanced and recurrent endometrial cancer: a systematic review. Int J Gynecol Cancer. 2007;17(5):964–78.
74. Tangen IL, et al. Loss of progesterone receptor links to high proliferation and increases from primary to metastatic endometrial cancer lesions. Eur J Cancer. 2014;50(17):3003–10.
75. Huvila J, et al. Progesterone receptor negativity is an independent risk factor for relapse in patients with early stage endometrioid endometrial adenocarcinoma. Gynecol Oncol. 2013;130(3):463–9.
76. Li M, et al. Clinical implications and prognostic value of single and combined biomarkers in endometrial carcinoma. Chin Med J (Engl). 2014;127(8):1459–63.
77. Ferrandina G, et al. Expression of cyclooxygenase-2 (COX-2), receptors for estrogen (ER), and progesterone (PR), p53, ki67, and neu protein in endometrial cancer. Gynecol Oncol. 2005;98(3):383–9.

78. Kitson S, et al. Ki-67 in endometrial cancer: scoring optimization and prognostic relevance for window studies. Mod Pathol. 2017;30(3):459–68.
79. Horree N, et al. The invasive front in endometrial carcinoma: higher proliferation and associated derailment of cell cycle regulators. Hum Pathol. 2007;38(8):1232–8.
80. Kosmas K, et al. Expression of Ki-67 as proliferation biomarker in imprint smears of endometrial carcinoma. Diagn Cytopathol. 2013;41(3):212–7.
81. Lax SF, et al. Clear cell carcinoma of the endometrium is characterized by a distinctive profile of p53, Ki-67, estrogen, and progesterone receptor expression. Hum Pathol. 1998;29(6):551–8.
82. Shih HC, et al. Immunohistochemical expression of cyclins, cyclin-dependent kinases, tumor-suppressor gene products, Ki-67, and sex steroid receptors in endometrial carcinoma: positive staining for cyclin A as a poor prognostic indicator. Hum Pathol. 2003;34(5):471–8.
83. Saraiva AL, et al. Immunohistochemical expression of cyclooxygenase-2 (COX-2) in feline endometrial adenocarcinoma and in normal and hyperplastic endometria. Reprod Domest Anim. 2015;50(2):333–40.
84. Ma X, et al. Clinical significance of COX-2, GLUT-1 and VEGF expressions in endometrial cancer tissues. Pak J Med Sci. 2015;31(2):280–4.
85. Ferrandina G, et al. Cyclooxygenase-2 expression in endometrial carcinoma: correlation with clinicopathologic parameters and clinical outcome. Cancer. 2002;95(4):801–7.
86. Werner HM, Salvesen HB. Current status of molecular biomarkers in endometrial cancer. Curr Oncol Rep. 2014;16(9):403.
87. Proctor L, et al. Assessment of DNA Ploidy in the ProMisE molecular subgroups of endometrial cancer. Gynecol Oncol. 2017;146(3):596–602.
88. Susini T, et al. Ten-year results of a prospective study on the prognostic role of ploidy in endometrial carcinoma: dNA aneuploidy identifies high-risk cases among the so-called 'low-risk' patients with well and moderately differentiated tumors. Cancer. 2007;109(5):882–90.
89. Dotters DJ. Preoperative CA 125 in endometrial cancer: is it useful? Am J Obstet Gynecol. 2000;182(6):1328–34.
90. Jiang T, Huang L, Zhang S. Preoperative serum CA125: a useful marker for surgical management of endometrial cancer. BMC Cancer. 2015;15:396.
91. Moore RG, et al. Utility of a novel serum tumor biomarker HE4 in patients with endometrioid adenocarcinoma of the uterus. Gynecol Oncol. 2008;110(2):196–201.
92. Bie Y, Zhang Z. Diagnostic value of serum HE4 in endometrial cancer: a meta-analysis. World J Surg Oncol. 2014;12:169.
93. Li X, et al. Expression of HE4 in endometrial cancer and its clinical significance. Biomed Res Int. 2015;2015:437468.
94. Dong C, Liu P, Li C. Value of HE4 combined with cancer antigen 125 in the diagnosis of endometrial cancer. Pak J Med Sci. 2017;33(4):1013–7.
95. Kunitomi H, et al. New use of microsatellite instability analysis in endometrial cancer. Oncol Lett. 2017;14(3):3297–301.
96. Popat S, Hubner R, Houlston RS. Systematic review of microsatellite instability and colorectal cancer prognosis. J Clin Oncol. 2005;23(3): 609–18.
97. An HJ, et al. Microsatellite instability in endometrioid type endometrial adenocarcinoma is associated with poor prognostic indicators. Am J Surg Pathol. 2007;31(6):846–53.
98. Kanopiene D, et al. Endometrial cancer and microsatellite instability status. Open Med (Wars). 2015;10(1):70–6.
99. Lee TS, et al. Aberrant microRNA expression in endometrial carcinoma using formalin-fixed paraffin-embedded (FFPE) tissues. PLoS One. 2013;8(12):e81421.
100. Jurcevic S, Olsson B, Klinga-Levan K. MicroRNA expression in human endometrial adenocarcinoma. Cancer Cell Int. 2014;14(1):88.
101. Widodo, Djati MS, Rifa'i M. Role of MicroRNAs in carcinogenesis that potential for biomarker of endometrial cancer. Ann Med Surg (Lond). 2016;7:9–13.
102. Banno K, et al. Candidate biomarkers for genetic and clinicopathological diagnosis of endometrial cancer. Int J Mol Sci. 2013;14(6):12123–37.
103. Panici PB, et al. Multiple serum markers in patients with endometrial cancer. Gynecol Obstet Invest. 1989;27(4):208–12.
104. Leslie KK, et al. Lapatinib and potential prognostic value of EGFR mutations in a Gynecologic Oncology Group phase II trial of persistent or recurrent endometrial cancer. Gynecol Oncol. 2012;127(2):345–50.
105. Fleming GF, et al. Phase II trial of trastuzumab in women with advanced or recurrent, HER2-positive endometrial carcinoma: a Gynecologic Oncology Group study. Gynecol Oncol. 2010;116(1):15–20.
106. Luque-Cabal M, et al. Mechanisms behind the resistance to trastuzumab in HER2-amplified breast cancer and strategies to overcome it. Clin Med Insights Oncol. 2016;10(Suppl 1):21–30.
107. Diver EJ, et al. The therapeutic challenge of targeting HER2 in endometrial cancer. Oncologist. 2015;20(9):1058–68.
108. Aghajanian C, et al. Phase II trial of bevacizumab in recurrent or persistent endometrial cancer: a Gynecologic Oncology Group study. J Clin Oncol. 2011;29(16):2259–65.
109. Carol Aghajanian VLF, Dizon DS, Carlson J, Powell MA, Secord AA, Tewari KS, Bender D, O'Malley DM, Stuckey A, Rotmensch J, Levine DA, Lankes HA, Moore KN. A randomized phase II study of paclitaxel/carboplatin/bevacizumab, paclitaxel/carboplatin/temsirolimus and ixabepilone/carboplatin/bevacizumab as initial therapy for measurable

stage III or IVA, stage IVB or recurrent endometrial cancer, GOG-86P. J Clin Oncol. 2015;33(15 Suppl):5500.
110. Lorusso D, Ferrandina G, Colombo N, Pignata S, Salutari V, Maltese G, Pisano C, Lapresa M, Savarese A, Tagliaferri P, Sorio R, Cinieri S, Breda E, Sabbatini R, Lepori S, Conte C, Cecere SC, Raspagliesi F, Scambia G. Randomized phase II trial of carboplatin-paclitaxel (CP) compared to carboplatin-paclitaxel-bevacizumab (CP-B) in advanced (stage III-IV) or recurrent endometrial cancer: the MITO END-2 trial. J Clin Oncol. 2015;33(15 Suppl):5502.
111. Dutt A, et al. Drug-sensitive FGFR2 mutations in endometrial carcinoma. Proc Natl Acad Sci U S A. 2008;105(25):8713–7.
112. Konecny GE, et al. Activity of the fibroblast growth factor receptor inhibitors dovitinib (TKI258) and NVP-BGJ398 in human endometrial cancer cells. Mol Cancer Ther. 2013;12(5):632–42.
113. Powell MA, et al. A phase II trial of brivanib in recurrent or persistent endometrial cancer: an NRG Oncology/Gynecologic Oncology Group Study. Gynecol Oncol. 2014;135(1):38–43.
114. Ignace Vergote MT, Powell MA, Miller DS, Garcia AA, Mikheeva ON, Pinter T, Bidzinski M, Cebotaru CL, Fan J, Ren M, Meneses N, Funahashi Y, Kadowaki T, O'Brien JP, Penson RT. A phase II trial of lenvatinib in patients with advanced or recurrent endometrial cancer: angiopoietin-2 as a predictive marker for clinical outcomes. J Clin Oncol. 2013;31(15 Suppl):5520.
115. Konecny GE, et al. Second-line dovitinib (TKI258) in patients with FGFR2-mutated or FGFR2-non-mutated advanced or metastatic endometrial cancer: a non-randomised, open-label, two-group, two-stage, phase 2 study. Lancet Oncol. 2015;16(6):686–94.
116. Meireles CG, et al. Effects of metformin on endometrial cancer: systematic review and meta-analysis. Gynecol Oncol. 2017;147(1):167–80.
117. Foretz M, et al. Metformin: from mechanisms of action to therapies. Cell Metab. 2014;20(6):953–66.
118. Wheaton WW, et al. Metformin inhibits mitochondrial complex I of cancer cells to reduce tumorigenesis. Elife. 2014;3:e02242.
119. Zhao Y, et al. Metformin is associated with reduced cell proliferation in human endometrial cancer by inbibiting PI3K/AKT/mTOR signaling. Gynecol Endocrinol. 2018;34(5):428–32.
120. Evans JM, et al. Metformin and reduced risk of cancer in diabetic patients. BMJ. 2005;330(7503):1304–5.

Molecular Diagnosis in Ovarian Carcinoma

19

Shailendra Dwivedi, Radhieka Misra, Purvi Purohit, Jeewan Ram Vishnoi, Puneet Pareek, Apul Goel, Sanjay Khattri, Praveen Sharma, Kamlesh Kumar Pant, and Sanjeev Misra

19.1 Introduction

Progression in screening of ovarian carcinoma has been influenced by the fact that ovarian cancer is neither a frequent nor a rare disease. The risk of developing ovarian cancer is 1 in 70 and the frequency is 1 in 2500 for postmenopausal women, patients generally diagnosed after crossing 50 years of age. It is fifth most common reason of cancer-linked death in women. The probable yearly incidence of this cancer globally is over 200,000 individuals, with about 125,000 deaths [1].

Persistent progress in the understanding of the natural history of the disease and thorough preliminary staging, along with surgical and chemotherapeutic interventions, has enriched the short-term course of ovarian carcinoma. Yet, despite such progresses, most patients revert after primary treatment and succumb to disease advancement.

Molecular diagnosis focusses on the designing of the medical treatment to the individual characteristics of each patient. Thus, it depends on the broad exploration of individual molecular database of genomic, epigenetics, proteomic and metabolomics, as well as in-silico tactics to acquire a thorough knowledge of the association between the control of gene(s) (functional protein) and disease status. This above progression depends on modern cutting edge technologies of genomics that includes real time PCR, microarray and next generation sequencing (NGS) having capabilities to explore the molecular characteristics in short time.

As we know, that any drug have its advantageous effects to only few individuals while others fail to show its response, now it is established that this fact is depend on molecular characteristics of individuals. Each and every living entity or group having exclusive phenotype (like disease) is primarily due to manifestation of its molecular characteristics i.e. variations (mutations) in gene make up or expression profile, so for screening any disease, our initial goal is to recognize such

S. Dwivedi (✉) · P. Purohit · P. Sharma
Department of Biochemistry, All India Institute of Medical Sciences, Jodhpur, India

R. Misra
Era's Lucknow Medical College and Hospital, Lucknow, India

J. R. Vishnoi · S. Misra
Department of Onco-surgery, All India Institute of Medical Sciences, Jodhpur, India

P. Pareek
Department of Radio-Therapy, All India Institute of Medical Sciences, Jodhpur, India

A. Goel
Department of Urology, King George Medical University, Lucknow, India

S. Khattri · K. K. Pant
Department of Pharmacology and Therapeutics, King George Medical University, Lucknow, India

K. K. Shukla et al. (eds.), *Molecular Diagnostics in Cancer Patients*,
https://doi.org/10.1007/978-981-13-5877-7_19

changes and on the behalf of which classify them in group then we can observe the suitability of any drug. Thus we will be able to sub-group them into beneficial or null or negative response group. The regulation of gene expression can also take place at the steps of translation and post-translation modification. Recent cutting-edge in genomics, transcriptome profiling, and epigenetic fingerprinting have been useful in screening ovarian cancer and that can probably be utilized for cultivating cancer medicine.

19.2 Progression of Cutting Edge Technology for Accurate Diagnosis

The oncology field is persistently growing primarily due to the use of huge funds and enhancements in the basic sciences. Modern molecular diagnostic techniques and tools of genomics, transcriptomics and proteomics have been widely exploited in diagnosis of various cancers. Nowadays automated and more advanced technologies like PCR real time PCR etc. have been upgraded the amplification and detection of nucleic acid sequences.

These automated and robotic platforms have provided precision of not only in assay efficiency but also in quality control of the tests and have added calibration of traditional biomarkers. It is known since Gregor Mendel that factors are accountable for expression of characters and after the launching of human genome the picture of genotype to phenotype connection seems more bright and dynamic. Thus, genetics has become the dynamic force in medical research and is now ready for amalgamation into medical practice.

19.2.1 Genomics

Genomics is an interdisciplinary branch of science focusing on genomes. A genome is actually the study of a whole set of DNA within a single cell of an organism, and as such genomics is a division of molecular biology related with the structure, function, evolution, and mapping of genomes. The genetics of humans basically elucidates their individual characteristics. Subtle variances found in the genetic makeup of a population generate the diverse characters perceived in community.

Moreover, variances in a genetic frame among a population result into diverse gene isoforms that may consequently alter gene function creating phenotypic variations in the form of characteristics either protective or make more susceptible for any disease. These are usually represented as mutated genes. Similarly like other several diseases, in ovarian cancer mutated genes inherited from a parent can make a person more predispose or susceptible of developing the disease in their lifespan. Though, inherited mutations only deduce for a small fraction of (20–25%) all diagnosed cases in ovarian cancer. So sporadic, scattered unpredictable gene alterations or deregulated gene expression would be the main sources for maximum ovarian cancer patients.

19.2.1.1 Genome and Genetic Characterization Tools and Techniques

In 2003 with the publication of human genome draft, a new innovatory phase of molecular biotechnology comes into existence but still the value of conventional tools and techniques is not obsolete. Confirmed mutations still screened by RFLP, probe based method or sybr green based methods on real time PCR based platform, or by micro-array. As discussed in previous paragraph, cancer has an extremely complex etiology and in the course of the development of the disease several number of mutations can occur. So, genomic sequencing has a great value but due to high charge still few laboratory process the sample by real time PCR, microarray or by sanger sequencing. Genomic sequencing has made possible to screen any mutation or variation if it has any pre-existence that would make them more susceptible to develop cancer in their lifetime. For instance, mutations found in the BRCA1 and BRCA2 genes upsurges a woman's susceptibility for developing ovarian cancer in her lifetime to approximately 40% and 18%, respectively.

Further, these high throughput sequencing platform have capacity to screen novel sporadic mutations in very short period and with more precision.

Genotyping or Mutation Analysis

Restriction Fragment Length Polymorphism (RFLP) is a technique capable to identify variation in homologous DNA sequences that can be screened by the presence of fragments of variable lengths after digestion of the DNA by using precise restriction endonucleases. These fragment of diverse length could be separated on the basis of molecular size in agarose gel electrophoresis.

Additionally, these fragments could be used in depicting unique blotting pattern after hybridization with complimentary probe labelled with some fluorescent dye. The RFLP probes are usually used in genome sequence mapping and in variation analysis (genotyping, hereditary disease diagnostics, etc.). These techniques can be categorized into following three sub-groups:

1. *Enzymatic methods*: Restriction Fragment Length Polymorphism analysis was conventionally the first technique mostly used, in exploring the variations in restriction enzyme sites, leading to the gain or loss of restriction events. Later, numerous enzymatic methods for mutation detection have been developed. These procedures use the activity of resolvase enzymes T4 endonuclease VII, and recently, T7 endonuclease I to digest heteroduplex DNA made by annealing wild type and mutant DNA. Digested fragments stipulate the presence and the position of any mutations. One more enzymatic method for mutation assessment is the oligonucleotide ligation assay. In this method, two oligonucleotides are hybridized to complementary DNA fragments at locations of probable mutations. The oligonucleotide primers are tailored such that the 3″ end of the one primer is instantly contiguous to the 5″ end of the other primer. Thus, if the first primer matches completely with the target DNA, then the primers can be ligated by DNA ligase. On the other hand, if a disparity happens at the 3″ end of the first primer, then no ligation products will be found.
2. *Electrophoretic-based techniques*. This class is renowned by many different methods planned for detection of known or unknown mutations, centered on the different electrophoretic mobility of the mutant alleles, under denaturing or non-denaturing conditions. Single strand conformation polymorphism (SSCP) and heteroduplex (HDA) techniques were among the main approaches considered to detect molecular defects in genomic loci. In arrangement with capillary electrophoresis, SSCP and HDA investigation now provide an excellent, modest, and fast mutation finding platform with low processing costs and, most fascinatingly, the capability of easily being automated, thus providing high-throughput analysis of patient's DNA. Likewise, Denaturing and Temperature Gradient Gel Electrophoresis (DGGE and TGGE, respectively) can be used for mutation screening. In this method, electrophoretic mobility differences between a wild type and mutant allele can be shown in a gradient of denaturing agents, such as urea and formamide, or of increasing temperature. Finally, a gradually utilized mutation screening technique is the two-dimensional gene scanning, based on two-dimensional electrophoretic separation of amplified DNA fragments, as per their size and base pair sequence. The concluding involves DGGE, following the size separation step.
3. *Solid phase-based techniques/hybridization or blotting techniques*. This established method uses the most contemporary mutation screening technologies, it does not require any extra effort as of being fully automated and therefore are extremely praised for high throughput mutation detection or screening. In 1970s there was advancement in nucleic acid hybridization techniques which is focused on the pairing of two complimentary nucleotide strands. This pairing is mainly due to envolvement of hydrogen thus duplex or hybrid results. The hybrids may be resultant of DNA-DNA, RNA-RNA, or DNA-RNA,

thus single stranded molecule may be DNA or RNA in which one nucleic acid strand (the probe) originates from an organism of recognized identity and the other strand (the target) originates from an unknown organism to be detected or identified.

A fast, precise, and suitable method for the discovery of known mutations is reverse dot-blot, originally established by Saiki and colleagues [2], and executed for the screening of b-thalassemia mutations. The crux of this technique is the application of oligonucleotides, bound to a membrane, as hybridization targets for amplified DNA. The extra benefit of this technique is that one membrane strip can be applied to screen many various known mutations in a single individual (a one strip-one patient type of assay), the potential of automation, and the ease of analysis of the results, using a classical avidin-biotin system.

Real-Time PCR: Semi-quantitative Approach

Higuchi first demonstrated procedural enhancement in the form of "real time PCR" approximately two decade earlier, which is modest, quantitative estimation for any amplifiable DNA sequence. This technique is established by using fluorescent labelled probes to detect, approve, and quantify the PCR yields as they are being produced in real time. The real time PCR, which is based on three novel characteristics as temperature cycling happens substantial faster than in standard PCR assays, hybridization of specific DNA probes take place continuously throughout the amplification reaction and a fluorescent dye is attached to the probe and fluoresces only when hybridization occurs. No post PCR handling of amplified products is desired. The generation of amplified products is observed automatically by continuous monitoring of fluorescence. Recently, several commercial automated real-time PCR systems have been available (Light Cycler & TaqMan). In these systems, such as the Light Cycler TM and the Smart Cycler®, these systems accomplish the real-time fluorescence monitoring by using fluorescent dyes such as SYBR-Green I, which binds non-specifically to double-stranded DNA produced during the PCR amplification. Others, such as the TaqMan, use florescent probes that bind exactly to amplification target sequences.

Microarrays

A microarray is actually a set of enriched characteristics of microscopic system, in which usually DNA is hybridized with target molecule for quantifiable (gene expression) or qualitative (diagnostic) of mammoth quantities of genes simultaneously or to genotype multiple loci of a genome. Each DNA spot contains approx. picomoles (10^{-12} moles) of a particular DNA sequence, known as probes (or reporters).

Normally due to advances in fabrication, robotics, and bioinformatics, microarray technology has relentless improvement in terms of efficiency, resolution power, robustness, sensitivity, and specificity. These improvements have allowed the transition of microarrays from strictly research bench site to bed site in clinical diagnostic applications. Microarrays can be differentiated on the basis of characteristics such as the nature of the probe, the solid-surface support applied, and the specific method utilized for probe addressing and/or target detection. An operative hybridization episode between the labeled target and the immobilized probe will accordingly lead to an increase of fluorescence intensity over a threshold level, which can be studied by using a fluorescent scanner [3]. Whole strength of the signal, from a spot (feature), be determined by the amount of target sample binding to the probes exist on that spot. Microarrays procedure works on relative quantization in which the intensity of characteristics is compared to the intensity of the same characteristics under a different condition, and the identity of the feature is known by its position. In situ-synthesized arrays are exceedingly high-density microarrays that usage oligonucleotide probes, of which Gene Chips (Affymetrix, Santa Clara, CA) are the most frequently known. Additionally, the oligonucleotide probes are blended directly on the surface of the microarray, which is typically a 1.2-cm^2 quartz wafer. As in situ-synthesized probes are usually short (20–25 bp), multiple probes per target are involved to improve sensitivity, specificity, and statistical accuracy. Like, above discussed microarrays, Bead Arrays (Illumina, San Diego, CA) provide a spotted substrate for the high-density detection of target nucleic acids. Though, instead of glass slides or silicon wafers as direct substrates, Bead Arrays rely on 3-μm silica beads that arbitrarily self-assemble onto one of two available substrates: the Sentrix Array Matrix (SAM) or the Sentrix Bead Chip [4, 5]. Nothing like the other array the special characteristics of Bead Arrays depend on passive transport for the hybridization of nucleic acids. One additional type of array, electronic microarrays exploits active hybridization via electric fields to control nucleic acid transport. Microelectronic cartridges (NanoChip 400; Nanogen, San Diego, CA) modify complementary metal oxide semiconductor technology for the electronic addressing of nucleic acids.

Traditional Methods and Next Generation Sequencing

Two different approaches for sequencing DNA were established in 1977, that is, the chain termination method and the chemical degradation method. In 1976–1977, A. Maxam and W. Gilbert developed a DNA sequencing technique based on chemical alteration of DNA and successive cleavage at specific bases. Maxam–Gilbert sequencing swiftly became more recognized, as purified DNA could be utilized directly, though the initial Sanger technique required that every read initiated be cloned for making of single-stranded DNA. Though, with the improvement of the chain-termination method, Maxam-Gilbert sequencing has dropped out of preferences due to its practical difficulty barring its utilization in standard molecular biology kits, wide use of harmful chemicals, and complications with scale-up. Each of four reactions (G, A + G, C, and C + T) labeled fragments are produced, from the radio labeled end to the first cut site in each molecule. The fragments in the four reactions are electrophoresed side by side in denaturing acrylamide gels for size separation. To visualize the fragments, the gel is visualized on to X-ray film for autoradiography, yielding a series of dark bands each corresponding to a radiolabeled DNA fragment, from which the sequence may be inferred, also sometimes known as "chemical sequencing" method.

Other method known as Sanger Sequencing Method, which is focused on the principle that single-stranded DNA molecules that vary in length by just a single nucleotide can be separated from by other, by using polyacrylamide gel electrophoresis. The stable laser beam stimulates the fluorescently labeled DNA bands and the light radiated is detected by sensitive photo detectors. Automated DNA-sequencing is easily automated by a variation of Sanger's sequencing method in which dideoxynucleosides castoff for each reaction is labeled with a differently colored fluorescent tag. Because the chain-terminator tactics or Frederick Sanger approach is more proficient and this procedure involves less toxic chemicals and lower amounts of radioactivity than the method of Maxam and Gilbert, it swiftly became the method of choice.

The announcement of the first draft sequence of the human genome in February 2001 [6, 7] and then with the genomic sequence of other organisms, molecular biology has move into a new era with exclusive opportunities and challenges. Technology has enhanced rapidly in last two decades and new mutation-detection techniques have been claimed, whereas old methodologies have cutting-edge to fit into the increasing need for automated and high throughput screening.

The chromatographic detection of polymorphic changes of disease-causing mutations by utilizing denaturing high performance liquid chromatography is one of the innovative technologies that occurred. DHPLC reveals the presence of a genetic variation by the differential retention of homo- and heteroduplex DNA on reversed-phase chromatography under partial denaturation. Single-base substitutions, deletions, and insertions can be identified effectively by UV or fluorescence monitoring within 2–3 min in unpurified PCR products as large as 1.5-kilo bases. These characteristics, together with its low cost, make DHPLC one of the most potent techniques for mutational analysis.

19.2.1.2 High-Throughput Sequencing Technologies

Sanger sequencing and other sequence analysis methods, have amplified sequencing outputs by orders of magnitude and driven down per base sequencing cost considerably [8, 9]. It is now usually estimated that NGS will allow the in-depth description of the cancer cell genome and further improvement in the fields of molecular pathology and personalized medicine for patients with cancer.

Illumina's Genome Analyzer

The vastly parallel signature sequencing advanced by Lynx Therapeutics was the second or next-generation approach to DNA sequencing. The elementary Lynx Therapeutics platform was a microsphere (bead)-based system that identify nucleotides in groups of 4 via an adapter ligation and adapter decoding strategy using reversible dye terminators [10]. Lynx Therapeutics (Hayward, CA) combined into Solexa, which was later acquired by Illumina. This short read sequencing technique is today incorporated into a fluidic flow cell design (HiSeq and Genome Analyzer systems, Illumina, San Diego, CA) with eight individual lanes. The flow cell surface is established with capture oligonucleotide anchors, which hybridize the properly modified DNA segments of a sequencing library generated from a genomic DNA sample. By a process called bridge amplification, engaged DNA templates are amplified in the flow cell by bending over and hybridizing to a contiguous anchor oligonucleotide primer [10]. Genuine sequencing is completed by hybridizing a primer complementary to the adapter sequence, then cyclically adding DNA polymerase and a mixture of four differently colored fluorescent reversible dye terminators to the captured DNA in the flow cell. By this technique, non-altered DNA fragments and unbounded nucleotides are washed away, while captured DNA fragments are extended 1 nucleotide at a time. After each nucleotide-coupling cycle, the flow cell is scanned, and digital images are developed to record the locations of fluorescently labeled nucleotide amalgamations. Next to imaging, the fluorescent dye and the terminal 3′ blocker are chemically detached from the DNA before the next nucleotide coupling cycle. The Illumina method is the most vastly used NGS platform, but it is limited by a relatively low multiplexing capability [11]. The Illumina system has been useful in programs for gene innovation, whole exome analysis, and SNP detection by resequencing [12].

Roche Second-Generation Sequencing

First offered in 2005, the 454 Genome Sequencer FLX Titanium System (Roche, Branford, CT) NGS platform controlled by highly parallel PCR reactions taking in minute emulsions consists of a primer-coated bead with a single captured DNA template covered with the DNA polymerase, oligonucleotide ligation after PCR amplification in an emulsion primers, and nucleoside triphosphates (NTPs) vital for PCR in an oil droplet. PCR amplification outcomes in each bead becoming covered with a single DNA amplicon. The emulsions are cracked, and the DNA-coated beads are loaded onto an array of Pico-liter wells for the sequencing reaction [13]. Pyrosequencing is accomplished over the picoliter well array and the nucleotide additions are visualized and located by a fiber-optic coupled imaging camera. The system provides longer read lengths than other NGS technologies, a strength of this system [12].

Helicos Heliscope: Single-Molecule Sequencing

The Heliscope platform includes fragmenting the sample DNA and performing polyadenylation at the 3′ ends of the fragments. Denatured polyadenylated strands are engaged by hybridization to poly (dT) oligonucleotides immobilized on a flow-cell surface. This technique was the first method to effectively perform single molecule sequencing [14]. The flow cell is cyclically swamped up with the fluorescently labeled deoxynucleoside triphosphates (dNTPs) in the existence of DNA polymerase, which incorporates nucleotides from the oligo-dT primer. The flow cell is imaged at each cycle using a CCD camera, allowing the documentation of the location of each nucleotide incorporation event. As in other systems, the fluorescent label is cut and washed away before each succeeding sequencing cycle [12, 14]. The Heliscope system is precise to provide the most nonbiased DNA sequence, which is its power, although relative to competing NGS platforms, it has relatively high NTP incorporation error rates [12].

SOLiD Sequencing: Sequencing-by-Ligation Approach

SOLiD sequencing (Supported Oligonucleotide Ligation and Detection) is constructed on DNA ligase–mediated oligonucleotide ligation after PCR amplification in an emulsion format. The primers in SOLiD NGS are progressively offset to allow the adapter bases to be sequenced when utilized in conjunction with the color-space coding for defining the template sequence by deconvolution. Fluorescent signals are taken by CCD camera imaging before enzymatic cleavage of the ligated probes and, after washing, repeating the sequencing process. The SOLiD method has been utilized in applications similar to the Illumina NGS, including whole genome sequencing, whole exome capture, and sequencing and SNP finding. Strengths of the SOLiD approach include reduction in sequencing error rates relative to the Illumina NGS by using 2-base encoding. A drawback of the SOLiD system has been it's relatively long run times and complex analysis requirements [12].

Ion Torrent Sequencing: Ion Semiconductor Sequencing

The present platform by Life Technologies, which suggests that this Post Light sequencing technology has the utmost significant benefit of being the first platform to eliminate the cost and effort associated with the four-color optical detection, currently used in all other NGS platforms. The Ion Torrent method relies on standard DNA polymerase sequencing with unchanged dNTPs but usages semiconductor based screening of hydrogen ions liberated during every cycle of DNA polymerization. Every nucleotide integrated into the budding complementary DNA strand causes the release of a hydrogen ion that is noticed by a hypersensitive ion sensor. The initial Ion Torrent system has relatively low parallelism, so it have a tendency to be concentrated on short sequence determination of mutation hot spots throughout the genome.

All NGS platforms have high entry costs, but all also have the probability to dramatically reduce the cost of comprehensive genomic profiling of cancer cells in the forthcoming years. Some techniques suggest speed, such as the 454 Pyro sequencing and Ion Torrent platforms, but, compared with the Illumina and SOLiD platforms, may not be as well suited for clinical somatic tumor DNA sequencing due to their relatively restricted capacities for supporting highly parallel, deep sequencing.

19.2.2 Somatic and Germ-Line Mutation/Variance Studied in Ovarian Carcinoma

Liede et al. [15] acknowledged 1 out of 8 of the ovarian cancer cases, the 185delAG mutation in the BRCA1 gene (113705.0003) segregated with the cancer. Liede et al. [15] established that site-specific ovarian cancer families perhaps signify a variant of the breast-ovarian cancer syndrome, have characteristic mutation in either BRCA1 or BRCA2 [15]. Stratton et al. [16] showed a population-based study to conclude the involvement of germ-line mutations, they reported two out of 101 women with invasive ovarian cancer had germ-line mutations in the MLH1 gene (120436), and no germ-line mutations were recognized in any of the other genes explored, including BRCA1, the ovarian cancer-cluster region (nucleotides 3139–7069) of BRCA2, and MSH2. This study concluded that germ-line mutations in BRCA1, BRCA2, MSH2, and MLH1 add to only a lesser of cases of early-onset epithelial ovarian cancer [16].

Cesari et al. [17] recognized the whole PARK2 gene (602544) within an LOH region on chromosome 6q25-q27. LOH investigation of 40 malignant breast and ovarian tumors showed a shared minimal region of loss, including the markers D6S305 (50%) and D6S1599 (32%), both of which are located within the PARK2 gene. Further, they found 2 somatic truncating deletions in the PARK2 gene (see, e.g., 602544.0016) in 3 of 20 ovarian cancers. This report proved that PARK2 may work as a tumor suppressor gene [17].

Sellar et al. [18] demonstrated that D11S4085 on 11q25 is positioned in the second intron of the OPCML gene (600632). OPCML was commonly somatically disabled in epithelial ovarian cancer tissue by allele loss and by CpG island methylation. OPCML behave like tumor suppressor gene as proved both in vitro and in vivo. A somatic missense mutation from an individual with epithelial ovarian cancer represent perfect proof of loss of function (600632.0001) [18].

The Cancer Genome Atlas Project has completed whole exome sequencing on ovarian cancer [19]. Screening DNA from 316 high-grade serous ovarian cancer patients and compared with normal for 19,356 somatic mutations (about 61 per tumor) were interpreted. High-grade serous ovarian cancer was recognized by TP53 mutations in almost all tissues (96%). BRCA1 and BRCA2 were mutated in 22% of tumors, as study have considered mixed type of germ-line and somatic mutations. Additional significant mutated genes including NF1, RB1, FAT3, CSMD3, GABRA6, and CDK12 occurred in 2–6% of cases. Mutational analysis also presented that mutations in BRAF, PIK3CA, KRAS, and NRAS may be central forces in high grade serous carcinoma. For instance, clear cell types have few TP53 mutations but have recurrent ARID1A and PIK3CA mutations. Although CTNNB1, ARID1A and PIK3CA mutations were commonly seen in endometrioid ovarian cancer histology, KRAS mutations were prevalent in mucinous types [20].

Bell et al. completed a study based on 316 HGS-OvCa samples and compared with normal samples for each individual (Supplementary Methods, section 2). Study was based on captured 180,000 exons from 18,500 genes totaling 33 mega-bases of non-redundant sequence. TP53 was mutated in 303 of 316 samples. BRCA1 and BRCA2 had germline mutations in 9% and 8% of cases, respectively, and showed somatic mutations in a further 3% of cases. Further this group also demonstrated the presence of other mutated genes: RB1, NF1, FAT3, CSMD3, GABRA6 and CDK12 [21].

Recently a study reported 11,479 somatic mutations in the 142 fresh TCGA cases. Entirely of these mutations were manually reviewed, resulting in a total of 27,280 mutations in 429 cases TP53, NF1, RB1, CDK12(CRKRS), and BRCA14, as well as the novel SMG, KRAS. BRCA2 and RB1CC1 were reported significantly associated. This group also identified 4 NRAS mutations, 3 NF2 mutations, and 3, 8, and 10 mutations in the identified tumor suppressor genes: ATR, ATM, and APC, respectively. Somatic truncation mutations were also detected in histone modifier genes including: ARID1A, ARID1B, ARID2, SETD2, SETD4, SETD6, JARID1C, MLL, MLL2, and MLL3 as well as the DNA excision repair gene ERCC6 [22]. Tables 19.1 and 19.2 have shown the various mutations as characterized by various researchers.

Table 19.1 Common mutations verified by various studies

Gene	No. of mutations detected	Studies
TP53	294	Bell et al. [21]; Nick et al. [23]
BRACA1	10	Bell et al. [21]; Couch et al. [24]
BRACA2	10	Bell et al. [21]; Kanchi et al. [22]
CSMD3	19	Bell et al. [21]; Kanchi et al. [22]
NF1	13	Bell et al. [21]; Sangha et al. [25]
CDK12	9	Bell et al. [21]; Dong et al. [26]
FAT3	18	Bell et al. [21]; Kanchi et al. [22]
GABRA6	6	Bell et al. [21]; Kanchi et al. [22]
RB1	6	Bell et al. [21]; Kanchi et al. [22]
CHEK2	24	Kurian et al. [27]
ATM	43	Kurian et al. [27]
RAD51C	32	Kurian et al. [27]
PALB2	21	Kurian et al. [27]
PMS2	21	Kurian et al. [27]
BRIP1	36	Kurian et al. [27]
MSH6	24	Kurian et al. [27]

Table 19.2 Somatic mutations prevalence in epithelial ovarian cancer

Gene mutation	Epithelial ovarian cancer overall	High grade serous (type II)	Low grade serous (type I)	Clear cell (type I)	Endometrioid (type I)	Mucinous (type I)
BRAF	11% [28]	<1% [21]	24–33% [29, 30]	1% [31, 32]	24% [30]	50–75% [33]
KRAS	11% [28]	<1% [21]	33% [29, 30]	<1–7% [30, 32]	<1% [30]	50–75% [33]
PIK3CA	6.7% [34, 35]	<1% [21]	5% [29, 36]	20–33% [32]	20–33% [37, 38]	Rare
PTEN	20% [28]	<1% mutation [21]	20% [39]	<1–5% [32, 40]	20–31% [28, 40, 41]	Rare [42]

19.2.3 Transcriptomics

For accurate functioning of our biological system, genes expression is required in definite quality and quantity so that smooth processing of all activities could be maintained. Modification or change that may happen in regulatory region of the particular gene so the product of that gene may be abnormal in quantity or quality, thus deregulation of governing function may occur. Commonly this unexpected regulations may manifest in two ways: Non-sense Mediated Decay (NMD) or Ubiquitin mediated decay and may cause carcinogenesis, further few studies suggested that this up-regulation of gene expression may advance the stage of the other cancer [43–47].

Exploring a large sample size of cancer specimen with environmental factors like tobacco exposure etc., can establish gene expression data base that can be used not only for molecular sub-typing but also for screening the advancement and survival of the disease, which ultimately could be very rewarding in management of these patients [48] Currently, one approach broadly utilized to assess the gene expression in terms of copy no., i.e. semi quantitative approach by the real time PCR. In this process initially, isolation of total RNA is prerequisite from any sample like blood or tissue and then convert into cDNA by reverse transcriptase. Thus the converted cDNA is quantified by using fluorescently labelled probe or sybr green based method.

This method allows researchers to examine expression of genes related to pathways or pathogenesis of patients and further help to compare the data with healthy individuals in very short time, like one study studied gene expression by quantifying the mRNA of the gene that have a role in the developmental and hormonal regulation of the trans membrane TJ protein, occludin (OCLN), and the cytoplasmic TJ proteins, TJ protein 1 (TJP1) and cingulin (CGN) in bovine granulosa cells (GC) and theca cells (TC) and found altered gene expression of these gene during ovarian cancer [49].

Further, standard technique for transcriptome profiling is microarray assays. Microarray exploration needs extracting the total RNA from sample and transforming it into cDNA as real time PCR. Though, microarrays dependent on in-situ hybridization of complementary nucleotide strands unlike gene polymerization in real-time PCR. DNA spots are fabricated on the microarray surface and every spot comprises a custom deliberated DNA sequence that works as a probe for specific gene detection. The sample with fluorescently labeled cDNA and when this combined with their corresponding spots on the microarray, a fluorescent signal is radiated based on the quantity of cDNA bound to the probe DNA. Microarray assays can be accomplished in a swift and economical manner that proves it a potent tool for medical transcriptome profiling of patient tumor biopsies and also to detect patient samples for distinctive subtype-specific gene sub types that can assist to forecast therapy response, tumor progression, and patient prognosis.

Recently, a study by Carrarelli et al. on Myostatin expression in endometrium in benign (endometriosis, polyps) and malignant (endometrial adenocarcinoma) patients and compared with healthy women during menstrual cycle. As Myostatin is a growth factor member of the transforming growth factor β superfamily, which is recognized to play main roles in cell proliferation and differentiation. The current data demonstrated for the first time the expression

Table 19.3 Study on exploration of gene expression in ovarian carcinoma

Gene	Expression	Diagnostic/prognostic/ therapeutics	Types of study	Study/researchers
E74-like factor 5 (ELF5)	Decreased	Therapeutics (gene therapy)	Human sample study	Yang et al. [52]
Receptor for advanced glycation end products (RAGE)	Increased	Diagnostic	Human sample study	Rahimi et al. [53]
RAP80 (HR-pathway-related gene)	Decreased	Poor prognosis	Human sample study	Romeo et al. [54]
Musashi-2 (MSI2)	Increased	Therapeutics (paclitaxel resistance), poor prognosis	Human sample study	Lee et al. [55]
DNA-PKcs, Akt3, and p53	Increased	Poor prognosis	Human sample study	Shin et al. [56]
aberrant ALK (anaplastic lymphoma kinase)	Present in ovarian serous carcinoma	Prognosis	Human sample study	Tang et al. [57]
YAP (autophagy related)	Present	Therapeutics (cisplatin-resistant; protective)	C13K cell line	Xiao et al. [58]
Urothelial carcinoma associated 1 (UCA1)	Increased	Poor prognosis and therapeutics	Human sample study	Zhang et al. [59]
Cyclin Y (CCNY)	Increased	Therapeutics	Cell line	Liu et al. [60]
Spalt-like transcription factor 4 (SALL4)	Increased	Poor prognosis	Cell line	Yang et al. [61]
Carnitine palmitoyltransferase 1A (CPT1)	Increased	Poor prognosis, therapeutics	Cell line	Shao et al. [62]
Galectin (Gal-9)	Increased	Positive prognostic factor	Human sample study	Schulz et al. [63]

of myostatin in healthy endometrium and aggravated copy no. expression in endometriosis and endometrial cancer, proposing myostatin involvement in human endometrial physiology and related pathologies [50].

Similarly, Wei et al. reported high expression of ITGA6 (Integrin subunit alpha 6) in 287 ovarian cancer patients of TCGA cohort was significantly associated with poorer progression-free survival. This study provide the basis of drug resistance in ovarian cancer, and integrins could be a probable biomarker for prognosis of ovarian cancer [51]. Table 19.3 have shown the recent studies which proved significant gene expression in ovarian carcinoma.

19.2.4 Epigenetic (DNA Methylation Analysis)

As previously mentioned, the role of mutations, copy number and gene expression in development and progression of ovarian carcinoma, but these factors alone are not responsible for carcinogenesis mechanism. So, it is now supposed that epigenetic modifications have role in carcinogenesis. Epigenetics can be defined as the potent permanent and inheritable alteration in gene expression that does not affect DNA sequence but alter the morphology of the gene or chromosome. Epigenetic modifications to the genome normally take place during normal cell cycle regulation. More remarkably, study has revealed these modifications tend to occur more commonly than mutations. Epigenetic modifications among cancer cells effect in abnormal gene expression via three process (1) DNA methylation, (2) histone modifications, and (3) non-coding microRNAs. These modifications have shown a significant association with initiation and progression of ovarian cancers.

Two main types of epigenetic regulations generally exist: first that results at the gene level and a second that occurs at the chromosomal level. The first is known as genomic methylation in which "Methyl" groups is added to definite locus of genes, which can either activate or inactivate gene expression. DNA methylation occurs among cytosine residues in cytosine–guanine (CpG) dinucleotides, which are frequently dispersed in the CpG-rich regions mentioned as "CpG islands". This type of methylation is accomplished by DNA methyltransferases (DNMTs), which are a family of enzymes that assist to transfer methyl groups onto DNA. In humans, DNMTs are classified into two groups: DNMT1 and DNMT3. Alterations in DNA methylation regulating gene expression are very common, appears in both normal and cancerous cells. As per assumptions, about 80% of CpG dinucleotides in the human genome get methylated during life-span [64].

19.2.4.1 Epigenetic Alterations in Cancer

DNA hyper-methylation has role in gene silencing whereas DNA hypo-methylation is known for alteration in gene expression, both have been reported in malignancy and cancer cells. Normally, hypermethylated CpG regions within the DNA cause silencing of tumor suppressor genes, demolishing the cell's capability to repair DNA damage, control cell growth, and inhibit proliferation. Whereas, DNA hypomethylation participates in oncogenesis when formerly silenced oncogenes become transcriptionally activated. Furthermore, DNA hypomethylation have role in triggering latent transposons and thus chromosomal instability take place in specific pericentromeric satellite regions [65].

19.2.4.2 Epigenetic Role in Ovarian Cancer

Epigenetic modifications have shown their strong promise to be employing as biomarkers not for early diagnosis but also to screen the advancement of the disease and prognosis. Epigenetic databases derived from the patient samples along with mutations and gene expression could be used in better management of the cancer. Table 19.4 represents the recent studies on epigenetic changes associated with ovarian cancer.

Table 19.4 Novel studies on exploration of epigenetic changes in ovarian carcinoma

Gene	Methylation/acetylation	Diagnostic/prognostic/therapeutics	Study/researchers
GATA	Hyper methylation	Better prognosis	Bubancova et al. [66]
miR-128-2	Methylation	Progression of the cancer	Jang et al. [67]
RGS2 (regulator of G-protein signaling 2)	Methylated	Therapeutics (chemo resistance)	Cacan [68]
4-1BB ligand (4-1BBL/CD157) and OX-40 ligand (OX-40L/CD252)	Histone deacetylation and DNA methylation	Therapeutics (chemo resistance)	Cacan [68]
Solute carrier family 6, member 12 (SLC6A12)	Methylation	Poor prognosis and advancement of the cancer	Sung et al. [69]
HNF1B	Methylation	Poor prognosis and advancement of the cancer	Ross-Adams et al. [70]
TBX15	Promoter methylation	Therapeutics	Gozzi et al. [71]
P16INK4a	Methylation	Risk, diagnosis	Xiao et al. [58]
DAPK1 and SOX1	Promoter methylation	Risk, diagnosis	Kaur et al. [72]
Cadherin 13 (CDH13), Dickkopf WNT signaling pathway inhibitor 3 (DKK3) and Forkhead box L2 (FOXL2)	Promoter hyper methylation	Diagnostic and advancement of the disease	Xu et al. [73]
ADAMTS12 and MGMT	Promoter hyper methylated in all type of cancer like endometrioid, mucinous, and germ cell tumors.	Diagnostic and advancement of the disease	Losi et al. [74]

19.2.5 Micro-RNAs Expression in Ovarian Cancer

The exclusive biomolecule miRNA was discovered by Victor Ambros et al. 2011, while working on lin-14 gene, which regulates the development of nematodes. Mature miRNA is a class of endogenous, noncoding, single-stranded small RNA, which is composed of about 20–22 nucleotides [75]. miRNA is involved in several physiological processes and is expressed aberrantly in many pathological conditions. These aberrant expressions of miRNA are meticulously linked to the manifestation, development, progression, diagnosis and prognosis of the human disease. The role for miRNAs in cancer was initially reported from the laboratory of Carlo Croce. A bicistronic miRNA cluster comprising *miR-15a* and *miR-16* at chromosome 13q14 was detected to be mutated, deleted or have reduced expression in chronic lymphocytic leukemia. Afterward, germline mutations in *miR-15a/-16* were screened and it was proved that both of these target anti-apoptotic *BCL-2* mRNA [76].

The alterations in miRNA expression can arise at both the DNA and RNA level. Modifications in Dicer1/Ago2 expression effects global changes in miRNA expression. Though, change of specific miRNAs in cancer is also very frequent. This may happen via one of many mechanisms, like by germline mutation, deletion or promoter methylation [77]. In current years, several novel micro-RNA as revealed in Table 19.5, have been interpreted and added into data-base, suggesting their immense potential in ovarian cancer diagnosis, prognosis and therapeutics.

19.2.6 Proteomics

The proteome is well-defined as the array of proteins expressed in a particular cell, at a fixed set of conditions. Like in human proteome more than million proteins formed. Initially, proteomic equipment has advanced from gel-based techniques (one- and two-dimensional SDS PAGE) to now gel-free techniques of mass spectrometry.

RPPA (Reversed-Phase Protein Array) is a high-throughput antibody-based method that deals with higher sensitivity, quantification, and multiplexing abilities than traditional immunoassay. TCGA (The Cancer Genome Atlas) used the RPPA practice in many tumor types, several proteins screened by RPPA method, but limitations due to unavailability of antibodies to detect isoform or phosphorylated antibodies with various distinct functions. So, MS (mass spectrometry) is now evolving as a technology of preference for screening various protein. Presently, electrospray ionization-MS and matrix-assisted laser desorption/ ionization (MALDI)-MS are the main systems utilized in exploring protein profiling, screening of posttranslational modifications, as well as for meticulous quantification. Nowadays, mass spectrometry-based proteomics created numerous milestones in terms of sensitivity, robustness, and consistency.

Moreover, the progression of quantitative strategies has opened new vistas for discovering the protein differential expression and posttranscriptional and posttranslational alterations in diverse conditions in an attempt to comprehend the functional significances of modified gene expression. Quantitative proteomics has observed major revolutions in precision and relative quantification methods: spectral counting, stable isotope labelling by amino acid in cell culture, isotope-coded affinity tags, and isobaric tags for relative and absolute quantification (iTRAQ) are the example of it. Proteomic approaches are now exclusively applied in several areas of ovarian cancer research not only in deciphering mechanism, characterization of the biomarkers (diagnostics and prognostics) but also in searching biomolecules involved in resistance of the therapy [65].

The ovarian cancer patients do not exhibit any definite symptoms during disease initiation and so when they diagnosed disease has progressed into advanced stage. Now for investigation in early stage, biomarker with higher sensitivity and specificity is warranted. Any standard biomarker can be DNA, RNA or protein that may show its presence in body fluids like blood, urine or saliva etc. Numerous biomarkers have been screened

Table 19.5 Recent study on exploration of miRNA expression and their role in ovarian carcinoma

miRNA	Increased/decreased expression	Involved mechanisms/pathway	Diagnostic/prognostic/therapeutics	Study/researchers
miR-125b	Repression	Cell migration by TGF-β	Therapeutic target	Yang et al. [52]
let-7a and miR-30c	Deregulation	Increased expression of high-mobility group AT-hook 2 protein (HMGA2) i	Therapeutic target	Agostini et al. [78]
miR-130b-3p	Increased	Cytidine monophosphate kinase inhibition by the TGF-β signalling pathway	Therapeutic target	Zou et al. [79]
miR-27b	Increased	Suppressed ovarian cancer cell migration and invasion by binding with VE-cadherin	Therapeutic target	Liu et al. [80]
miR-196b	Increased	Invasion activities in recurrent Epithelial Ovarian Carcinoma by regulating the HOXA9 gene	Prognosis/therapeutic target	Chong et al. [81]
miR-429	Increased	Suppress zinc finger E-box binding homeobox1 (ZEB1) and increased cisplatin sensitivity	Prognosis/therapeutic target	Zou et al. [79]
miR-490-3p	Increased	Increased Cisplatin (CDDP) sensitivity by downregulating ABCC2 expression	Prognosis/therapeutic target	Tian et al. [82]
let-7e	Decreased	Activation of BRCA1 and Rad51 expression and enhancement of DSB repair, which in turn results in cisplatin-resistance	Therapeutic target	Xiao et al. [83]
miR-221	Increased	Promotes cell proliferation by targeting the apoptotic protease activating factor-1	Diagnostic/prognostic/therapeutics	Li et al. [84]
miR-28-5p	Increased	Progression of ovarian cancer cell cycle, proliferation, migration and invasion, inhibited apoptosis, and induced the process of EMT through inhibition of N4BP1	Diagnostic/prognostic/therapeutics	Xu et al. [85]
miR-3129	Increased	Suppresses epithelial ovarian cancer through CD44	Diagnostic/prognostic/therapeutics	Sun et al. [86]

for a few types of cancer, but ovarian cancer is fails to show robustness that correlate with ovarian tumor formation and progression.

One such recognized biomarker is the CA-125 glycoprotein, many researchers have claimed that several patients with ovarian cancer showed increased levels of CA-125 [65]. In fact, various results showed that approximately 78% (70–90%) of patients with ovarian cancer have elevated levels of this glycoprotein. Thus due to its higher specificity in comparison to other biomarkers known, this biomarker is recommended initially to pre-symptomatic women. Though, the strength of CA-125 as a biomarker for screening ovarian cancer is doubtful. There are several others conditions, diseases like some other cancers where the levels of CA-125 shoots up like all inflammatory diseases, cirrhosis, and liver diseases, Diabetes mellitus and in cancers of endometrial, fallopian, lung cancers. False positive outcomes weakens CA-125 to be used as a standard biomarker. Therefore there is need of some other potent biomarker that could differentiate ovarian cancer from normal conditions with a higher specificity and sensitivity [87]. The following Table 19.6 have summarized the current progress in proteomics based biomarker that showed some potency to be act like a better biomarker.

19.3 Future Prospects

The upcoming era of precision medicine [98, 99] in ovarian cancer treatment looks exciting. With the progressions in the field of genomics and integration of the basic science and clinical databases, novel therapeutics can be developed targeted to specific onco-proteins responsible for multidrug resistance, tumour progression and anti-apoptotic cellular defense in ovarian cancer cells or getting overexpressed in tumour cells compared to adjoining tissue. One such forthcoming field is the nanotechnology based deliver of therapeutics. One such method has been discussed by Sapiezynski J et al. 2016 as in Fig. 19.1, they used nanotechnology-based targeted delivery systems (NTD). This is exact personalized treatment, where tumour proteins of specific patient are recognized and targeted using NTDs. The NTDS encompasses only one protein inhibitor (siRNA) to suppress one targeted protein or

Table 19.6 Current progress in proteomics based biomarker

Subtype	Markers	Method	Reference
Serous	Wilm's tumor 1 (WT-1)	MALDI-TOF	Zhu et al. [88]
	Ras-related protein (Rab-3D)	MALDI-TOF	Zhu et al. [88]
	Mesothelin	LC-MS/MS	Tian et al. [89]
	ICAM3, CTAG2, p53, STYXL1, PVR, POMC, NUDT11, TRIM39, UHMK1, KSR1, and NXF3	Protein microarrays	Katchman et al. [90]
Endometroid	Estrogen receptor α (ERα)	RPPA	Sereni et al. [91]
Clear cell	Annexin-A4 (ANXA4)	2-DE, MALDI-TOF	Toyama et al. [92]; Zhu et al. [88]
	Napsin A	Immuno-histochemistry and tissue microarrays	Alshenawy and Radi [93]; Skirnisdottir et al. [94]
	Phosphoserine aminotransferase (PSAT1)	2-DE	Toyama et al. [92]
Mucinous	Serpin B5 (SPB5)	2-DE	Toyama et al. [92]
	FOXA1	Immuno-histochemistry	Karpathiou et al. [95]
	REG4	Immuno-histochemistry tissue microarrays	Lehtinen et al. [96]
	CEA5	LC-MS/MS	Tian et al. [89]
	CEA6	LC-MS/MS	Tian et al. [89]
Early diagnosis marker	Transthyretin (TTR)	ELISA	Zheng et al. [97]

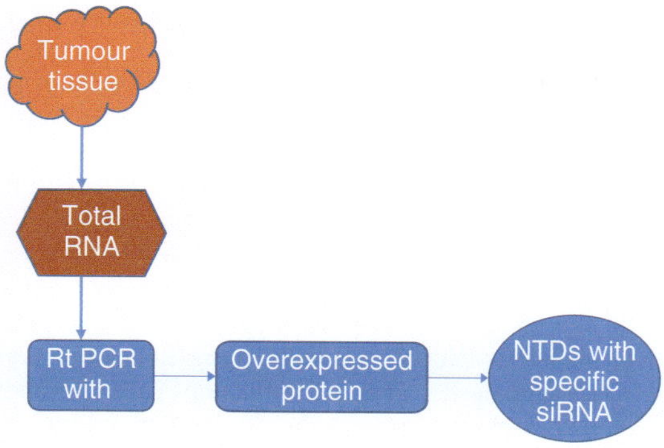

Fig. 19.1 Procedure for personalized treatment using NTDs

an anticancer drug. These NTDSs can be used in any combination with each other.

The researchers reported encouraging invitro and invivo results at preliminary stage, since their data showed that such a personalized treatment method is much more effective in comparison of a standard treatment protocol. In mice model they selected five genes which were over expressing (*BCL2, MDR1, CD44, MMP9, PGR*) and caused metastases. The NTDs were intended accordingly. The NTDs (siRNAs) were delivered along with paclitaxel using dendrimer-based delivery system. The combination therapy reduced the expression of the target genes. This is because of significantly enhanced cell death induction, imposed tumor shrinkage and preventing the development of intraperitoneal metastases.

One more nanotechnology based treatment regimen for ovarian cancer has been aimed in mice model for delivery of folate conjugates. It has been stated that Nanoceria (NCe), nanoparticles of cerium oxide when conjugated to folic acid (NCe-FA), it increased the cellular NCe internalization and inhibited cell proliferation. A combination therapy of NCe-FA and cisplatinum lowered the tumor burden significantly and NCe-FA significantly reduced proliferation and angiogenesis in the xenograft mouse model [100]. The efforts in other field like nutrigenomics and nutri-genetics along with molecular medicine will definitely help in resolving the cancer [101, 102]. In coming era of medicine, the thrilling field of precision medicine shall become a beneficial arena not just for research but the advances that may be translated into clinical practice benefitting hundreds of ovarian cancer patients with early diagnosis and effective treatment.

References

1. Sankaranarayanan R, Ferlay J. Worldwide burden of gynaecological cancer: the size of the problem. Best Pract Res Clin Obstet Gynaecol. 2006;20(2):207–25. https://doi.org/10.1016/j.bpobgyn.2005.10.007.
2. Saiki RK, Walsh PS, Levenson CH, Erlich HA. Genetic analysis of amplified DNA with immobilized sequence-specific oligonucleotide probes. Proc Natl Acad Sci U S A. 1989;86(16):6230–4.
3. Miller MB, Tang YW. Basic concepts of microarrays and potential applications in clinical microbiology. Clin Microbiol Rev. 2009;22(4):611–33.
4. Fan J-B, Gunderson KL, Bibikova M, Yeakley JM, Chen J, Wickham Garcia E, et al. Illumina universal bead arrays. Methods Enzymol. 2006;410:57–73.
5. Oliphant A, Barker DL, Stuelpnagel JR, Chee MS. BeadArray technology: enabling an accurate, cost-effective approach to high-throughput genotyping. Biotechniques. 2002;32:S56.
6. International Human Genome Sequencing Consortium. Initial sequencing and analysis of the human genome. Nature. 2001;409:860–921.
7. Venter JC, Adams MD, Myers EW, Li PW, Mural RJ, Sutton GG, et al. The sequence of the human genome. Science. 2001;291:1304–51.
8. Roukos DH. Personalized cancer diagnostics and therapeutics. Expert Rev Mol Diagn. 2009;9(3):227–9.
9. Church GM. The personal genome project. Mol Syst Biol. 2005;1:2005.0030.
10. Mardis ER. Next-generation DNA sequencing methods. Annu Rev Genomics Hum Genet. 2008;9:387–402. https://doi.org/10.1146/annurev.genom.9.081307.164359.
11. Erlich H, Valdes AM, Noble J, Carlson JA, Varney M, Concannon P, et al. HLA DR-DQ haplotypes and genotypes and type 1 diabetes risk: analysis of the type 1 diabetes genetics consortium families. Diabetes. 2008;57(4):1084–92. https://doi.org/10.2337/db07-1331.
12. Margulies M, Egholm M, Altman WE, Attiya S, Bader JS, Bemben LA, et al. Genome sequencing in microfabricated high-density picolitre reactors. Nature. 2005;437(7057):376–80.
13. Tawfik DS, Griffiths AD. Man-made cell-like compartments for molecular evolution. Nat Biotechnol. 1998;16:652–6.
14. Braslavsky I, Hebert B, Kartalov E, Quake SR. Sequence information can be obtained from single DNA molecules. Proc Natl Acad Sci U S A. 2003;100:3960–4.

15. Liede A, Tonin PN, Sun CC, Serruya C, Daly MB, Narod SA, Foulkes WD. Is hereditary site-specific ovarian cancer a distinct genetic condition? Am J Med Genet. 1998;75(1):55–8.
16. Stratton JF, Thompson D, Bobrow L, Dalal N, Gore M, Bishop DT, Scott I, et al. The genetic epidemiology of early-onset epithelial ovarian cancer: a population-based study. Am J Hum Genet. 1999;65(6):1725–32. https://doi.org/10.1086/302671.
17. Cesari R, Martin ES, Calin GA, Pentimalli F, Bichi R, McAdams H, Trapasso F, et al. Parkin, a gene implicated in autosomal recessive juvenile parkinsonism, is a candidate tumor suppressor gene on chromosome 6q25-q27. Proc Natl Acad Sci U S A. 2003;100(10):5956–61. https://doi.org/10.1073/pnas.0931262100.
18. Sellar GC, Watt KP, Rabiasz GJ, Stronach EA, Li L, Miller EP, Massie CE, et al. OPCML at 11q25 is epigenetically inactivated and has tumor-suppressor function in epithelial ovarian cancer. Nature Genetics. 2003;34(3):337–43. https://doi.org/10.1038/ng1183.
19. Cancer Genome Atlas Research Network. Integrated genomic analyses of ovarian carcinoma. Nature. 2011;474(7353):609–15. https://doi.org/10.1038/nature10166.
20. Wiegand KC, Shah SP, Al-Agha OM, Zhao Y, Tse K, et al. ARID1A mutations in endometriosis-associated ovarian carcinomas. N Engl J Med. 2010;363:1532–43.
21. Bell D, Berchuck A, Birrer M, Chien J, Cramer DW, Dao F, Dhir R, et al. Integrated genomic analyses of ovarian carcinoma. Nature. 2011;474(7353):609–15. https://doi.org/10.1038/nature10166.
22. Kanchi KL, Johnson KJ, Lu C, McLellan MD, Leiserson MD, Wendl MC, Zhang Q, et al. Integrated analysis of germline and somatic variants in ovarian cancer. Nature Communications. 2014;5:3156. https://doi.org/10.1038/ncomms4156.
23. Nick AM, Coleman RL, Ramirez PT, Sood AK. A framework for a personalized surgical approach to ovarian cancer. Nat Rev Clin Oncol. 2015;12(4):239–45. https://doi.org/10.1038/nrclinonc.2015.26.
24. Couch FJ, Wang X, McGuffog L, Lee A, Olswold C, Kuchenbaecker KB, Soucy P, et al. Genome-wide association study in BRCA1 mutation carriers identifies novel loci associated with breast and ovarian cancer risk. PLoS Genet. 2013;9(3):e1003212.
25. Sangha N, Wu R, Kuick R, Powers S, Mu D, Fiander D, Yuen K, et al. Neurofibromin 1 (NF1) defects are common in human ovarian serous carcinomas and co-occur with TP53 mutations. Neoplasia (New York, NY). 2008;10(12):1362–72, following 1372.
26. Dong A, Lu Y, Lu B. Genomic/epigenomic alterations in ovarian carcinoma: translational insight into clinical practice. J Cancer. 2016;7(11):1441–51. https://doi.org/10.7150/jca.15556.
27. Kurian AW, Hughes E, Handorf EA, Gutin A, Allen B, Hartman A-R, Hall MJ. Breast and ovarian cancer penetrance estimates derived from germline multiple-gene sequencing results in women. JCO Precis Oncol. 2017;1:1–12.
28. Kurman RJ, Shih I-M. Molecular pathogenesis and extraovarian origin of epithelial ovarian cancer—shifting the paradigm. Hum Pathol. 2011;42(7):918–31. https://doi.org/10.1016/j.humpath.2011.03.003.
29. Nakayama K, Nakayama N, Kurman RJ, Cope L, Pohl G, Samuels Y. Cancer Biol Ther. 2006;5(7):779–85.
30. Singer G, Oldt R, Cohen Y, Wang BG, Sidransky D, Kurman RJ, Shih I-M. Mutations in BRAF and KRAS characterize the development of low-grade ovarian serous carcinoma. J Natl Cancer Inst. 2003;95(6):484–6.
31. Zannoni GF, Improta G, Pettinato A, Brunelli C, Troncone G, Scambia G, Fraggetta F. Molecular status of PI3KCA, KRAS and BRAF in ovarian clear cell carcinoma: an analysis of 63 patients. J Clin Pathol. 2016;69(12):1088–92. https://doi.org/10.1136/jclinpath-2016-203776.
32. Kuo K-T, Mao T-L, Jones S, Veras E, Ayhan A, Wang T-L, Glas R, et al. Frequent activating mutations of PIK3CA in ovarian clear cell carcinoma. Am J Pathol. 2009;174(5):1597–601. https://doi.org/10.2353/ajpath.2009.081000.
33. Gemignani F, Perra C, Landi S, Canzian F, Kurg A, Tonisson N, Galanello R, Cao A, Metspalu A, Romeo G. Reliable detection of beta-thalassemia and G6PD mutations by a DNA microarray. Clin Chem. 2002;48:2051–4.
34. Levine DA, Bogomolniy F, Yee CJ, Lash A, Barakat RR, Borgen PI, Boyd J. Frequent mutation of the PIK3CA gene in ovarian and breast cancers. Clin Cancer Res. 2005;11(8):2875–8.
35. Campbell IG, Russell SE, Phillips WA. PIK3CA mutations in ovarian cancer. Clin Cancer Res. 2005;11(19 Pt 1):7042. https://doi.org/10.1158/1078-0432.CCR-05-1024; author reply 7042–7043.
36. Wu R, Baker SJ, Hu TC, Norman KM, Fearon ER, Cho KR. Type I to Type II ovarian carcinoma progression: mutant Trp53 or Pik3ca confers a more aggressive tumor phenotype in a mouse model of ovarian cancer. Am J Pathol. 2013;182(4):1391–9. https://doi.org/10.1016/j.ajpath.2012.12.031.
37. Cho KR, Shih I-M. Ovarian cancer. Annu Rev Pathol. 2009;4:287–313. https://doi.org/10.1146/annurev.pathol.4.110807.092246.
38. Samuels Y, Waldman T. Oncogenic mutations of PIK3CA in human cancers. Curr Top Microbiol Immunol. 2010;347:21–41. https://doi.org/10.1007/82_2010_68.
39. Landen CN, Birrer MJ, Sood AK. Early events in the pathogenesis of epithelial ovarian cancer. J Clin Oncol. 2008;26(6):995–1005. https://doi.org/10.1200/JCO.2006.07.9970.
40. Willner J, Wurz K, Allison KH, Galic V, Garcia RL, Goff BA, Swisher EM. Alternate molecular genetic pathways in ovarian carcinomas of common

histological types. Hum Pathol. 2007;38(4):607–13. https://doi.org/10.1016/j.humpath.2006.10.007.
41. McConechy MK, Ding J, Senz J, Yang W, Melnyk N, Tone AA, Prentice LM, et al. Ovarian and endometrial endometrioid carcinomas have distinct CTNNB1 and PTEN mutation profiles. Mod Pathol. 2014;27(1):128–34. https://doi.org/10.1038/modpathol.2013.107.
42. Obata K, Morland SJ, Watson RH, Hitchcock A, Chenevix-Trench G, Thomas EJ, Campbell IG. Cancer Res. 1998;58(10):2095–7.
43. Dwivedi S, Goel A, Khattri S, Mandhani A, Sharma P, Misra S, Pant KK. Genetic variability at promoters of IL-18 (pro-) and IL-10 (anti-) inflammatory gene affects susceptibility and their circulating serum levels: an explorative study of prostate cancer patients in North Indian populations. Cytokine. 2015;74(1):117–22. https://doi.org/10.1016/j.cyto.2015.04.001.
44. Dwivedi S, Goel A, Mandhani A, Khattri S, Sharma P, Misra S, Pant KK. Functional genetic variability at promoters of pro-(IL-18) and anti-(IL-10) inflammatory affects their mRNA expression and survival in prostate carcinoma patients: five year follow-up study. Prostate. 2015;75(15):1737–46. https://doi.org/10.1002/pros.23055.
45. Dwivedi S, Singh S, Goel A, Khattri S, Mandhani A, Sharma P, Misra S, Pant KK. Pro-(IL-18) and anti-(IL-10) inflammatory promoter genetic variants (intrinsic factors) with tobacco exposure (extrinsic factors) may influence susceptibility and severity of prostate carcinoma: a prospective study. Asian Pac J Cancer Prev. 2015;16(8):3173–81.
46. Dwivedi S, Goel A, Khattri S, Sharma P, Pant KK. Aggravation of inflammation by smokeless tobacco in comparison of smoked tobacco. Indian J Clin Biochem. 2015;30(1):117–9. PMID: 25646053.
47. Dwivedi S, Goel A, Mandhani A, Khattri S, Pant KK. Tobacco exposure may enhance inflammation in prostate carcinoma patients: an explorative study in north Indian population. Toxicol Int. 2012;19(3):310–8. PMID: 2329347.
48. Dwivedi S, Shukla KK, Gupta G, Sharma P. Non-invasive biomarker in prostate carcinoma: a novel approach. Indian J Clin Biochem. 2013;28(2):107–9. https://doi.org/10.1007/s12291-013-0312-5.
49. Zhang T, Xu J, Deng S, Zhou F, Li J, Zhang L, et al. Core signaling pathways in ovarian cancer stem cell revealed by integrative analysis of multi-marker genomics data. PLoS One. 2018;13(5):e0196351. https://doi.org/10.1371/journal.pone.0196351.
50. Carrarelli P, Funghi L, Ciarmela P, Centini G, Reis FM, Dela Cruz C, Mattei A, Vannuccini S, Petraglia F. Deep infiltrating endometriosis and endometrial adenocarcinoma express high levels of myostatin and its receptors messenger RNAs. Reprod Sci (Thousand Oaks, CA). 2017;24(12):1577–82. https://doi.org/10.1177/1933719117698579.
51. Wei L, Yin F, Zhang W, Li L. STROBE-compliant integrin through focal adhesion involve in cancer stem cell and multidrug resistance of ovarian cancer. Medicine. 2017;96(12):e6345. https://doi.org/10.1097/MD.0000000000006345.
52. Yang L, Zhang X, Ma Y, Zhao X, Li B, Wang H. Ascites promotes cell migration through the repression of miR-125b in ovarian cancer. Oncotarget. 2017;8(31):51008–15. https://doi.org/10.18632/oncotarget.16846.
53. Rahimi F, Karimi J, Goodarzi MT, Saidijam M, Khodadadi I, Razavi AN, Nankali M. Overexpression of receptor for advanced glycation end products (RAGE) in ovarian cancer. Cancer Biomark. 2017;18(1):61–8. https://doi.org/10.3233/CBM-160674.
54. Romeo M, Karachaliou N, Chaid I, Queralt C, De Aguirre I, Del Carmen Gómez M, Sanchez-Ronco M, Radua J, Ramírez JL, Rosell R. Low RAP80 mRNA expression correlates with shorter survival in sporadic high-grade serous ovarian carcinoma. Int J Biol Marker. 2017;32(1):90–5. https://doi.org/10.5301/jbm.5000223.
55. Lee J, An S, Choi YM, Lee J, Ahn KJ, Lee JH, et al. Musashi-2 is a novel regulator of paclitaxel sensitivity in ovarian cancer cells. Int J Oncol. 2016;49(5):1945–52.
56. Shin K, Kim KH, Yoon MS, Suh DS, Lee JY, Kim A, Eo W. Expression of interactive genes associated with apoptosis and their prognostic value for ovarian serous adenocarcinoma. Adv Clin Exp Med. 2016;25(3):513–21. https://doi.org/10.17219/acem/62540.
57. Tang S, Yang F, Du X, Lu Y, Zhang L, Zhou X. Aberrant expression of anaplastic lymphoma kinase in ovarian carcinoma independent of gene rearrangement. Int J Gynecol Pathol. 2016;35(4):337–47.
58. Xiao L, Shi X-Y, Zhang Y, Zhu Y, Zhu L, Tian W, Zhu B-K, Wei Z-L. YAP induces cisplatin resistance through activation of autophagy in human ovarian carcinoma cells. Onco Targets Ther. 2016;9:1105–14. https://doi.org/10.2147/OTT.S102837.
59. Zhang L, Cao X, Zhang L, Zhang X, Sheng H, Tao K. UCA1 overexpression predicts clinical outcome of patients with ovarian cancer receiving adjuvant chemotherapy. Cancer Chemother Pharmacol. 2016;77(3):629–34.
60. Liu H, Shi H, Fan Q, Sun X. Cyclin Y regulates the proliferation, migration, and invasion of ovarian cancer cells via Wnt signaling pathway. Tumour Biol. 2016;37(8):10161–75. https://doi.org/10.1007/s13277-016-4818-3.
61. Yang M, Xie X, Ding Y. SALL4 is a marker of poor prognosis in serous ovarian carcinoma promoting invasion and metastasis. Oncol Rep. 2016;35(3):1796–806.
62. Shao H, Mohamed EM, Xu GG, Waters M, Jing K, Ma Y. Carnitine palmitoyltransferase 1A functions to repress FoxO transcription factors to allow cell cycle progression in ovarian cancer. Oncotarget. 2016;7(4):3832–46.

63. Schulz H, Kuhn C, Hofmann S, Mayr D, Mahner S, Jeschke U, Schmoeckel E. Overall survival of ovarian cancer patients is determined by expression of galectins-8 and -9. Int J Mol Sci. 2018;19(1). pii: E323. https://doi.org/10.3390/ijms19010323.
64. Nguyen HT, Tian G, Murph MM. Molecular epigenetics in the management of ovarian cancer: are we investigating a rational clinical promise? Front Oncol. 2014;4:71. https://doi.org/10.3389/fonc.2014.00071.
65. Sapiezynski J, Taratula O, Rodriguez-Rodriguez L, Minko T. Precision targeted therapy of ovarian cancer. J Control Release. 2016;243:250–68. https://doi.org/10.1016/j.jconrel.2016.10.014.
66. Bubancova I, Kovarikova H, Laco J, Ruszova E, Dvorak O, Palicka V, Chmelarova M. Next-generation sequencing approach in methylation analysis of HNF1B and GATA4 genes: searching for biomarkers in ovarian cancer. Int J Mol Sci. 2017;18(2). https://doi.org/10.3390/ijms18020474.
67. Jang K, Kim M, Gilbert CA, Simpkins F, Ince TA, Slingerland JM. VEGFA activates an epigenetic pathway upregulating ovarian cancer-initiating cells. EMBO Mol Med. 2017;9(3):304–18. https://doi.org/10.15252/emmm.201606840.
68. Cacan E. Epigenetic regulation of RGS2 (Regulator of G-protein signaling 2) in chemoresistant ovarian cancer cells. J Chemother. 2017;29(3):173–8.
69. Sung HY, Yang SD, Park AK, Ju W, Ahn JH. Aberrant hypomethylation of solute carrier family 6 member 12 promoter induces metastasis of ovarian cancer. Yonsei Med J. 2017;58(1):27–34. https://doi.org/10.3349/ymj.2017.58.1.27.
70. Ross-Adams H, Ball S, Lawrenson K, Halim S, Russell R, Wells C. HNF1B variants associate with promoter methylation and regulate gene networks activated in prostate and ovarian cancer. Oncotarget. 2016;7(46):74734–46.
71. Gozzi G, Chelbi ST, Manni P, Alberti L, Fonda S, Saponaro S, Fabbiani L, Rivasi F, Benhattar J, Losi L. Promoter methylation and downregulated expression of the TBX15 gene in ovarian carcinoma. Oncol Lett. 2016;12(4):2811–9. https://doi.org/10.3892/ol.2016.5019.
72. Kaur M, Singh A, Singh K, Gupta S, Sachan M. Development of a multiplex MethyLight assay for the detection of DAPK1 and SOX1 methylation in epithelial ovarian cancer in a north Indian population. Genes Genet Syst. 2016;91(3):175–81. https://doi.org/10.1266/ggs.15-00051.
73. Xu Y, Li X, Wang H, Xie P, Yan X, Bai Y, Zhang T. Hypermethylation of CDH13, DKK3 and FOXL2 promoters and the expression of EZH2 in ovary granulosa cell tumors. Mol Med Rep. 2016;14(3):2739–45. https://doi.org/10.3892/mmr.2016.5521.
74. Losi L, Fonda S, Saponaro S, et al. Distinct DNA methylation profiles in ovarian tumors: opportunities for novel biomarkers. Int J Mol Sci. 2018;19(6):1559. https://doi.org/10.3390/ijms19061559.
75. Lehrbach NJ, Miska EA. Functional genomic, computational and proteomic analysis of C. elegans microRNAs. Brief Funct Genomic Proteomic. 2008;7(3):228–35. https://doi.org/10.1093/bfgp/eln024.
76. Calin GA, Garzon R, Cimmino A, Fabbri M, Croce CM. MicroRNAs and leukemias: how strong is the connection? Leuk Res. 2006;30(6):653–5. https://doi.org/10.1016/j.leukres.2005.10.017.
77. Calin GA, Ferracin M, Cimmino A, Di Leva G, Shimizu M, Wojcik SE, Iorio MV, et al. A microRNA signature associated with prognosis and progression in chronic lymphocytic leukemia. N Engl J Med. 2005;353(17):1793–801. https://doi.org/10.1056/NEJMoa050995.
78. Agostini A, Brunetti M, Davidson B, Tropé CG, Heim S, Panagopoulos I, et al. Genomic imbalances are involved in miR-30c and let-7a deregulation in ovarian tumors: implications for HMGA2 expression. Oncotarget. 2017;8(13):21554–60.
79. Zou J, Liu L, Wang Q, Yin F, Yang Z, Zhang W, Li L. Downregulation of miR-429 contributes to the development of drug resistance in epithelial ovarian cancer by targeting ZEB1. Am J Transl Res. 2017;9(3):1357–68.
80. Liu W, Lv C, Zhang B, Zhou Q, Cao Z. MicroRNA-27b functions as a new inhibitor of ovarian cancer-mediated vasculogenic mimicry through suppression of VE-cadherin expression. RNA (New York, NY). 2017;23(7):1019–27. https://doi.org/10.1261/rna.059592.116.
81. Chong GO, Jeon H-S, Han HS, Son JW, Lee YH, Hong DG, Park HJ, Lee YS, Cho YL. Overexpression of microRNA-196b accelerates invasiveness of cancer cells in recurrent epithelial ovarian cancer through regulation of homeobox A9. Cancer Genomics Proteomics. 2017;14(2):137–41. https://doi.org/10.21873/cgp.20026.
82. Tian J, Xu Y-Y, Li L, Hao Q. MiR-490-3p sensitizes ovarian cancer cells to cisplatin by directly targeting ABCC2. Am J Transl Res. 2017;9(3):1127–38.
83. Xiao M, Cai J, Cai L, Jia J, Xie L, Zhu Y, Huang B, Jin D, Wang Z. Let-7e sensitizes epithelial ovarian cancer to cisplatin through repressing DNA double strand break repair. J Ovarian Res. 2017;10(1):24. https://doi.org/10.1186/s13048-017-0321-8.
84. Li J, Li Q, Huang H, Li Y, Li L, Hou W, You Z. Overexpression of miRNA-221 promotes cell proliferation by targeting the apoptotic protease activating factor-1 and indicates a poor prognosis in ovarian cancer. Int J Oncol. 2017;50(4):1087–96. https://doi.org/10.3892/ijo.2017.3898.
85. Xu J, Jiang N, Shi H, Zhao S, Yao S, Shen H. miR-28-5p promotes the development and progression of ovarian cancer through inhibition of N4BP1. Int J Oncol. 2017;50(4):1383–91. https://doi.org/10.3892/ijo.2017.3915. [Epub ahead of print].
86. Sun X, Cui M, Tong L, Zhang A, Wang K. Upregulation of microRNA-3129 suppresses

epithelial ovarian cancer through CD44. Cancer Gene Ther. 2018;25(11–12):317–25. https://doi.org/10.1038/s41417-018-0026-1.
87. Elzek MA, Rodland KD. Proteomics of ovarian cancer: functional insights and clinical applications. Cancer Metastasis Rev. 2015;34(1):83–96. https://doi.org/10.1007/s10555-014-9547-8.
88. Zhu Y, Wu R, Sangha N, Yoo C, Cho KR, Shedden KA, Katabuchi H, Lubman DM. Classifications of ovarian cancer tissues by proteomic patterns. Proteomics. 2006;6(21):5846–56. https://doi.org/10.1002/pmic.200600165.
89. Tian Y, Yao Z, Roden RBS, Zhang H. Identification of glycoproteins associated with different histological subtypes of ovarian tumors using quantitative glycoproteomics. Proteomics. 2011;11(24):4677–87. https://doi.org/10.1002/pmic.201000811.
90. Katchman BA, Chowell D, Wallstrom G, Vitonis AF, LaBaer J, Cramer DW, Anderson KS. Autoantibody biomarkers for the detection of serous ovarian cancer. Gynecol Oncol. 2017;146(1):129–36. https://doi.org/10.1016/j.ygyno.2017.04.005.
91. Sereni MI, Baldelli E, Gambara G, Deng J, Zanotti L, Bandiera E, Bignotti E, et al. Functional characterization of epithelial ovarian cancer histotypes by drug target based protein signaling activation mapping: implications for personalized cancer therapy. Proteomics. 2015;15(2–3):365–73. https://doi.org/10.1002/pmic.201400214.
92. Toyama A, Suzuki A, Shimada T, Aoki C, Aoki Y, Umino Y, et al. Proteomic characterization of ovarian cancers identifying annexin-A4, phosphoserine aminotransferase, cellular retinoic acid-binding protein 2, and serpin B5 as histology-specific biomarkers. Cancer Sci. 2012;103(4):747–55.
93. Alshenawy HA, Radi DA. Napsin-A, a possible diagnostic marker for differentiating clear cell ovarian carcinoma from other high-grade ovarian carcinomas. Appl Immunohistochem Mol Morphol. 2018;26(8):605–10. https://doi.org/10.1097/PAI.0000000000000510.
94. Skirnisdottir I, Bjersand K, Akerud H, Seidal T. Napsin A as a marker of clear cell ovarian carcinoma. BMC Cancer. 2013;13:524. https://doi.org/10.1186/1471-2407-13-524.
95. Karpathiou G, Venet M, Mobarki M, Forest F, Chauleur C, Peoc'h M. FOXA1 is expressed in ovarian mucinous neoplasms. Pathology. 2017;49(3):271–6. https://doi.org/10.1016/j.pathol.2016.11.009.
96. Lehtinen L, Vesterkvist P, Roering P, Korpela T, Hattara L, Kaipio K, Mpindi J-P, et al. REG4 is highly expressed in mucinous ovarian cancer: a potential novel serum biomarker. PLoS One. 2016;11(3):e0151590. https://doi.org/10.1371/journal.pone.0151590.
97. Zheng X, Chen S, Li L, Liu X, Liu X, Dai S, Zhang P, Lu H, Lin Z, Yu Y, Li G. Evaluation of HE4 and TTR for diagnosis of ovarian cancer: comparison with CA-125. J Gynecol Obstet Hum Reprod. 2018;47(6):227–30.
98. Sharma P, Dwivedi S. Prospects of molecular biotechnology in diagnostics: step towards precision medicine. Indian J Clin Biochem. 2017;32(2):121–3. PMID: 28428685.
99. Sharma P, Dwivedi S. Nutrigenomics and nutrigenetics: new insight in disease prevention and cure. Indian J Clin Biochem. 2017;32(4):371–3. https://doi.org/10.1007/s12291-017-0699-5. PMID: 29062169.
100. Hijaz M, Das S, Mert I, Gupta A, Al-Wahab Z, Tebbe C, Dar S, et al. Folic acid tagged nanoceria as a novel therapeutic agent in ovarian cancer. BMC Cancer. 2016;16:220. https://doi.org/10.1186/s12885-016-2206-4.
101. Dwivedi S, Purohit P, Misra R , Pareek P, Vishnoi JR, Sharma P, Misra S. Methods for isolation of high quality and quantity of RNA and single cell suspension for flow-cytometry from cancer tissue: a comparative analysis. Indian J Clin Biochem. 2017. https://doi.org/10.1007/s12291-017-0719-5. (Online available).
102. Gupta G, Dwivedi S, Shukla KK, Sharma P. Tissue-resident memory cells: new marked shield to fight cancers. Indian J Clin Biochem. 2018;33(2):119–20. https://doi.org/10.1007/s12291-018-0745-y.

MIX
Papier aus verantwortungsvollen Quellen
Paper from responsible sources
FSC® C105338

If you have any concerns about our products,
you can contact us on
ProductSafety@springernature.com

In case Publisher is established outside the EU,
the EU authorized representative is:
Springer Nature Customer Service Center GmbH
Europaplatz 3, 69115 Heidelberg, Germany

Printed by Libri Plureos GmbH
in Hamburg, Germany